COLOR TEXTBOOK OF
Histology

COLOR TEXTBOOK OF
Histology

Leslie P. Gartner, Ph.D.

Associate Professor
 of Anatomy
Department of OCBS
Baltimore College of
 Dental Surgery
Dental School
University of Maryland
Baltimore, Maryland

James L. Hiatt, Ph.D.

Associate Professor
 of Anatomy
Department of OCBS
Baltimore College of
 Dental Surgery
Dental School
University of Maryland
Baltimore, Maryland

W.B. SAUNDERS COMPANY
A *Harcourt Health Sciences Company*
Philadelphia   London   New York   St. Louis   Sydney   Toronto

W.B. Saunders Company
A *Harcourt Health Sciences Company*

The Curtis Center
Independence Square West
Philadelphia, Pennsylvania 19106

Library of Congress Cataloging-in-Publication Data

Color textbook of histology/Leslie P. Gartner, James L. Hiatt.

p.   cm.

ISBN 0–7216–5124–0

1. Histology.   I. Hiatt, James L.   II. Title.
    [DNLM: 1. Histology—atlases.   QS 517 G244h*ca* 1997]

QM551.G373 1997   611'.018—dc20

DNLM/DLC   96–16721

Illustration Development and Production:
J/B Woolsey Associates

COLOR TEXTBOOK OF HISTOLOGY   ISBN 0–7216–5124–0

Printed in the United States of America

Last digit is the print number: 9   8   7   6   5

To my wife Roseann,
my daughter Jennifer,
and my mother Mary.

LPG

To my grandchildren
Nathan David,
James Mallary,
Hanna Elisabeth,
Alexandra Renate,
and Eric James.

JLH

Preface

Histology, as a subject, stands at the crossroads between gross anatomy and physiology and acts as an integrative element between them. As our knowledge of biology has progressed, new disciplines such as cell and molecular biology have developed. These have exerted a great impact on the classical body of knowledge of Histology, which has expanded to incorporate vast amounts of newly discovered information. Unfortunately, the curricular time allotted to Histology has not expanded; instead, in most medical and dental schools it has been reduced. However, students need to know Histology if they are to understand the normal and abnormal processes that occur in the human organism. Hence, this text was written to present the subject of Histology in such a manner that it not only incorporates newly discovered information but also attempts to present the discipline concisely so that it fits into current curricular time frames.

One of the most difficult aspects of Histology is that it is presented from the perspectives of light and electron microscopy from which the student is expected to infer the material's three-dimensional reality. For most students the ability to extrapolate the three-dimensional aspect from two-dimensional information is a quantum jump that takes about five weeks of hard work. In view of this, we have labored to make this book readable, conveying the information as efficiently as possible, and supplementing the textual material with three-dimensional full-color conceptual illustrations. Additionally, many of the schematic diagrams are didactic in nature. We believe that this will help in emphasizing the important tenet of modern-day Histology: that structure and function are intimately related.

Numerous electron micrographs and full-color light micrographs are presented to illustrate the morphology of cells, tissues, and organs. These will assist the student in correlating information gained in the didactic and laboratory portions of the course.

Much of the information is summarized in the form of tables to promote the acquisition of knowledge. Frequently, the text is interrupted by bulleted inserts that not only organize important aspects of functional histology but also alert the reader to their significance. Important words are presented in **bold face** type to focus attention to them as well as to permit a quick review of important words as the student prepares for examinations. Finally, throughout the text the reader will find important clinical correlations, inset in blocks, illustrating the relevance of Histology to students of the health professions.

While we have made every effort to present a complete and accurate account of the subject matter, we realize that there are omissions and errors in any undertaking of this magnitude. Therefore, we encourage and welcome suggestions, advice, and criticism that will facilitate the improvement of this text.

LESLIE P. GARTNER
JAMES L. HIATT

Acknowledgments

We would like to thank the following individuals for the help and support that they have provided in the preparation of this book. Special thanks go to Dr. William A. Falkler, Jr., for reviewing the chapter on the Lymphoid System. Additionally, we wish to thank our graduate students Ms. Kendall Donaldson and Ms. Sharon Liu for helping in so many ways.

Because Histology is a visual subject, it is imperative to have excellent graphic illustrations. For that we are indebted to the following individuals at J/B Woolsey: Koji Shimizu, Mark Desman, Birck Cox, and John Woolsey: special thanks go to Todd Smith for his careful attention to detail and for his devotion to the project. We also thank our many colleagues from around the world and their publishers, who generously permitted us to borrow illustrative materials from their publications.

Additionally, we wish to express our gratitude to Carol-Lynn Brown and especially Ruth Steyn for their careful attention to editing. Finally, our thanks go to the project team at W.B. Saunders for all their help, namely Kimberly Kist, formerly Senior Medical Editor; William R. Schmitt, Editorial Manager; Edna Dick, Copy Editor; Gene Harris, Designer; Peg Shaw, Senior Illustrations Specialist; and especially our two Developmental Editors, Faith Voit and Elizabeth A. Hatter.

LESLIE P. GARTNER
JAMES L. HIATT

Contents

Introduction to Histology and Basic Histological Techniques

1

Histology is that branch of anatomy that studies tissues of animals and plants. This textbook, however, addresses only animal, and more specifically human, tissues. In its broader aspect, the word *histology* is used as if it were a synonym for microscopic anatomy, because its subject matter encompasses not only the microscopic structure of tissues but also that of the cell, organs, and organ systems.

It should be understood that the body is composed of cells, intercellular matrix, and a fluid substance, tissue fluid (extracellular fluid), which bathes these components. Tissue fluid, which is derived from plasma of blood, carries nutrients, oxygen, and signaling molecules to cells of the body. Conversely, signaling molecules, waste products, and carbon dioxide released by cells of the body reach blood and lymph vessels by way of the tissue fluid. Tissue fluid as well as much of the intercellular matrix are not visible in routine histological preparations, yet their invisible presence must be appreciated by the student of histology.

Histology no longer deals merely with the structure of the body; it also deals with its function. In fact, the subject matter of histology has a direct relationship to other disciplines and is essential for their understanding. This textbook, therefore, intertwines the disciplines of cell biology, biochemistry, physiology, and, as appropriate, pathology. The student will recognize the importance of this subject as he/she refers to the text later in his/her career. An excellent example of this relationship will be evident when the reader learns about the histology of the kidney and realizes it is the intricate and almost sublime structure of that organ (down to the molecular level) that is responsible for its ability to perform its function. Alterations of the kidney's structure is responsible for a great number of life-threatening conditions.

In the remainder of this chapter the methods histologists use to study the microscopic anatomy of the body are discussed.

Light Microscopy

Steps in Tissue Preparation

Various techniques have been developed to prepare tissues for study so that they closely resemble their natural, living state. The steps involved are **fixation, embedding** in a suitable medium, **sectioning** into thin slices to permit viewing by transillumination, **mounting** onto a surface for ease of handling, and **staining** so that the various tissue and cell components may be differentiated.

Fixation

Fixation refers to treatment of the tissue with chemical agents that not only retard the alterations of tissue subsequent to death (or after removal from the body) but also maintain its normal architecture. The most common fixative agents used in light microscopy are neutral buffered **formalin** and **Bouin's fluid.** Both of these substances cross-link proteins, thus maintaining a lifelike image of the tissue.

Dehydration and Clearing

Because a large fraction of the tissue is composed of water, a graded series of alcohol baths beginning with 50% alcohol and progressing in graded steps to 100% alcohol, are utilized to remove the water (**dehydration**). Then the tissue is treated with xylene, a chemical that is miscible with melted paraffin. This process is known as **clearing,** since the tissue becomes transparent in xylene.

Embedding

In order to distinguish the overlapping cells in a tissue and the extracellular matrix from one another, tissues must be **embedded** in a proper medium and then sliced into thin sections. For light microscopy the usual embedding medium is paraffin. The tissue is placed in a suitable container of melted paraffin until it is completely **infiltrated.** Once the tissue is impregnated with paraffin it is placed into a small receptacle, covered with melted paraffin, and then allowed to harden, forming a paraffin block containing the tissue.

Sectioning

After the blocks of tissue are trimmed of excess embedding material, they are mounted for **sectioning** with a microtome. This machine is equipped with a blade and an arm that advances the tissue block in specific equal increments. For light microscopy the thickness of each section is about 5 to 10 μm.

Sectioning can also be performed on specimens frozen either in liquid nitrogen or on the rapid-freeze bar of a cryostat. These sections are mounted by the use of a quick freezing mounting medium and sectioned at subzero temperatures using a precooled steel blade. The sections are placed on precooled glass slides, permitted to come to room temperature, and stained with specific dyes (or treated for histochemistry).

Mounting and Staining

Paraffin sections for conventional light microscopy, cut by stainless steel blades, are placed (**mounted**) on adhesive-coated glass slides. Since many tissue constituents have approximately the same optical densities, they must be stained for light microscopy. **Staining** for light microscopy is performed mostly with water-soluble stains. Therefore, the paraffin first is removed from the section, then the tissue is rehydrated and stained. Subsequent to staining, the section is again dehydrated so that the coverslip may be permanently affixed by the use of a suitable mounting medium. The coverslip not only protects the tissue from damage but also is necessary for viewing the section with the microscope.

Although there are various types of stains that have been developed to visualize many components of cells and tissues, they may be grouped into three classes: stains that differentiate between acidic and basic components of the cell; specialized stains that differentiate the fibrous components of the extracellular matrix; and metallic salts that precipitate on tissues, forming metal deposits on them.

The most commonly used stains in histology are hematoxylin and eosin, commonly referred to as H and E. Hematoxylin is a base that preferentially colors acidic components of the cell a bluish tint. Because the most acidic components are DNA and RNA, the nucleus and regions of the cytoplasm stain dark blue. These components are referred to as **basophilic.** Eosin is an acid that dyes the basic components of the cell a pinkish color. Because many cytoplasmic constituents have a basic pH, regions of the cyto-

plasm stain pink. These elements are said to be **acidophilic.** Many other stains are also utilized in preparing specimens for histological study (Table 1–1).

Molecules of some stains, such as **toluidine blue,** polymerize with each other when exposed to high concentrations of polyanions in tissue. These aggregates are of different color than their individual molecules. For example, toluidine blue stains tissues blue except for those that are rich in polyanions (e.g., cartilage matrix and granules of mast

Table 1–1. Common Histological Stains and Reactions

Reagent	Result
Hematoxylin	*Blue:* nucleus; acidic regions of the cytoplasm; cartilage matrix
Eosin	*Pink:* basic regions of the cytoplasm; collagen fibers
Masson's trichrome	*Dark blue:* nuclei *Red:* muscle, keratin, cytoplasm *Light blue:* mucinogen, collagen
Orcein's elastic stain	*Brown:* elastic fibers
Weigert's elastic stain	*Blue:* elastic fibers
Silver stain	*Black:* reticular fibers
Iron hematoxylin	*Black:* striations of muscle, nuclei, erythrocytes
Periodic acid–Schiff	*Magenta:* glycogen and carbohydrate rich molecules
Wright and Giemsa stains	Used for differential staining of blood cells *Pink:* erythrocytes, eosinophil granules *Purple:* leukocyte nuclei, basophil granules *Blue:* cytoplasm of monocytes and lymphocytes

cells), which are stained purple. A tissue or cell component that stains purple with this stain is said to be **metachromatic,** and toluidine blue is said to exhibit **metachromasia.**

Light Microscope

The present-day light microscope utilizes a specific arrangement of groups of lenses to magnify an image (Fig. 1–1). Due to the use of more than just a single lens, this instrument is known as a compound microscope. The light source is an electric bulb with a tungsten filament whose light is gathered into a focused beam by the **condenser lens.**

The light beam is located below and is focused on the specimen. Light passing through the specimen enters one of the objective lenses; these lenses sit on a movable turret located just above the specimen. Usually four objective lenses are available on a single turret, providing low, medium, high, and oil magnifications. The first 3 lenses magnify 4, 10, and 40 times, respectively, and are used without oil; the oil lens magnifies the image 100 times.

The image from the objective lens is gathered and further magnified by the ocular lens of the eyepiece. This lens usually magnifies the image by a factor of 10—for total magnifications of 40, 100, 400, and 1000—and focuses the resulting image on the retina of the eye.

Focusing of the image is performed by the use of knurled knobs that move the objective lenses up or down above the specimen. The coarse-focus knob moves it in larger increments than does the fine-focus knob. It is interesting to note that the image projected on the retina is reversed from right to left and is upside down.

The quality of an image depends not only on the capability of a lens to magnify but also on its **resolution**—its ability to show that two distinct objects are separated by a distance. The quality of a lens depends on how close its resolution approaches the theoretical limit of 0.25 μm, determined by the wavelength of visible light.

There are several types of light microscopes depending on the type of light they use as a light source and the manner in which they use the light source. However, most students of histology are required to recognize only images obtained from compound light microscopy, transmission electron microscopy, and scanning electron microscopy; therefore, the other types of microscopy will not be discussed.

Interpretation of Microscopic Sections

One of the most difficult, frustrating, and time-consuming histological skills to learn is the interpretation of what a two-dimensional section looks like in three dimensions. If

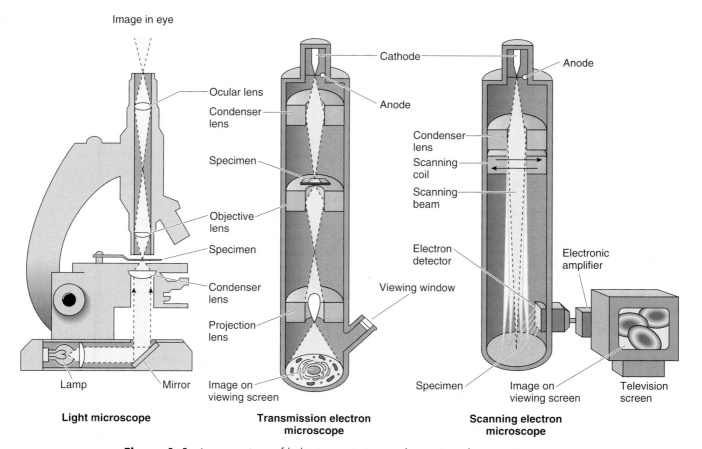

Figure 1-1. A comparison of light, transmission, and scanning electron microscopes.

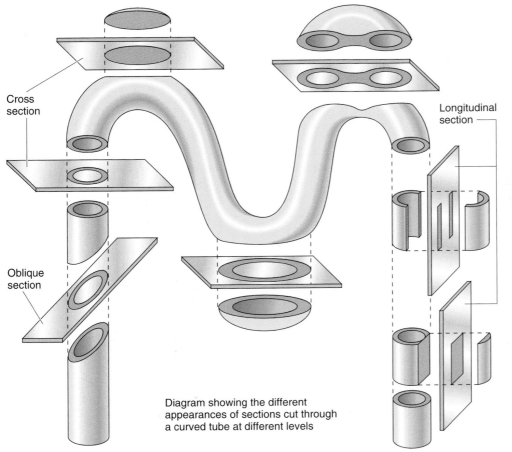

Diagram showing the different
appearances of sections cut through
a curved tube at different levels

Figure 1–2. Histology requires a mental reconstruction of two-dimensional images into the three-dimensional solid from which they were sectioned. In this diagram, a curved tube is sectioned in various planes to illustrate the relationship between a series of two-dimensional sections and the three-dimensional structure.

one imagines a garden hose coiled as in Figure 1–2 and then takes the indicated thin sections from that hose, it becomes clear that the three-dimensional object is not necessarily discerned from any *one* of the two dimensional depictions. However, by viewing all of the sections drawn from the coiled tube, one can mentally reconstruct the correct three-dimensional image.

Advanced Visualization Procedures

Histochemistry

Specific chemical constituents of tissues and cells can be localized by the method of **histochemistry** and **cytochemistry.** These methods capitalize on the enzyme activity, chemical reactivity, or other physicochemical phenomena associated with the constituent of interest. Reactions of interest are monitored by the formation of an insoluble precipitate that takes on a certain color. Frequently, histochemistry is performed on frozen tissues and can be applied to both light and electron microscopy.

A common histochemical reaction uses the periodic acid–Schiff reagent, which forms a magenta-colored precipitate with glycogen and carbohydrate rich molecules. In order to ensure that the reaction is specific for glycogen,

consecutive sections are treated with amylase. Thus sections not treated with amylase will display a magenta-colored deposit, whereas amylase-treated sections display a lack of staining in the same region.

Enzymes can be localized by histochemical procedures. Actually, the product of enzymatic reaction—not the enzyme itself—is visualized. The reagent is designed so that the product precipitates at the site of the reaction and is visible either as a metallic or colored deposit.

Immunocytochemistry

Although histochemical procedures permit fairly good localization of some enzymes and macromolecules in cells and tissues, more precise localization can be achieved by the use of **immunocytochemistry.** This procedure requires the development of an antibody against the particular macromolecule to be localized and labeling the antibody with a fluorescent dye such as fluorescein or rhodamine.

There are two methods of antibody labeling, **direct** and **indirect.** In the direct method (Fig. 1–3) the antibody against the macromolecule is labeled with a fluorescent dye. The antibody is then permitted to react with the macromolecule and the resultant complex may be viewed with a fluo-

Figure 1–3. Direct and indirect methods of immunocytochemistry. **Left on Figure,** An antibody against the antigen was labeled with a fluorescent dye and viewed with a fluorescent microscope. The fluorescence occurs only over the location of the antibody. **Right on Figure,** Fluorescent-labeled antibodies are prepared against an antibody that reacts with a particular antigen. When viewed with fluorescent microscopy, the region of fluorescence represents the location of the antibody.

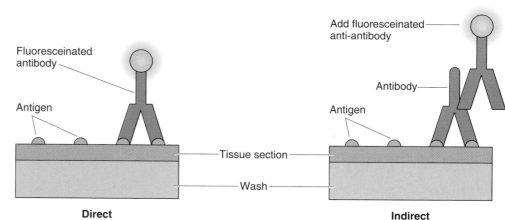

Direct   **Indirect**

rescent microscope (Fig. 1–4). In the indirect method (see Fig. 1–3) a fluorescent-labeled antibody is prepared against the primary antibody specific for the macromolecule of interest. After the primary antibody reacts with the antigen, the preparation is washed to remove unbound primary antibody; the labeled antibody is then added and reacts with the original antigen–antibody complex, forming a secondary complex visible by fluorescent microscopy (Fig. 1–5). The indirect method is more sensitive than the direct method because multiple-labeled anti-antibodies bind to the primary antibody, making them easier to visualize. In addition, the indirect method does not require labeling of the primary antibody, which often is available only in limited quantities.

Immunocytochemistry can be used with specimens for electron microscopy by labeling the antibody with ferritin, an electron-dense molecule, instead of a fluorescent dye. Ferritin labeling can be applied to both the direct and indirect methods.

Autoradiography

Autoradiography (radioautography) is a particularly useful method for localizing and investigating a specific temporal sequence of events. The method requires incorporation of a radioactive isotope—most commonly tritium (^{3}H)—into the compound being studied (Fig. 1–6). An example would be the use of tritiated amino acid to follow the synthesis and packaging of proteins. Subsequent to the injection of the radiolabeled compound into an animal, tissue specimens are taken at selected time intervals. The tissue is processed as usual and placed on a glass slide, but instead of the tissue being sealed with a coverslip, a thin layer of photographic emulsion is placed over it. The tissue is placed in a dark box for a few days or weeks, during which time particles emitted from the radioactive isotope expose the emulsion over the cell sites where the isotope is located. The emulsion is developed and fixed using photographic techniques, leaving small silver grains over the exposed portions

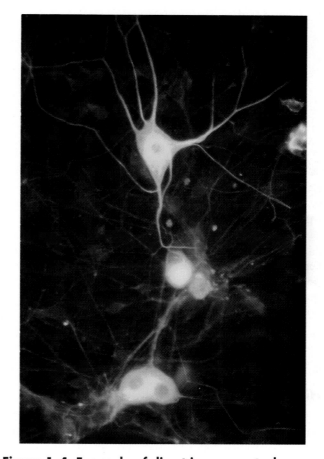

Figure 1–4. Example of direct immunocytochemistry. Cultured neurons from rat superior cervical ganglion were immunostained with fluorescent-labeled antibody specific for the insulin receptor. The bright areas correspond to sites where the antibody has bound to insulin receptors. The staining pattern indicates that receptors are located throughout the cytoplasm of the soma and processes but are missing from the nucleus. (From James, S., Patel, N., Thomas, P., and Burnstock, G.: Immunocytochemical localisation of insulin receptors on rat superior cervical ganglion neurons in dissociated cell culture. J. Anat. **182:**95–100, 1993.)

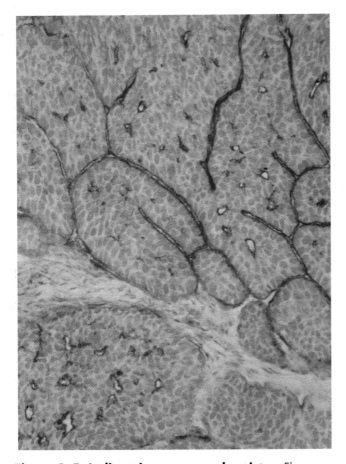

Figure 1–5. Indirect immunocytochemistry. Fluorescent antibodies were prepared against primary antibodies against type IV collagen, to demonstrate the presence of a continuous basal lamina at the interface between malignant clusters of cells and the surrounding connective tissue. (From Kopf-Maier, P. and Schroter-Kermani, C.: Distribution of type VII collagen in xenografted human carcinomas. Cell Tissue Res. **272:**395–405, 1993. Copyright Springer-Verlag.)

of the emulsion. The specimen then is sealed with a coverslip and viewed microscopically.

This method has been used to follow the time course of incorporation of tritiated proline into the basement membrane underlying endodermal cells of the yolk sac (see Fig. 1–6). An adaptation of autoradiography method for electron microscopy was used to show that the tritiated proline first appears in the cytosol of the endodermal cells, then travels to the rough endoplasmic reticulum, then to the Golgi apparatus, then into vesicles, and finally into the extracellular matrix (Fig. 1–7). In this manner the sequence of events occurring in the synthesis of collagen—the main protein in the basement membrane—was visually demonstrated.

Electron Microscopy

In light microscopes, optical lenses focus visible light (photon beam). In electron microscopes, electromagnets focus a

beam of electrons. Because the wavelength of an electron beam is much shorter than that of visible light, electron microscopes theoretically are capable of resolving two objects separated by 0.005 nm. In practice, the resolution of the **transmission electron microscope** is about 0.2 nm, more than a thousandfold greater than the resolution of the compound light microscope. The resolution of the **scanning**

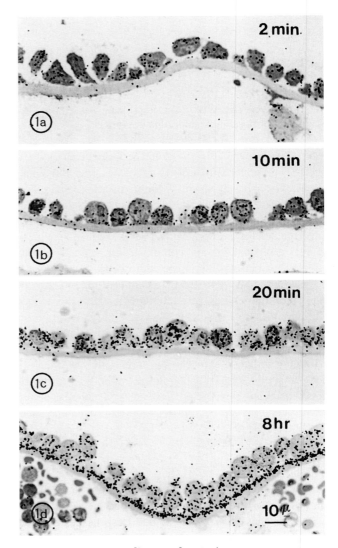

Figure 1–6. Autoradiography. Light microscopic examination of tritiated proline incorporation into the basement membrane as a function of time subsequent to tritiated proline injection. Observe that in photomicrographs 1a, 1b, and 1c the silver grains (black dots) are localized mostly in the endodermal cells, but after eight hours (1d), the silver grains are also localized in the basement membrane. The presence of silver grains indicates the location of tritiated proline. (From Mazariegos, M.R., Leblond, C.P., and van der Rest, M.: Radioautographic tracing of ³H-proline in endodermal cells of the parietal yolk sac as an indicator of the biogenesis of basement membrane components. Am. J. Anat. **179:**79–93, 1987. Copyright 1987. Reprinted by permission of John Wiley & Sons, Inc.)

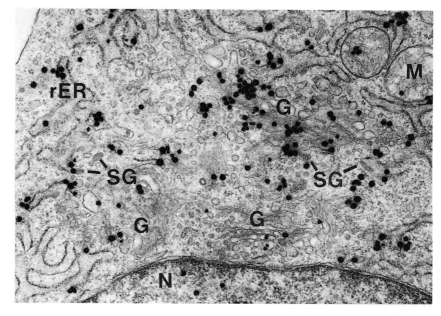

Figure 1–7. Autoradiography. In this electron micrograph of a yolk sac endodermal cell, similar to those of Figure 1–6, silver grains, representing the presence of tritiated proline, are evident overlying the rough endoplasmic reticulum (rER), Golgi apparatus (G), and secretory granules (SG). Type IV collagen, which is rich in proline, is synthesized in endodermal cells and released into the basement membrane. The tritiated proline is most concentrated in organelles involved in protein synthesis. (From Mazariegos, M.R., Leblond, C.P., and van der Rest, M.: Radioautographic tracing of ^{3}H-proline in endodermal cells of the parietal yolk sac as an indicator of the biogenesis of basement membrane components. Am. J. Anat. **179:** 79–93, 1987. Copyright 1987. Reprinted by permission of John Wiley & Sons, Inc.)

electron microscope is about 10 nm, considerably less than that of transmission instruments. Moreover, modern electron microscopes can magnify an object as much as 150,000 times; this magnification is powerful enough for visualization of individual macromolecules such as DNA and myosin.

Transmission Electron Microscopy

Preparation of tissue specimens for **transmission electron microscopy (TEM)** involves the same basic steps as in light microscopy. Special fixatives have been developed for use with TEM, since the greater resolving power of the electron microscope requires finer and more specific cross linking of proteins. These fixatives, which include buffered solutions of **glutaraldehyde, paraformaldehyde, osmium tetroxide,** and **potassium permanganate,** not only preserve fine structural details but also act as electron-dense stains, which permit observation of the tissue with the electron beam.

Because these fixatives penetrate fresh tissues even less than those for light microscopy, relatively small pieces of tissues are infiltrated in large volumes of fixatives. Tissue blocks for TEM are usually no larger than 1 mm³. Suitable embedding media has been developed, such as epoxy resin; plastic-embedded tissues may be cut into ultrathin sections (25 to 100 nm), which do not absorb the beam of electrons.

Electron beams are produced in an evacuated chamber by heating a tungsten filament, the **cathode.** The electrons then are attracted to the positively charged **anode,** a donut-shaped metal plate with a central hole. By placing a charge differential of about 60,000 volts between the cathode and the anode, the electrons that pass through the hole in the anode have high kinetic energy.

The electron beam is focused on the specimen by the use of electromagnets, which are analogous to the condenser lens of a light microscope (see Fig. 1–1). Because the tissue is stained with heavy metals that preferentially precipitate on lipid membranes, the electrons lose some of their kinetic energy as they interact with the tissue. The more heavy metal an electron encounters the less energy it will retain.

The electrons leaving the specimen are subjected to the electromagnetic fields of several additional electromagnets, which focus the beam on a fluorescent plate. As the electrons hit the plate their kinetic energy is converted into points of light, whose intensity is a direct function of the electron's kinetic energy. A permanent record is made of the resultant image by substituting an electron sensitive film in place of the fluorescent plate and producing a negative from which a black and white photomicrograph can be printed.

Scanning Electron Microscopy

Unlike transmission electron microscopy, **scanning electron microscopy (SEM)** is utilized to view the surface of a solid specimen. This technique provides a three-dimensional image of the object being viewed. Usually the object to be viewed is prepared in a special manner that permits a thin layer of heavy metal, such as gold or palladium, to be deposited on the specimen's surface.

As a beam of electrons scans the surface of the object, some are reflected (backscatter electrons) and others are ejected (secondary electrons) from the heavy metal coat. The backscatter and secondary electrons are captured by electron detectors that are interpreted, collated, and displayed on a monitor as a three dimensional image (see Fig. 1–1). The image may be made permanent either by photographing it or digitizing it for storage in a computer.

Freeze-Fracture Technique

The macromolecular structure of the internal aspects of membranes is revealed by the method of **freeze fracture** (Fig. 1–8). Quick-frozen specimens that have been treated with cryopreservatives do not develop ice crystals during the freezing process, hence the tissue does not suffer mechanical damage. As the frozen specimen is hit by a super-cooled razor blade, it fractures along cleavage planes, which are regions of least molecular bonding; in cells, fracture occurs between the inner and outer leaflets of membranes.

The fracture face is coated at an angle by evaporated platinum and carbon, forming accumulations of platinum on one side of a projection and no accumulation on the opposite side next to the projection, thus generating a replica of the surface. The tissue is then digested away and the replica is examined by transmission electron microscopy. This method displays the transmembrane proteins of cellular membranes (see Fig. 1–8).

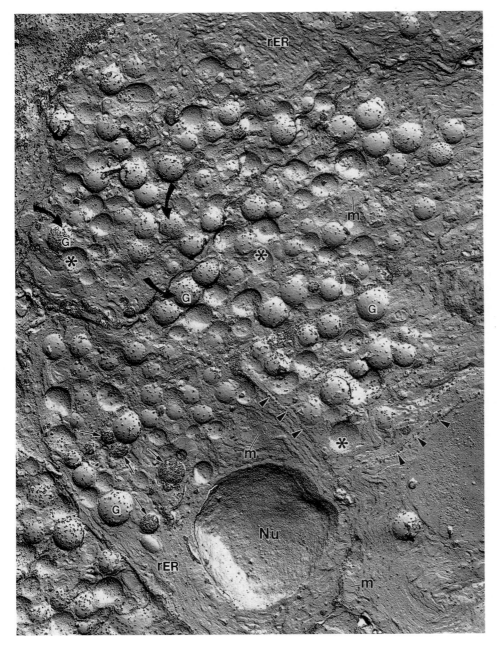

Figure 1–8. Cytochemistry and freeze etching. Fracture-label replica of an acinar cell of the rat pancreas. *N*-Acetyl-*D*-galactosamine residues were localized by the use of *Helix pomatia* lectin-gold complex, which appears as black dots in the image. Note that the nucleus (Nu) appears as a depression, the rER as parallel lines, and secretory granules (G) as small elevations or depressions. The elevations (labeled G) represent the E face half and the depressions (labeled *) represent the P face of the membrane of the secretory granule. (From Kan, F.W.K., and Bendayan, M.: Topographical and planar distribution of *Helix pomatia* lectin-binding glycoconjugates in secretory granules and plasma membrane of pancreatic acinar cells of the rat: Demonstration of membrane heterogeneity. Am. J. Anat. **185:**165–176, 1989. Copyright 1989. Reprinted by permission of John Wiley & Sons, Inc.)

Cytoplasm

2

Cells are the basic units of complex organisms. Similar or related cells that function in a particular manner or serve a common purpose are grouped together to form **tissues.** The four basic tissues (epithelium, connective tissues, muscle, and nervous tissue) that compose the body are assembled to form **organs** which, in turn, are collected into **organ systems.** The task of each organ system is specific in that it performs a collection of associated functions, such as digestion, reproduction, or respiration.

Although the human body comprises more than 200 different types of cells, each performing a different function, all cells possess certain unifying characteristics, and thus can be described in general terms. Every cell is surrounded by a bilipid plasma membrane, possesses organelles that permit it to discharge its functions, synthesizes macromolecules for its own use or for export, produces energy, and is

capable of communicating with other cells (Figs. 2–1 through 2–4).

Protoplasm, the living substance of the cell, is subdivided into two compartments, the **cytoplasm,** extending from the plasma membrane to the nuclear envelope, and the **karyoplasm,** the substance forming the contents of the nucleus. The cytoplasm will be detailed in this chapter, whereas the nucleus is discussed in Chapter 3.

The bulk of the cytoplasm is **water,** in which various inorganic and organic chemicals are dissolved and suspended. This fluid component of the cell is referred to as the **cytosol.** The cytosol contains **organelles,** metabolically active structures that perform distinctive functions (Figs. 2–5 and 2–6). Additionally, the shapes of cells, their ability to move, as well as the intracellular pathways within cells, are maintained by a system of tubules and filaments known as the

Figure 2–1. Light photomicrograph of typical cells from a monkey (× 1024). Note the blue nucleus and the pink cytoplasm. The boundaries of individual cells may be easily distinguished.

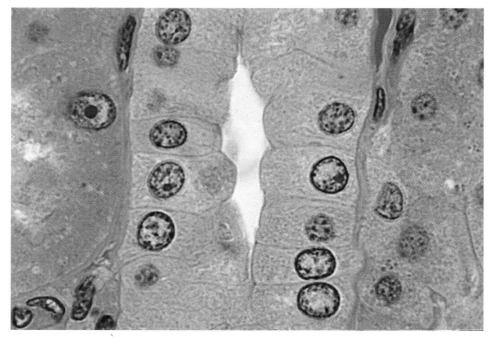

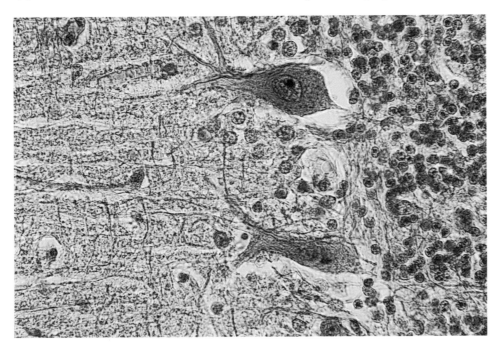

Figure 2-2. Purkinje cells from the cerebellum of a monkey (× 540). Observe the long, branching processes (dendrites) of these cells. The nucleus is located in the widest portion of the cell.

cytoskeleton. Finally, cells also contain **inclusions,** which consist of metabolic byproducts, storage forms of various nutrients, or inert crystals and pigments. The following sections cover the structure and functions of the major constituents of organelles, cytoskeleton, and inclusions.

Organelles

Although some organelles were discovered by light microscopists, their structure and function were not elucidated until the advent of electron microscopy, separation tech-

niques, and sensitive biochemical and histochemical procedures. Due to the application of these methods, it is now known that the membranes of organelles are composed of a phospholipid bilayer, which not only partitions the cell into compartments but also provides large surface areas for the biochemical reactions essential for the maintenance of life.

Cell Membrane

Each cell is bounded by a **cell membrane** (also known as the **plasma membrane** or **plasmalemma**) that functions in:

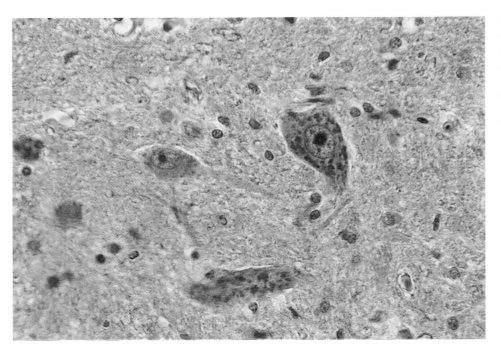

Figure 2-3. Motoneurons from the human spinal cord (× 540). Note that these nerve cells have numerous processes (axons and dendrites). The centrally placed nucleus and the single large nucleolus are clearly visible. The Nissl bodies (rough endoplasmic reticulum) are the most conspicuous features of the cytoplasm.

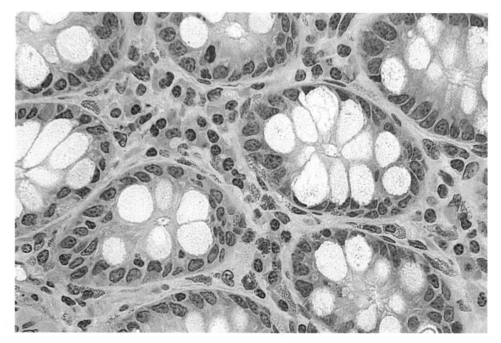

Figure 2–4. Goblet cells from the monkey colon (× 540). Some cells, such as the goblet cell, specialize in secreting materials. These cells accumulate mucinogen, which occupies much of the cell's volume, and then release it into the lumen of the intestine. During the processing of the tissue the mucinogen was extracted, leaving behind empty spaces.

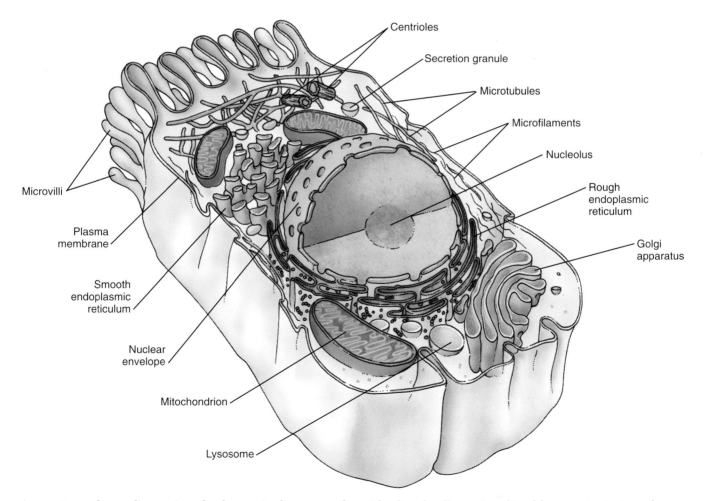

Figure 2–5. Three-dimensional schematic diagram of an idealized cell as visualized by transmission electron microscopy. Various organelles and cytoskeletal elements are displayed.

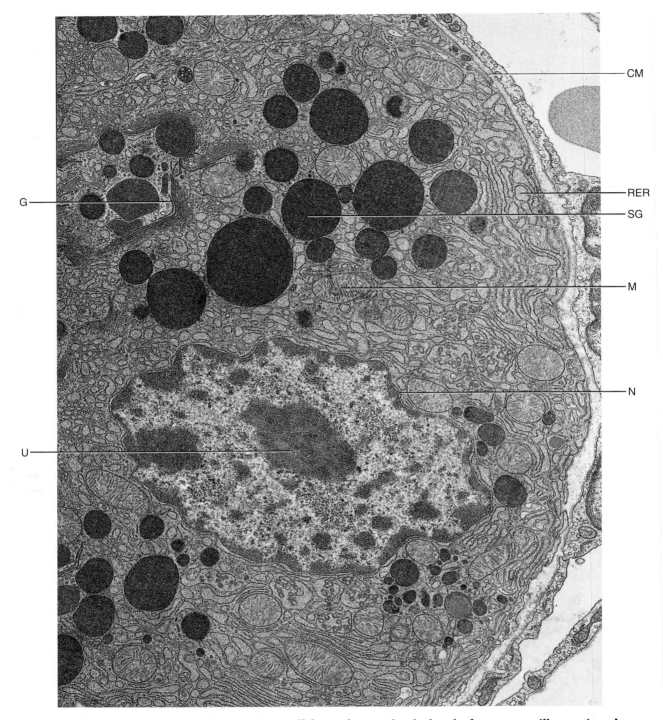

Figure 2–6. Electron micrograph of an acinar cell from the urethral gland of a mouse, illustrating the appearance of some organelles. M, mitochondria; G, Golgi apparatus; N, nucleus; U, nucleolus; SG, secretory granules; RER, rough endoplasmic reticulum; CM, cell membrane (× 15,500). (From Parr, M.B., Ren, H.P., Kepple, L., et al.: Ultrastructure and morphometry of the urethral glands in normal, castrated, and testosterone-treated castrated mice. Anat. Rec. **236**:449–458, 1993. Copyright 1993. Reprinted by permission of Wiley-Liss, Inc., a subsidiary of John Wiley & Sons, Inc.)

1. Maintaining the structural integrity of the cell
2. Controlling movements of substances in and out of the cell (selective permeability)
3. Regulating cell–cell interactions
4. Recognition (via receptors) of antigens, foreign cells, as well as altered cells
5. Acting as an interface between the cytoplasm and the external milieu
6. Establishing transport systems for specific molecules
7. Transducing extracellular physical and/or chemical signals into intracellular events.

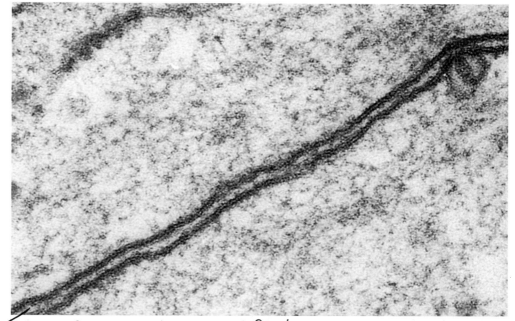

Figure 2–7. A junction between two cells demonstrates the trilaminar structures of the two cell membranes (×240,000). (From Leeson, T.S., Leeson, C.R., and Papparo, A.A.: Text/Atlas of Histology. Philadelphia, W.B. Saunders Company, 1988.)

fatty residues from outer & inner leaflet

Cell membranes are not visible with the light microscope. In electron micrographs, the plasmalemma is about 7.5 nm thick and appears as a trilaminar structure of two thin, dense lines with an intervening light area. Each layer is about 2.5 nm in width and the entire structure is known as the **unit membrane** (Fig. 2–7). The inner (cytoplasmic) dense line is its **inner leaflet,** whereas the outer dense line is its **outer leaflet.**

Molecular Composition

Each leaflet is composed of a single layer of **phospholipids** and associated **proteins,** usually in a 1:1 proportion by weight. However, in certain cases, such as myelin sheaths, the lipid component outweighs the protein component by a ratio of 4:1. The two leaflets, composing a **lipid bilayer** in which **proteins** are suspended, constitute the basic structure of all membranes of the cell (Fig. 2–8).

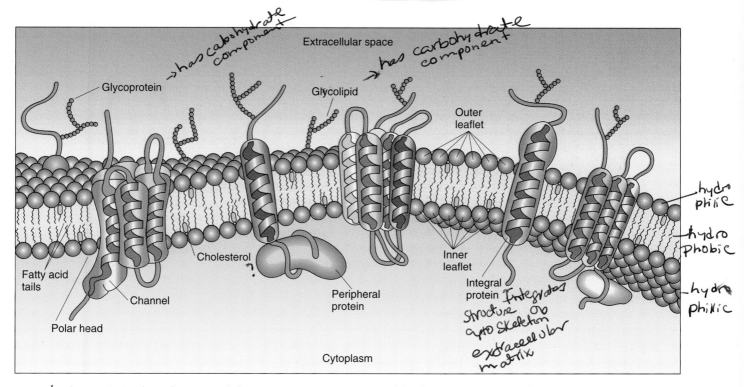

→ has carbohydrate component

→ has carbohydrate component

Extracellular space

Glycoprotein

Glycolipid

Outer leaflet

Inner leaflet

Fatty acid tails

Cholesterol ?

Channel

Peripheral protein

Integral protein *Integrates structure of cyto Skeleton to extracellular matrix*

Polar head

Cytoplasm

hydro philic

hydro phobic

hydro philic

Figure 2–8. Three-dimensional diagrammatic representation of the fluid mosaic model of the cell membrane.

Each **phospholipid molecule** of the lipid bilayer is composed of a **polar head,** located at the surface of the membrane, and two long **nonpolar** fatty acyl tails projecting into the center of the plasmalemma (see Fig. 2–8). The nonpolar fatty acyl tails of the two layers face each other within the membrane and form weak noncovalent bonds with each other, holding the bilayer together. Because the phospholipid molecule is composed of a **hydrophilic** head and a **hydrophobic** tail, the molecule is said to be **amphipathic.**

The polar heads are composed of **glycerol,** to which a positively charged nitrogenous group is attached by a negatively charged **phosphate group.** The two fatty acyl tails, only one of which is usually saturated, are covalently bound to glycerol. Other amphipathic molecules, such as **glycolipids** and **cholesterol,** are also present in the cell membrane. The unsaturated fatty acyl molecules increase membrane fluidity, whereas cholesterol decreases it.

The protein components of the plasmalemma either span the entire lipid bilayer as **integral proteins** or are attached to the cytoplasmic aspect of the lipid bilayer as **peripheral proteins.** Because most integral proteins pass through the thickness of the membrane, they are also referred to as **transmembrane proteins.** Those regions of transmembrane proteins that project into the cytoplasm or the extracellular space are composed of hydrophilic amino acids, whereas the intramembrane region consists of hydrophobic amino acids. Transmembrane proteins frequently form ion channels and carrier proteins that facilitate the passage of specific ions and molecules across the cell membrane.

Many of these proteins are quite long and are folded so that they make several passes through the membrane and thus are known as **multipass proteins** (see Fig. 2–8). Frequently the cytoplasmic and extracytoplasmic aspects of these proteins possess receptor sites that are specific for particular **signaling molecules.** Once these molecules are recognized at these receptor sites, the integral proteins can alter their conformation and perform a specific function.

Because the same integral membrane proteins have the ability to float like icebergs in the sea of phospholipids, this model is referred to as the **fluid mosaic model** of membrane structure. However, the integral proteins frequently possess only limited mobility, especially in polarized cells, in which particular regions of the cell serve specialized functions.

Peripheral proteins do not usually form covalent bonds with either the integral proteins or the phospholipid components of the cell membrane. Although they are usually located on the cytoplasmic aspect of the cell membrane, occasionally they may be on the extracellular surface. These proteins may form bonds either with the phospholipid molecules or with the transmembrane proteins. Frequently they are associated with the secondary messenger system of the cell (see later) or with the cytoskeletal apparatus.

Utilizing freeze-fracture techniques, the plasma membrane can be cleaved into its two leaflets in order to view the hydrophobic surfaces (Figs. 2–9 and 2–10). The outer sur-

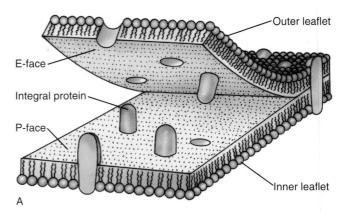

Figure 2–9. Schematic diagram of the E face and P face of the cell membrane.

face of the inner leaflet is referred to as the **P face** (closer to the protoplasm) and the inner surface of the outer leaflet is known as the **E face** (closer to the extracellular space). Electron micrographs of freeze-fractured plasma membranes show that the integral proteins, visualized by shadowing replica, are more numerous on the P face than on the E face (see Fig. 2–10).

Glycocalyx

A fuzzy coat, referred to as the **cell coat** or **glycocalyx,** is frequently evident in electron micrographs of the cell membrane. This coat is usually composed of carbohydrate chains that are covalently attached to transmembrane proteins and/or phospholipid molecules of the outer leaflet (see Fig. 2–8). Additionally, some of the extracellular matrix molecules, adsorbed to the cell surface, also contribute to its formation. Its intensity and thickness vary but it may be as thick as 50 nm on some epithelial sheaths, such as those lining regions of the digestive system.

Due to its numerous negatively charged sulfate and carboxyl groups, the glycocalyx stains intensely with lectins and dyes such as ruthenium red and Alcian blue, permitting its visualization with light microscopy. The most important function of the glycocalyx is protection of the cell from interaction with inappropriate proteins, from chemical injury, and from physical injury. Other cell coat functions include cell–cell recognition and adhesion, as occurs between endothelial cells and neutrophils, in blood clotting, and in inflammatory responses.

Membrane Transport Proteins

Although the hydrophobic components of the plasma membrane limit the movement of polar molecules across it, the presence and activities of specialized transmembrane proteins facilitate the transfer of these hydrophilic molecules across this barrier. These transmembrane proteins and pro-

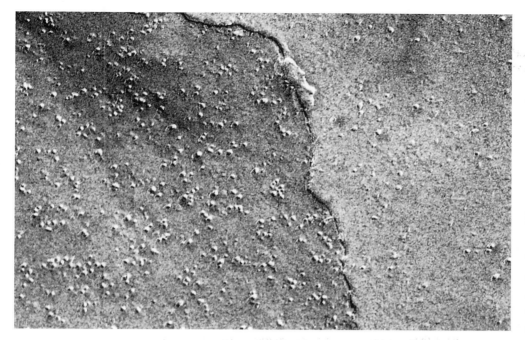

Figure 2–10. Freeze-fracture replica of a cell membrane. E face is on the right, P face is on the left (× 168,000). (From Leeson, T.S., Leeson, C.R., and Papparo, A.A.:Text/Atlas of Histology. Philadelphia, W.B. Saunders Company, 1988.)

tein complexes form **channel proteins** and **carrier proteins,** which are specifically concerned with the transfer of ions and small molecules across the plasma membrane. An ion or molecule traversing the membrane does not form a bond with channel proteins, whereas it does bind to carrier proteins.

A few nonpolar molecules (e.g., benzene, O_2, N_2) and uncharged polar molecules (e.g., H_2O, glycerol) can move across the cell membrane by simple diffusion down their concentration gradients. Even when driven by a concentration gradient, however, movement of most ions and small molecules across a membrane requires the aid of membrane transport proteins, either channel proteins or carrier proteins. This process is referred to as **facilitated diffusion.** Because both types of diffusion occur without any input of energy other than that inherent in the concentration gradient, they represent **passive transport** (Fig. 2–11). By expending energy, cells can transport ions and small molecules against their concentration gradients. Only carrier proteins can mediate such energy-requiring **active transport.** The several channel proteins involved in facilitated diffusion are discussed first and then the more versatile carrier proteins are considered.

Channel Proteins

Channel proteins participate in the formation of hydrophilic pores, called **ion channels,** across the plasmalemma. In order to form hydrophilic channels, the proteins are folded so that the hydrophobic amino acids are positioned peripherally, interacting with the fatty acyl tails of the phospholipid molecules of the lipid bilayer, and the hydrophilic

amino acids face inward, forming a polar inner lining for the channel.

Of the more than 100 different types of ion channels, some are specific for one particular ion, whereas others permit the passage of several different ions and small water-soluble molecules. Although these ions and small molecules follow chemical or electrochemical concentration gradients for the direction of their passage, cells possess methods of preventing these substances from entering these hydrophilic tunnels by means of controllable **gates** that block their opening. Most channels are **gated channels;** only a few are **ungated.** Gated channels are classified according to the control mechanism required to open the gate.

VOLTAGE-GATED CHANNELS. Voltage-gated channels go from the closed to the open position, permitting the passage of ions from one side of the membrane to the other, the most common example being depolarization in the transmission of nerve impulses. However, the open position is unstable and the channel goes from an open to an **inactive** position, where the passage of the ion is not only blocked but for a short period of time (a few milliseconds) the gate cannot be opened again. This is the **refractory period,** discussed in more detail in Chapter 9 on the nervous system. The velocity of response to depolarization may also vary, and channels that are slower to open are referred to as **delayed voltage-gated channels.**

LIGAND-GATED CHANNELS. Channels that require the binding of a **ligand** (signaling molecule) to their gate are known as **ligand-gated channels.** Unlike voltage-gated channels, these channels remain open until the ligand disso-

A   Passive Transport

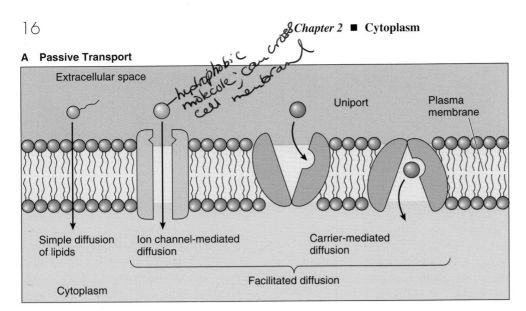

hydrophobic molecule; can cross cell membrane

Extracellular space

Uniport

Plasma membrane

Simple diffusion of lipids

Ion channel-mediated diffusion

Carrier-mediated diffusion

Facilitated diffusion

Cytoplasm

B   Active Transport

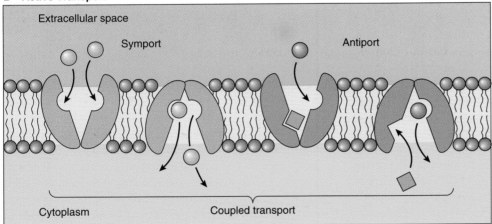

Extracellular space

Symport

Antiport

Cytoplasm

Coupled transport

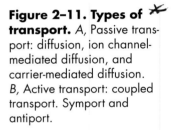

Figure 2–11. Types of transport. *A,* Passive transport: diffusion, ion channel-mediated diffusion, and carrier-mediated diffusion. *B,* Active transport: coupled transport. Symport and antiport.

ciates from the gate. The gate possesses the qualities of a **receptor molecule** because the binding of a signaling molecule causes conformational alterations of the gate. These gates are frequently referred to as **ion channel–linked receptors.** Some of the ligands controlling these gates are neurotransmitters, whereas others are nucleotides.

Neurotransmitter-gated channels are usually located on the postsynaptic membrane. The neurotransmitter binds to a specific site on the gate, altering its molecular conformation, thus opening it and permitting the influx of a specific ion into the cell. Some neurotransmitters are **excitatory,** regulating cation (positive ion) channels, whereas others are **inhibitory,** regulating anion (negative ion) channels. Excitatory neurotransmitters (e.g., acetylcholine) facilitate depolarization, whereas inhibitory neurotransmitters facilitate hyperpolarization of the membrane.

In **nucleotide-gated channels** the signal molecule is a nucleotide (e.g., cyclic AMP in olfactory receptors and cyclic GMP in rods of the retina) that binds to a site on the gate and, by altering the protein complex's conformation, permits the flow of a particular ion through the ion channel.

MECHANICALLY GATED CHANNELS. In **mechanically gated channels** an actual physical manipulation is required to open the gate. An example of this is found in the hair cells of the inner ear. These cells, located on the basilar membrane, possess **stereocilia** that are embedded in a matrix known as the **tectorial membrane.** Movement of the basilar membrane causes a shift in the positions of the hair cells resulting in the bending of the stereocilia. This physical distortion opens the mechanically gated channels of the stereocilia located in the inner ear, permitting the entry of cations into the cell, depolarizing it. This event generates impulses that the brain interprets as sound.

G-PROTEIN–GATED ION CHANNELS. Certain gated ion channels (e.g., muscarinic acetylcholine receptors of cardiac muscle cells) require the interaction between a receptor molecule and a G-protein complex (discussed later) with the resultant activation of the G protein. The activated G protein then interacts with the gate of the ion channel, opening it so that ions can gain access to and traverse the channel.

UNGATED CHANNELS. The most common form of an ungated channel is the **K+ leak channel** that permits the movement of K+ across it and is instrumental in the creation of an **electrical potential (voltage) difference** between the two sides of the cell membrane. Because this channel is ungated, the transit of K+ ions is not under the cell's control; rather, the direction of ion movement reflects its concentration on the two sides of the membrane.

Carrier Proteins

Carrier proteins are multipass membrane transport proteins that possess binding sites for specific ions or molecules on both sides of the lipid bilayer. When a solute binds to the binding site, the carrier protein undergoes *reversible* conformational changes; as the molecule is released on the other side of the membrane, the carrier protein returns to its previous conformation. As stated earlier, transport by carrier proteins may be **passive,** along an electrochemical concentration gradient, or **active,** against a gradient. Transport may be **uniport,** a single molecule moving in one direction, or **coupled,** two different molecules moving in the same (**symport**) or opposite (**antiport**) directions (see Fig. 2–11). Coupled transporters convey the solutes either simultaneously or sequentially.

PRIMARY ACTIVE TRANSPORT BY NA+-K+ PUMP. Normally, Na+ concentration is much greater outside the cell than inside, and the concentration of K+ is much greater inside the cell than outside. The cell maintains this concentration differential by expending ATP to drive a coupled antiport carrier protein known as the **Na+-K+ pump.** This pump transports K+ ions into and Na+ ions out of the cell, each against a steep concentration gradient. Because this concentration differential is essential for the survival and normal functioning of practically every animal cell, the plasma membrane of all animal cells possesses a large number of these pumps.

The Na+-K+ pump possesses two binding sites for K+ on its external aspect and three binding sites for Na+ on its cytoplasmic aspect; thus for every two K+ ions conveyed into the cell, three Na+ ions are transported out of the cell.

Na+-K+ ATPase has been shown to be associated with the Na+-K+ pump. When three Na+ ions bind on the cytosolic aspect of the pump, ATP is hydrolyzed to ADP and the released phosphate ion is used to phosphorylate the ATPase, resulting in alteration of the conformation of the pump, with the consequent transfer of Na+ ions out of the cell. Binding of two K+ ions on the external aspect of the pump causes dephosphorylation of the ATPase with an ensuing return of the carrier protein to its previous conformation, resulting in the transfer of the K+ ions into the cell.

The constant operation of this pump reduces the intracellular ion concentration that results in decreased intracellular osmotic pressure. If the osmotic pressure within the cell were not reduced by the Na+-K+ pump, water would enter the cell in large quantities, causing the cell to swell and eventually to succumb to osmotic lysis (i.e., burst). Hence, it is through the operation of this pump that the cell is able to regulate its osmolarity and, consequently, its volume. Additionally, this pump assists the K+ leak channels in the maintenance of the cell membrane potential.

Because the binding sites on the external aspect of the pump bind not only K+ but also the glycoside **ouabain,** this glycoside inhibits the Na+-K+ pump.

SECONDARY ACTIVE TRANSPORT BY COUPLED CARRIER PROTEINS. The ATP-driven transport of Na+ out of the cell establishes a high extracellular concentration of that ion. The energy reservoir inherent in this ion gradient can be utilized by carrier proteins to transport ions or other molecules against a concentration gradient. Frequently, this mode of active transport is referred to as **secondary active transport**, distinct from the **primary active transport** that utilizes the energy released from the hydrolysis of ATP.

The carrier proteins that participate in secondary active transport are either symports or antiports. As a Na+ ion binds to the extracellular aspect of the carrier protein, another ion or small molecule (e.g., **glucose**) also binds to a region on the same aspect of the carrier protein, inducing in it a conformational alteration. The change in conformation results in the transfer and subsequent release of both molecules on the other side of the membrane.

Cell Signaling

When cells communicate with each other, the one that sends the signal is referred to as the **signaling cell** and the cell receiving the signal is the **target cell.** Transmission of the information may occur either by the secretion or presentation of **signaling molecules,** which contact **receptors** on the target cell membrane (or intracellularly), or by the formation of intercellular pores known as **gap junctions,** which permit the movement of ions and small molecules (e.g., cyclic AMP) between the two cells. Gap junctions are discussed in Chapter 5 on epithelium and glands.

The signaling molecule, or **ligand,** may either be secreted and released by the signaling cell, or it may remain bound to its surface and be presented by the signaling cell to the target cell. A cell-surface receptor usually is a transmembrane protein, whereas an intracellular receptor is a protein in the cytosol or in the nucleus. Ligands that bind to cell-surface receptors usually are polar molecules; those that bind to intracellular receptors are **hydrophobic** and thus are able to diffuse through the cell membrane.

In the most selective signaling process, **synaptic signaling,** the signaling molecule, a **neurotransmitter,** is released so close to the target cell that only a single cell is affected by the ligand. A more generalized but still local form of signaling, **paracrine signaling,** occurs when the signaling molecule is released into the intercellular environment and affects cells in its immediate vicinity. Occasionally, the signaling cell is also the target cell, resulting in a specialized type of paracrine signaling known as **autocrine signaling.** The most widespread form of signaling is **endocrine signaling;** in this case the signaling molecule enters the bloodstream to be ferried to cells situated at a distance from the signaling cell.

Signaling Molecules

Most signaling molecules are hydrophilic (e.g., **acetylcholine**) and cannot penetrate the cell membrane. Therefore, they require receptors on the cell surface. Other signaling molecules are either hydrophobic, such as **steroid hormones,** or they are small nonpolar molecules, such as **nitric oxide (NO),** which have the capability of diffusing through the lipid bilayer. These ligands require the presence of an intracellular receptor. Hydrophilic ligands have a very short lifespan (a few milliseconds to minutes at most), whereas steroid hormones last for extended time periods (several hours to days).

Frequently, signaling molecules act in concert, in that several different ligands are required before a specific cellular response is elicited. Moreover, the same ligand or combination of ligands may elicit different responses from different cells. For instance, acetylcholine causes skeletal muscle cells to contract, cardiac muscle cells to relax, endothelial cells of blood vessels to release nitric oxide, and parenchymal cells of some glands to release the contents of their secretory granules.

Binding of signaling molecules to their receptors activates an intracellular **second messenger system,** initiating a cascade of reactions that result in the required response. A hormone, for example, binds to its receptors on the cell membrane of its target cell. The receptor alters its conformation, with the resultant activation of **adenylate cyclase,** a transmembrane protein, whose cytoplasmic region catalyses the transformation of ATP to **cyclic adenosine monophosphate (cAMP),** one of the most common **second messengers.**

Cyclic AMP activates a cascade of enzymes within the cell, thus multiplying the effects of a very few molecules of hormones on the cell surface. The specific intracellular event depends on the enzymes located within the cell—thus cAMP will activate one set of enzymes within an endothelial cell and an other set of enzymes within a follicular cell of the thyroid gland. Therefore, the same molecule can have a different effect in different cells. The system is known as a secondary messenger system because the hormone is the first messenger that activates the formation of cAMP, the second messenger.

Other second messengers include Ca^{2+}, cyclic guanosine monophosphate (cGMP), inositol triphosphate, and diacylglycerol.

Steroid hormones (e.g., cortisol) are also capable of diffusing through the cell membrane. Once in the cytosol they bind to **steroid hormone receptors** (members of the **intracellular receptor family**), and the ligand-receptor complex activates gene expression, that is **transcription** (the formation of messenger RNA [mRNA]). Transcription may be induced directly, resulting in a fast **primary response,** or indirectly, effecting a slower, **secondary response.** In the secondary response the mRNA codes for the protein that is necessary to activate the expression of additional genes.

Cell-Surface Receptors

Most cell-surface receptors are integral **glycoproteins** that function in recognizing signaling molecules and **transducing** the signal into an intracellular action. There are three main classes of receptor molecules: ion channel–linked receptors (discussed earlier), enzyme-linked receptors, and G-protein–linked receptors.

ENZYME-LINKED RECEPTORS. Enzyme-linked receptors are transmembrane proteins whose extracellular regions act as receptors for specific ligands. When a signaling molecule binds to the receptor site, the receptor's intracellular domain becomes activated so that it now possesses enzymatic capabilities. These enzymes then function to either induce the formation of second messengers, such as cyclic GMP, or permit the assembly of intracellular signaling molecules that relay the signal intracellularly. This signal then elicits the required response by activating additional enzyme systems or by stimulating gene regulatory proteins to initiate the transcription of specific genes.

G-PROTEIN–LINKED RECEPTORS. G-protein–linked receptors are multipass proteins whose extracellular domains act as receptor sites for ligands. Their intracellular regions have two separate sites, one that binds to G proteins and another that becomes phosphorylated during the process of receptor desensitization.

Most cells possess two types of GTPases, monomeric and trimeric, each of which has the capability of binding guanosine triphosphate (GTP) and guanosine diphosphate (GDP). Trimeric GTPases, **G proteins,** are composed of a large α **subunit** and two small β and γ **subunits,** and are able to associate with G-protein–linked receptors. There are several types of G proteins, including stimulatory ($\mathbf{G_s}$), inhibitory ($\mathbf{G_i}$), phospholipase C activator ($\mathbf{G_p}$), and transducin ($\mathbf{G_t}$). G proteins act by linking receptors with enzymes that modulate the levels of the intracellular signaling molecules (second messengers) cAMP or Ca^{2+}.

Signaling Via G_S and G_I Proteins. G_s proteins (Fig. 2–12) are usually present in the **inactive** state, in which a GDP molecule is bound to the α subunit. When a ligand binds to the G-protein–linked receptor, it alters the receptor's confor-

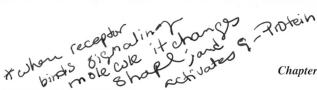

when receptor binds signaling molecule it changes shape, and activates G-Protein

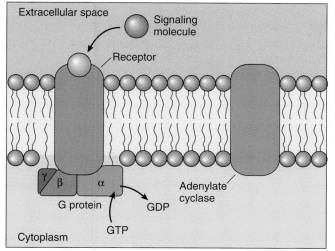

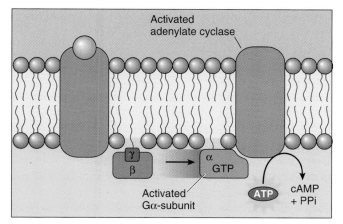

Figure 2–12. G-protein–linked receptor. When the signaling molecule contacts its receptor, the α subunit dissociates from the G protein and contacts and activates adenylate cyclase, which converts ATP to cyclic AMP. ✗

mation, permitting it to bind to the α subunit of the G_s protein, which in turn exchanges its GDP for a **GTP.** The binding of GTP causes the **α subunit** to dissociate not only from the receptor but also from the other two subunits and to bind with **adenylate cyclase,** a transmembrane protein. This binding activates adenylate cyclase to form many molecules of cAMP from ATP molecules. As the activation of adenylate cyclase is occurring, the ligand uncouples from the G-protein–linked receptor, returning the receptor to its original conformation without affecting the activity of the α subunit. Within a few seconds, the α subunit hydrolyzes its GTP to GDP, detaches from adenylate cyclase (thus deactivating it), and reassociates the β and γ subunits.

G_i behaves similarly to G_s, except that instead of activating adenylate cyclase, it inhibits it, so that cAMP is not being produced. The lack of cAMP prevents the phosphorylation—thus activation—of enzymes that would elicit a particular response. Hence, a particular ligand binding to a particular receptor may activate or inactivate the cell, de-

pending on the type of G protein that couples it to adenylate cyclase.

Cyclic AMP and its Role as a Secondary Messenger. Cyclic AMP is an intracellular signaling molecule which activates cAMP-dependent protein kinase (A-kinase) by binding to it. The activated **A-kinase** dissociates into its **regulatory component** and two **active catalytic subunits.** The active catalytic subunits perform either of two functions: they either phosphorylate other enzymes in the cytosol, thus initiating a cascade of phosphorylations and resulting in a specific response, or they travel to the nucleus, where they phosphorylate gene regulatory proteins, resulting in the transcription of the requisite genes.

As long as cAMP is present at a high enough concentration, a particular response is elicited from the target cell. In order to prevent responses of unduly long duration, cAMP is quickly degraded by **cyclic AMP phosphodiesterases** to 5′-AMP, which is unable to activate A-kinase. Moreover, the enzymes phosphorylated during the cascade of phosphorylations become deactivated by becoming dephosphorylated by another series of enzymes (**serine/threonine phosphoprotein phosphatases**).

Signaling via G_p Protein. When a ligand becomes bound to G_p-protein–linked receptor, the receptor alters its conformation and binds with G_p. This trimeric protein dissociates and its α subunit activates **phospholipase C,** the enzyme responsible for cleaving the membrane phospholipid **phosphatidylinositol biphosphate (PIP₂)** into **inositol triphosphate (IP₃)** and **diacylglycerol.** IP_3 leaves the membrane and diffuses to the endoplasmic reticulum, where it causes the release of Ca^{2+}—another second messenger—into the cytosol. Diacylglycerol remains attached to the inner leaflet of the plasma membrane and, with the assistance of Ca^{2+}, activates the enzyme **protein kinase C (C-kinase).** C-kinase in turn initiates a phosphorylation cascade, whose end result is the activation of gene regulatory proteins that initiate transcription of specific genes.

IP_3 is rapidly inactivated by being dephosphorylated, and diacylglycerol is catabolized within a few seconds of being formed. These actions ensure that responses to a ligand are of limited duration.

Ca^{2+} and Calmodulin. Because cytosolic Ca^{2+} acts as an important second messenger, its cytosolic concentration must be carefully controlled by the cell. These control mechanisms include the sequestering of Ca^{2+} by the endoplasmic reticulum, specific Ca^{2+}-binding molecules in the cytosol and mitochondria, and the active transport of this ion out of the cell.

When IP_3 causes an elevation of cytosolic Ca^{2+} levels, the excess ions bind to **calmodulin,** a protein found in high concentration in most animal cells. The Ca^{2+}-calmodulin complex activates a group of enzymes known as **Ca^{2+}-**

calmodulin–dependent protein kinases (CaM-kinases). CaM-kinases have numerous regulatory functions in the cell, such as the initiation of glycogenolysis, synthesis of catecholamines, and contraction of smooth muscle.

Protein Synthetic and Packaging Machinery of the Cell

Primary Components

RIBOSOMES. Ribosomes are small particles, approximately 12 nm wide and 25 nm long, composed of proteins and ribosomal RNA (rRNA). They function as a surface for the synthesis of proteins. Each ribosome is composed of a **large** and a **small subunit,** which are manufactured in the nucleolus and released as separate entities into the cytosol. The small subunit has a sedimentation value of 40S and is composed of 33 proteins and an 18S rRNA. The sedimentation value of the large subunit is 60S, and it consists of 49 proteins and 3 rRNAs. The sedimentation values of the RNAs are 5S, 5.8S, and 28S.

The small subunit has a site for binding mRNA, a **P-site** for binding peptidyl tRNA, and an **A-site** for binding aminoacyl tRNAs. The small and large subunits are present in the cytosol individually and will not form a ribosome until protein synthesis begins.

ENDOPLASMIC RETICULUM. The **endoplasmic reticulum (ER)** is the largest membranous system of the cell, comprising approximately half of the total membrane volume. It is a system of interconnected tubules and vesicles whose lumen is referred to as the **cistern.** The metabolic processes that occur on the surface of and within the ER are protein synthesis and modification, lipid and steroid synthesis, and detoxification of certain toxic compounds, as well as the manufacture of all membranes of the cell. The ER has two components, named smooth and rough endoplasmic reticulum.

Smooth Endoplasmic Reticulum. A system of anastomosing tubules and occasional flattened membrane-bound vesicles constitute the **smooth endoplasmic reticulum (SER)** (Fig. 2–13). The lumen of the SER is assumed to be continuous with that of the rough endoplasmic reticulum. Except for cells active in synthesis of steroids, cholesterol, and triglycerides, and cells that function in detoxification of toxic materials (e.g., alcohol and barbiturates), most cells do not possess an abundance of SER. The SER has become specialized in some cells such as skeletal muscle cells, where it is known as the sarcoplasmic reticulum. Here it functions in sequestering calcium ions from the cytosol, assisting in the control of muscle contraction.

Rough Endoplasmic Reticulum. Cells that function in the synthesis of proteins that are to be exported are richly endowed with **rough endoplasmic reticulum (RER)** (see Fig.

2–6). The membranes of this organelle are somewhat different from those of its smooth counterpart, because it possesses integral proteins that function in recognizing and binding ribosomes to its cytosolic surface as well as maintaining the flattened morphology of the RER. The integral proteins of interest for the purposes of this textbook are **signal recognition particle receptor (docking protein), ribosome receptor protein** (ribophorin I and ribophorin II), and **pore protein.** Their functions are discussed later.

Rough endoplasmic reticulum functions in the synthesis of all proteins that are to be packaged or delivered to the plasma membrane. It also performs post-translational modifications of these proteins, including sulfation, folding, and glycosylation. Additionally, lipids and integral proteins of all membranes of the cell are manufactured by the RER. The cisterna of the RER is continuous with the perinuclear cistern, the space between the inner and outer nuclear membranes.

POLYRIBOSOMES. Proteins to be packaged are synthesized on the RER surface, whereas proteins destined for the cytosol are manufactured within the cytosol. The information for the primary structure of a protein (sequence of amino acids) is housed in the DNA of the nucleus. This information is **transcribed** into a strand of mRNA, which leaves the nucleus and enters the cytoplasm. The sequence of **codons** of the mRNA thus represents the chain of amino acids, in which each codon is composed of three consecutive nucleotides. Because any three consecutive nucleotides constitute a codon, it is essential that the protein synthetic machinery recognize the beginning and the end of the message, otherwise an incorrect protein will be manufactured.

The three types of RNA play distinctive roles in protein synthesis. **Messenger RNA (mRNA)** carries the coded instructions specifying the sequence of amino acids. **Transfer RNAs (tRNAs)** form covalent bonds with amino acids, forming **aminoacyl tRNAs.** These enzyme-catalyzed reactions are specific; that is, each tRNA reacts with its own corresponding amino acid. Each tRNA also contains the **anticodon** that recognizes the codon in mRNA corresponding to the amino acid it carries. Finally, several **ribosomal RNAs (rRNAs)** associate with a large number of proteins to form the small and large ribosomal subunits.

Protein Synthesis (Translation)

The requirements for this process are:

1. **Messenger RNA (mRNA)** strand
2. **Transfer RNAs (tRNAs),** each of which carries an amino acid and possesses the **anticodon** that recognizes the codon of the mRNA coding for that particular amino acid;
3. Small and large **ribosomal subunits.**

It is interesting that the approximate time of synthesis of a protein composed of 400 amino acids is about 20 seconds.

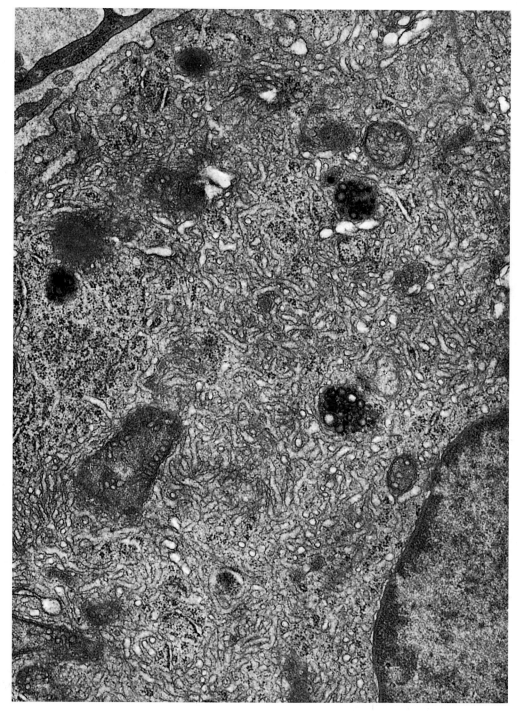

Figure 2–13. Electron micrograph of the smooth endoplasmic reticulum of the human suprarenal cortex. (From Leeson, T.S., Leeson, C.R., and Papparo, A.A.:Text/Atlas of Histology. Philadelphia, W.B. Saunders Company, 1988.)

Because a single strand of mRNA may have as many as 15 ribosomes translating it simultaneously, a large number of protein molecules may be synthesized in a short period of time. This conglomeration of mRNA-ribosome complex, which usually has a spiral form, is referred to as a **polyribosome,** or **polysome.**

SYNTHESIS OF CYTOSOLIC PROTEINS. The general process of protein synthesis in the cytosol is outlined in Figure 2–14.

STEP 1

a. The process begins when the P site of the small ribosomal subunit is occupied by an **initiator tRNA,** whose **anticodon** recognizes the triplet **codon AUG,** coding for the amino acid **methionine.**

b. An **mRNA** binds to the small subunit.

c. The small subunit assists the anticodon of the tRNA molecule to recognize the **start codon AUG** on the mRNA molecule. This step acts as a registration step so

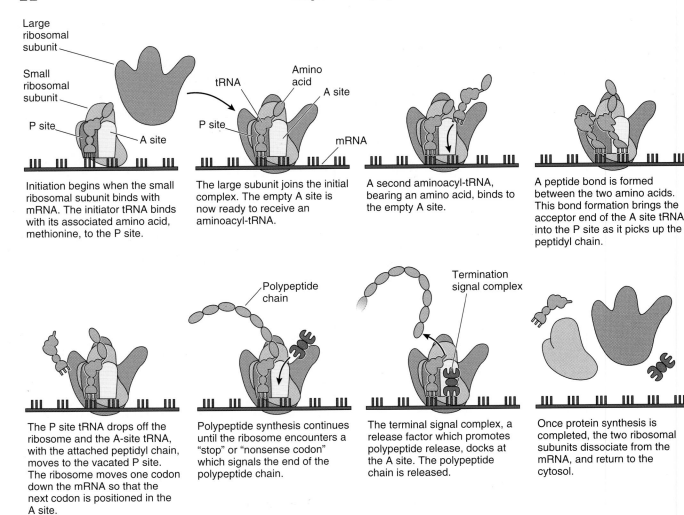

Figure 2–14. Schematic diagram of protein synthesis in the cytosol.

that the next three nucleotides of the mRNA molecule may be recognized as the next codon.

STEP 2

The large ribosomal subunit binds to the small subunit and the ribosome moves along the mRNA chain, in a 5′ to 3′ direction, until the next codon lines up with the A site of the small subunit.

STEP 3

An acylated tRNA (tRNA bearing an amino acid) compares its anticodon with the codon of the mRNA; if they match, the tRNA binds to the A site.

STEP 4

a. The amino acids at the A and P sites form a peptide bond.

b. The tRNA on the P site yields its amino acid to the tRNA at the A site, which now has two amino acids attached to it. These reactions are catalyzed by the enzyme **peptidyl transferase.**

STEP 5

The deaminated tRNA leaves the P site and the tRNA with its two amino acids attached moves from the A site to the P site. Concurrently, the ribosome moves along the mRNA chain until the next codon lines up with the A site of the small ribosomal subunit. The energy required by this step is derived from the hydrolysis of GTP.

STEP 6

a. Steps 3 through 5 are repeated, elongating the polypeptide chain until the **stop codon** is reached.

b. There are three stop codons (**UAG, UAA,** and **UGA**), each one of which may halt translation.

STEP 7

a. When the A site of the small ribosomal subunit reaches a stop codon, a **release factor** binds to the A site.

b. This factor is responsible for releasing the newly formed polypeptide chain from the tRNA of the P site into the cytosol.

STEP 8

The tRNA is released from the P site, the release factor is released from the A site, and the small and large ribosomal subunits leave the mRNA.

SYNTHESIS OF PROTEINS ON THE ROUGH ENDO-PLASTIC RETICULUM. Proteins that need to be packaged either for delivery to the outside of the cell or merely isolated from the cytosol must be identified and be delivered **cotranslationally** (during the process of synthesis) into the RER cistern. The mode of identification resides in a small segment of the mRNA, located immediately following the start codon, which codes for a sequence of amino acids, known as the **signal peptide.**

Employing the sequence just outlined for the synthesis of protein in the cytosol, the mRNA begins to be translated, forming the signal peptide (Fig. 2–15). This peptide is recognized by a protein–RNA complex located in the cytosol, the **signal recognition particle** (**SRP**). The SRP attached to the signal peptide and by occupying the P site on the small subunit of the ribosome halts translation; it then directs the polysome to migrate to the RER.

The SRP receptor protein (docking protein) in the RER membrane contacts the SRP, and the ribosome receptor protein contacts the large subunit of the ribosome, attaching the polysome to the cytosolic surface of the RER. The following events then occur almost simultaneously:

1. The pore proteins assemble, forming a **pore** through the lipid bilayer of the RER.

2. The signal peptide contacts the pore protein and begins to be translocated (amino terminus first) into the cistern of the RER.

3. The SRP is dislodged, reenters the cytosol, and frees the P site on the small ribosomal subunit. The ribosome remains on the RER surface.

4. As translation resumes, the nascent protein continues to be channeled into the cistern of the RER.

5. An enzyme attached to the cisternal aspect of the RER membrane, known as **signal peptidase,** cleaves the signal peptide from the forming protein. The signal peptide becomes degraded into its amino acid components.

6. As detailed previously, when the stop codon is reached, protein synthesis is completed, and the small and large ribosomal subunits dissociate and reenter the cytosol to join the pool of ribosomal subunits.

7. The newly formed proteins are folded, glycosylated, and undergo additional post-translational modifications within the RER cistern.

8. The modified proteins leave the cistern via small **transport vesicles** (without a clathrin coat) at regions of the RER devoid of ribosomes.

Golgi Apparatus

The Golgi apparatus functions in the synthesis of carbohydrates—specifically polysaccharides—as well as the modification and sorting of proteins manufactured on the RER.

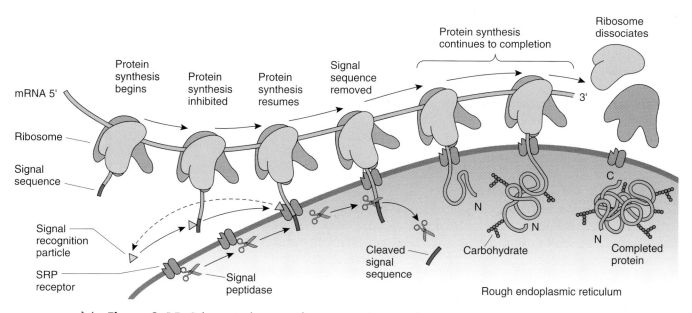

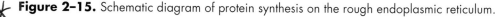

Figure 2–15. Schematic diagram of protein synthesis on the rough endoplasmic reticulum.

Proteins manufactured and packaged in the RER follow a **default pathway** to the Golgi apparatus for post-translational modification and packaging. Proteins destined to remain in the RER or to go to a compartment other than the Golgi apparatus possess a signal that will divert them from the default pathway.

The Golgi apparatus is composed of one or more series of flattened, slightly curved membrane-bounded **cisternae,** the **Golgi stack,** which resemble a stack of pita breads that do not quite contact each other (Figs. 2–16 and 2–17). The periphery of each cisterna is dilated and is rimmed by vesicles that are in the process of either fusing with or budding off that particular compartment.

Each stack has a region closest to the RER, the *cis*-face (convex) or entry face, and the opposite aspect, the *trans*-face (concave) or exit face. Between the two faces are two or more **medial compartments.** It has been shown recently that associated with each face is a corresponding cisternal network, the *cis* **Golgi network (CGN)** and the *trans* **Golgi network (TGN).**

Transport vesicles arriving from the RER fuse, via a mechanism requiring energy, with the membranes of the CGN and release their protein content into its cisterna. It is in the CGN that proteins destined to remain in the RER are selectively returned to the RER along a microtubule-mediated pathway.

Small spherical vesicles that bud off the rim of the CGN transport the nascent protein to the *cis*-face of the Golgi stack. Some investigators suggest that there is a direct connection between the CGN and the *cis*-face so that the protein does not necessarily have to be ferried by vesicles.

Proteins are transferred from the *cis* to the medial and fi-nally to the *trans* cisternae via nonclathrin-coated vesicles that bud off and fuse with the rims of the particular compartment (Fig. 2–18). As the proteins pass through the Golgi apparatus they are modified within the Golgi stack. Proteins that form the cores of glycoprotein molecules become heavily glycosylated, whereas other proteins acquire or lose sugar moieties.

Mannose phosphorylation occurs within the CGN and the *cis* cisterna, whereas the removal of mannose from certain proteins takes place within the *cis* and medial compartments of the Golgi stack. *N*-acetylglucosamine is added to the protein within the medial cisternae. Addition of sialic acid (*N*-acetylneuraminic acid) and galactose as well as phosphorylation and sulfation of amino acids occurs in the *trans* face.

SORTING IN THE *TRANS* GOLGI NETWORK. Proteins that leave the TGN are enclosed in vesicles that may do one of the following (see Fig. 2–18).

- Insert into the cell membrane as membrane proteins and lipids
- Fuse with the cell membrane such that the protein they carry is *immediately* released into the extracellular space
- Congregate in the cytoplasm near the apical cell membrane as **secretory granules (vesicles),** and, upon a given signal, fuse with the cell membrane for *eventual* release of the protein outside the cell
- Fuse with **late endosomes** (discussed later), releasing their content into that organelle, which then becomes a **lysosome**

The first three processes are known as **exocytosis,** because material leaves the cytoplasm proper. Neither immedi-

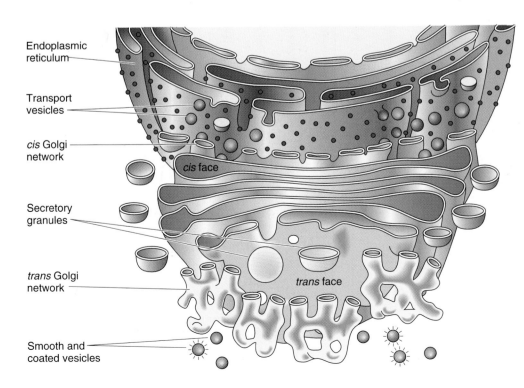

Endoplasmic reticulum

Transport vesicles

cis Golgi network

cis face

Secretory granules

trans Golgi network

trans face

Smooth and coated vesicles

Figure 2–16. Schematic diagram illustrating the rough endoplasmic reticulum and the Golgi apparatus. Note that transfer vesicles contain newly synthesized protein and are ferried to the *cis* Golgi network of the Golgi apparatus. The protein is modified in the various faces of the Golgi complex and enters the *trans* Golgi network for packaging.

Figure 2–17. Electron micrograph of the Golgi apparatus of the rat epididymis. ER, endoplasmic reticulum; TGN, trans Golgi network; m, mitochondrion; numbers, represent the saccules of the Golgi apparatus. (From Hermo, L., Green, H., and Clermont, Y.: Golgi apparatus of epithelial principal cells of the ependymal initial segment of the rat: Structure, relationship with endoplasmic reticulum, and role in the formation of secretory vesicles. Anat. Rec. **229:**159–176, 1991. Copyright 1991. Reprinted by permission of John Wiley & Sons, Inc.)

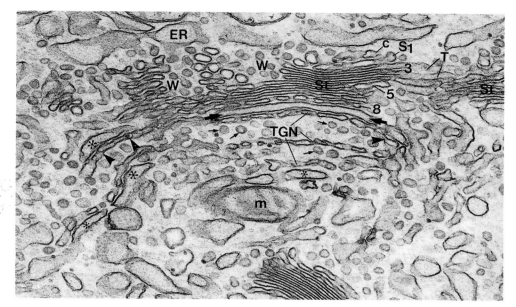

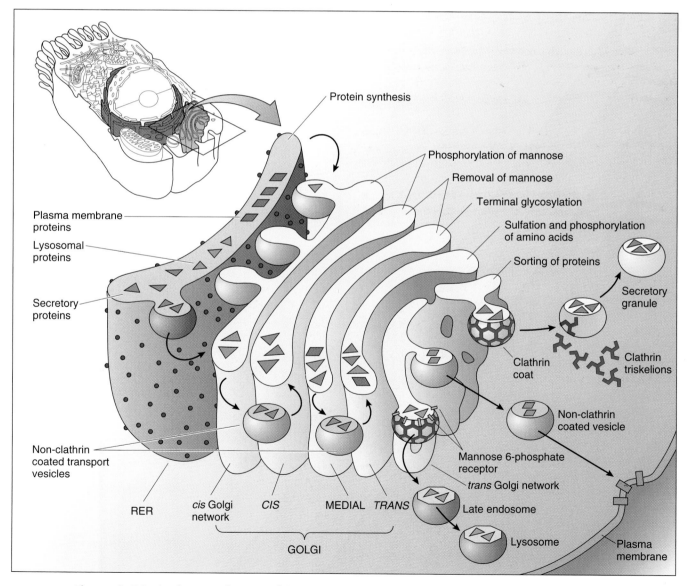

Figure 2–18. A schematic diagram of the Golgi apparatus and packaging in the *trans* Golgi network.

ate release into the extracellular space nor insertion into the cell membrane requires a particular regulatory process; thus both are said to follow the **constitutive secretory pathway (default pathway).** In contrast, the pathways to lysosomes and to secretory vesicles are known as the **regulated secretory pathway.**

TRANSPORT OF LYSOSOMAL PROTEINS. The sorting process begins with the phosphorylation of mannose residues of the lysosomal proteins (lysosomal hydrolases) in the *cis* Golgi network and in the *cis* cisterna of the Golgi stack. When these proteins reach the *trans* Golgi network, their mannose-6-phosphate (M6P) is recognized as a signal, and they become bound to mannose-6-phosphate receptors, transmembrane proteins of the TGN membrane.

A small pit is formed with the assistance of **clathrin triskelions,** protein complexes composed of three heavy and three light chains forming a structure with three arms that radiate from a central point (see Fig. 2–18). The triskelions self-assemble, coating the cytoplasmic aspect of the TGN rich in M6P receptors to which M6P is bound. As the pit deepens, it pinches off the TGN and forms a **clathrin-coated vesicle.** The clathrin coat is also referred to as the **clathrin basket.**

The clathrin-coated vesicle quickly loses its clathrin coat, which, unlike the formation of the clathrin basket, is an energy-requiring process. The uncoated vesicle reaches, fuses with, and releases its contents into the late endosome (discussed later).

Because clathrin coats are utilized for many other types of vesicles, there is an intermediary protein, **adaptin,** that is interposed between the cytoplasmic aspect of the receptor molecule and the clathrin. Many different types of adaptins exist, each of which has a binding site for a particular receptor as well as a binding site for clathrin.

TRANSPORT OF REGULATED SECRETORY PROTEINS. Proteins that are to be released into the extracellular space in a discontinuous manner also require the formation of clathrin-coated vesicles. The signal for their formation is not known; however, the mechanism is believed to be similar to that for lysosomal proteins.

Unlike vesicles that ferry lysosomal enzymes, secretory granules are quite large and carry many more proteins than there are receptors on the vesicle surface. Additionally, the contents of the secretory granules become condensed with time due to the loss of fluid from the secretory granules (see Figs. 2–6 and 2–18). During this process of increasing concentration, these vesicles are frequently referred to as **condensing vesicles.** Moreover, secretory granules of polarized cells remain localized in a particular region of the cell. They remain as clusters of secretory granules that, in reaction to a particular signal (e.g., neurotransmitter or hormone), fuse with the cell membrane to release their contents into the intercellular space.

TRANSPORT ALONG THE CONSTITUTIVE PATHWAY. All vesicles that participate in nonselective transport, such as those passing between the RER and the *cis* Golgi network, or among the cisternae of the Golgi stack, or those utilizing the constitutive pathway between the TGN and the plasma membrane, also require a coated vesicle (see Fig. 2–18). However, the coating is composed of a seven-unit protein complex known as **coatomer,** rather than of clathrin. Each protein of the coatomer complex is referred to as a **coat protein subunit (COPS),** whose assembly, unlike that of clathrin, is energy-requiring and remains with the vesicle until it reaches its intended target.

Endocytosis, Endosomes, and Lysosomes

The process whereby a cell ingests macromolecules, particulate matter, and other substances from the extracellular space is referred to as **endocytosis.** The endocytosed material is engulfed in a vesicle appropriate for its volume. If the vesicle is large (>250 nm in diameter), the method is referred to as **phagocytosis** (cell eating) and the vesicle is a **phagosome.** If the vesicle is small (<150 nm in diameter), the type of endocytosis is known as **pinocytosis** (cell drinking) and the vesicle is a **pinocytotic vesicle.**

Endocytotic Mechanisms

PHAGOCYTOSIS. The process of engulfing large particulate matter, such as microorganisms, cell fragments, and cells (e.g., defunct red blood cells), is usually performed by specialized cells known as **phagocytes.** The most common phagocytes are the white blood cells, **neutrophils** and **monocytes.** When monocytes leave the bloodstream to perform their task of phagocytosis, they become known as **macrophages.**

Phagocytes are able to internalize particulate matter because they possess receptors that recognize certain surface features of the material to be engulfed. Two of the better understood of these surface features come from the study of immunology and are the constant regions (Fc regions) of antibodies and a blood-borne series of proteins known as **complement.** Because the variable region of the antibody binds to the surface of a microorganism, the Fc region projects away from its surface.

Macrophages and neutrophils possess Fc receptors that bind the Fc regions of the antibody upon contact. This relationship acts as a signal for the cell to extend pseudopods, surround the microorganism, and internalize the microorganism by forming a **phagosome.** Complement on the surface of the microorganism probably assists phagocytosis in a similar manner, because macrophages also possess complement receptors on their surface. Interaction between complement and its receptor presumably activates the cell to form pseudopods and engulf the offending microorganism.

PINOCYTOSIS. Because most cells export substances into the intercellular space, they continually add the membranes of vesicles that transport those substances from the *trans* Golgi network to the plasma membrane. These cells, in order to maintain their shape and size, must continually remove the excess membrane and return it for recycling. This cycle of exocytosis/endocytosis is known as **membrane trafficking,** referring to the movement of membranes to and from various compartments of the cell. In most cells, **pinocytosis** is the most active transporting process, contributing most to the recapturing of membranes (Fig. 2–19).

RECEPTOR-MEDIATED ENDOCYTOSIS. Many cells specialize in the pinocytosis of several types of macromolecules. The most efficient form of capturing these substances depends on the presence of receptor proteins (**cargo receptors**) in the cell membrane. Cargo receptors are transmembrane proteins that become associated with the particular macromolecule (**ligand**) extracellularly and with a **clathrin coat** intracellularly (see Fig. 2–19).

The assembly of clathrin triskelions beneath the cargo receptors forms a **clathrin-coated pit** (Figs. 2–20 and 2–21), which eventually becomes a **pinocytotic vesicle,** enclosing the ligand and ferrying it inside the cell. This method is known as **receptor-mediated endocytosis.** It permits the cell to increase the concentration of the ligand (such as low-density lipoprotein) within the pinocytotic vesicle.

It is interesting to note that a typical pinocytotic vesicle may have as many as 1000 cargo receptors of several types, for they may bind different macromolecules. Each cargo receptor is linked to its own **adaptin,** the protein with a binding site for the cytoplasmic aspect of the receptor, and a binding site for the clathrin triskelion.

Endosomes

Shortly after their formation, pinocytotic vesicles lose their clathrin coats (which return to the pool of clathrin triskelions in the cytosol) and fuse with **early endosomes** (see Figs. 2–19 and 2–22), a system of vesicles and tubules lo-

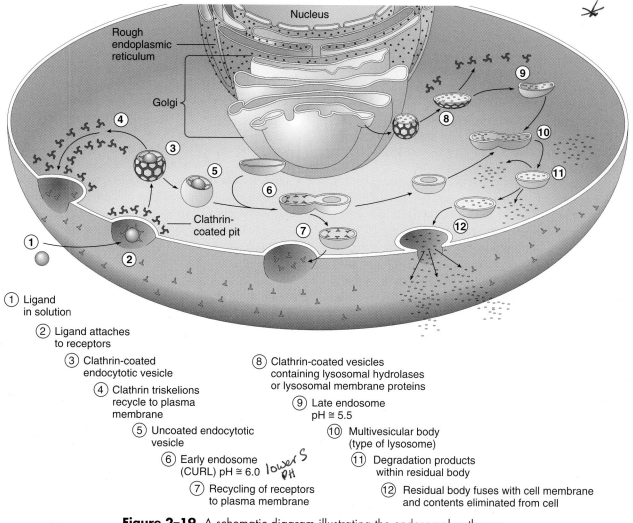

① Ligand in solution

② Ligand attaches to receptors

③ Clathrin-coated endocytotic vesicle

④ Clathrin triskelions recycle to plasma membrane

⑤ Uncoated endocytotic vesicle

⑥ Early endosome (CURL) pH ≅ 6.0 *lower pH*

⑦ Recycling of receptors to plasma membrane

⑧ Clathrin-coated vesicles containing lysosomal hydrolases or lysosomal membrane proteins

⑨ Late endosome pH ≅ 5.5

⑩ Multivesicular body (type of lysosome)

⑪ Degradation products within residual body

⑫ Residual body fuses with cell membrane and contents eliminated from cell

Figure 2–19. A schematic diagram illustrating the endosomal pathways.

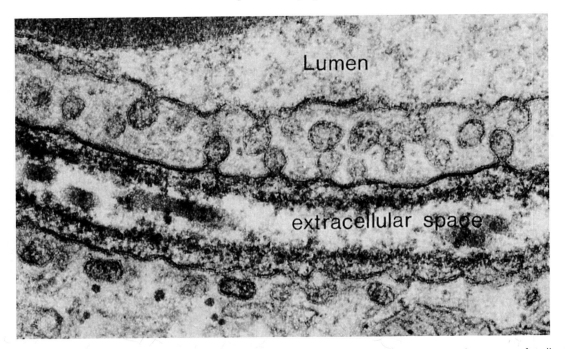

Figure 2–20. Electron micrograph of endocytosis in a capillary. (From Hopkins, C.R.:Structure and Function of Cells. Philadelphia, W.B. Saunders Company, 1978.)

cated near the plasma membrane. If the entire contents of the pinocytotic vesicle requires degradation, then the material from the early endosome will be transferred to a **late endosome.** This similar set of tubules and vesicles, located deeper in the cytoplasm near the Golgi apparatus, functions to prepare its contents for eventual destruction by lysosomes.

Early and late endosomes, collectively, constitute the **endosomal compartment.** The membranes of all endosomes contain ATP-linked H^+ pumps that acidify the interior of the endosomes by actively pumping H^+ ions into the interior of the endosome, so that the early endosome has a pH of 6.0, whereas the late endosome has a pH of 5.5.

Material entering the early endosome may be retrieved from that compartment and returned to its earlier location. This happens with cargo receptors that need to be recycled. When the pinocytotic vesicle fuses with the early endosome, the acidic environment causes an uncoupling of the ligand from its receptor molecule. The ligand remains within the lumen of the early endosome, whereas the receptor molecules (e.g., low-density lipoprotein receptors) are returned to the plasma membrane. Some authors refer to this type of an early endosome as a **CURL** (*c*ompartment for *u*ncoupling of *r*eceptor and *l*igand) (see Figs. 2–19 and 2–22).

Within a few minutes of entering the early endosome, the ligand either is transferred to a late endosome (as in the case of low-density lipoprotein) or is packaged to be returned to the cell membrane, where it is released (e.g., transferrin) into the extracellular space. Occasionally both the receptor and the ligand (e.g., epidermal growth factor and its receptor) are transferred to the late endosome for eventual degradation.

The transport between early and late endosomes has not been elucidated. Some authors suggest that early endosomes migrate into a deeper location within the cell and become late endosomes. Others suggest that these are two separate compartments, and that specific **endosomal carrier vesicles** ferry material from early to late endosomes. These are believed to be large vesicles containing numerous small vesicles that have been noted in electron micrographs as **multivesicular bodies.** Both concepts recognize the presence of a system of microtubules along which either the early endosome or the endosomal carrier vesicle negotiates its way to the late endosome.

Lysosomes

The contents of late endosomes are delivered for enzymatic digestion into the lumina of specialized organelles known as **lysosomes** (see Figs. 2–22 and 2–23). Each lysosome is round to polymorphous in shape. Its average diameter is 0.3 to 0.8 μm, and it contains at least 40 different types of **acid hydrolases,** such as sulfatases, proteases, nucleases, lipases, and glycosidases, among others. Because all of these enzymes require an acid environment for optimal function, lysosomal membranes possess proton pumps that actively transport H^+ ions into the lysosome, maintaining its lumen at a pH of 5.0 (see Fig. 2–19).

Lysosomes function in digesting not only macromolecules, phagocytosed microorganisms, cellular debris, and cells but also excess or senescent organelles such as mitochondria and RER. The various enzymes digest the engulfed

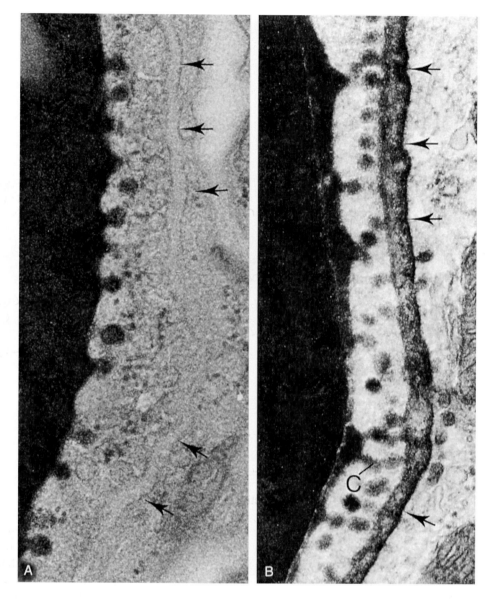

Figure 2–21. Electron microscopy of transport of microperoxidase, a trace molecule, across the endothelial cell of a capillary (× 42,000). *A,* The lumen of the capillary is filled with the tracer; note its uptake by pinocytotic vesicles on the luminal aspect. *B,* One minute later the tracer has been conveyed across the endothelial cell and exocytosed on the connective tissue side into the extracellular space (*demarcated by arrows*). Note that the letter C indicates a region of fused vesicles, forming a temporary channel between the lumen of the capillary and the extracellular space. (From Hopkins, C.R.: Structure and Function of Cells. Philadelphia, W.B. Saunders Company, 1978.)

material into small, soluble end products that are transported by carrier proteins in the lysosomal membrane from the lysosomes into the cytosol and are either reused by the cell or exported from the cell into the extracellular space. Additionally, certain cells, especially during embryogenesis, are programmed to die; the lysosomes of these cells release their hydrolytic enzymes and the cell undergoes **autolysis.**

FORMATION OF LYSOSOMES. Lysosomes receive their hydrolytic enzymes as well as their membranes from the *trans* Golgi network; however, they arrive in different vesicles. Although both types of vesicles possess a clathrin coat as they pinch off the TGN, it is lost shortly after formation. The uncoated vesicles then fuse with late endosomes.

Vesicles ferrying lysosomal enzymes possess **mannose-6-phosphate receptors,** to which these enzymes are bound.

In the acidic environment of the late endosome, the lysosomal enzymes dissociate from their receptors, their mannose residue becomes dephosphorylated, and the receptors are recycled by being returned to the TGN. It should be understood that the dephosphorylated lysosomal hydrolases can no longer bind to the mannose-6-phosphate receptors and therefore stay in the late endosome (see Figs. 2–18 and 2–19).

When late endosomes possess both enzymatic and membrane components, then, according to some authors, the late endosome fuses with a lysosome. However, others suggest that it matures to become a lysosome.

Transport of Substances into Lysosomes. Substances destined for degradation within lysosomes reach these organelles in one of three ways: through phagosomes, pinocytotic vesicles, or autophagosomes (see Fig. 2–19).

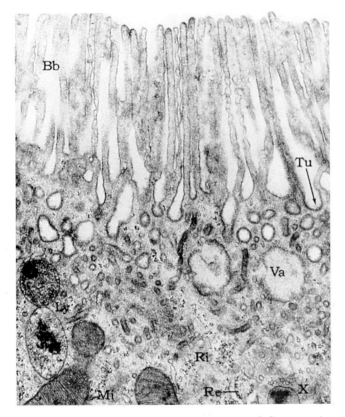

Figure 2–22. Endocytotic vesicles (Tu) of the proximal tubule cell of the kidney cortex. Note the presence of microvilli (Bb), lysosome (Ly), mitochondria (Mi), rough endoplasmic reticulum (Re), free ribosomes (Ri), and possibly, early endosomes (Va) (× 25,000). (From Rhodin, J.A.G.: An Atlas of Ultrastructure. Philadelphia, W.B. Saunders Company, 1963.)

Phagocytosed material, contained within **phagosomes,** moves toward the interior of the cell. The phagosome either joins a lysosome or a late endosome. The hydrolytic enzymes digest most of the contents of the phagosome, especially the protein and carbohydrate components. Lipids, however, are more resistant to complete digestion, and they remain enclosed within the spent lysosome, now referred to as a **residual body.**

Senescent organelles, such as mitochodria and organelles no longer required by the cell, or the RER of a quiescent fibroblast, need to be degraded. The organelles in question become surrounded by elements of the endoplasmic reticulum, and are enclosed in vesicles known as **autophagosomes.** These structures fuse with either late endosomes or with lysosomes, and share the same subsequent fate as the phagosome.

CLINICAL CORRELATIONS

Lysosomal Storage Disorders

Certain individuals have hereditary enzyme deficiencies, so that they are incapable of completely degrading various macromolecules into soluble byproducts. As the insoluble intermediaries of these substances become amassed within the lysosomes of their cells, the size of these lysosomes increases sufficiently to interfere with the abilities of these cells to perform their function (Table 2–1).

Probably the most commonly known of these conditions is **Tay-Sachs disease,** occurring mostly in children of Northeast European Jewish ancestry. These children display a deficiency in the enzyme hexosaminidase and are

Figure 2–23. Lysosomes of rat cultured alveolar macrophages (× 45,000). (From Sakai, M., Araki, N., and Ogawa, K.: Lysosomal movements during heterophagy and autophagy: With special reference to nematolysosome and wrapping lysosome. J. Electron Microscopy Tech. **12:**101–131, 1989. Copyright 1989. Reprinted by permission of John Wiley & Sons, Inc.)

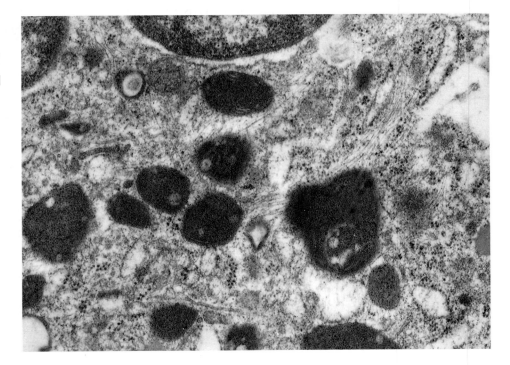

incapable of catabolizing GM$_2$ gangliosides. Although most cells of these children accumulate GM$_2$ ganglioside in their lysosomes, it is the neurons in their central and peripheral nervous systems that are the most problematic. Lysosomes of these cells become so engorged that they interfere with neuronal function, causing the children to become vegetative within the first year or two and die by the third year of life.

Peroxisomes

Peroxisomes (microbodies) are small (0.2 to 1.0 μm in diameter), spherical to ovoid membrane-bound organelles that contain more than 40 oxidative enzymes, especially **urate oxidase, catalase,** and **D-amino acid oxidase** (Fig. 2–24). They are present in almost all animal cells and function in the catabolism of long-chained fatty acids **(beta oxidation),** forming acetyl CoA as well as **H$_2$O$_2$ (hydrogen peroxide)** by combining hydrogen from the fatty acid with molecular oxygen. Acetyl CoA is used by the cell for its own metabolic needs or is exported into the intercellular space to be utilized by neighboring cells. Hydrogen peroxide detoxifies various noxious agents (e.g., ethanol) and kills microorganisms. Excess **H$_2$O$_2$** is destroyed by the enzyme **catalase.**

Proteins destined for peroxisomes are not manufactured on the RER but in the cytosol and are transported into the peroxisomes. As these peroxisomes increase in size, they undergo fission to form new peroxisomes.

Mitochondria

Mitochondria are flexible, rod-shaped organelles that are about 0.5 to 1 μm in girth and may be as much as 7 μm in length. Most animal cells possess a large number of mitochondria (as many as 2000 in each liver cell) because, via **oxidative phosphorylation,** they produce **adenosine triphosphate (ATP),** a stable storage form of energy that can be utilized by the cell for its various energy-requiring activities.

Each mitochondrion possesses a smooth **outer** and a folded **inner membrane** (see Figs. 2–6 and 2–25). The folds of the inner membrane, known as **cristae,** greatly increase the surface area of the inner membrane. The number of cristae a mitochondrion possesses is directly related to the energy requirement of the cell; thus, a cardiac muscle cell mitochondrion has more cristae than has an osteocyte mitochondrion. The narrow space (10 to 20 nm in width) between the inner and outer membranes is referred to as the **intermembrane space,** whereas the large space enclosed by the inner membrane is known as the **matrix space (intercristal space).** The contents of the two spaces are quite different and are discussed later.

Table 2–1. Major Lysosomal Storage Diseases

Disease Type	Disease Name	Enzyme Deficiency	Metabolite Buildup
Glycogenosis	Pompe's disease (Type II)	Lysosomal glucosidase	Glycogen
Sphingolipidosis	GM$_1$-gangliosidoses	GM$_1$-ganglioside beta-galactosidase	GM$_1$ ganglioside; oligosaccharides containing galactose
Sphingolipidosis	GM$_2$-gangliosidoses (Tay-Sachs disease)	Hexosaminidase A	GM$_2$-ganglioside
Sphingolipidosis	GM$_2$-gangliosidoses (Gaucher's disease)	Glucocerebrosidase	Glucocerebroside
Sphingolipidosis	GM$_2$-gangliosidoses (Neimann-Pick disease)	Sphingomyelinase	Sphingomyelin
Mucopolysaccharidosis	MPS I H (Hurler)	α-L-iduronidase	Heparan and dermatan sulfate
Mucopolysaccharidosis	MPS II (Hunter)	L-iduronosulfate sulfatase	Heparan and dermatan sulfate
Glycoproteinosis		Enzymes that degrade polysaccharide side chains of glycoproteins	Several, depending on enzyme

Modified from Kumar V, Cotran RS, and Robbins SL. Basic Pathology, 5th ed. Philadelphia, W.B. Saunders Company, 1992.

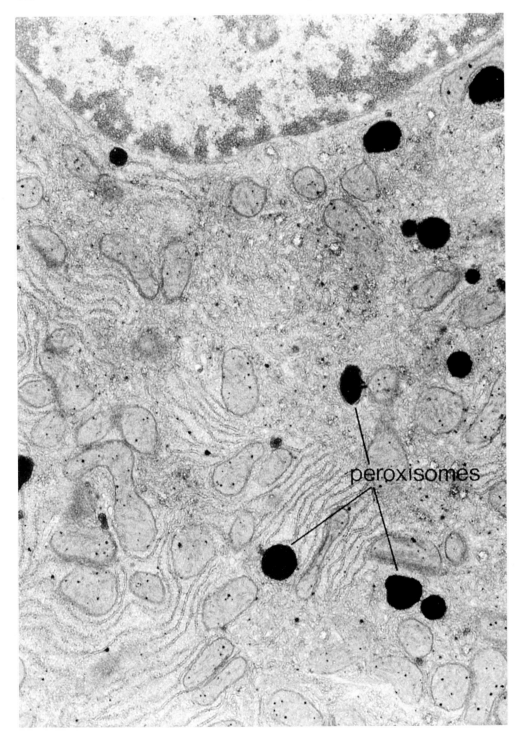

Figure 2–24. Peroxisomes in hepatocytes (× 12,500). The cells were treated with 3′, 3′-diaminobenzidine and osmium tetroxide, yielding a black reaction product due to the enzyme catalase located within peroxisomes. (From Hopkins, C.R.: Structure and Function of Cells. Philadelphia, W.B. Saunders Company, 1978.)

Outer Mitochondrial Membrane and Intermembrane Space

The outer mitochondrial membrane possesses a large number of **porins,** multipass transmembrane proteins. Each porin forms a large aqueous channel through which water-soluble molecules as large as 10 kilodaltons may pass. Because this membrane is relatively permeable to small molecules, including proteins, the contents of the intermem-

brane space resembles the cytosol. Additional proteins located in the outer membrane are responsible for the formation of mitochondrial lipids.

Inner Mitochondrial Membrane

The inner mitochondrial membrane, which encloses the matrix space, is folded to form cristae. This membrane is richly

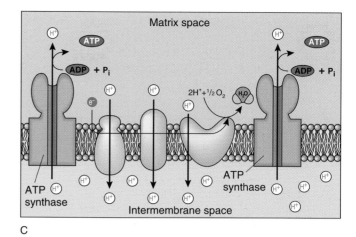

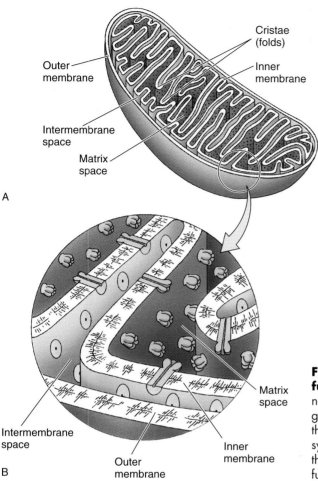

Figure 2–25. Diagrams illustrating the structure and function of mitochondria. *A,* Mitochondrion sectioned longitudinally to demonstrate its outer and folded inner membranes. *B,* Diagram of a negatively stained preparation at higher magnification of the region circled in *A,* displaying the inner membrane subunits, ATP synthase. *C,* Diagram displaying two ATP synthase complexes and three of the five members of the electron transport chain that also function to pump H+ from the matrix into the intermembrane space.

endowed with **cardiolipin,** a phospholipid that possesses four, rather than the usual two, fatty acyl chains. The presence of this phospholipid in high concentration makes the inner membrane nearly impermeable to ions, electrons, and protons.

In certain regions the outer and inner mitochondrial membranes contact each other; these **contact sites** act as pathways for proteins and small molecules to enter and leave the matrix space. These contact sites are composed of carrier proteins for the transport and regulatory proteins for the recognition of markers denoting the transportability of the specific macromolecules. These same contact sites are utilized also for the transport of proteins into the intermembrane space, provided that the proteins bear markers specific for entry into that space.

Viewed in negatively stained preparations, this membrane displays the presence of a large number of lollipop-like inner membrane subunits, protein complexes known as **ATP synthase** that are responsible for the generation of ATP from ADP and inorganic phosphate. The globular head of the subunit, about 10 nm in diameter, is attached to a narrow

flattened cylinder-like stalk, 4 nm wide and 5 nm long, projecting from the inner membrane into the matrix space (see Fig. 2–25).

Additionally, a large number of protein complexes, the **respiratory chains,** are present in the inner membrane. Each respiratory chain is composed of three respiratory enzyme complexes, **NADH dehydrogenase complex, cytochrome b-c₁ complex,** and **cytochrome oxidase complex.** These complexes form an **electron transport chain** that is responsible for the passage of electrons along this chain and, more importantly, function as proton pumps that transport H+ from the matrix into the intermembrane space, establishing an **electrochemical gradient** that provides energy for the ATP-generating action of ATP synthase.

Matrix

The **matrix space** is filled with a dense fluid composed of at least 50% protein, which accounts for its viscosity. Much of the protein component of the matrix is enzymes responsible for the stepwise degradation of fatty acids and pyruvate to the metabolic intermediate **acetyl CoA** and the subsequent oxidation of this intermediate in the **tricarboxylic acid (Krebs) cycle.** Mitochondrial ribosomes, tRNA, mRNA, and dense spherical **matrix granules** (30 to 50 nm in diameter) are also present in the matrix.

The function of matrix granules is not understood. They are composed of phospholipoprotein, although in some cells, especially of bone and cartilage, they may bind magnesium and calcium. Moreover, in injured cells whose cytosolic Ca^{2+} levels are dangerously high, matrix granules may sequester calcium, to protect the cell from calcium toxicity.

The matrix also contains the double-stranded mitochondrial circular DNA and the enzymes necessary for the expression of the mitochondrial genome. The cDNA contains information for the formation of only 13 mitochondrial proteins, 16S and 12S rRNA, and genes for 22 tRNAs. Therefore, most of the codes necessary for the formation and functioning of mitochondria are located in the genome of the nucleus.

Oxidative Phosphorylation

Acetyl CoA, formed through the β-oxidation of fatty acids and the degradation of glucose, is oxidized in the citric acid cycle to produce, in addition to CO_2, large quantities of the reduced cofactors NADH (nicotineamide adenine dinucleotide) and $FADH_2$ (flavin adenine dinucleotide). Each of these cofactors releases a hydride ion (H^-) which is stripped of its two high-energy electrons and becomes a proton (H^+). The electrons are transferred to the electron transport chain and during mitochondrial respiration reduce O_2 to form H_2O.

According to the **chemiosmotic theory,** the energy released by the sequential transfer of the electrons is utilized to transport H^+ from the matrix into the intermembrane space, establishing a high proton concentration in that space which exerts a **proton motive force** (see Fig. 2–25). It is only through ATP synthase that these protons may leave the intermembrane space and reenter the matrix. As the protons pass down this electrochemical gradient, the energy differential in the proton motive force is transformed into the stable high-energy bond of ATP by the globular head of the inner membrane subunit, which catalyzes the formation of ATP from ADP + P_i. The newly formed ATP is either utilized by the mitochondrion or is transported, through an ADP-ATP antiport system, into the cytosol. During the entire process of glycolysis, tricarboxylic acid cycle, and electron transport, each glucose molecule yields 36 molecules of ATP.

In some cells, such as brown fat of hibernating animals, oxidation is uncoupled from phosphorylation, resulting not in the formation of ATP but of heat. This uncoupling is dependent on the presence of proton shunts, known as **thermogenins,** that resemble ATP synthase but do not have the capability of generating ATP. As the protons pass through thermogenins to reenter the matrix, the energy of the proton motive force is transformed into heat. It is this heat that awakens the animal from its state of hibernation.

Origin and Replication of Mitochondria

Due to the presence of the mitochondrial genetic apparatus, it is believed that mitochondria were free-living organisms that either invaded or were phagocytosed by anaerobic eukaryotic cells, developing a **symbiotic relationship.** The mitochondrion-like organism received protection and nutrients from its host and provided its host with the capability of reducing its O_2 content and simultaneously supplying it with a stable form of chemical energy.

Mitochondria are self-replicating, in that they are generated from preexisting mitochondria. These organelles enlarge in size, replicate their DNA, and undergo fission. The division usually occurs through the intracristal space of one of the centrally located cristae. The outer mitochondrial membrane of the opposing halves extends through that intracristal space; the halves meet and fuse with each other, thus dividing the mitochondria into two nearly equal halves. The two new mitochondria move away from each other. The average lifespan of a mitochondrion is about 10 days.

Annulate Lamella

Annulate lamellae are parallel aggregates of membranes that enclose cistern-like spaces, thus resembling multiple copies, usually six to ten, of nuclear envelopes. They possess nuclear pore complex–like regions, known as **annuli,** that are in register with those of neighboring membranes. The cisternae of these organelles are relatively evenly spaced, separated by about 80 to 100 nm, and are continuous with the cisternae of the rough endoplasmic reticulum.

These organelles are normally present only in cells that have high mitotic indices, such as oocytes, tumor cells, and embryonic cells. Because of their resemblance to the nuclear envelope, it has been suggested that they act as reserves for the nuclear envelope in these rapidly dividing cells. However, immunocytochemical studies of annulate lamellae do not lend support to that supposition, and neither their function nor their significance is understood.

Inclusions

Inclusions are considered to be nonliving components of the cell that neither possess metabolic activity nor are bounded by membranes. The most common inclusions are glycogen, lipid droplets, pigments, and crystals.

Glycogen

Glycogen is the most common storage form of glucose in animals and is especially abundant in cells of muscle and liver. It appears in electron micrographs as clusters, or

rosettes, of β particles (and larger α particles in the liver) that resemble ribosomes, located in the vicinity of the smooth endoplasmic reticulum. On demand, enzymes responsible for glycogenolysis degrade glycogen into individual molecules of glucose.

CLINICAL CORRELATIONS

Some individuals suffer from **glycogen storage disorders,** due to their inability to degrade glycogen, resulting in excess accumulation of this substance in their cells. There are three forms of this disease, **hepatic, myopathic,** and **miscellaneous.** The lack or malfunction of one of the enzymes responsible for the degradation is responsible for these disorders (Table 2–2).

Lipids

Lipids, storage forms of triglycerides, are stored not only in specialized cells, **adipocytes,** but they also are located as individual droplets in various cell types, especially those of the liver. Most solvents used in histological preparations extract triglycerides from cells, leaving empty spaces indicative of the locations of lipids. However, utilizing osmium and glutaraldehyde, the lipids (and cholesterol) may be fixed in position as gray-to-black intracellular droplets. Lipids are very efficient forms of energy reserves; twice as many ATPs are derived from 1 gram of fat as from 1 gram of glycogen.

Pigments

The most common pigment in the body, aside from **hemoglobin** of red blood cells, is **melanin** manufactured by melanocytes of skin and hair, pigment cells of the retina, and specialized nerve cells in the substantia nigra of the brain. These pigments have protective functions in skin and aid in the sense of sight in the retina, but their role in hair and neurons is not understood. Additionally, in long-lived cells, such as neurons of the central nervous system and cardiac muscle cells, a yellow-to-brown pigment, **lipofuscin,** has been demonstrated. Unlike other inclusions, lipofuscin pigments are membrane-bound and are believed to represent the undigestable remnants of lysosomal activity. They are formed from fusion of several **residual bodies.**

Crystals

Crystals are not commonly found in cells, with the exception of Sertoli cells (**crystals of Charcot-Böttcher**), interstitial cells (**crystals of Reinke**) of the testes, and occasionally in macrophages (Fig. 2–26). It is believed that these structures are crystalline forms of certain proteins.

Cytoskeleton

The cytoplasm of animal cells contains a **cytoskeleton,** an intricate three-dimensional meshwork of protein filaments that are responsible for the maintenance of cellular morphology. Additionally, the cytoskeleton is an active participant in cellular motion, whether of organelles or vesicles within the cytoplasm, regions of the cell, or the entire cell. The cytoskeleton has three components: thin filaments (microfilaments), intermediate filaments, and microtubules.

Thin Filaments

Thin filaments (microfilaments) are composed of two chains of globular subunits, **G-actin,** coiled around each

Table 2–2. Major Subgroups of Glycogen Storage Disorders

Type	Deficient Enzyme	Tissue Changes	Clinical Signs
Hepatic Hepatorenal (von Gierke's disease)	Glucose-6-phosphatase	Intracellular accumulation of glycogen in hepatocytes and cortical tubules of kidneys	Enlarged liver and kidneys; hypoglycemia with subsequent convulsions; gout; bleeding; 50% mortality
Myopathic McArdle's syndrome	Muscle phosphorylase	Glycogen accumulation in skeletal muscle cells	Cramps following vigorous exercise; adult onset
Miscellaneous Pompe's disease	Lysosomal acid maltase	Glycogen accumulation Enlarged lysosomes in hepatocytes	Massively enlarged heart; cardiac and respiratory failure within two years of onset; adult has a milder form involving only skeletal muscle

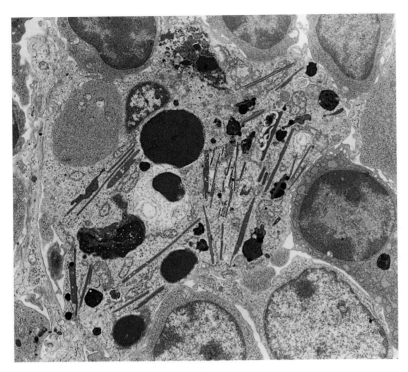

Figure 2–26. Electron micrograph of crystalloid inclusions in a macrophage (× 5100). (From Yamazaki, K.: Isolated cilia and crystalloid inclusions in murine bone marrow stromal cells. Blood Cells **13:**407–416, 1988.)

other to form a filamentous protein, **F-actin** (Figs. 2–27 and 2–28). Actin constitutes about 15% of the total protein content of nonmuscle cells. Only about half of their total actin is in the filamentous form, because the monomeric G-actin form is bound by small proteins, such as **profilin** and **thymosin,** that prevent their polymerization. Actin molecules present in the cells of many different vertebrate and invertebrate species are very similar to each other in their amino acid sequence, attesting to their highly conserved nature.

Thin filaments are 6 nm thick and possess a faster growing **plus end** and a slower growing **minus end.** When the actin filament reaches its desired length, members of a family of small proteins, **capping proteins,** attach to the plus end, terminating the lengthening of the filament. The process of shortening of actin filaments is regulated in the presence of ATP, ADP, and Ca^{2+} by capping proteins, such as **gelsolin,** which prevent polymerization of the filament. The cell membrane phospholipid **polyphosphoinositide** has the opposite effect, in that it removes the gelsolin cap, permitting elongation of the actin filament.

Depending on their isoelectric point, there are three classes of actin: **α actin** of muscle, and **β actin** and **γ actin** of nonmuscle cells. Although actin participates in the formation of various cellular extensions as well as in assembling structures responsible for motility, its basic composition is unaltered. It is capable of fulfilling its many roles via its association with different actin binding proteins. The most commonly known of these proteins is **myosin,** but numerous other proteins, such as α-actinin, spectrin, fimbrin, filamin, gelsolin, and talin, also bind to actin to perform essential cellular functions (Table 2–3).

Actin filaments form bundles of varied lengths, depending on the function that they perform in nonmuscle cells. These bundles form three types of associations: contractile bundles, gel-like networks, and parallel bundles.

Contractile bundles, such as those responsible for the formation of cleavage furrows (contractile rings) during mitotic division, are usually associated with myosin. Their actin filaments are arranged loosely, parallel to each other, with the plus and minus ends alternating in direction. These assemblies are responsible for movement not only of organelles and vesicles within the cell but also for cellular activities such as exocytosis and endocytosis, as well as the extension of filopodia and cell migration. The myosin associated with these contractile bundles may be one of two types, **myosin-I** or **myosin-II.** Myosin-II forms **thick filaments** (15 nm in diameter) and moves only actin filaments. Myosin-I has the capability of binding not only to actin filaments but also to other cytoplasmic components, such as vesicles, moving them along an actin filament from one position in the cell to another.

Gel-like networks provide the structural foundation of much of the cell cortex. Their stiffness is due to the protein **filamin,** which assists in the establishment of a loosely organized network of actin filaments resulting in localized high viscosity. During the formation of filopodia the gel is liquefied by proteins such as **gelsolin,** which, in the presence of ATP and high Ca^{2+}, cleaves the actin filaments and, by forming a cap over their plus end, prevents them from lengthening.

The proteins **fimbrin** and **villin** are responsible for forming actin filaments into closely packed **parallel bundles** that form the core of microspikes and microvilli, respectively. These bundles of actin filaments are anchored in the **terminal web,** a region of the cell cortex composed of a network of intermediate filaments and the protein **spectrin.** Spectrin molecules are flexible, rod-like tetramers that assist the cell in maintaining the structural integrity of the cortex.

Actin also plays an important role in the establishment and maintenance of **focal contacts** of the cell with extracellular matrix (Fig. 2–29). At focal contacts the **integrin** (a transmembrane protein) of the cell membrane binds to structural glycoproteins, such as **fibronectin,** of the extracellular matrix, permitting the cell to maintain its attachment. Simultaneously, the intracellular region of the integrin contacts the cytoskeleton via intermediary proteins that attach it to actin filaments. The mode of attachment involves integrin binding to **talin,** which contacts both **vinculin** and the actin filament. Vinculin binds to α-actinin, the actin-binding protein that assembles actin into contractile bundles. These contractile bundles, referred to as **stress fibers** in fibroblasts maintained in tissue culture, resemble myofibrils of striated muscle. Stress fibers may extend between two focal points or a focal point and intermediate filaments and assist the cell in exerting a tensile force on the extracellular matrix (as in the wound contraction function of fibroblasts).

Intermediate Filaments

Electron micrographs display a category of filaments in the cytoskeleton whose diameter of 8 to 10 nm places them between thick and thin filaments and are consequently named **intermediate filaments** (see Fig. 2–27). The major function of these filaments is to provide structural support for the cell. Their great tensile strength is important in protecting cells from stresses and strains.

Biochemical investigations have determined that there are several categories of intermediate filaments that share the same morphological and structural characteristics. These rope-like intermediate filaments are constructed of tetramers of rod-like proteins that are tightly bundled into long helical arrays. The individual subunit of each tetramer differs considerably for each type of intermediate filament. The categories of intermediate filaments include keratins, desmin, vimentin, glial fibrillary acidic protein, neurofilaments, and nuclear lamins (Table 2–4).

Several intermediate filament-binding proteins have been discovered. As they bind to intermediate filaments, they link them into a three-dimensional network that facilitates the formation of the cytoskeleton. Three of the best known of these proteins are filaggrin, synamin, and plectin. Filaggrin binds keratin filaments into bundles, whereas synamin and plectin bind desmin and vimentin, respectively, into three-dimensional intracellular meshworks.

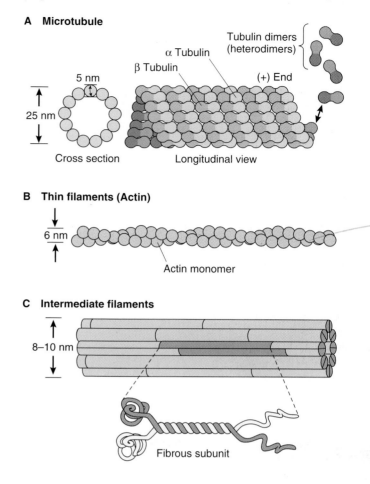

A   Microtubule

5 nm

25 nm

Cross section   Longitudinal view

α Tubulin

β Tubulin

Tubulin dimers (heterodimers)

(+) End

B   Thin filaments (Actin)

6 nm

Actin monomer

C   Intermediate filaments

8–10 nm

Fibrous subunit

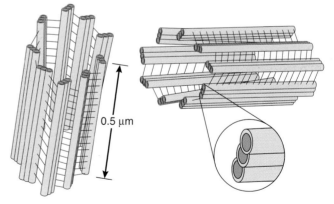

D   Centriole

0.5 μm

Figure 2–27. Diagram of the elements of the cytoskeleton and centriole. ✕

CLINICAL CORRELATIONS

Immunocytochemical methods, utilizing specific immunofluorescent antibodies, are employed to distinguish intermediate filament types in tumors of unknown origin. Knowledge of the source of these tumors assists not only in their diagnosis but also in devising effective treatment plans.

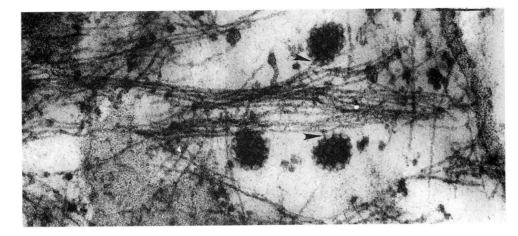

Figure 2–28. Electron micrograph of clathrin-coated vesicles contacting filaments (*arrowheads*) in granulosa cells of the rat ovary (× 35,000). (From Batten, B.E. and Anderson, E.: The distribution of actin in cultured ovarian granulosa cells. Am. J. Anat. **167:**395–404, 1983. Copyright 1983. Reprinted by permission of John Wiley & Sons, Inc.)

Microtubules

Microtubules are long, straight, rigid, hollow-appearing cylindrical structures 25 nm in outer diameter, with a lumen whose diameter is 15 nm (see Figs. 2–27 and 2–30). They are polarized, having a rapidly growing **plus end** as well as a **minus end,** which must be stabilized or will depolymerize, thus shortening the microtubule. The minus end is stabilized by being embedded in the **centrosome,** the region of the cell in the vicinity of the nucleus that houses the centrioles (discussed later).

Table 2–3. Actin-Binding Proteins

Actin-Binding Protein	Molecular Mass of Each Subunit (D)	Number of Subunits	Function
α-actinin	100,000	2	Bundling actin filaments for contractile bundles
fimbrin	68,000	1	Bundling actin filaments for parallel bundles
filamin	270,000	2	Cross link actin filaments into gel-like network
myosin-I	150,000	1	Movement of vesicles along actin filaments
myosin-II	260,000	2	Contraction by sliding actin filaments
spectrin α β	265,000 260,000	2 2	Forms supporting network for plasma membrane of RBC
gelsolin	90,000	1	Cleaves and caps actin filaments
thymosin	5,000	1	Binds to G-actin subunits, maintaining them in monomeric form

Table 2–4. Predominant Types of Intermediate Filaments

Filament	Polypeptide Component Size (D)	Cell Type	Function
Keratins (30 variations) Type I (acidic) Type II (neutral/basic)	40,000–70,000 40,000–70,000	Epithelial cells and cells of hair and nails	Support cell assemblies by providing tensile strength to cytoskeleton.
Tonofilaments	40,000–70,000	Epithelial cells, especially stratified squamous keratinized	Assist in the formation of desmosomes and hemidesmosomes.
Desmin	53,000	All types of muscle cells	Links myofibrils in striated muscle (around Z disks); attaches to cytoplasmic densities in smooth muscle.
Vimentin	54,000	Cells of embryo as well as cells of mesenchymal origin: fibroblasts, leukocytes, endothelial cells	Surrounds nuclear envelope and is associated with cytoplasmic aspect of nuclear pore complex.
Glial fibrillary acidic protein (GFAP)	50,000	Astrocytes, Schwann cells, oligodendroglia	Supports glial cell structure.
Neurofilaments [three types: low (L), medium (M), and high (H) molecular weight] NF-L NF-M NF-H	68,000 160,000 210,000	Neurons	Form the cytoskeleton of axons and dendrites; assist in the formation of the gel state of the cytoplasm; cross linking is responsible for great tensile strength.
Nuclear lamins A B C	65,000–75,000	Lining the nuclear envelopes of all cells	Control and assembly of the nuclear envelope; organization of the perinuclear chromatin.

The centrosome, which in electron micrographs displays a fibrillar image, is considered to be the **microtubule-organizing center (MTOC)** of the cell, from which most of the cell's microtubules emanate. Microtubules are dynamic structures that frequently change their length by undergoing growth spurts and then becoming shorter, both processes occurring at the plus ends, so that the average half-life of a microtubule is only about 10 minutes. The main functions of microtubules are providing rigidity and maintaining cell shape, regulating intracellular movement of organelles and vesicles, establishing intracellular compartments, and providing the capability of ciliary (and flagellar) motion.

Each microtubule consists of 13 parallel **protofilaments** composed of heterodimers of the globular polypeptide α- and β-tubulin subunits, each having a molecular mass of about 50,000 daltons (see Fig. 2–27). Polymerization of the heterodimers requires the presence of Mg^{2+} and GTP. During cell division, rapid polymerization of existing as well as new microtubules is responsible for the formation of the spindle apparatus.

CLINICAL CORRELATIONS

Disruption of the polymerization process by antimitotic drugs, such as **colchicine,** blocks the mitotic event by binding to the tubulin molecules, preventing their assembly into the protofilament.

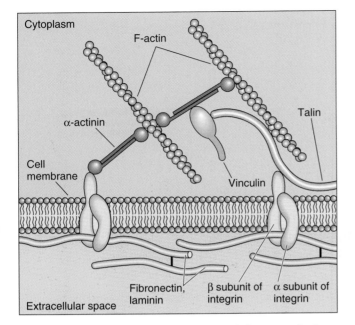

Figure 2–29. Schematic diagram of the cytoskeleton. Fibronectin or laminin receptor regions of integrin molecules bind to fibronectin or laminin, respectively, in the extracellular space. Intracellular talin or α-actinin binding regions of integrin molecules bind to talin or α-actinin, respectively. Thus integrin molecules bridge the cytoskeleton to an extracellular support framework.

Microtubule-associated Proteins

In addition to tubulin heterodimers, microtubules also possess **microtubule-associated proteins (MAPs)** bound to their periphery at 32-nm intervals. There are various types of MAPs, ranging in molecular weight from about 50,000 to more than 300,000. Their primary functions are to prevent depolymerization of microtubules and to assist in the intracellular movement of organelles and vesicles.

Movement along a microtubule occurs in both directions, that is both toward the plus and minus ends. The two major types of microtubule motor proteins, the MAPs **dynein** and **kinesin,** both bind to the microtubule as well as to vesicles (and organelles). In the presence of ATP, dynein moves the vesicle toward the minus end of the microtubule. Kinesin effects vesicular (and organelle) transport in the opposite direction, toward the plus end. The mechanism of ATP utilization by these MAPs is not understood. The vesicles to be transported include those derived from the RER, the *trans* Golgi network, and endosomes.

Centrioles

Centrioles are small, cylindrical structures, 0.2 μm in diameter and 0.5 μm in length (see Fig. 2–27). Usually they are paired structures, arranged perpendicular to each other, and are located in the centrosome (cytocenter) in the vicinity of the Golgi apparatus.

They are composed of a specific arrangement of nine triplets of microtubules arranged around a central axis. Each microtubule triplet consists of one complete and two incomplete microtubules fused to each other, so that the incomplete ones share three protofilaments. The complete microtubule, referred to as "A," is positioned closest to the center of the cylinder, whereas C is the farthest away. Adjacent triplets are connected to each other by a fibrous substance of unknown composition, extending from microtubule A to microtubule C. Each triplet is arranged so that it forms an oblique angle with the adjacent and a straight angle with the fifth triplet.

During the S phase of the cell cycle, each centriole of the pair replicates, forming a procentriole in some unknown manner, at 90 degrees to itself. This procentriole initially possesses no microtubules, but tubulin molecules begin to polymerize closest to the parent centriole, with the plus end growing away from the parent. Although the suggestion has not been verified because these organelles self-replicate, it has been suggested that they may possess centriolar DNA.

Centrioles appear to have an important association with the microtubule-organizing center of the cell. During mitotic activity, the centrioles are responsible for the formation of the spindle apparatus. Additionally, the **basal bodies** of cilia and flagella are identical to individual (unpaired) centrioles.

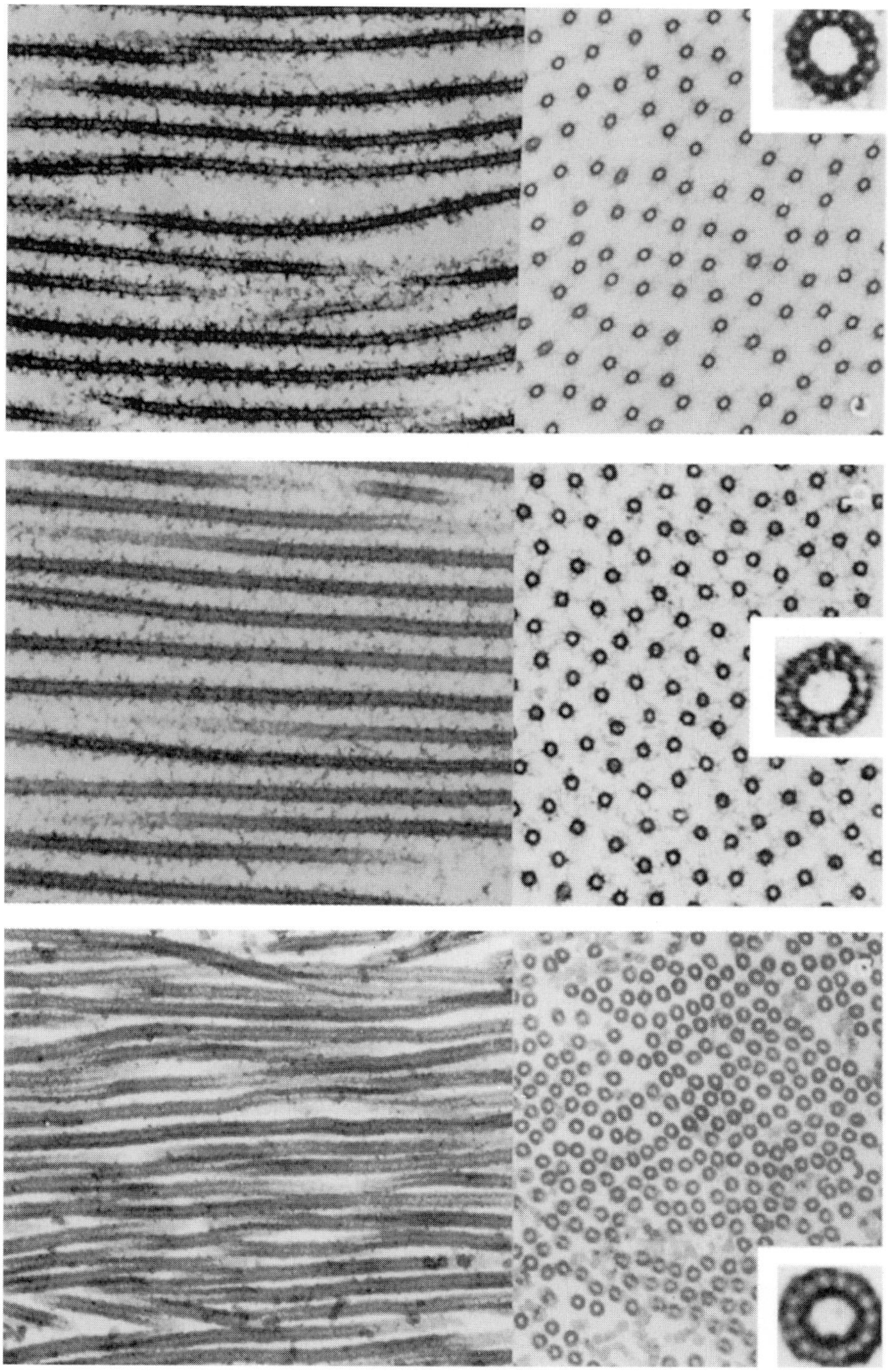

Figure 2–30. Electron micrograph of microtubules assembled with and without microtubule associated proteins (MAPs)(× 76,400).
Top, Microtubules assembled without MAPs; *center,* microtubules assembled from unfractionated MAPs; *bottom,* microtubules assembled in the presence of MAP₂ subfraction, only. (From Leeson, T.S., Leeson, C.R., and Papparo, A.A.: Text/Atlas of Histology. Philadelphia, W.B. Saunders Company, 1988.)

Nucleus

3

The **nucleus** is the largest organelle of the cell (Fig. 3–1). It contains nearly all of the DNA possessed by the cell, the mechanisms for RNA synthesis, and is the location for the assembly of ribosomal subunits. The nucleus, bounded by two lipid membranes, houses three major components: **chromatin,** the genetic material of the cell, **nucleolus,** the center for ribosomal RNA synthesis, and **nucleoplasm,** containing macromolecules and nuclear particles involved in the maintenance of the cell.

The nucleus is usually spherical and centrally located in the cell; however, in some cells it may be spindle- to oblong-shaped, twisted, lobulated, or even disk-shaped. Although usually each cell has a single nucleus, some cells such as osteoclasts possess several nuclei, whereas mature red blood cells have extruded their nuclei. The size, shape, and form of the nucleus are generally constant for a particular cell type,

a fact useful in clinical diagnoses of the degree of malignancy of certain cancerous cells.

Nuclear Envelope

The nucleus is surrounded by the **nuclear envelope,** composed of two parallel unit membranes, the **inner** and **outer nuclear membranes,** separated from each other by a 10- to 30-nm space, the **perinuclear cisterna** (Figs. 3–2 and 3–3). The nuclear envelope is perforated at various intervals by **nuclear pores** (to be discussed later) that permit communication between the cytoplasm and the nucleus. At these pores the inner and outer nuclear membranes are continuous with one another. The nuclear envelope helps control movement of macromolecules between the nucleus and the cytoplasm and assists in organizing the chromatin.

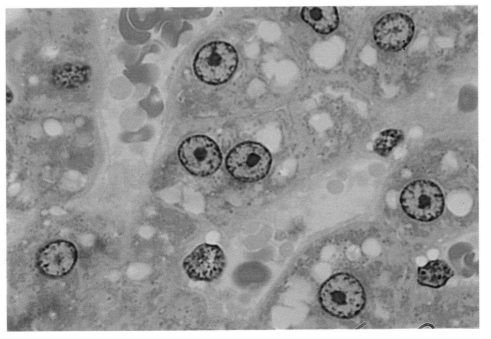

Figure 3–1. Cell Nuclei. Light micrograph (× 1323). Typical cells, each containing a spherical nucleus. Observe the chromatin granules and the nucleolus.

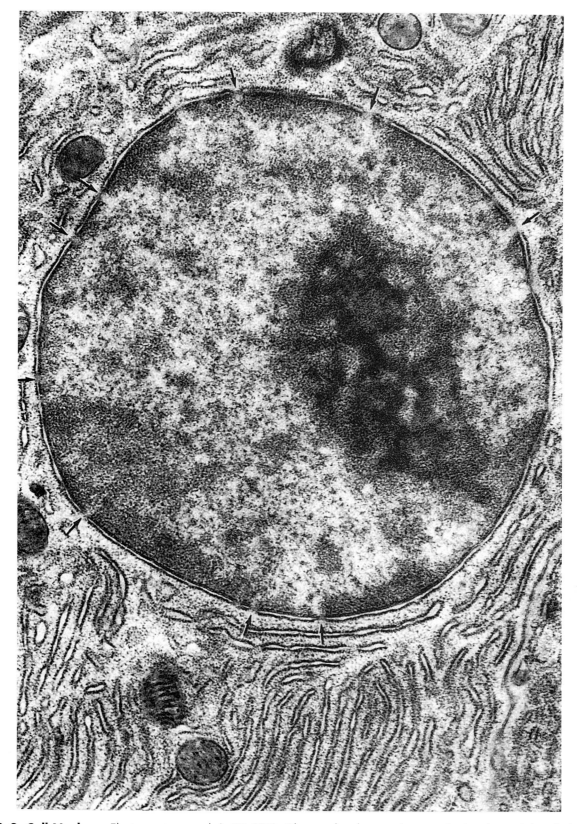

Figure 3–2. Cell Nucleus. Electron micrograph (× 22,000). Observe the electron dense nucleolus, the peripherally located dense heterochromatin, and the light euchromatin. The nuclear envelope surrounding the nucleus is composed of an inner and outer nuclear membrane that is interrupted by the nuclear pores *(arrows)*. (From Fawcett, D.W.: The Cell. Philadelphia, W.B. Saunders Company, 1981.)

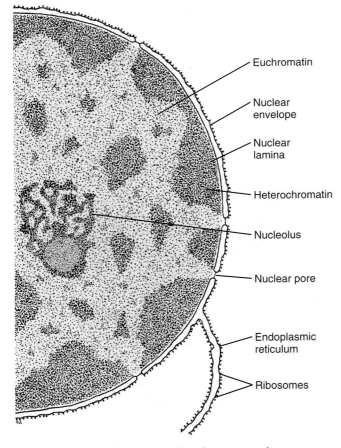

Figure 3–3. Nucleus. Note that the outer nuclear membrane is studded with ribosomes on its cytoplasmic surface and that it is continuous with the rough endoplasmic reticulum. The space between the inner and outer nuclear membranes is the perinuclear cistern. Observe that the two membranes are united at the nuclear pores.

Inner Nuclear Membrane

The **inner nuclear membrane** is about 6 nm thick and faces the nuclear contents. It is in close contact with the **nuclear lamina,** an interwoven meshwork of intermediate filaments, 80- to 100-nm thick, composed of **lamins A, B,** and **C** and located at the periphery of the nucleoplasm. The nuclear lamina functions to help organize and provide support to the lipid bilayer membrane and the perinuclear chromatin. Certain integral proteins of the inner nuclear membrane act either directly or via other nuclear matrix proteins as contact sites for nuclear RNAs and chromosomes.

Outer Nuclear Membrane

The **outer nuclear membrane** is also about 6 nm thick, faces the cytoplasm, and is continuous with the rough endoplasmic reticulum (RER) and is considered by some authors

as a specialized region of the RER (see Figs. 3–2 and 3–3). Its cytoplasmic surface is surrounded by a thin loose meshwork of the intermediate filaments, **vimentin**. Its cytoplasmic surface usually possesses ribosomes actively synthesizing transmembrane proteins that are destined for the outer or inner nuclear membranes.

Nuclear Pores

At certain locations on the surface of the nuclear envelope the outer and inner nuclear membranes are continuous with each other, creating openings known as **nuclear pores,** which permit communication between the nuclear compartment and the cytoplasm (Fig. 3–4). The number of nuclear pores ranges between a few dozen to several thousand, correlated directly with the metabolic activity of the cell.

High-resolution electron microscopy has revealed that the nuclear pore is surrounded by nonmembranous structures embedded in its rim. These structures and the pore are referred to as the **nuclear pore complex,** which selectively guards passage through the pore (Fig. 3–5). Recent evidence suggests that each of the nuclear pore complexes is in communication with the others via the nuclear lamina and certain pore-connecting fibers.

Nuclear Pore Complex

The **nuclear pore complex** is about 80 to 100 nm in diameter and spans the two nuclear membranes. It is thought to be composed of four elements: the scaffold, transporter subunit (central hub), thick filaments, and a basket (Fig. 3–6).

The **scaffold,** representing the major mass of the pore complex, surrounds and entwines the periphery of the pore, forming a cytoplasmic ring and a nucleoplasmic ring. Additionally, the scaffold is attached to and maintains the fusion of the nuclear membranes, supports the transporter, and provides diffusion channels.

The **transporter (hub)** is a proteinaceous ring that occupies the center of the pore and is supported by the scaffold. It was previously termed the **central granule** and was believed to be preribosomal subunits or other particulate materials caught in transit between the nuclear compartment and the cytoplasm. The current understanding is that the transporter functions in transport of material into and out of the nucleus. Nuclear proteins synthesized in the cytoplasm bind to the periphery of the transporter ring and dock at its central channel, inducing it to open, then enter the nucleus through the open channel.

Thick filaments (about 3 nm in diameter) radiate out into the cytoplasm from the cytoplasmic ring of the scaffold. It is suggested that these filaments may act as a staging area for the binding of proteins that are to be transported into the nucleus.

Eight filaments (about 100 nm in length) extend from the nucleoplasmic ring of the scaffold to a smaller ring located

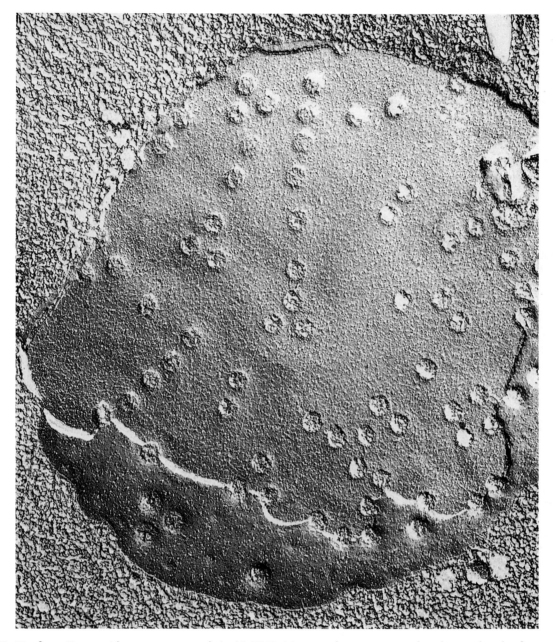

Figure 3–4. Nuclear Pores. Electron micrograph (× 60,000). Many nuclear pores may be observed in this freeze-fractured preparation of a nucleus. (From Leeson, T.S., Leeson, C.R., and Paparo, A.A.: *Text*/Atlas of Histology. Philadelphia, W.B. Saunders Company, 1988.)

in the nucleus. This configuration gives the impression of a **basket,** which has been shown to disassemble in the absence and reassemble in the presence of Ca^{2+}. The precise function of the basket is yet unclear, but it is believed to be related to RNA transport.

Nuclear Pore Transport

Although the nuclear pore is fairly large, it is nearly filled with the structures constituting the nuclear pore complex.

Due to the structural conformation of those subunits, there are several 9- to 11-nm wide channels available for simple diffusion of ions and small molecules.

Substances and particles larger than 11 nm are unable to reach or leave the nuclear compartment via simple diffusion; instead they are selectively transported via a **receptor-mediated transport** process. Signal sequences of molecules to be transported through the nuclear pores must be recognized by one of the many receptor sites of the nuclear pore complex. Subsequent to recognition the actual traversing of the pore is an energy requiring process.

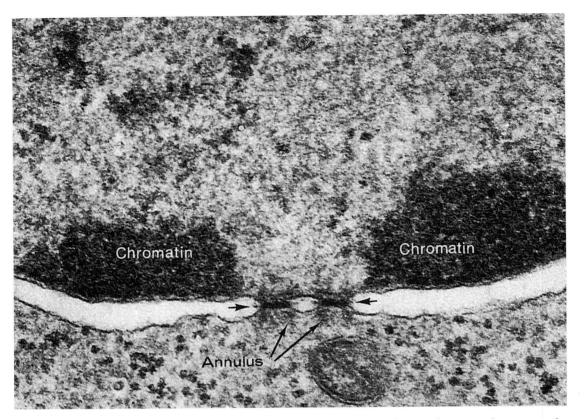

Figure 3–5. Nuclear Pore. Electron micrograph (× 30,000). Note the heterochromatin adjacent to the inner nuclear membrane and that the inner and outer nuclear membranes are continuous at the nuclear pore. (From Fawcett, D.W.: The Cell. Philadelphia, W.B. Saunders Company, 1981.)

Chromatin

DNA, the genetic material of the cell, resides in the nucleus in the form of chromosomes that are clearly visible during cell division. In the interval between cell divisions the chromosomes are unwound in the form of chromatin (see Figs. 3–2 and 3–3). Depending on its transcriptional activity, chromatin may be condensed as heterochromatin or extended as euchromatin.

Heterochromatin, a condensed inactive form that stains deeply with Feulgen stains making it visible with the light microscope, is located mostly at the periphery of the nucleus. The remainder of the chromatin scattered throughout the nucleus and not visible with the light microscope is **euchromatin.** This represents the active form of chromatin where the genetic material of the DNA molecules is being transcribed into RNA.

When euchromatin is examined with electron microscopy, it is noted to be composed of a thread-like material 30 nm thick. More careful evaluation indicates that these threads may be unwound, resulting in an 11-nm wide structure resembling "beads on a string." The beads are termed **nucleosomes,** and the string, which is the **DNA** molecule, appears as a thin filament 2 nm in diameter (Fig. 3–7).

Each nucleosome is made up of an octomer of proteins, duplicates of each of four types of **histones (H_2A, H_2B, H_3,**

and **H_4).** The nucleosome is also wrapped with two complete turns (about 150 nucleotide pairs) of the DNA molecule that continues as **linker DNA** extending to the next "bead." The spacing between each nucleosome is about 200 base

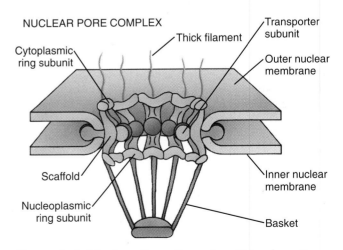

Figure 3–6. Nuclear Pore Complex. This schematic representation of the current understanding of the structure of the nuclear pore complex demonstrates that it is made up of several combinations of eight units each. (Modified from Alberts, B., Bray, D., Lewis, J., et al.: Molecular Biology of the Cell, 3rd ed., New York, Garland Publishing, 1994.)

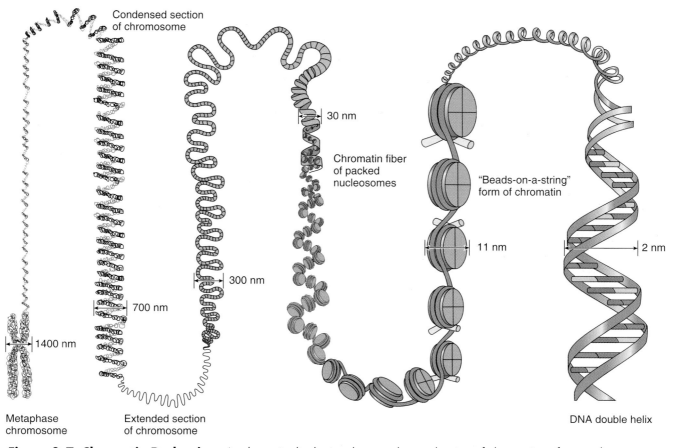

Figure 3–7. Chromatin Packaging. A schematic displaying the complex packaging of chromatin to form a chromosome.

pairs. This configuration of the nucleosome with its coils of DNA represents the simplest arrangement of chromatin packaging in the nucleus. Because only a small amount of the chromatin in the cell is in this configuration, it is thought to represent regions where the DNA is being transcribed.

Electron microscopic studies of the nuclear contents subsequent to more careful manipulation has revealed chromatin fibers exhibiting diameters of 30 nm. Packaging of chromatin into 30-nm threads is believed to occur by helical coiling of consecutive nucleosomes at six nucleosomes per turn of the coil and cooperatively bound there with **histone H_1** (Fig. 3–7). It should be noted that there are also nonhistone proteins associated with the chromatin, but their function is not clear.

Chromosomes

As the cell leaves the interphase stage and prepares to undergo mitotic or meiotic activity, the chromatin fibers are extensively condensed to form **chromosomes,** structures that are visible with the light microscope. Tighter condensing of the chromatin material is accomplished by looping the coiled 30-nm fibers into 300-nm loops held together by specific protein/DNA bound complexes located at their bases. Further coiling of the 300-nm loops into tightly woven

700-nm helical loops forms the maximally condensed chromosomes observed in the metaphase stage of mitosis or meiosis (see Fig. 3–7).

The number of chromosomes in somatic cells is specific for the species and is called the **genome,** the total genetic makeup. In humans the genome is made up of 46 chromosomes representing 23 homologous pairs of chromosomes. One member of each of the chromosome pairs is derived from the maternal parent, whereas the other comes from the paternal parent. Of the 23 pairs, 22 are called **autosomes,** whereas the remaining pair that determines gender are the sex chromosomes. The **sex chromosomes** of the female are two X chromosomes (**XX**) and those of a male are made up of the X and Y chromosomes (**XY**) (Fig. 3–8).

Sex Chromatin

Microscopic study of interphase nuclei of cells from females displays a very tightly coiled clump of chromatin, the **sex chromatin (Barr body),** the inactive counterpart of the two X chromosomes. Epithelial cells obtained from the lining of the cheek and neutrophils from blood smears are especially useful for studying sex chromatin. The sex chromatin is observed at the edge of the nuclear envelope in smears of the oral epithelial cells and as a small drumstick-

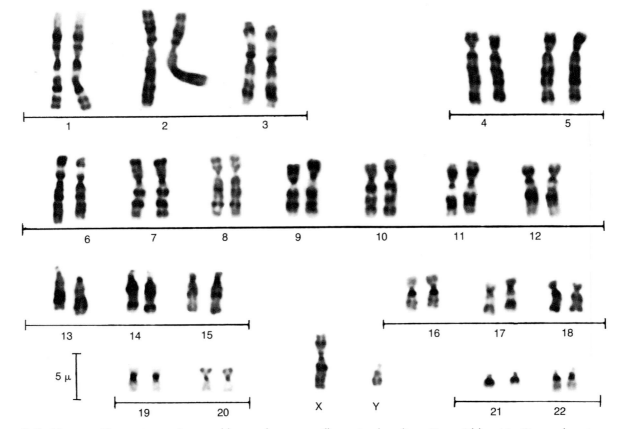

Figure 3-8. Human Karyotype. A normal human karyotype illustrating banding. (From Bibbo, M.: Comprehensive Cytopathology. Philadelphia, W.B. Saunders Company, 1991.)

like evagination of the nuclei of the neutrophils. It should be noted that a number of cells must be examined to observe sex chromatin because the X chromosome must be in the proper orientation to be displayed for observation.

Ploidy

Cells containing the full complement of chromosomes (46) are said to be **diploid (2n)**. Germ cells (mature ova or spermatozoa) are said to be **haploid (1n)**—that is, only one member of each of the homologous pairs of chromosomes is present. Upon fertilization, the chromosomal number is restored to the diploid (2n) amount as the nuclei of the two germ cells unite.

Certain alkaloids, such as colchicine, a plant derivative, arrest a dividing cell in the metaphase stage of mitosis when the chromosomes are maximally condensed, thus permitting the pairing and numbering of the chromosomes via a conventional system of **karyotyping,** an analysis of chromosome number (see Fig. 3-8).

CLINICAL CORRELATIONS

One of the items that may be observed from the karyotype is **aneuploidy,** an abnormal chromosome number.

Down's syndrome is an example of this, in which analysis of the karyotype reveals an extra chromosome 21 **(trisomy 21).** Persons with this syndrome exhibit mental retardation, stubby hands, and many congenital malformations, especially of the heart, among other manifestations.

Certain syndromes are associated with abnormalities in the number of sex chromosomes. **Kleinfelter's syndrome** results when an individual possesses three sex chromosomes **(XXY).** These persons exhibit the male phenotype, but they do not develop secondary sexual characteristics and are usually sterile. **Turner's syndrome** is another example of aneuploidy called **monosomy** of the sex chromosomes. The karyotype of these individuals exhibits only one sex chromosome **(XO).** These individuals are females who never develop ovaries, have undeveloped breasts and a small uterus, and mental retardation.

Giemsa reagent stains the adenine-thymine–rich regions of chromosomes, producing a pattern of **G bands** that is unique for each chromosome pair and is characteristic for each species. Careful analysis of the G bands can help reveal deletions of certain portions of the chromosome, nondisjunctions, translocations, and so on, that may assist in diagnosing certain genetic disorders and/or diseases resulting from chromosomal anomalies.

Deoxyribonucleic acid (DNA) and Genes

Nearly all of the **DNA,** a double-stranded polynucleotide chain wound into a double helix, is housed in the nucleus of the cell. Each nucleotide is composed of a nitrogenous base, a deoxyribose sugar, and a phosphate molecule, and the nucleotides are linked to one another by phosphodiester bonds formed between the sugar molecules. There are two types of bases, purines (adenine and guanine) and the pyrimidines (cytosine and thymine). A double helix is established by the formation of hydrogen bonds between complementary bases on each strand of the DNA molecule. These bonds are formed between adenine (A) and thymine (T) and between guanine (G) and cytosine (C).

GENES. The biological information that is passed from one cell generation to the next, the units of heredity, are located at specific regions on the DNA molecule called **genes.** Each gene represents a specific segment of the DNA molecule that codes for the synthesis of a particular protein. The sequential arrangement of bases constituting the gene represents the sequence of amino acids of the protein. The genetic code is designed in such a manner that a triplet of consecutive bases, a **codon,** denotes a particular amino acid. Each amino acid is represented by a different codon. There is a concerted effort under way presently to research the human genome and map the various genes at each chromosome locus. This is a very long and complicated study whose results will be of tremendous value in medicine. Several findings from the study have already added to the understanding of certain disease entities.

Ribonucleic acid (RNA)

Ribonucleic acid (RNA) is similar to DNA, in that it too is composed of a linear sequence of nucleotides. However, it is single-stranded (Fig. 3–9), and the sugar in RNA is ribose instead of deoxyribose. One of the bases, thymine, is replaced by uracil (U), which, like thymine, is complementary to adenine.

The DNA in the nucleus serves as a template for synthesis of a complementary strand of RNA, a process called **transcription.** Synthesis of the three types of RNA is catalyzed by three different **RNA polymerases: messenger RNA**

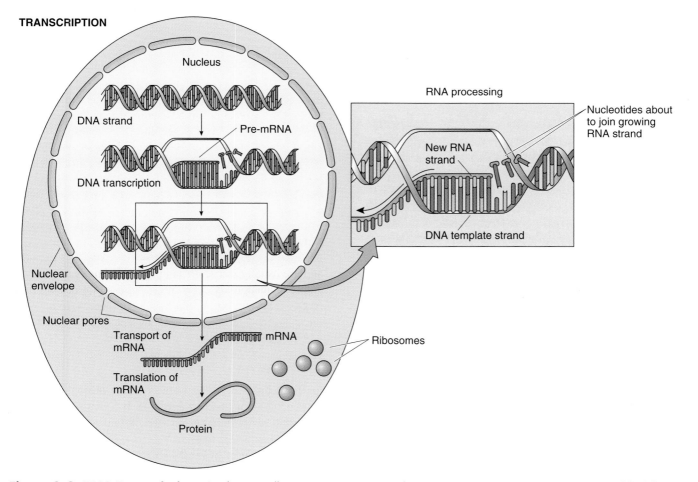

Figure 3–9. DNA Transcription. A schematic illustrating transcription of DNA into messenger RNA (mRNA). (Modified from Alberts, B., Bray, D., Lewis, J., et al.: Molecular Biology of the Cell, 3rd ed., New York, Garland Publishing, 1994.)

(mRNA) by RNA polymerase II, **transfer RNA (tRNA)** by RNA polymerase III, and **ribosomal RNA (rRNA)** by RNA polymerase I. The mechanism of transcription is generally the same for all three types of RNA.

Messenger RNA

Messenger RNA (mRNA) serves as an intermediary for carrying the genetic information encoded in DNA that specifies the primary sequence of proteins from the nucleus to the protein-synthesizing machinery in the cytoplasm (see Fig. 3–9). Each mRNA is a complementary copy of the region of the DNA molecule that constitutes one gene. An mRNA molecule thus consists of a series of codons corresponding to particular amino acids. It also contains a **start codon (AUG)**, which is necessary for initiating protein synthesis, and one or more **stop codons (UAA, UAG, or UGA)**, which act to terminate protein synthesis. Once formed in the nucleus, mRNA is transported to the cytoplasm, where it is translated into protein, as described in Chapter 2.

TRANSCRIPTION. Transcription of DNA into mRNA begins with attachment of RNA polymerase II to a **core promoter,** a specific DNA sequence located adjacent to a gene. In the presence of a series of cofactors, RNA polymerase II initiates transcription by unwinding the double helix of the DNA two turns, thus exposing the nucleotides on the DNA strand. The enzyme uses one of the exposed DNA strands as a template on which to assemble and polymerize complementary bases of the RNA molecule. The process repeats as a new region of the DNA double helix is unwound and more nucleotides are polymerized into the growing mRNA chain. As the enzyme moves along the DNA molecule, the polymerized mRNA chain is separated from the template DNA strand, permitting the two DNA strands to re-form into the double helix configuration (see Fig. 3–9). Transcription begins at a DNA triplet corresponding to the start codon AUG and is concluded when the RNA polymerase II recognizes a **chain-terminator** site complementary to the stop codons UAA, UAG, or UGA. When the enzyme reaches the chain terminator, it is released from the DNA molecule, permitting it to repeat the process of transcription. Simultaneously, the newly formed RNA strand (primary transcript) is released from the DNA molecule, leaving it free in the nucleoplasm.

The primary transcript is a long, single-stranded RNA molecule, called **precursor messenger RNA (pre-mRNA).** It contains both coding segments **(exons)** and noncoding segments **(introns).** The introns must be removed and the exons have to be spliced together. For that to occur, pre-mRNA and nuclear processing proteins form complexes of **heterogenous nuclear ribonucleoprotein particles (hnRNPs)** that begin **RNA splicing,** thus reducing the length of the pre-mRNA molecule. Other processing proteins, such as **small nuclear ribonucleoprotein particles (snRNPs),** also assist in the splicing to produce **messenger ribonucleoprotein (mRNP).** Finally, the nuclear processing proteins are removed from the complex, leaving mRNA ready to be transported out of the nucleus via the nuclear pores (see Fig. 3–9).

This description of mRNA synthesis is only a brief overview and omits many details. Readers desiring more information should consult texts in molecular and cellular biology.

Transfer RNA

Transfer RNA (tRNA) is a small RNA molecule produced from DNA by RNA polymerase III. It is about 80 nucleotides in length and is folded upon itself to resemble a cloverleaf with base pairing between some of the nucleotides. Two regions of the tRNA are of special significance. One of these, the **anticodon,** recognizes the codon of the mRNA, whereas the other is the amino acid–bearing region residing at the 3′ end of the molecule. The function of the tRNA then is to transfer activated amino acids to the ribosome-mRNA complex where they are incorporated into the polypeptide chain forming the protein, as described in Chapter 2.

Ribosomal RNA

Ribosomal RNA (rRNA) is synthesized in the fibrillar (pars fibrosa) region of the nucleolus by RNA polymerase I (Fig. 3–10). The primary transcript is called **45S rRNA (pre-rRNA),** a huge molecule of about 13,000 nucleotides. A 5S rRNA molecule synthesized in the nucleus as well as ribosomal proteins synthesized in the cytoplasm are transported into the nucleolus. Here they will associate with the 45S rRNA molecule, forming a very large **ribonucleoprotein particle (RNP).** This ribonucleoprotein particle is processed by several resident molecules into precursors of the large and small ribosomal subunits in the pars granulosa region of the nucleolus. Thereafter, assembled small ribosomal subunits, made up of 18S rRNAs and other ribosomal proteins, make their way from the nucleolus to the cytoplasm by transport via the nuclear pore complexes. The remaining 28S, 5.8S, and 5S rRNAs are assembled into large ribosomal subunits and transported out of the nucleus to the cytoplasm by way of the nuclear pore complexes.

Nucleoplasm

The **nucleoplasm** is that portion of the protoplasm that is surrounded by the nuclear envelope. It consists of interchromatin and perichromatin granules, ribonucleoprotein particles, and the nuclear matrix.

Interchromatin granules (IGs), which are 20 to 25 nm in diameter, contain ribonucleoprotein particles and several enzymes, including ATPase, GTPase, ß-glycerophosphatase, and NAD-pyrophosphatase. They are located in clusters

RIBOSOME FORMATION

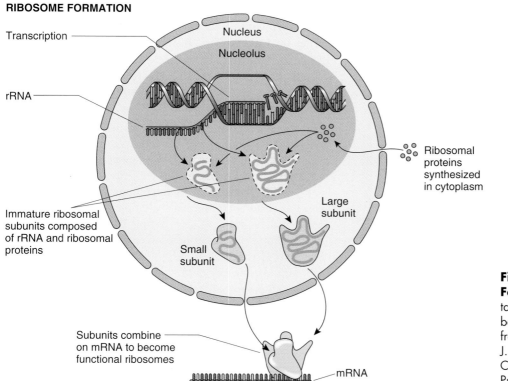

Figure 3–10. Ribosome Formation. A schematic presentation of the nuclear events in ribosome formation. (Modified from Alberts, B., Bray, D., Lewis, J., et al.: Molecular Biology of the Cell, 3rd ed., New York, Garland Publishing, 1994.)

scattered throughout the nucleus among the chromatin material and appear to be connected to each other by thin fibrils. Their function is unclear.

Perichromatin granules (PCGs) are 30 to 50 nm in diameter and located at the margins of the heterochromatin. These electron-dense particles are surrounded by a 25-nm wide halo of a less dense region. They are composed of densely packed fibrils of 4.7S low-molecular-weight RNA complexed to two peptides, resembling **heterogeneous nuclear ribonucleoproteins (hnRNPs).**

Small nuclear ribonucleoprotein particles (snRNPs) function in splicing, cleaving, and transporting hnRNPs. Although most snRNPs are located in the nucleus, some are limited to nucleoli. Several minor subgroups of these particles have been discovered recently, but their function has yet to be elucidated.

NUCLEAR MATRIX. The **nuclear matrix** is defined both in structural and biochemical terms. It appears that differences reported in its components may be due to the extraction methods employed in studying its contents. Biochemically, the matrix contains about 10% of the total protein, 30% of the RNA, 1% to 3% of the total DNA, and 2% to 5% of the total nuclear phosphate. The structural components include the nuclear pore–nuclear lamina complex, residual nucleoli, residual RNP networks, and fibrillar elements.

Functionally, the nuclear matrix has been shown to be associated with DNA replication sites, rRNA and mRNA transcription and processing, steroid receptor binding, heat shock proteins, carcinogen binding, DNA viruses, and viral proteins. This list is neither inclusive nor does it address the functional natures of each of these associations because they are as yet unclear.

Nucleolus

The **nucleolus,** a dense nonmembranous structure located in the nucleus, is observed only during interphase because it dissipates during cell division. It stains basophilic with hematoxylin and eosin, being rich in rRNA and protein. The nucleolus contains only small amounts of DNA, which is also inactive, so it does not stain with Feulgen stains. Usually there are no more that two or three nucleoli per cell; however, their number, size, and shape are generally related to the species and the synthetic activity of the cell. In cells that are actively synthesizing protein, the nucleolus may occupy up to 25% of the nuclear volume. Densely staining regions are the **nucleolus-associated chromatin,** which is being transcribed into rRNA (see Figs. 3–2 and 3–3). In malignant cells the nucleolus may become hypertrophic.

Four distinct areas of the nucleolus have been described: the **pale-staining fibrillar center,** containing inactive DNA (not being transcribed), **pars fibrosa,** containing nucleolar RNAs being transcribed, **pars granulosa,** in which maturing ribosomal subunits are assembled, and the **nucleolar**

matrix, a network of fibers that participates in nucleolar organization.

Also located in the pale-staining regions are the tips of chromosomes 13, 14, 15, 21, and 22 (in humans), containing the **nucleolar organizer regions (NORs),** where gene loci encoding rRNA are located.

Cell Cycle

The **cell cycle** is divided into two major events: **mitosis,** the short period of time when the cell divides its nucleus and cytoplasm, giving rise to two daughter cells, and **interphase,** a longer period of time during which the cell increases its size and content and replicates its genetic material (Fig. 3–11). The cell cycle may be thought of as beginning at the conclusion of the telophase stage in **mitosis (M),** after which the cell enters interphase. Interphase is subdivided into three phases: **G_1 (gap) phase,** when the synthesis of macromolecules essential for DNA duplication begins; **S phase,** when the DNA is duplicated; and **G_2 phase,** when the cell undergoes preparations for mitosis.

Cells that become highly differentiated after the last mitotic event may cease to undergo mitosis either permanently (e.g., neurons, muscle cells), or temporarily (e.g., peripheral lymphocytes) and return to the cell cycle at a later time. Cells that have left the cell cycle are said to be in a resting stage, the **G_0 (outside) phase.**

Interphase

G_1 Phase

The daughter cells formed during mitosis enter the **G_1 phase.** During this phase the cells synthesize RNA, regulatory proteins essential to DNA replication, and enzymes necessary to carry out these synthetic activities. Thus the cell volume, reduced by dividing the cell in half during mitosis, is restored to normal. Additionally, the nucleoli are reestablished during G_1. It is during this time that the centrioles begin to duplicate themselves, a process that is completed by G_2.

It appears that key events in the cell cycle are controlled by certain protein kinases. One of these, **p34,** possibly the **"trigger" protein** that functions to initiate mitosis, is produced during G_1. Also a small group of proteins called **cyclins,** which influence the activity of these kinases, are produced at this time. It is speculated that once a kinase has been activated by a cyclin, it phosphorylates a target protein, driving the cell into another phase. Recently, other cyclin-like proteins have been found that either activate p34 or p34-like kinases that may trigger or drive the cell to enter the S phase. Perhaps other of these kinase reactions may include the **S-phase activator, M-phase delaying factor,** and the **M-phase promoting factor** previously described.

Cells that produce these cyclins reach a certain **restriction point** physiologically, and may proceed to the next phase in the cell cycle. Cells that do not produce the proper cyclins or kinases do not reach the restriction point and are incapable of progressing through the cell cycle and become resting cells in the **G_0 phase.**

S phase

During the **S phase,** the synthetic phase of the cell cycle, the genome is duplicated. All of the requisite nucleoproteins including the histones are imported and incorporated into the DNA molecule forming the chromatin material. The cell now contains twice the normal complement of its DNA. The amount of DNA present in autosomal and germ cells varies also. Autosomal cells contain the diploid (2n) amount of DNA before the synthetic (S) phase of the cell cycle when the (2n) amount of DNA is doubled (4n) in preparation for cell division. In contrast, germ cells produced by meiosis possess the haploid (1n) number of chromosomes and also the (1n) amount of DNA.

G2 phase

During **G_2 phase** the RNA and proteins essential to cell division are synthesized. Also the energy for mitosis is stored.

CELL CYCLE

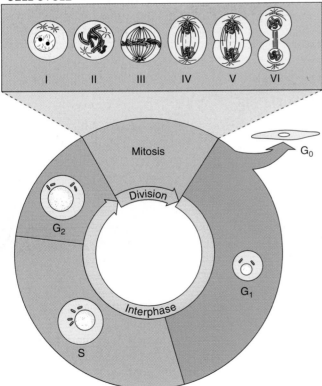

Figure 3–11. Cell Cycle. A diagram illustrating the cell cycle in actively dividing cells. Nondividing cells such as neurons leave the cycle to enter the **G_0 phase** (resting stage). Other cells such as lymphocytes may return to the cell cycle.

Additionally, tubulin is synthesized for assembly into microtubules required for mitosis.

Mitosis

Mitosis (M) is the process whereby the cytoplasm and the nucleus of the cell are divided equally into two identical daughter cells (Fig. 3–12). First, the nuclear material is divided, a process called **karyokinesis,** followed by division of the cytoplasm, called **cytokinesis.** The process of mitosis is divided into five distinct stages: **prophase, prometaphase, metaphase, anaphase,** and **telophase** (Fig. 3–13).

Prophase

At the beginning of prophase the chromosomes are condensing to become visible microscopically. Each chromosome consists of two parallel **sister chromatids** joined together at one point along their length, the **centromere.** As chromosomes condense, the nucleolus disappears. The **centrosome** also divides into two regions, each half containing a pair of **centrioles** and a **microtubule-organizing center (MTOC),** which migrate away from each other to opposite poles of the cell.

From each MTOC develop **astral rays** and **spindle fibers** that will give rise to the **mitotic spindle apparatus.** It is thought that the astral rays—microtubules that radiate out from the pole of the spindle—may function in orienting the MTOC at the pole of the cell. Those microtubules that attach to the centromere region of the chromosome are the spindle fibers that assist in directing the chromosome migration to the pole.

At the centromere region of each chromatid a new microtubule organizing center, the **kinetochore,** develops. **Spindle fibers** bind to the kinetochore in preparation for chromatid migration to effect karyokinesis.

Prometaphase

Prometaphase begins as the nuclear lamins are phosphorylated, resulting in the breakdown and disappearance of the nuclear envelope. The chromosomes are arranged randomly throughout the cytoplasm during this phase. Microtubules that become attached to the kinetochores are known as **mitotic spindle microtubules,** whereas microtubules that do not become incorporated into the spindle apparatus are called **polar microtubules.** Some believe that the polar microtubules are responsible for maintaining the spacing between the two poles during the mitotic event. The mitotic spindle microtubules assist in migration of the chromosomes so that they become oriented into an alignment with the mitotic spindle.

Metaphase

During **metaphase** the chromosomes become maximally condensed and the chromosomes are lined up at the equator of the mitotic spindle (**metaphase plate** configuration). Each chromatid parallels the equator and spindle microtubules are attached to its kinetochore, radiating to the spindle pole.

Anaphase

Anaphase begins when sister chromatids, located at the equator of the metaphase plate, pull apart and begin their

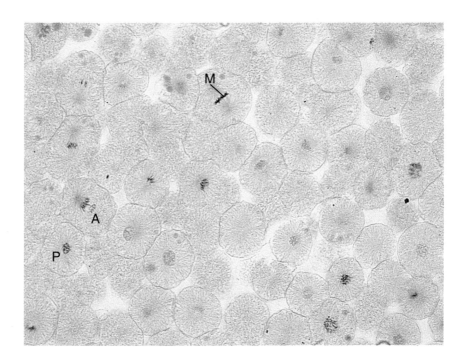

Figure 3–12. Stages of Mitosis. Light micrograph (× 270). Note the various stages of mitosis: A, anaphase; M, metaphase; P, prophase.

MITOSIS

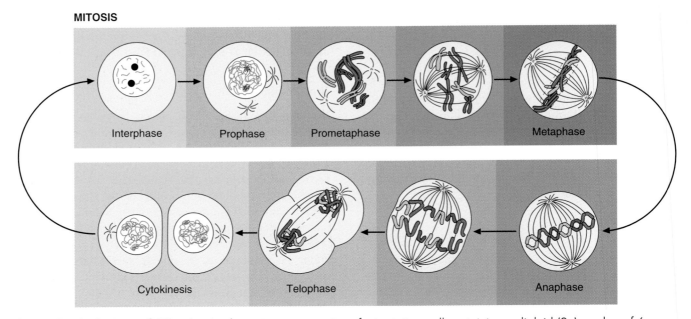

Figure 3–13. Stages of Mitosis. A schematic representation of mitosis in a cell containing a diploid (2n) number of 6 chromosomes.

migration toward the opposite poles of the mitotic spindle. The spindle/kinetochore attachment site leads the way, with the arms of the chromatids simply trailing, contributing nothing to the migration or its pathway.

It has been postulated that the observed movement of the chromatids toward the pole in anaphase is the result of shortening of the microtubules via depolymerization at the kinetochore end. This, coupled with the recent discovery of dynein associated with the kinetochore, may be analogous to vesicle transport along microtubules. In late anaphase a cleavage furrow begins to form at the plasmalemma, indicating the region where the cell will be divided during cytokinesis.

Telophase

At **telophase** each set of chromosomes has reached its respective pole, the nuclear lamins are dephosphorylated, and the nuclear envelope is reconstituted. The chromosomes uncoil and become organized into heterochromatin and euchromatin of the interphase cell. The nucleolus is developed during this phase from the nucleolus-organizing regions (NORs) on each of five pairs of chromosomes.

Cytokinesis

The cleavage furrow continues to deepen until only the **midbody,** a small bridge of cytoplasm, and remaining polar microtubules connect the two daughter cells (Fig 3–14). The polar microtubules are surrounded by a **contractile ring** lying just inside the plasma membrane. The contractile ring is composed of **actin** and **myosin filaments** attached to the plasma membrane. Constriction of the ring is followed by

depolymerization of the remaining spindle microtubules separating the two **daughter cells.** During separation of the daughter cells and shortly thereafter, the elements of the contractile ring and the remaining microtubules of the mitotic apparatus are disassembled, concluding cytokinesis.

Each daughter cell resulting from mitosis is identical in every respect including the entire genome, and each daughter cell possesses a diploid (2n) number of chromosomes.

CLINICAL CORRELATIONS

A more complete understanding of mitosis and the cell cycle has greatly aided cancer chemotherapy, making it possible to use drugs at a time when the cells are in a particular stage of the cell cycle. For example, **vincristine** and similar drugs disrupt the mitotic spindle, arresting the cell in mitosis. **Colchicine,** another plant alkaloid that produces the same effect, has been used extensively for studying individual chromosomes and karyotyping. **Methotrexate,** which inhibits purine synthesis, and **5-fluorouracil,** which inhibits pyrimidine synthesis, both halt the cell cycle in the S phase, preventing cell division; both are common chemotherapy agents.

Oncogenes are mutated forms of normal genes called proto-oncogens that code for proteins that control cell division. Oncogenes may result from a viral infection or random genetic accidents. When present in a cell, oncogenes dominate genes over the normal proto-oncogene alleles, causing unregulated cell division and proliferation. Examples of cancer cells arising from oncogenes include **bladder cancer** and **acute myelogenous leukemia.**

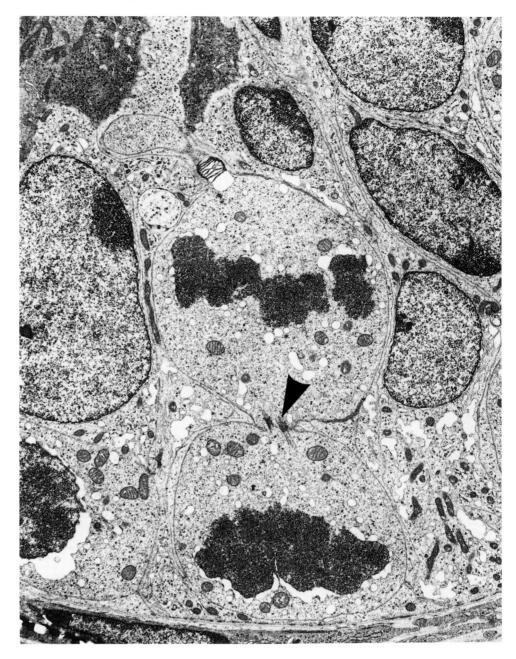

Figure 3–14. Cytokinesis.
Electron micrograph (× 9200).
A spermatogonium in late
telophase demonstrating the
forming **midbody** *(arrowhead)*. Note that the chromosomes in the daughter nuclei
are beginning to uncoil. (From
Miething, A.: Intercellular
bridges between germ cells in
the immature golden hamster
testis: evidence for clonal and
nonclonal mode of prolifera-
ton. Cell Tissue Res.
262:559–567, 1990.)

Meiosis

Meiosis is a specialized type of cell division that produces
the germ cells—ova and spermatozoa. This process has two
crucial results: (1) reduction in the number of chromosomes
from the **diploid (2n)** to the **haploid (1n)** number, ensuring
that each gamete carries the haploid amount of DNA and the
haploid number of chromosomes, and (2) recombination of
genes, ensuring genetic variability and diversity of the gene
pool.

Meiosis is divided into two separate events or divisions.
Meiosis I, the first division, is called **reductional division.**
In this event homologous pairs of chromosomes line up,
members of each pair separate and go to opposite poles, and
the cell divides; thus each daughter cell receives half the
number of chromosomes (haploid number). **Meiosis II,** the
second division, is called **equatorial division.** In this event
the two **chromatids** of each chromosome are separated, as
in mitosis, followed by migration of the chromatids to opposite poles and the formation of two daughter cells. These
two events produce four cells (gametes), each with the haploid number of chromosomes and haploid DNA content.

Meiosis I (Reductional division)

Meiosis begins at the conclusion of interphase in the cell
cycle. In gametogenesis, when the germ cells are in the
S phase of the cell cycle preceding meiosis, the amount of
DNA is doubled to **4n** and the chromosome number is also
doubled to **4n.** Meiosis I proceeds as outlined in Figure 3–15.

MEIOSIS I

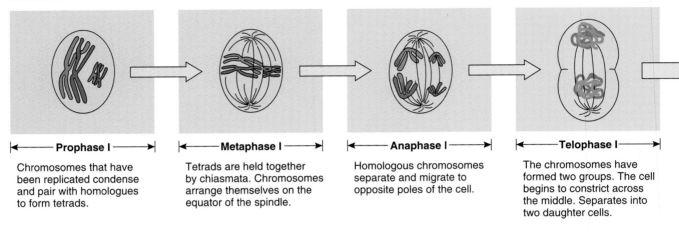

|←——— **Prophase I** ———→| |←——— **Metaphase I** ———→| |←——— **Anaphase I** ———→| |←——— **Telophase I** ———→|

Chromosomes that have been replicated condense and pair with homologues to form tetrads.

Tetrads are held together by chiasmata. Chromosomes arrange themselves on the equator of the spindle.

Homologous chromosomes separate and migrate to opposite poles of the cell.

The chromosomes have formed two groups. The cell begins to constrict across the middle. Separates into two daughter cells.

Figure 3–15. Stages of Meiosis. A schematic presentation of the events in meiosis in an idealized cell containing a diploid (2n) number of 4 chromosomes.

Prophase I

Prophase of meiosis I lasts a long time and is subdivided into the following five phases.

1. *Leptotene.* Individual chromosomes, composed of two chromatids joined at the centromere, begin to condense, forming long strands in the nucleus.
2. *Zygotene.* Homologous pairs of chromosomes approximate each other, lining up in register (gene locus to gene locus), and make synapses via the **synaptonemal complex,** forming a tetrad.
3. *Pachytene.* Chromosomes continue to condense, becoming thicker and shorter; **chiasmata** (crossing over sites) are formed as random exchange of genetic material occurs between homologous chromosomes.
4. *Diplotene.* Chromosomes continue to condense and then begin to separate, revealing chiasmata.
5. *Diakinesis.* Chromosomes condense maximally and the nucleolus disappears, as does the nuclear envelope, freeing the chromosomes into the cytoplasm.

Metaphase I

During **metaphase I** homologous chromosomes align as pairs on the equatorial plate of the spindle apparatus in random order, ensuring a subsequent reshuffling of the mater-

nal and paternal chromosomes. Spindle fibers become attached to the kinetochores of the chromosomes.

Anaphase I

In **anaphase I** homologous chromosomes migrate away from each other, going to opposite poles. Each chromosome still consists of two chromatids.

Telophase I

Telophase I is similar to telophase of mitosis. The chromosomes reach the opposing poles, nuclei are reformed and cytokinesis occurs, giving rise to two daughter cells. Each cell possesses 23 chromosomes, the haploid (**1n**) number, but because each chromosome is composed of two chromatids, the DNA content is still diploid. Each of the two newly formed daughter cells enters meiosis II.

Meiosis II (Equatorial Division)

The **equatorial division** is not preceded by an **S** phase. It is very much like mitosis and is subdivided into **prophase II, metaphase II, anaphase II, telophase II,** and **cytokinesis** (Fig. 3–15). The chromosomes line up on the equator, the kinetochores attach to spindle fibers, followed by the chro-

MEIOSIS II

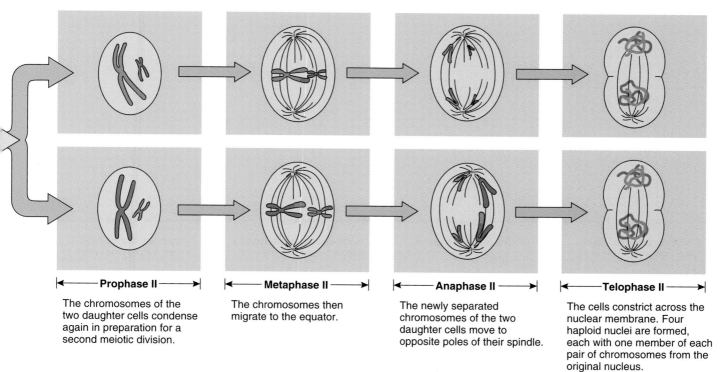

|←————Prophase II————→| |←————Metaphase II————→| |←————Anaphase II————→| |←————Telophase II————→|

The chromosomes of the two daughter cells condense again in preparation for a second meiotic division.

The chromosomes then migrate to the equator.

The newly separated chromosomes of the two daughter cells move to opposite poles of their spindle.

The cells constrict across the nuclear membrane. Four haploid nuclei are formed, each with one member of each pair of chromosomes from the original nucleus.

matids migrating to opposite poles, and cytokinesis divides each of the two cells, giving a total of four daughter cells from the original diploid germ cell. Each of the four cells contains a haploid amount of DNA content and a haploid chromosome number.

Unlike the daughter cells resulting from mitosis, each of which contains the diploid number of chromosomes and is an identical copy of the other, the four cells resulting from meiosis contain the haploid number of chromosomes and are genetically distinct because of reshuffling of the chromosomes and crossing over. Thus every gamete contains its own unique genetic complement.

Extracellular Matrix

4

Cells of multicellular organisms congregate to form structural and functional associations, known as tissues. Each of the four basic tissues of the body—epithelium, connective tissue, muscle, and nervous tissue—possesses specific, defined characteristics, which will be detailed in subsequent chapters. However, it should be understood that all tissues are composed of **cells** and an **extracellular matrix,** a complex of nonliving macromolecules manufactured by the cells and exported by them into the intercellular space.

Some tissues, such as epithelia, form sheets of cells with only a scant amount of extracellular matrix. At the opposite extreme is connective tissue, composed mostly of extracellular matrix with a limited number of cells scattered throughout the matrix. Cells maintain their associations with the extracellular matrix by forming specialized junctions that hold them to the surrounding macromolecules. This chapter explores the nature of the extracellular matrix and the junctional associations that cells form with it.

The extracellular matrix of connective tissue proper, the most ubiquitous connective tissue of the body, is composed of a hydrated gel-like **ground substance** with **fibers** embedded in it. The former resists forces of compression and the latter withstands tensile forces. The water of hydration permits the rapid exchange of nutrients and waste products carried by the tissue fluid as it percolates through the ground substance (Fig. 4–1).

Ground Substance

Ground substance is composed of **glycosaminoglycans, proteoglycans,** and **adhesive glycoproteins.** These three families of macromolecules form various interactions with each other, with fibers, and with the cells of connective tissue and epithelia (Fig. 4–2).

Glycosaminoglycans

Glycosaminoglycans (GAGs) are long, inflexible, unbranched polysaccharides, composed of chains of repeating disaccharide units. One of the two repeating disaccharides is always an **amino sugar** (N-acetylglucosamine or N-acetylgalactosamine); the other one is typically a **uronic acid** (iduronic or glucuronic) (Table 4–1). Because the amino

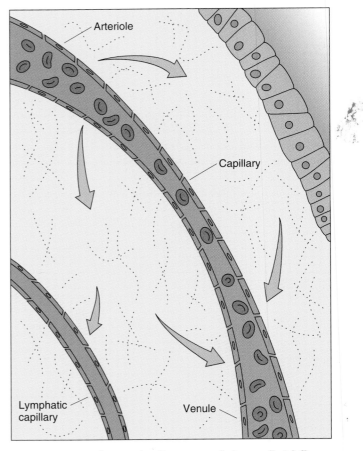

Figure 4–1. Schematic diagram of tissue fluid flow. Plasma from capillaries and venules enters the connective tissue spaces as tissue fluid which percolates through the ground substance. Tissue fluid reenters the venule as well as lymphatic capillaries.

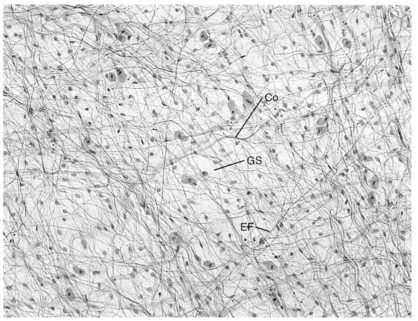

Figure 4–2. Light micrograph of areolar connective tissue, displaying cells, collagen fibers (Co) and elastic fibers (EF) and ground substance (GS) (×132).

[handwritten notes] glycosal amino glycans; type of carbohydrate that absorbs a lot of H2O

Table 4–1. Types of Glycosaminoglycans

GAG	Molecular Mass (Da)	Repeating Disaccharides	Sulfated Amino Sugar	Covalent Linkage to Protein	Location in Body
Hyaluronic acid	10^7–10^8	Glucuronate and N-acetyl-glucosamine	None	No	Most connective tissue, synovial fluid, cartilage, dermis
Keratan sulfate	10,000–30,000	Galactose and N-acetyl-glucosamine	N-acetyl-glucosamine	Yes	Cartilage, cornea, intervertebral disk
Heparan sulfate	15,000–20,000	Glucuronate (or iduronate) and N-acetyl-galactosamine	N-acetyl-galactosamine	Yes	Blood vessels, lung, basal lamina
Heparin	15,000–20,000	Glucuronate (or iduronate) and N-acetyl-glucosamine	N-acetyl-glucosamine	No	Mast cell granule, liver, lung, skin
Chondroitin-4-sulfate	10,000–30,000	Glucuronate and N-acetyl-galactosamine	N-acetyl-galactosamine	Yes	Cartilage, bone, cornea, blood vessels
Chondroitin-6-sulfate	10,000–30,000	Glucuronate and N-acetyl-galactosamine	N-acetyl-galactosamine	Yes	Cartilage, Wharton's jelly, blood vessels
Dermatan sulfate	10,000–30,000	Glucuronate (or iduronate) and N-acetyl-galactosamine	N-acetyl-galactosamine	Yes	Heart valves, skin, blood vessels

sugar is usually sulfated and these sugars also have carboxyl groups projecting from them, they are negatively charged and thus attract cations, such as Na+. High sodium concentration in the ground substance attracts tissue fluid, which (by hydrating the intercellular matrix) assists in the resistance to forces of compression.

All but one of the major glycosaminoglycans of extracellular matrix are sulfated, each consisting of less than 300 repeating disaccharide units (Table 4–1). The sulfated glycosaminoglycans include keratan sulfate, heparan sulfate, heparin, chondroitin-4-sulfate, chondroitin-6-sulfate, and dermatan sulfate. These GAGs are usually linked covalently to protein molecules to form proteoglycans. The only nonsulfated glycosaminoglycan is hyaluronic acid, which may possess as many as 25,000 repeating disaccharide units. It is a huge macromolecule that does not form covalent links to protein molecules (although proteoglycans do become attached to it).

Proteoglycans

When sulfated GAGs form covalent bonds with a protein core, they form a family of macromolecules known as **proteoglycans,** many of which occupy huge domains. These large structures look like a bottle brush, with the protein core resembling the wire stem and the various sulfated GAGs projecting from its surface in three-dimensional space, as do the bristles of the brush (Fig. 4–3).

Proteoglycans may be of various sizes, ranging from about 50,000 daltons (decorin and betaglycan) to as many as 3 million daltons (aggrecan). The protein cores of proteoglycans are manufactured on the rough endoplasmic reticulum (RER), and the glycosaminoglycan groups are covalently bound to the protein in the Golgi apparatus. Sulfation and epimerization (rearrangement of various groups around the carbon atoms of the sugar units) also occur in the Golgi apparatus.

Many proteoglycans, especially **aggrecan,** a macromolecule found in cartilage and connective tissue proper, attach to hyaluronic acid (Fig. 4–3). The mode of attachment involves link proteins that form bonds both with the core protein of aggrecan and the sugar groups of hyaluronic acids. Because hyaluronic acid may be 20 μm in length, the result of this association is an aggrecan composite that occupies a huge volume and may have as large a molecular mass as several hundred million daltons. This immense molecule is responsible for the gel state of the extracellular matrix and acts as a barrier to fast diffusion of aqueous deposits, as is evident when one observes the slow disappearance of an aqueous bubble subsequent to its subdermal injection.

CLINICAL CORRELATIONS

Many pathogenic bacteria, such as *Staphylococcus aureus,* secrete **hyaluronidase,** an enzyme that cleaves

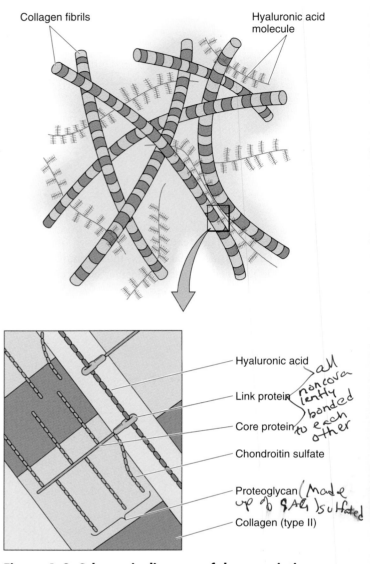

Collagen fibrils   Hyaluronic acid molecule

Hyaluronic acid   *all noncovalently bonded to each other*

Link protein

Core protein

Chondroitin sulfate

Proteoglycan *(Made up of GAG) sulfated*

Collagen (type II)

Figure 4–3. Schematic diagram of the association of aggrecan molecules with collagen fibers. The inset displays a higher magnification of the aggrecan molecule, indicating the core protein of the proteoglycan molecule to which glycosaminoglycans are attached. The core protein is attached to the hyaluronic acid by link proteins. (Adapted from Fawcett, D.W.: Bloom and Fawcett's A Textbook of Histology, 11th ed. Philadelphia, W.B. Saunders Company, 1986.)

hyaluronic acid into numerous small fragments, thus converting the gel state of the extracellular matrix to a sol state. The consequence of this reaction is to permit the rapid spread of the bacteria through the connective tissue spaces.

Functions of Proteoglycans

Proteoglycans have numerous functions. By occupying a large volume, they resist compression and retard the rapid movement of microorganisms and metastatic cells. Additionally, in association with the basal lamina, they form molecular filters of varying pore sizes and charge distributions that selectively screen and retard macromolecules as they pass through them. Proteoglycans also possess binding sites for certain signaling molecules, such as transforming growth factor-β (TGF-β). By binding these signaling molecules, proteoglycans can either impede their function by preventing the molecules from reaching their destinations or enhance their function by concentrating them in a specific location.

Some proteoglycans, such as **syndecans,** instead of being released into the extracellular matrix, remain attached to the cell membrane. The core proteins of syndecans act as transmembrane proteins and are attached to the actin filaments of the cytoskeleton. Their extracellular moieties bind to components of the extracellular matrix, thus permitting the cell to become attached to macromolecular components of the matrix. Additionally, syndecans of fibroblasts function as co-receptors because they bind fibroblast growth factor (FGF) and present it to cell membrane FGF receptors in their vicinity.

Adhesive Glycoproteins

The ability of cells to adhere to components of the intercellular matrix is mediated to a great extent by **adhesive glycoproteins.** These large macromolecules have several domains, at least one of which usually binds to cell surface proteins called **integrins,** one to collagen fibers, and one to proteoglycans. In this manner adhesive glycoproteins fasten the various components of tissues to each other. The major types of adhesive proteoglycans are fibronectin, laminin, entactin, tenascin, chondronectin, and osteonectin.

Fibronectin is a large dimer, composed of two similar polypeptide subunits, each about 220,000 daltons, attached to one another at their carboxyl ends by disulfide bonds. Each arm of this V-shaped macromolecule possesses binding sites for various extracellular components (e.g., collagen, heparin, heparan sulfate, and hyaluronic acid), and for integrins of the cell membrane. The region of the fibronectin that is specific for adhering to the cell membrane possesses the three residue sequence arginine, glycine, and aspartate, referred to as the **RGD sequence.** This sequence of amino acids is characteristic of the integrin-binding site in many adhesive glycoproteins. Although fibronectin is produced mainly by connective tissue cells known as **fibroblasts,** it is also present in blood as **plasma fibronectin.** In addition, it may be temporarily attached to the plasma membrane as **cell surface fibronectin.** Fibronectin has also been demonstrated to mark migratory pathways for embryonic cells, so that the migrating cells of the developing organism can reach their destination.

Laminin is a very large glycoprotein (950,000 daltons) composed of three large polypeptide chains A, B₁, and B₂. The B chains wrap around the A chain, forming a cross-like pattern of one long and three short chains. The three chains are held in position by disulfide bonds. The location of laminin is almost strictly limited to the basal lamina; therefore, this glycoprotein has binding sites for heparan sulfate, type IV collagen, entactin, and the cell membrane.

The sulfated glycoprotein **entactin** binds to the laminin molecule where the three short arms of that molecule meet each other. Entactin also binds to type IV collagen, thus facilitating the binding of laminin to the collagen meshwork.

Tenascin is a large glycoprotein, composed of six polypeptide chains held together by disulfide bonds. This macromolecule, which resembles a bug whose six legs project radially from a central body, has binding sites for the transmembrane proteoglycan syndecans and for fibronectin. Tenascin's distribution is usually limited to embryonic tissue, where it is used to mark migratory pathways for specific cells.

Chondronectin and **osteonectin** are similar to fibronectin. The former has binding sites for type II collagen, chondroitin sulfates, hyaluronic acid, and integrins of chondroblasts and chondrocytes. Osteonectin possesses domains for type I collagen, proteoglycans, and integrins of osteoblasts and osteocytes. Additionally, it may facilitate the binding of calcium hydroxyapatite crystals to type I collagen in bone.

Fibers

The fibers of the extracellular matrix provide tensile strength and elasticity to this substance. Classical histologists have described three types of fibers, based on their morphology and reactivity with histological stains. The three fiber types include **collagen, reticular,** and **elastic** (Fig. 4–2). Although it is now known that reticular fibers are composed of collagen, many histologists retain the term *reticular fibers* not only for historical reasons but also for the sake of convenience when describing organs that possess large quantities of this particular collagen type.

Collagen Fibers: Structure and Function

The capability of the extracellular matrix to withstand compressive forces is due to the presence of the hydrated matrix formed by glycosaminoglycans and proteoglycans, whereas tensile forces are resisted by fibers of the tough inelastic protein **collagen.** This family of proteins is very abundant, constituting about 20% of all the proteins in the body. Collagen forms a flexible fiber (Fig. 4–4) whose tensile strength is greater than that of stainless steel of comparable diameter.

Large collections of collagen fibers appear glistening white in the living individual; therefore, collagen fiber bundles are also referred to as *white fibers.* Collagen fibers of connective tissue are usually less than 10 μm in diameter and are colorless when unstained. Stained with hematoxylin and eosin, they appear as long, wavy pink fiber bundles.

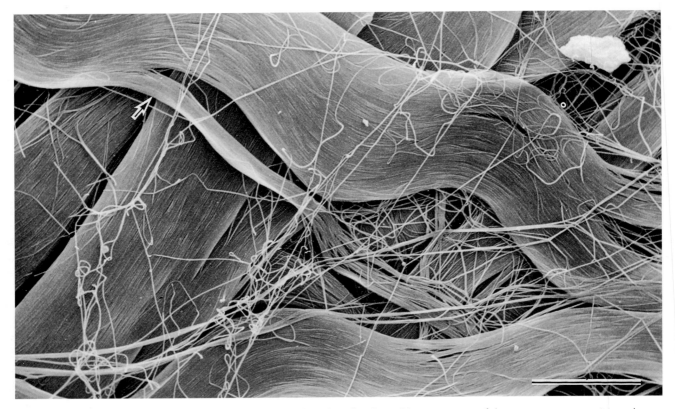

Figure 4–4. Scanning electron micrograph of collagen fiber bundles from the epineurium of the rat sciatic nerve. Note that the collagen bundle is composed of finer fiber bundles (× 2900). (From Ushiki, T. and Ide, C.: Three-dimensional organization of the collagen fibrils in the rat sciatic nerve as revealed by transmission and scanning electron microscopy. Cell Tissue Res. **260:**175–184, 1990. Copyright Springer-Verlag.)

Electron micrographs of collagen fibers stained with heavy metals display cross-banding at regular intervals of 67 nm, an identifying characteristic of these fibers. These fibers are formed from parallel aggregates of thinner fibrils 10 to 300 nm in diameter (Fig. 4–5). The fibrils themselves are fashioned from a highly regular assembly of even smaller subunits, **tropocollagen molecules,** each about 280 nm long and 1.5 nm in diameter. Individual tropocollagen molecules are composed of three polypeptide chains, called **α chains,** wrapped around each other in a triple helical configuration.

Each α chain possesses about 1000 amino acid residues, where every third amino acid is glycine, and the majority of the remaining amino acids is composed of proline, hydroxyproline, and hydroxylysine. It is believed that glycine, because of its small size, permits the close association of the three α chains; the hydrogen bonds of hydroxyproline hold the three α chains together; and hydroxylysine permits the formation of fibrils by binding the collagen molecules to each other.

Although there are at least 15 different types of collagen known, depending on the amino acid sequence of their α chains, only six of them are of interest in this textbook. Each α chain is coded by a separate mRNA. These different collagen types are located in specific regions of the body where they serve various functions (Table 4–2).

Type I, the most common type of collagen, forms thick fibers and is present in connective tissue proper, bone, dentin, and cementum (Fig. 4–6). **Type II** forms slender fibers and is almost exclusively found in the matrices of hyaline and elastic cartilage. **Type III collagen** is also referred to as **reticular fiber** because it was believed to differ from collagen. It is now known that reticular fiber is a type of collagen that becomes highly glycosylated and forms thin fibers 0.5 to 2.0 μm in diameter. Because of the rich coating of sugar groups, type III collagen fibers are preferentially stained by silver salts or by the periodic acid–Schiff (PAS) reaction.

Type IV collagen does not form fibers and does not display the 67 nm periodicity. Instead, type IV collagen forms a meshwork of procollagen molecules matted together to form a supporting carpet of basal lamina.

Type V collagen forms very thin fibrils, possesses a 67 nm periodicity, and is found in association with type I collagen. **Type VII collagen** forms small aggregates, known as **anchoring fibrils,** which secure the basal lamina to the underlying type I and type III collagen fiber bundles.

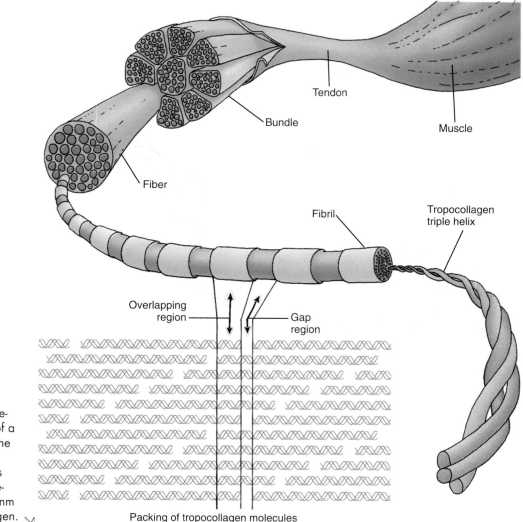

Figure 4–5. Schematic representation of the components of a collagen fiber. Observe that the ordered arrangement of the tropocollagen molecules gives rise to the gap and overlap regions, responsible for the 67 nm cross banding of Type I collagen.

Packing of tropocollagen molecules

CLINICAL CORRELATIONS

At the end of surgery, the cut surfaces of skin are carefully sutured and usually a week later the sutures are removed. The tensile strength of the dermis at that point is only about 10% that of normal skin. Within the next four weeks, the tensile strength increases to about 80% of normal, but in many cases it never reaches 100%. The initial weakness is attributed to the formation of type III collagen formed during early wound healing, whereas the later improvement in tensile strength is due to scar maturation, when type III collagen is replaced by type I collagen.

Some individuals, especially blacks, are predisposed to an excessive accumulation of collagen during wound healing. In these patients the scar forms an elevated growth known as a **keloid.**

Synthesis of Collagen

The synthesis of collagen occurs on the RER as individual **preprocollagen** chains (Fig. 4–7), which are α chains pos-

sessing additional amino acid sequences, known as **propeptides,** at the amino and carboxyl ends. As a preprocollagen molecule is being synthesized, it enters the cisterna of the RER, where it is modified. First, the signal sequence directing the molecule to the RER is removed; then some of the proline and lysine residues are hydroxylated (by the enzymes peptidyl proline hydroxylase and peptidyl lysine hydroxylase) to form hydroxyproline and hydroxylysine, respectively. Subsequently, selected hydroxylysines are glycosylated.

Three preprocollagen molecules align with each other and assemble to form a tight helical configuration, known as a **procollagen molecule.** It is believed that the precision of their alignment is accomplished by the propeptides. These propeptides do not wrap around each other, so that the procollagen molecule resembles a tightly wound rope with frayed ends. The propeptides apparently have the additional function of keeping the procollagen molecules soluble, thus preventing their spontaneous aggregation into collagen fibers within the cell.

The procollagen molecules leave the RER via transfer

Table 4–2. Major Types and Characteristics of Collagen

Molecular Type	Molecular Formula	Synthesizing Cells	Function	Location in Body
I	$[\alpha 1(I)]_2\alpha 2(I)$	Fibroblast, osteoblast, odontoblast, cementoblast	Resists tension	Dermis, tendon, ligaments, capsules of organs, bone, dentin, cementum
II	$[\alpha 1(II)]_3$	Chondroblasts	Resists pressure	Hyaline cartilage, elastic cartilage
III	$[\alpha 1(III)]_3$	Fibroblast, reticular cell, smooth muscle cell, Schwann cell, hepatocyte	Forms structural framework of spleen, liver, lymph nodes, smooth muscle, adipose tissue	Lymphatic system, spleen, liver, cardiovascular system, lung, skin
IV	$[\alpha 1(IV)]_2\alpha 2(IV)]$	Epithelial cells, muscle cells, Schwann cells	Forms the meshwork of the lamina densa of the basal lamina to provide support and filtration	Basal lamina
V	$[\alpha 1(V)]_2\alpha 2(V)$	Fibroblasts, mesenchymal cells	Associated with type I collagen, also with placental ground substance	Dermis, tendon, ligaments, capsules of organs, bone, cementum, placenta
VII	$[\alpha 1(VII)]_3$	Epidermal cells	Forms anchoring fibrils that fasten the lamina densa to the underlying lamina reticularis	Junction of the epidermis and the dermis

vesicles that transport them to the Golgi apparatus, where they are further modified by the addition of oligosaccharides. The modified procollagen molecules are packaged in the *trans* Golgi network and are immediately ferried out of the cell.

As procollagen enters the extracellular environment, proteolytic enzymes, **procollagen peptidases,** cleave the propeptides (removing the frayed ends) from both amino and carboxyl ends (Fig. 4–7). The newly formed molecule is shorter (280 nm in length) and is known as a **tropocollagen (collagen) molecule.** Tropocollagen molecules spontaneously self-assemble (Fig. 4–7), in specific head to tail direction, into a regularly staggered array, fashioning fibrils that display a 67 nm banding representative of collagen types I, II, III, V, and VII (see Fig. 4–5). The formation and maintenance of the fibrillar structure is augmented by covalent bonds formed between lysine and hydroxylysine residues of neighboring tropocollagen molecules.

As the tropocollagen molecules self-assemble in a three-dimensional array, the spaces between the heads and tails of successive molecules in a single row, line up as repeating

gap regions (every 67 nm), not in adjoining but in neighboring rows (Figs. 4–5 and 4–7). Similarly, the overlaps of heads and tails in neighboring rows also are in register with one another as the **overlap regions.** Heavy metal stains used in electron microscopy preferentially deposit in the gap regions. Consequently, viewed in the electron microscope, collagen displays alternating dark and light bands, where the dark bands represent the gap region, filled with heavy metal, and light bands, overlap regions, where the heavy metal cannot be deposited (Fig. 4–6).

The alignment of the collagen fibrils and fiber bundles is determined by the cells that synthesize them. The procollagen is released into folds and furrows of the plasmalemma, which act as molds that arrange the forming fibrils in the proper direction. The fibril orientation is further enhanced as the cells tug on the fibrils and physically drag them to fit the required pattern.

Fibrillar structure is absent in **type IV collagen,** because the propeptides are not removed from the procollagen molecule. Its procollagen molecules assemble into dimers, which then form a felt-like meshwork.

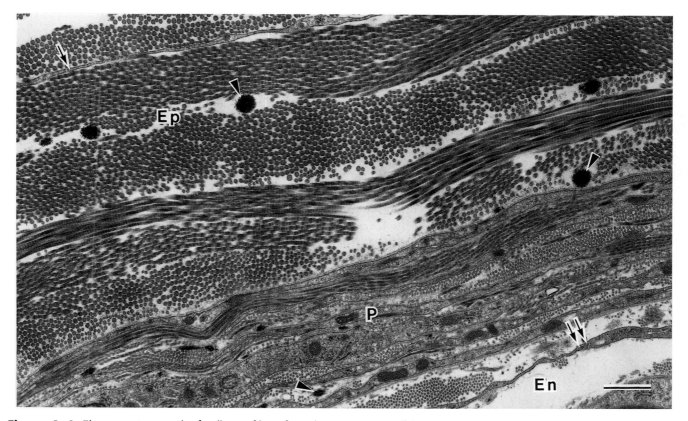

Figure 4–6. Electron micrograph of collagen fibers from the perineurium of the rat sciatic nerve; Ep, epineurium; En, endoneurium; P, perineurium (× 32,500). (From Ushiki, T. and Ide, C.: Three-dimensional organization of the collagen fibrils in the rat sciatic nerve as revealed by transmission and scanning electron microscopy. Cell Tissue Res. **260:**175–184, 1990. Copyright Springer-Verlag.)

CLINICAL CORRELATIONS

Hydroxylation of proline residues requires the presence of vitamin C. In individuals who suffer from the deficiency of this vitamin, the α chains of the tropocollagen molecules are unable to form stable helices, and the tropocollagen molecules are incapable of aggregating into fibrils. This condition, known as **scurvy,** first affects connective tissues with high turnover of collagen, such as the periodontal ligament and gingiva (Fig. 4–8). Because these two structures are responsible for maintaining teeth in their sockets, the symptoms of scurvy include bleeding gums and loose teeth. If the vitamin C deficiency is prolonged, then other sites will also be affected. These symptoms may be alleviated by eating foods rich in vitamin C.

Deficiency of the enzyme **lysyl hydroxylase,** a genetic disorder known as **Ehlers-Danlos syndrome,** results in abnormal cross-links among tropocollagen molecules. Individuals afflicted by this anomalous condition possess abnormal collagen fibers that result in hypermobile joints and hyperextensive skin. In many instances the skin of affected patients is readily traumatized and they are subject to dislocation of the affected joints.

Elastic Fibers

The elasticity of connective tissue is due in great part to the presence of **elastic fibers** in the extracellular matrix (Figs. 4–2 and 4–9). These fibers are usually slender, long, and branching in loose connective tissue, but they may form coarser bundles in ligaments and fenestrated sheets. Such bundles are found in the ligamentum flava of the vertebral column, and concentric sheets occur in the walls of larger blood vessels.

Elastic fibers are manufactured by fibroblasts of connective tissue as well as by smooth muscle cells of blood vessels. They are composed of **elastin,** a protein rich in glycine and proline, and also contain the unusual amino acids **desmosine** and **isodesmosine.** These two amino acids form considerable cross-linking of the elastin molecules, imparting a high degree of elasticity to elastic fibers, so much so that these fibers may be stretched to about 150% of their resting lengths prior to breakage. After being stretched, elastic fibers return to their resting length.

The core of elastic fibers is composed of elastin and is surrounded by a sheath of **microfibrils,** each of which is about 10 nm in diameter and is composed of the glycopro-

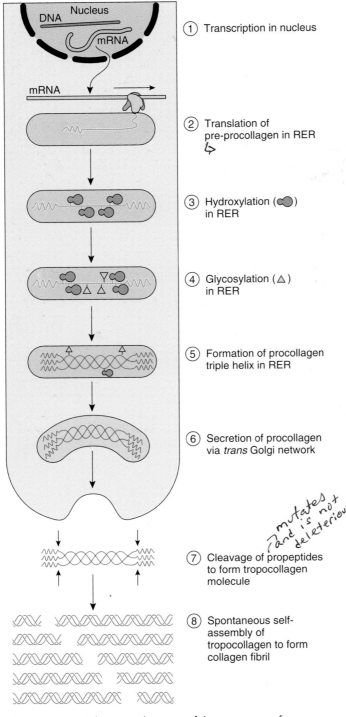

1. Transcription in nucleus

2. Translation of pre-procollagen in RER

3. Hydroxylation (⬤⬤) in RER

4. Glycosylation (△) in RER

5. Formation of procollagen triple helix in RER

6. Secretion of procollagen via *trans* Golgi network

7. Cleavage of propeptides to form tropocollagen molecule

8. Spontaneous self-assembly of tropocollagen to form collagen fibril

Figure 4-7. Schematic diagram of the sequence of events in the synthesis of type I collagen.

tein **fibrillin** (Fig. 4–10). During the formation of elastic fibers, the microfibrils are elaborated first and the elastin is deposited into the space surrounded by the microfibrils (Fig. 4–11).

CLINICAL CORRELATIONS

The integrity of elastic fibers depends on the presence of microfibrils. Patients with **Marfan's syndrome** possess a genetic defect in the gene on chromosome 15 that codes for fibrillin; therefore, their elastic fibers do not develop normally. Individuals who are severely affected with this condition are predisposed to fatal rupture of the aorta.

Basement Membrane

The interface between epithelium and connective tissue is occupied by a narrow, acellular region, the **basement membrane,** that is well stained by the PAS reaction and by other histological stains that detect glycosaminoglycans. A structure similar to the basement membrane, the **external lamina,** surrounds smooth and skeletal muscle cells, adipocytes, and Schwann cells.

The basement membrane visible by light microscopy is better defined by electron microscopy into two constituents: the **basal lamina,** elaborated by epithelial cells, and the **lamina reticularis,** manufactured by cells of the connective tissue (Fig 4–12).

Basal Lamina

Electron micrographs of the **basal lamina** display its two regions, the lamina lucida, a 50-nm thick electron-lucent region just beneath the epithelium, and the lamina densa, a 50-nm thick electron-dense region (Fig. 4–13).

The **lamina lucida** consists mainly of the extracellular glycoproteins laminin and entactin, as well as the **integrins** (discussed below) that project from the epithelial cell membrane into the basal lamina.

The **lamina densa** comprises a meshwork of type IV collagen, which is coated on both the lamina lucida and lamina reticularis sides by the proteoglycan **perlacan.** The **heparan sulfate** sidechains projecting from the protein core of perlacan form a polyanion. The lamina reticularis aspect of the lamina densa also possesses **fibronectin.**

Laminin has domains that bind to type IV collagen, heparan sulfate, and to the integrins of the epithelial cell membrane, thus anchoring the epithelial cell to the basal lamina. The basal lamina appears to be well anchored to the reticular lamina by several substances, including fibronectin, anchoring fibrils (type VII collagen), and microfibrils (fibrillin), all elaborated by fibroblasts of connective tissue (Fig. 4–14).

The basal lamina functions both as a molecular filter and as a flexible, firm support for the overlying epithelium. The filtering aspect is due not only to the type IV collagen whose interwoven meshwork forms a physical filter of specific pore size but also to the negative charges of its heparan sulfate constituent, which preferentially restricts the passage of negatively charged molecules. An additional function of the basal lamina is to direct the migration of cells along its sur-

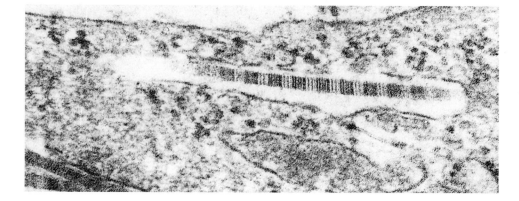

Figure 4–8. Degradation of type I collagen by fibroblasts. (From Ten Cate, A. R.: Oral Histology. Development, Structure, and Function, 4th ed. St. Louis, Mosby-Year Book, 1994.)

face, as in reepithelialization during wound repair or in the reestablishment of myoneural junctions during regeneration of motor nerves.

Lamina reticularis

The **lamina reticularis** (see Figs. 4–12 and 4–13), a region of varying thickness, is manufactured by fibroblasts, and is composed of type I and type III collagen. It is the interface between the basal lamina and the underlying connective tis-

sue, and its thickness varies with the amount of frictional forces attendant on the overlying epithelium. Thus, it is quite thick in skin and very thin beneath the epithelial lining of the alveolus of the lung.

Type I and type III collagen fibers of the connective tissue loop into the lamina reticularis, where they interact with and are bound to the microfibrils and anchoring fibrils of the lamina reticularis. Moreover, the basic groups of the collagen fibers form bonds with the acidic groups of the glycosaminoglycans of the lamina densa. Additionally, collagen-binding domains and glycosaminoglycan domains of fibronectin further assist in achoring the basal lamina to the lamina reticularis. Thus the epithelial sheath is bound to the underlying connective tissue by these resilient, acellular interfaces, the basal lamina and lamina reticularis.

Integrins

Integrins are transmembrane proteins that are similar to cell membrane receptors in that they form bonds with ligands. However, unlike receptors, their cytoplasmic regions are linked to the cytoskeleton, and their ligands are not signaling molecules but structural members of the extracellular

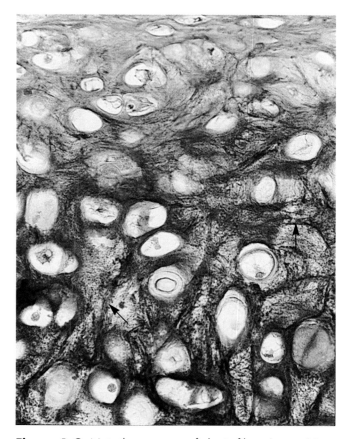

Figure 4–9. Note the presence of elastic fibers (*arrows*) in the matrix of this photomicrograph of elastic cartilage (× 270).

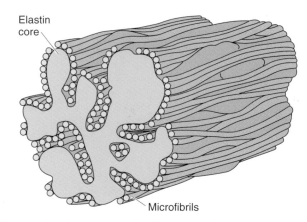

Elastin core

Microfibrils

Figure 4–10. Schematic diagram of elastic fiber. Microfibrils surround the amorphous elastin.

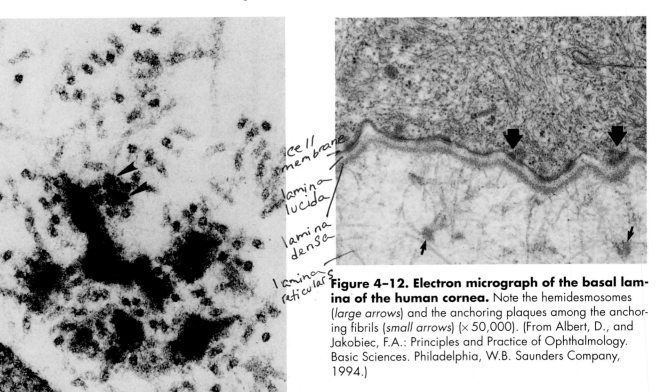

cell membrane

lamina lucida

lamina densa

lamina reticularis

Figure 4–12. Electron micrograph of the basal lamina of the human cornea. Note the hemidesmosomes (*large arrows*) and the anchoring plaques among the anchoring fibrils (*small arrows*) (× 50,000). (From Albert, D., and Jakobiec, F.A.: Principles and Practice of Ophthalmology. Basic Sciences. Philadelphia, W.B. Saunders Company, 1994.)

Figure 4–11. Electron micrograph of elastic fiber development. Note the presence of microfibrils surrounding the amorphous matrix of elastin (*arrowheads*). (From Fukuda., Y., Ferrans, V.J., and Crystal, R.G.: Development of elastic fibers of nuchal ligament, aorta, and lung of fetal and postnatal sheep: An ultrastructural and electron microscopic immunohistochemical study. Am. J. Anat. **170:**597–629, 1984. Copyright 1984. Reprinted with permission of Springer-Verlag.)

matrix such as collagen, laminin, and fibronectin. Moreover, the association between an integrin and its ligand is much weaker than that between a receptor and its ligand. Integrins are much more numerous than receptors, thus compensating for the bond weakness and also permitting the migration of cells along a surface of extracellular matrix.

Integrins are heterodimers (about 250,000 daltons) composed of α and β glycoprotein chains whose carboxyl ends are linked to talin and α-actinin of the cytoskeleton. Their amino ends possess binding sites for macromolecules of the extracellular matrix (see Fig. 2–29). Because integrins link

Figure 4–13. Schematic diagram of the basal lamina and the lamina reticularis. (Adapted from Fawcett, D.W.: Bloom and Fawcett's A Textbook of Histology, 12th ed. New York, Chapman and Hall, 1994.)

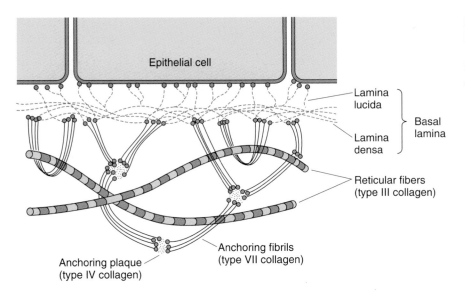

Epithelial cell

Lamina lucida

Lamina densa

Basal lamina

Reticular fibers (type III collagen)

Anchoring fibrils (type VII collagen)

Anchoring plaque (type IV collagen)

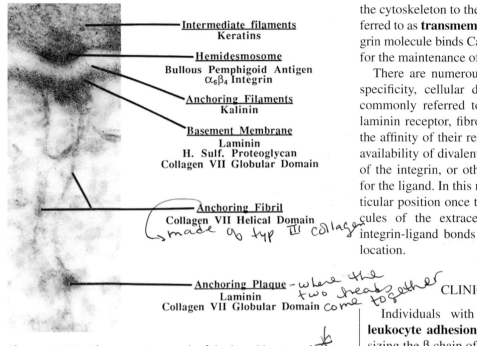

Intermediate filaments
Keratins

Hemidesmosome
Bullous Pemphigoid Antigen
$\alpha_6\beta_4$ Integrin

Anchoring Filaments
Kalinin

Basement Membrane
Laminin
H. Sulf. Proteoglycan
Collagen VII Globular Domain

Anchoring Fibril
Collagen VII Helical Domain
(→ made of typ III collagen)

Anchoring Plaque — where the two areas come together
Laminin
Collagen VII Globular Domain

Figure 4–14. Electron micrograph of the basal lamina of the corneal epithelium (× 165,000). (From Albert, D., and Jakobiec, F.A.: Principles and Practice of Ophthalmology. Basic Sciences. Philadelphia, W.B. Saunders Company, 1994.)

the cytoskeleton to the extracellular matrix, they are also referred to as **transmembrane linkers.** The α chain of the integrin molecule binds Ca^{2+} or Mg^{2+}, divalent cations necessary for the maintenance of proper binding with the ligand.

There are numerous integrins that differ in their ligand specificity, cellular distribution, and function. Some are commonly referred to as *receptors* for their ligand (e.g., laminin receptor, fibronectin receptor). Cells can modulate the affinity of their receptor for its ligand by regulating the availability of divalent cations, modifying the conformation of the integrin, or otherwise altering the integrin's affinity for the ligand. In this manner cells are not locked into a particular position once their integrins bind to the macromolecules of the extracellular matrix but can release their integrin-ligand bonds and move away from that particular location.

CLINICAL CORRELATIONS

Individuals with the autosomal recessive disorder, **leukocyte adhesion deficiency,** are incapable of synthesizing the β chain of their white blood cell integrins. Their leukocytes are incapable of adhering to the endothelial cells of blood vessels and thus cannot migrate to the site of inflammation. Individuals with this disease have difficulties in fighting bacterial infections.

Epithelium and Glands

5

The approximately 200 distinctly different types of cells composing the human body are arranged and cooperatively organized into four basic **tissues.** Groups of these tissues are assembled in various organizational and functional arrangements into **organs,** which carry out functions of the body. The four basic tissue types are **epithelium, connective tissue, muscle,** and **nervous tissue.** This and the next few chapters will discuss each of these tissues and the cells that constitute them.

Epithelial Tissue

Epithelial tissue is present in two forms: (1) as sheets of contiguous cells—**epithelia**—that cover the body on its external surface and line the body on its internal surface, and (2) glands, which originate from invaginated epithelial cells. Epithelia are derived from all three embryonic germ layers, although most of the epithelia are derived from ectoderm and endoderm. The ectoderm gives rise to the oral and nasal mucosae, cornea, and epidermis of skin. Glands of the skin and the mammary glands are also derived from ectoderm. The liver, pancreas, and lining of the respiratory and gastrointestinal tract are derived from the endoderm. The uriniferous tubules of the kidney, the lining of the male and female reproductive systems, the endothelial lining of the circulatory system, and the mesothelium of the body cavities develop from the mesodermal germ layer.

Epithelial tissues have numerous functions:

- **Protection** of underlying tissues of the body from abrasion and injury
- **Transcellular transport** of molecules across epithelial layers
- **Secretion** of mucus, hormones, enzymes, etc., from various glands
- **Absorption** of material from a lumen (e.g., intestinal tract or certain kidney tubules)
- Control of movement of materials between body compartments via **selective permeability** of intercellular junctions between epithelial cells
- Detection of **sensations** via taste buds, retina of eye, and specialized hair cells in the ear

Epithelium

The sheet of contiguous cells in the epithelium are tightly bound together by junctional complexes. Epithelia display little intercellular space and little extracellular matrix. They are separated from the underlying connective tissue by an extracellular matrix, the basal lamina, synthesized by the epithelial cells. Because epithelium is avascular, the adjacent supporting connective tissue through its capillary beds supplies nourishment and oxygen via diffusion through the basal lamina.

Classification of Epithelial Membranes

Epithelial membranes are classified according to the number of cell layers between the basal lamina and the free surface and by the morphology of the epithelial cells (Table 5–1). If the membrane is composed of a single layer of cells it is called **simple epithelium;** if it is composed of more than one cell layer it is called **stratified epithelium** (Fig. 5–1). The morphology of the cells may be squamous (flat), cuboidal, or columnar when viewed in sections taken perpendicular to the basement membrane. Stratified epithelia are classified by the morphology of the cells in their superficial layer only. In addition to these two major classes of epithelia, which are further identified by cellular morphology, there are two other distinct types: pseudostratified epithelium and transitional epithelium (see Fig. 5–1).

Simple Squamous Epithelium

This epithelium is composed of a single layer of tightly packed, thin, or low-profile polygonal cells. When viewed

Table 5–1. Classification of Epithelia

Type	Shape of Surface Cells	Sample Locations	Functions
Simple			
Simple squamous	Flattened	*Lining:* pulmonary alveoli, loop of Henle, parietal layer of Bowman's capsule, inner and middle ear, blood and lymphatic vessels, pleural and peritoneal cavities	Limiting membrane, fluid transport, gaseous exchange, lubrication, reducing friction (thus aiding movement of viscera), lining membrane
Simple cuboidal	Cuboidal	Ducts of many glands, covering of ovary, form kidney tubules	Secretion, absorption, protection
Simple columnar	Columnar	*Lining:* paranasal sinuses, oviducts, ductuli efferentes of testis, uterus, small bronchi, much of digestive tract, gall bladder, and large ducts of some glands	Transportation, absorption, secretion, protection
Pseudostratified	All cells rest on basal lamina but not all reach epithelial surface; surface cells are columnar	*Lining:* most of trachea, primary bronchi, epididymis and ductus deferens, auditory tube, part of tympanic cavity, nasal cavity, lacrimal sac, male urethra, large excretory ducts	Secretion, absorption lubrication, protection, transportation
Stratified			
Stratified squamous (nonkeratinized)	Flattened (with nuclei)	*Forms:* mouth, epiglottis, esophagus, vocal folds, vagina	Protection, secretion
Stratified squamous (keratinized) ← *no nucleus*	Flattened (without nuclei)	Epidermis of skin	Protection
Stratified cuboidal	Cuboidal	*Lining:* ducts of sweat glands	Absorption, secretion
Stratified columnar	Columnar	Conjunctiva of eye, some large excretory ducts, portions of male urethra	Secretion, absorption, protection
Transitional	Dome-shaped (relaxed), flattened (distended)	*Lining:* urinary tract from renal calyces to urethra	Protection, distensible

from the surface, the epithelial sheet looks much like a tile floor with a centrally placed bulging nucleus in each cell (Fig. 5–2A). However, viewed in section, only some cells display nuclei because the plane of section frequently does not encounter the nucleus. Simple squamous epithelia line pulmonary alveoli, compose the loop of Henle and the parietal layer of Bowman's capsule in the kidney, and form the endothelial lining of blood and lymph vessels, as well as the mesothelium of the pleural and peritoneal cavities.

Simple Cuboidal Epithelium

A single layer of polygonal-shaped cells constitute **simple cuboidal epithelia** (Fig. 5–2A). When viewed in section cut perpendicular to the surface, the cells present a square profile, with a centrally placed round nucleus. Simple cuboidal epithelia make up the ducts of many glands of the body, form the covering of the ovary, and compose some kidney tubules.

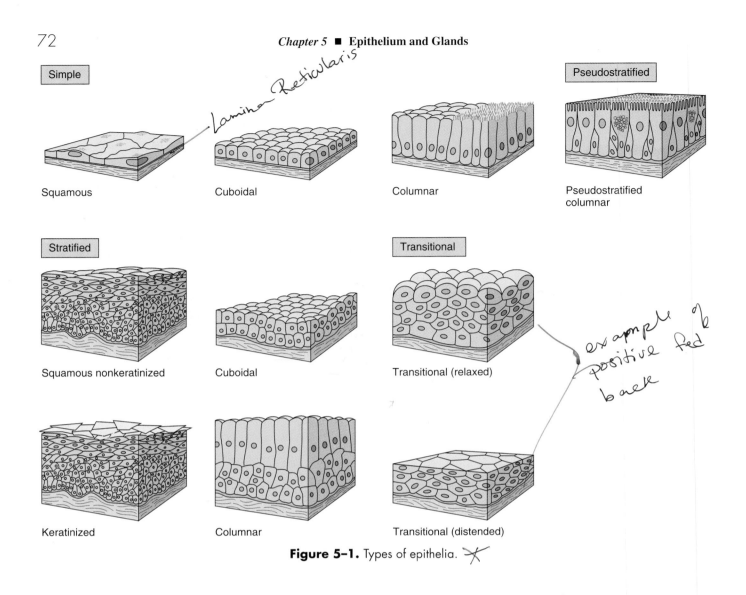

Figure 5–1. Types of epithelia.

Simple Columnar Epithelium

The cells of **simple columnar epithelium** appear much like those of simple cuboidal epithelium in a surface view, but when viewed in longitudinal section they are tall, rectangular cells whose ovoid nuclei are usually located at the same level in the basal half of the cell (Fig. 5–2B). Simple columnar epithelium is found in the lining of much of the digestive tract, gall bladder, and large ducts of glands. Simple columnar epithelium may exhibit a striated border, or **microvilli,** projecting from the apical surface of the cells. The simple columnar epithelium that lines the uterus, oviducts, ductuli efferentes, small bronchi, and paranasal sinuses is **ciliated.** In these organs, cilia project from the apical surface of the columnar cells into the lumen.

Stratified Squamous (Nonkeratinized) Epithelium

Stratified squamous (nonkeratinized) epithelium is thick; because it is composed of several layers of cells, only the

deepest layer is in contact with the basal lamina (Fig. 5–3A). The basal-most (deepest) cells of this epithelium are cuboidal in shape; those located in the middle of the epithelium are polymorphous; and the cells composing the free surface of the epithelium are flattened (squamous), hence the name stratified squamous. Because the surface cells are nucleated, this epithelium is called **nonkeratinized epithelium.** This type of epithelium is usually wet and is found lining the mouth, oral pharynx, esophagus, true vocal cords, and vagina.

Stratified Squamous (Keratinized) Epithelium

Stratified squamous (keratinized) epithelium is similar to stratified squamous (nonkeratinized) epithelium except that the superficial layers of the epithelium are composed of dead cells whose nuclei and the cytoplasm has been replaced with **keratin** (Fig. 5–3B). This epithelium constitutes the epidermis of skin, a tough layer that resists friction and is impermeable to water.

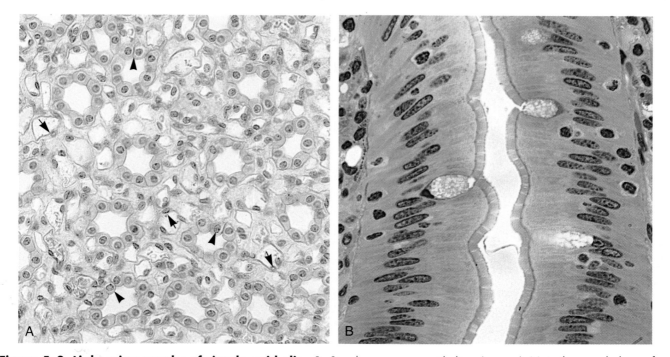

Figure 5–2. Light micrographs of simple epithelia. A, Simple squamous epithelium (*arrows*). Note the morphology of the cells and their nuclei. Simple cuboidal epithelium (*arrowheads*). Note the round, centrally placed nuclei (× 270). **B,** Simple columnar epithelium. Observe the oblong nuclei and the striated border (× 540).

Stratified Cuboidal Epithelium

Stratified cuboidal epithelium, which contains only two layers of cuboidal cells, lines the ducts of sweat glands (Fig. 5–3*C*).

Stratified Columnar Epithelium

Stratified columnar epithelium is composed of a low polyhedral to cuboidal deeper layer in contact with the basal lamina and a superficial layer of columnar cells. This epithelium is found only in a few places in the body—the conjunctiva of the eye, some large excretory ducts, and regions of the male urethra.

Transitional Epithelium

Transitional epithelium received its name because it was erroneously believed to be in transition between stratified columnar and stratified squamous epithelia. This epithelium is now known to be a distinct type located exclusively in the urinary system, where it lines the urinary tract from the renal calyces to the urethra. Transitional epithelium is composed of many layers of cells: those located basally are either low columnar or cuboidal cells. Polyhedral cells compose several layers above the basal cells. The most superficial cells of the empty bladder are large, are occasionally binucleated, and exhibit rounded dome tops that bulge

into the lumen (Fig. 5–3*D*). These dome-shaped cells become flattened and the epithelium becomes thinner when the bladder is distended.

Pseudostratified Columnar Epithelium

As the name implies, **pseudostratified columnar epithelium** appears to be stratified but is really composed of a single layer of cells. All of the cells in pseudostratified columnar epithelium are in contact with the basal lamina, but only some cells reach the surface of the epithelium (Fig. 5–4). Cells not extending to the surface usually have a broad base and become narrow at their apical end. Taller cells reach the surface and possess a narrow base in contact with the basal lamina and a broadened apical surface. Because the cells of this epithelium are of different heights, their nuclei are located at different levels, giving the impression of a stratified epithelium even though it is composed of a single layer of cells. Pseudostratified columnar epithelium is found in the male urethra, epididymis, and larger excretory ducts of glands.

The most widespread type of pseudostratified columnar epithelium is **ciliated,** possessing cilia on the apical surface of those cells that reach the epithelial surface. Pseudostratified ciliated columnar epithelium is found lining most of the trachea and primary bronchi, the auditory tube, part of the tympanic cavity, the nasal cavity, and the lacrimal sac.

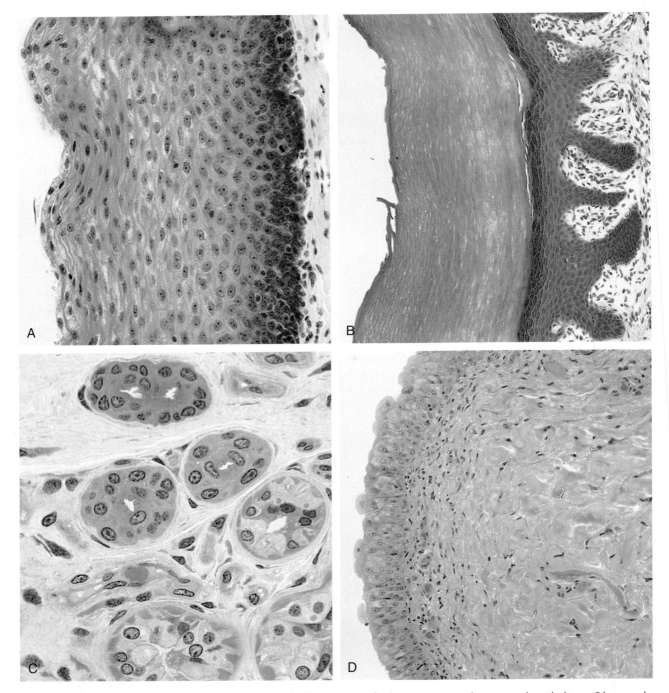

Figure 5–3. Light micrographs of stratified epithelia. A, Stratified squamous nonkeratinized epithelium. Observe the many layers of cells and flattened (squamous), nucleated cells in the top layer (× 540). **B,** Stratified squamous keratinized epithelium (× 132). **C,** Stratified cuboidal epithelium of the duct of a sweat gland (× 540). **D,** Transitional epithelium. Observe that the surface cells facing the lumen of the bladder are dome-shaped, which characterizes transitional epithelium (× 132).

Polarity and Cell-Surface Specializations

Most epithelial cells have distinct morphological, biochemical, and functional domains and thus commonly display a polarity that may be related to one or all of these differences. Such polarized cells, for instance, possess an **apical domain**

that faces a lumen and a **basolateral domain** whose basal component is in contact with the basal lamina. Because these regions are distinct functionally, each may possess surface modifications and specializations related to that function. For example, the apical surfaces of many epithelial cells possess microvilli or cilia, whereas their basolateral regions may exhibit many types of junctional specializations and intercellular interdigitations. The apical and basolateral domains are separated from each other by tight junctions that encircle the apical aspect of the cell.

Apical Domain

The **apical domain,** the region of the epithelial cell facing the lumen, is rich in ion channels, carrier proteins, H$^+$ ATPase, glycoproteins, and hydrolytic enzymes; it also is the site where regulated secretory products are delivered for release. Several surface modifications are necessary for the apical domain of an epithelium to carry out its many functions. These include microvilli with associated glycocalyx and, in some cases, stereocilia, cilia, and flagella.

MICROVILLI. When observed by electron microscopy, absorptive columnar epithelial cells exhibit closely packed **microvilli,** which are cylindrical, membrane-bound projections of the cytoplasm emanating from the apical (luminal) surface of these cells (Fig. 5–5). Microvilli represent the **striated border** of the intestinal absorptive cells and the **brush border** of the kidney proximal tubule cells observed by light microscopy.

In less active cells, microvilli may be sparse and short, but in intestinal epithelia, where major function is transport and absorption, they are crowded and 1 to 2 μm in length, thus greatly increasing the surface area of the cells. Each microvillus contains a core of 25 to 30 **actin filaments,** cross-linked by **villin,** attached to an amorphous region at its tip and extending into the cytoplasm, where the actin filaments are embedded into the **terminal web,** a complex of **actin** and **spectrin** molecules as well as intermediate filaments lo-

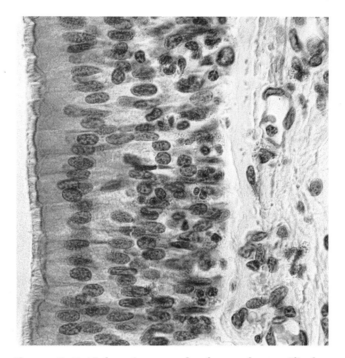

Figure 5–4. Light micrograph of pseudostratified epithelia. This type of epithelium appears to be stratified; however, all of the epithelial cells in this figure stand on the basal lamina (× 540).

cated at the cortex of the epithelial cells (Figs. 5–6, 5–7, 5–8). At regular intervals **myosin-I** and **calmodulin** connect the actin filaments to the plasma membrane of the microvillus, giving it support. It should be noted that epithelia not functioning in absorption or transport may exhibit microvilli without cores of actin filaments.

Figure 5–5. Electron micrograph of microvilli of epithelial cells from the small intestine (× 2800). (From Hopkins, C.R.: Structure and Function of Cells. Philadelphia, W.B. Saunders Company, 1978.)

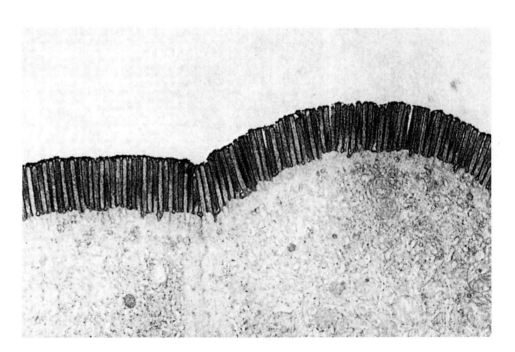

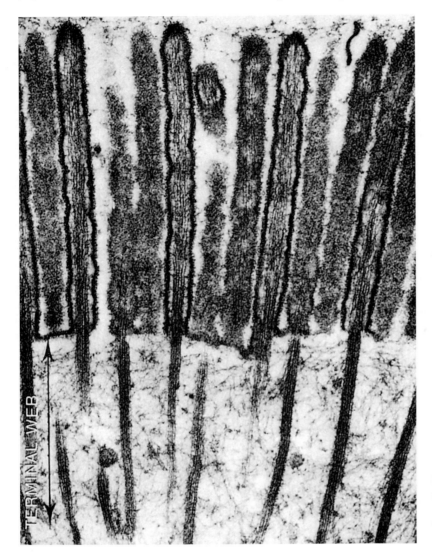

Figure 5-6. High-magnification electron micrograph of microvilli (× 60,800).
(From Hopkins, C.R.: Structure and Function of Cells. Philadelphia, W.B. Saunders Company, 1978.)

Light microscopy of epithelia stained for carbohydrates reveals the **glycocalyx,** evident in electron micrographs as an amorphous fuzzy coating over the luminal surface of the microvilli. The glycocalyx represents carbohydrate residues attached to the transmembrane proteins of the plasmalemma. These glycoproteins function in protection and cell recognition as discussed in Chapter 2.

Stereocilia are long microvilli found only in the epididymis and on the sensory hair cells of the cochlea (inner ear). They should not be confused with cilia. It is believed that these nonmotile structures are unusually rigid because of their core of actin filaments. In the epididymis they probably function in increasing the surface area, whereas in the hair cells of the ear they function in signal generation.

CILIA. Cilia are motile, hair-like projections with a diameter of 0.2 μm and a length of 7 to 10 μm emanating from the surface of certain epithelial cells. In the ciliated epithelia of the respiratory system (e.g., trachea and bronchi) and in the oviduct, there may be hundreds of cilia in orderly arrays on the luminal surface of the cells. However, other epithelial cells, such as the hair cells of the vestibular apparatus in the inner ear, possess only a single cilium, which functions in a sensory mechanism.

Cilia are specialized to function in propelling mucus and other substances over the surface of the epithelium via rapid rhythmic oscillations. Cilia of the respiratory tree, for example, move mucus and debris toward the oropharynx, where it may be swallowed or expectorated. Cilia of the oviduct move the fertilized ovum toward the uterus.

Electron microscopy reveals that cilia possess a specific internal structure that is consistently conserved throughout the plant and animal kingdoms (Figs. 5–9, 5–10). The core of the cilium contains a complex of uniformly arranged microtubules called the **axoneme.** The axoneme is composed of a constant number of longitudinal microtubules arranged in a consistent 9 + 2 organization (see Fig. 5–10B). Two centrally placed microtubules **(singlets)** are evenly surrounded

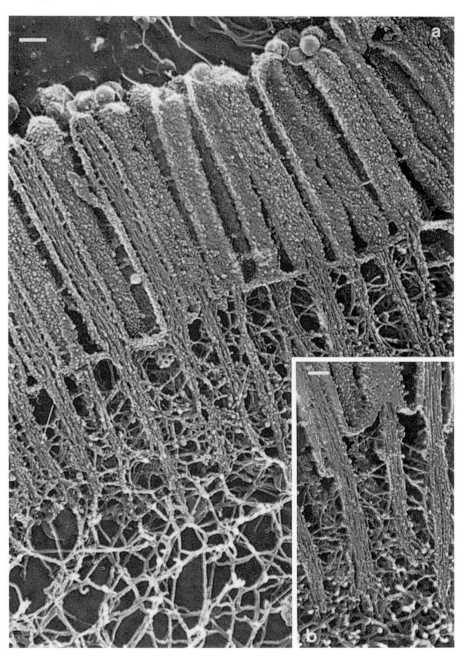

Figure 5–7. Electron micrograph of the terminal web and microvillus. Observe that the actin filaments of the microvilli are attached to the terminal web (× 97,000, inset × 77,000). (From Hirokana, N., Tilney, L.G., Fujiwara, K., and Heuser, J.E.: Organization of actin, myosin, and intermediate filaments in the brush border of intestinal epithelial cells. J. Cell Biol. **94:**425–443, 1982. Reproduced with the permission of The Rockefeller University Press.)

by nine **doublets** of microtubules. The two microtubules located in the center of the core are separated from each other, each displaying a circular profile in cross-section, composed of 13 protofilaments. Each of the nine doublets is composed of two subunits. In cross-section, **subunit A** is a microtubule composed of 13 protofilaments, exhibiting a circular profile. **Subunit B** possesses 10 protofilaments, exhibits an incomplete circular profile in cross-section, and shares three protofilaments of subunit A.

Several elastic protein complexes are associated with the axoneme. **Radial spokes** project from subunit A of each doublet inward toward the **central sheath** surrounding the two singlets. Neighboring doublets are connected by **nexin**

extending from subunit A of one doublet to subunit B of the adjacent doublet (see Fig. 5–9).

The microtubule-associated protein, **dynein,** which has ATPase activity, radiates from subunit A of one doublet toward subunit B of the neighboring doublet. These dynein arms are arranged at 24-nm intervals along the length of subunit A. Dynein ATPase, by hydrolyzing ATP, provides the energy for the ciliary bending. Movement of the cilia is initiated by the dynein arms transiently attaching to specific sites on the protofilaments of the adjacent doublets, sliding them toward the tip of the cilium. However, nexin, an elastic protein extending between adjacent doublets, restrains this action to some degree, translating the sliding movement into

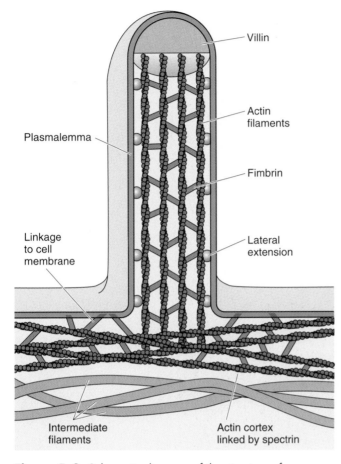

Figure 5–8. Schematic diagram of the structure of a microvillus.

a bending motion. As the cilium bends, an energy-requiring process, the elastic protein complex is stretched. When the dynein arms release their hold on the B subunit, the elastic protein complex returns to its original length, snapping the cilium back to its straight position (which does not require energy), effecting movement of material at the tip of the cilium.

The 9 + 2 microtubule arrangement within the axoneme continues throughout most of the length of the cilium except at its base, where it is attached to the **basal body** (see Fig. 5–9). The morphology of the basal body is similar to that of a centriole, in that it is composed of nine triplets and no singlets.

Basal bodies develop from **procentriole organizers.** As tubulin dimers are added, the procentriole lengthens to form the nine triplet microtubules characteristic of the basal body. After formation, the basal body migrates to the apical plasmalemma and gives rise to a cilium. Nine doublet microtubules develop from the nine triplets of the basal body, and a single pair of microtubules form to give the cilium its characteristic 9 + 2 microtubule arrangement.

FLAGELLA. The only cells in the human body that possess **flagella** are the spermatozoa. The structure of flagella is discussed in Chapter 21 on the male reproductive system.

Basolateral Domain

The **basolateral domain** may be subdivided into two regions: the lateral plasma membrane and the basal plasma membrane. Each region possesses its own junctional specializations and receptors for hormones and neurotransmitters. Additionally, these regions are rich in Na+-K+ ATPase and ion channels and are sites for constitutive secretion.

Lateral Membrane Specializations

Light microscopy reveals zones, called **terminal bars,** where epithelial cells contact and presumably attach to each other. Especially notable in the apical region of the simple columnar epithelium lining the gut, terminal bars once were thought to be composed of an amorphous intercellular ce-

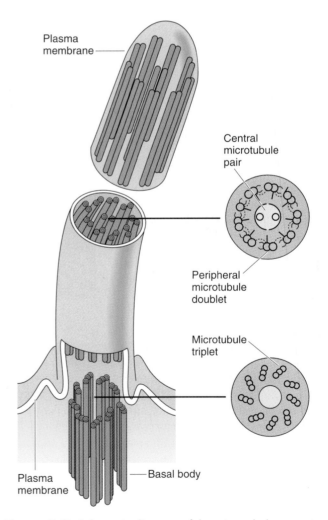

Figure 5–9. Schematic diagram of the microtubular arrangement of the axoneme in the cilium.

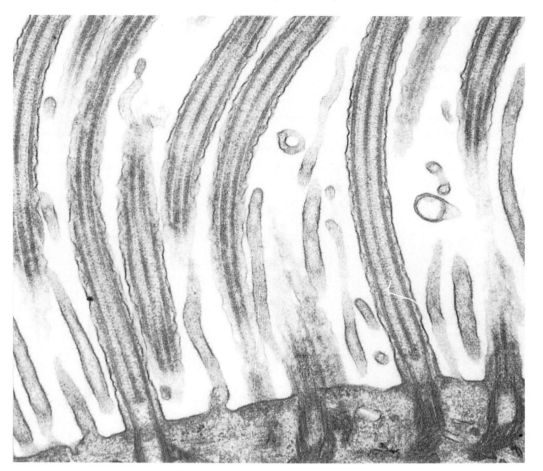

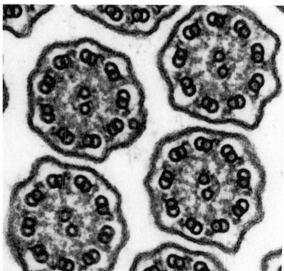

Figure 5–10. Electron micrographs of cilia. A, Longitudinal section of cilia (× 36,000). **B,** Cross-sectional view demonstrating microtubular arrangement in cilia (× 88,000). (From Leeson, T.S., Leeson, C.R., Paparo, A.A.: Text/Atlas of Histology. Philadelphia, W.B. Saunders Company, 1988.)

ment substance. Horizontal sections through the terminal bars demonstrated them to be continuous around the entire circumference of each cell, indicating that these cells were attached to every adjacent cell. Electron microscopy has revealed that terminal bars are in fact composed of complex **junctional complexes.** These complexes, which hold con-

tiguous epithelial cells together, may be classified into three types, schematically depicted in Figure 5–11:

• **Occluding junctions** function in joining cells to form an impermeable barrier, preventing material from taking an intercellular route in passing across the epithelial sheath

- **Anchoring junctions** function in maintaining cell-to-cell or cell-to–basal lamina adherence
- **Communicating junctions** function in permitting movement of ions or signaling molecules between cells, thus coupling adjacent cells both electrically and metabolically

ZONULAE OCCLUDENTES. Also known as **tight junctions, zonulae occludentes** are located between adjacent plasma membranes and are the most apically located junction between the cells of the epithelia. They form a "belt-like" junction that encircles the entire circumference

of the cell. In electron micrographs, the adjoining cell membranes approximate each other; their outer leaflets fuse, then diverge, then fuse again several times within a distance of 0.1 to 0.3 μm (Fig. 5–12). At the fusion sites, thin strands of **transmembrane junctional proteins** of the two membranes bond to each other, thus forming a seal occluding the intercellular space. Freeze-fracture analysis of cell membranes at the zonulae occludentes displays a **"quilted" appearance** of anastomosing strands of transmembrane proteins on the P face and a corresponding network of grooves on the E face (Fig. 5–13).

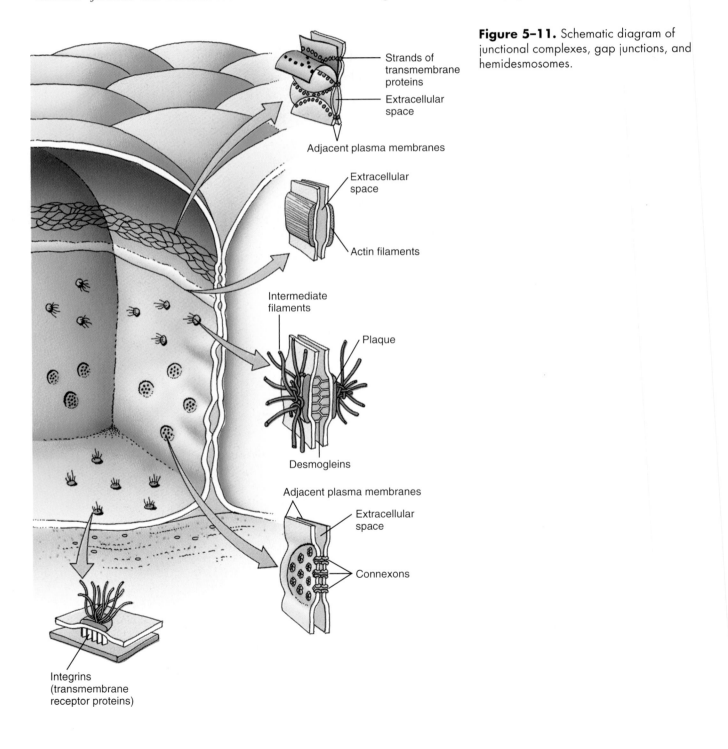

Figure 5–11. Schematic diagram of junctional complexes, gap junctions, and hemidesmosomes.

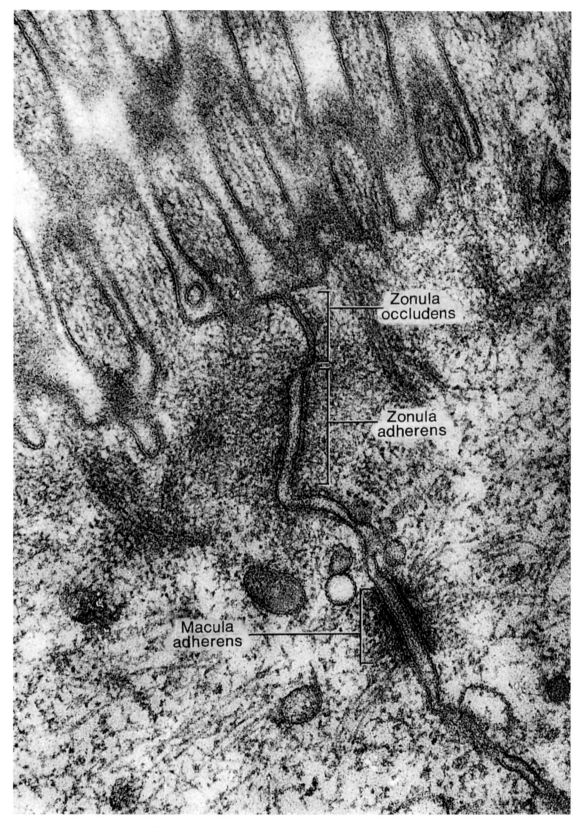

Figure 5–12. Electron micrograph of the junctional complex. (From Fawcett, D.W.: The Cell. 2nd ed. Philadelphia, W.B. Saunders Company, 1981.)

Tight junctions function in two ways: (1) to prevent the movement of membrane proteins from the apical domain to the basolateral domain, and (2) to fuse plasma membranes of adjacent cells to prohibit water-soluble molecules from passing between cells. Depending on the numbers and patterns of the strands in the zonula, some tight junctions are said to be tight, whereas others are "leaky." These terms reflect the efficiency of the cells in maintaining the integrity of the epithelial barrier between two adjacent body compartments.

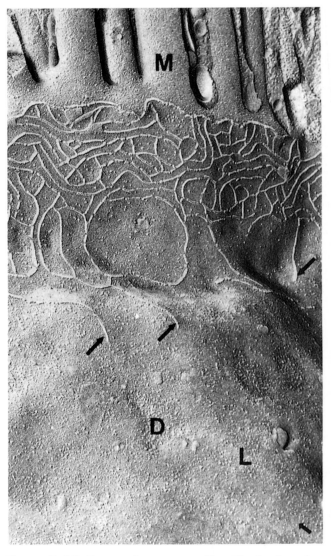

Figure 5–13. Freeze fracture replica displaying the tight junction (zonula occludens) in guinea pig small intestine. Note that the P face of the microvillar membrane (M) possesses fewer intramembrane particles than the P face of the lateral cell membrane (L). The *arrows* point to free terminal ridge-shaped protrusions. A desmosome is shown (D) (× 60,000). (From Trier, J.S., Allan, C.H., Marcial, M.A., and Madara, J.L.: Structural features of the apical and tubulovesicular membranes of rodent small intestinal tuft cells. Anat. Rec. **219:**69–77, 1987. Copyright © 1987. Reprinted by permission of John Wiley & Sons, Inc.)

ZONULAE ADHERENTES. Zonulae adherentes of the junctional complex are located just basal to the zonulae occludentes and also encircle the cell. The intercellular space of 15 to 20 nm between the outer leaflets of the two adjacent cell membranes is occupied by the extracellular moieties of **cadherins** (see Fig. 5–12). These Ca^+-dependent integral proteins of the cell membrane are **transmembrane linker proteins.** Their intracytoplasmic aspect binds to a specialized region of the cell web, specifically a bundle of actin filaments that run parallel to and along the cytoplasmic aspect of the cell membrane. The actin filaments are attached to each other and to the cell membrane by **vinculin** and **α-actinin.** The extracellular region of the cadherins of one cell forms bonds with those of the adjoining cell participating in the formation of the zonula adherens. This junction then not only joins the cell membranes to each other but also links the cytoskeleton of the two cells via the transmembrane linker proteins.

Fascia adherens is similar to zonula adherens, except that it does not go around the entire circumference of the cell. Instead of being belt-like, it is "ribbon-like." Cardiac muscle cells, for example, are attached to each other at their longitudinal terminals via the fascia adherens.

DESMOSOMES (MACULAE ADHERENTES). Desmosomes are the last of the three components of the junctional complex. These "spot weld–like" junctions also appear to be randomly distributed along the lateral cell membranes of simple epithelia and throughout the cell membranes of stratified squamous epithelia, especially in the epidermis.

Disk-shaped **attachment plaques** (about $400 \times 250 \times 10$ nm) are located opposite each other on the cytoplasmic aspects of the plasma membranes of adjacent epithelial cells (Fig. 5–14). Each plaque is composed of a series of attachment proteins, the best characterized of which are **desmoplakins** and **pakoglobins.**

Intermediate filaments of cytokeratin are observed to insert into the plaque, where they make a hairpin turn, then extend back out into the cytoplasm. These filaments are thought to be responsible for dispersing the shearing forces on the cell.

In the region of the opposing attachment plaques, the intercellular space measures up to 30 nm in width and contains filamentous materials with a thin, dense, vertical line located in the middle of the intercellular space. High-resolution electron microscopy reveals the filamentous material to be **desmoglein,** the extracellular components of the Ca^{2+}-dependent **transmembrane linker proteins** of the cadherin family. In the presence of Ca^{2+}, they bond with transmembrane linker proteins from the adjoining cell. In the presence of a calcium-chelating agent, the desmosomes will break into two halves, and the cells will separate. Thus, it should be noted that two cells are required for the formation of a desmosome. The cytoplasmic aspect of the transmembrane linker proteins bind to the desmoplakins and pakoglobins constituting the plaque.

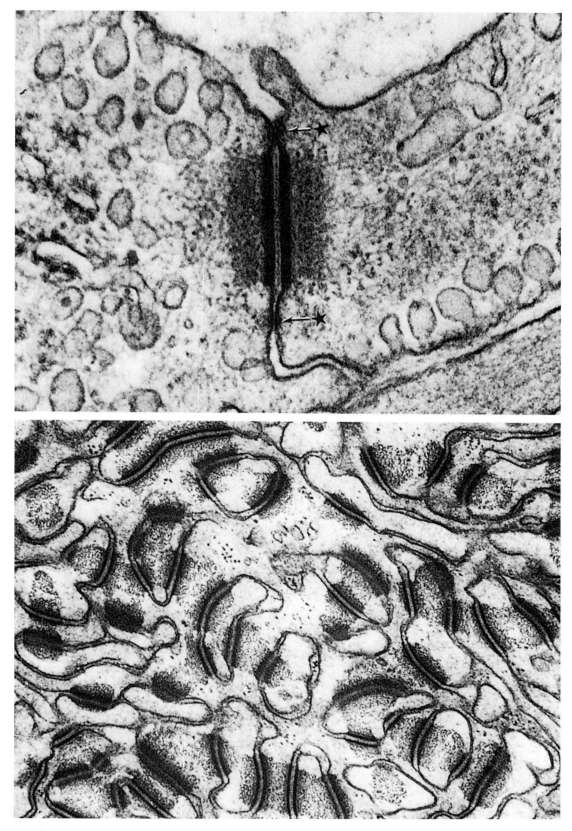

Figure 5–14. Electron micrograph of a desmosome. Observe the dense accumulation of intracellular intermediate filaments inserting into the plaque of each cell. (From Fawcett, D.W.: The Cell. 2nd ed. Philadelphia, W.B. Saunders Company, 1981.)

CLINICAL CORRELATIONS

Some persons produce autoantibodies against desmosomal proteins, especially those in the skin, producing a skin disease called **pemphigus vulgaris.** Binding of the autoantibodies to desmosomal proteins disrupts cell adhesion, resulting in widespread blistering and consequent loss of tissue fluids; if untreated, this condition leads to death. Treatment with systemic steroids and immunosuppressive agents usually controls the condition.

GAP JUNCTIONS. Gap junctions, also called **nexus** or **communicating junctions,** are widespread in epithelial tissues throughout the body as well as in cardiac muscle cells, smooth muscle cells, and neurons.

Gap junctions differ from the occluding and anchoring junctions just described in that they mediate intercellular communication by permitting the passage of ions and small molecules between adjacent cells. The intercellular cleft at the gap junction is narrow and constant at about 2 to 3 nm. Gap junctions are built by six closely packed transmembrane proteins (**connexins**) that form structures called **connexons,** aqueous pores through the plasma membrane and extending into the intercellular space (Fig. 5–15). When a connexon of one plasma membrane is in register with its counterpart from an adjacent plasma membrane, each connexon will jut out of the plasma membrane about 1.5 nm into the intercellular space. The two connexons fuse, forming the functional intercellular communication channel. With a diameter of 1.5 to 2.0 nm, the hydrophilic channel permits the passage of ions, amino acids, cyclic AMP, and some hormones.

It should be noted, however, that gap junctions are regulated, so they may be opened or closed. Although the opening and closing mechanism is not understood, it has been shown experimentally that a decrease in cytosolic pH or an increase in cytosolic Ca^{2+} concentrations closes channels. Conversely, high pH or low Ca^{2+} concentration opens the channels. Additionally, different gap junctions have different properties with diverse channel permeabilities in different cells. Gap junctions are important during embryogenesis in coupling the cells of the developing embryo electrically and in distributing informational molecules throughout the migrating cell masses.

Basal Surface Specializations

Three important features mark the basal surface of epithelia: the basal lamina, plasma membrane enfoldings, and hemidesmosomes, which anchor the basal plasma membrane to the basal lamina. An extracellular supporting struc-

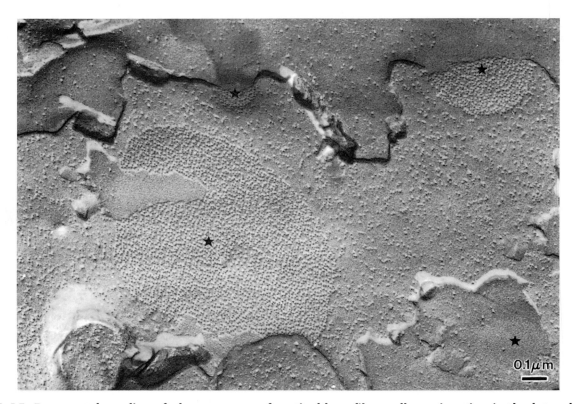

Figure 5–15. Freeze etch replica of ultrastructure of cortical lens fiber cell gap junction in the lateral cell membrane. The *stars* indicate the presence of closely packed transmembrane proteins (connexons) of the gap junction. (From Albert, D.M., and Jakobiec, F.A.: Principles and Practice of Ophthalmology. Philadelphia, W.B. Saunders Company, 1994.)

ture secreted by an epithelium, the **basal lamina** is located at the boundary between the epithelium and the underlying connective tissue. The structure and appearance of the basal lamina are covered in Chapter 4.

PLASMA MEMBRANE ENFOLDINGS. The basal surface of some epithelia, especially those involved in ion transport, possesses multiple enfoldings of the basal plasma membranes. These enfoldings, which increase the surface area of the plasma membrane, partition the basal cytoplasm and many mitochondria into the finger-like enfoldings. The mitochondria provide the energy required for active transport of ions in establishing osmotic gradients to ensure the movement of water across the epithelium, such as those of the kidney tubules. The compactness of the infolded plasma membranes coupled with the arrangement of the mitochondria within the enfoldings give a striated appearance when viewed with the light microscope—thus the origin of the term **striated ducts** for certain duct cells of the pancreas and salivary glands.

HEMIDESMOSOMES. Hemidesmosomes resemble half desmosomes and serve to attach the basal cell membrane to the basal lamina (Fig. 5–16). **Attachment plaques** composed of desmoplakins and other associated proteins are present on the cytoplasmic aspect of the plasma membrane. **Keratin tonofilaments** insert into these plaques, unlike those in the desmosome, where the filaments enter the plaque, then make a sharp turn to exit it. The cytoplasmic aspects of **transmembrane linker proteins** are attached to the plaque, whereas their extracellular moieties bind to **laminin** and **type**

IV collagen of the basal lamina. The transmembrane linker proteins of hemidesmosomes are **integrins,** a family of extracellular matrix receptors, whereas those of desmosomes belong to the cadherin family of cell-to-cell adhesion proteins.

Renewal of Epithelial Cells

Cells making up the epithelial tissues generally exhibit a high turnover rate, which is related to their location and function. The time frame for cell renewal remains constant for a particular epithelium. Cells of the epidermis, for example, are constantly being renewed at the basal layer by cell division. From here the cells begin their migration from the germinal layer to the surface, being keratinized on their route until they reach the surface, die, and are sloughed, the total event taking approximately 28 days. Other epithelial cells are renewed in less time. Cells lining the small intestine are replaced every 4 to 6 days by regenerative cells in the base of the crypts. The new cells then migrate to the tips of the villi, die, and are sloughed. Still other epithelia, for example, are renewed periodically until adulthood is reached, then the cell population remains for life. However, even in this instance, when a large number of cells are lost because of injury or acute toxic destruction, cell proliferation is triggered and the cell population is restored.

CLINICAL CORRELATIONS

Each epithelium within the body has its own unique characteristics, location, cell morphology, etc., all of

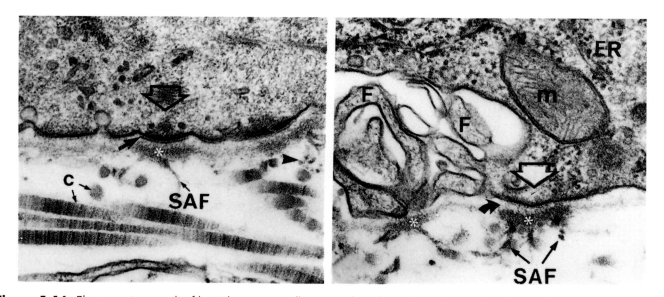

Figure 5-16. Electron micrograph of hemidesmosomes illustrating the relationship of striated anchoring fibers (SAF), composed of type VII collagen, with the lamina densa and type III collagen of the lamina reticularis; Collagen fibers (C); rough endoplasmic reticulum (ER); cell extensions (F); open *arrowheads* indicate the cytoplasmic aspect of hemidesmosomes. (From Clermont, Y., Xia, L., Turner, J.D., and Hermo, L.: Striated anchoring fibrils—anchoring plaque complexes and their relation to hemidesmosomes of myoepithelial and secretory cells in mammary glands of lactating rats. Anat. Rec. **237:**318–325, 1993. Copyright 1993. Reprinted by permission of John Wiley & Sons, Inc.)

which are related to function. In certain pathological conditions the cell population of an epithelium may undergo **metaplasia,** transforming it into another epithelial type.

Pseudostratified ciliated columnar epithelium of the bronchi of heavy smokers may undergo **squamous metaplasia,** transforming it into stratified squamous epithelium. This change impairs function, but the process may be reversed when the pathological insult is removed.

Tumors that arise from epithelial cells may be **benign** (nonmalignant) or **malignant.** Malignant tumors arising from epithelia are called **carcinomas;** those arising from glandular epithelial cells are called **adenocarcinomas.**

Glands

Glands originate from epithelial cells that leave the surface from where they developed and penetrate into the underlying connective tissue, manufacturing a basal lamina around themselves. The secretory units, along with their ducts, are the **parenchyma** of the gland; the **stroma** of the gland represents the elements of the connective tissue that invade and support the parenchyma.

Glandular epithelia manufacture their product intracellularly by synthesis of macromolecules that are usually packaged and stored in vesicles called **secretory granules.** The secretory product may be a polypeptide hormone (e.g., from the pituitary gland); a waxy substance (e.g., from the ceruminous glands of the ear canal); mucin (e.g., from the goblet cells); or a combination of protein, lipid, and carbohydrates (e.g., from the mammary glands). Other glands such as the sweat glands secrete little beside the exudate they receive from the bloodstream. Additionally, striated ducts—for example, those of the major salivary glands—act as ion pumps that modify the substances produced by the secretory units.

Glands fall into two major groups based on the method of distribution of their secretory products. **Exocrine glands** secrete their products via ducts onto the external or internal epithelial surface from which they originated. **Endocrine glands** are **ductless,** having lost their connections to the originating epithelium, and thus secrete their products into the blood or lymphatic vessels for distribution. Many cell types secrete signaling molecules called **cytokines** that perform the function of cell-to-cell communication. Cytokines are released by **signaling cells** and act on **target cells** possessing receptors for the specific signaling molecule. (Hormone signaling is detailed in Chapter 2.)

Depending on the distance the cytokine must travel to reach its target cell, its effect is referred to as **autocrine, paracrine,** or **endocrine:**

- **Autocrine:** the signaling cell is its own target, so the cell stimulates itself
- **Paracrine:** the target cell is located in the vicinity of the signaling cell, so the cytokine does not have to enter the vascular system

- **Endocrine:** the target cell and signaling cell are far from each other, so the cytokine has to be transported either by the blood or by the lymph vascular system

Glands that secrete their products via a **constitutive secretory pathway** do so continuously, releasing their secretory products immediately without storage and without requiring a prompt by signaling molecules. Glands that exhibit a **regulated secretory pathway** concentrate and store their secretory products until the proper signaling molecule for its release is received (see Chapter 2, Figs. 2–18, 2–19).

Exocrine Glands

Exocrine glands are classified according to the nature of their secretion, their mode of secretion and the number of cells (unicellular or multicellular). Many exocrine glands in the digestive, respiratory, and urogenital systems secrete substances that are described as mucous, serous, or mixed (both) types. **Mucous glands** secrete **mucinogens,** large glycosylated proteins that, upon hydration, swell to become a thick, viscous, gel-like protective lubricant known as **mucin,** a major component of **mucus.** Examples of mucous glands include goblet cells and the minor salivary glands of the tongue and palate. **Serous glands,** such as the pancreas, secrete an enzyme-rich watery fluid. **Mixed glands** contain acini (secretory units) that produce mucous secretions as well as acini that produce serous secretions; in addition, some of their mucous acini possess **serous demilunes,** a group of cells that secrete a serous fluid. The sublingual and submandibular glands are examples of mixed glands (Fig. 5–17).

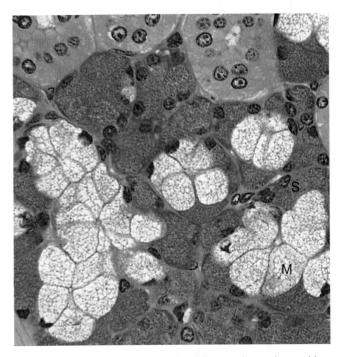

Figure 5–17. Light micrograph of the monkey submandibular gland; mucous acini (M); serous demilunes (S) (× 540).

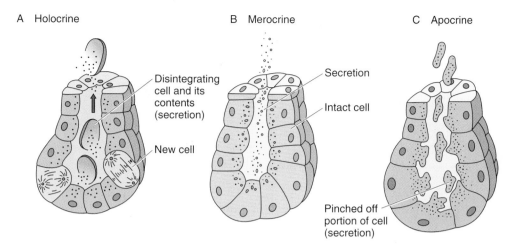

A Holocrine   B Merocrine   C Apocrine

Disintegrating cell and its contents (secretion)

New cell

Secretion

Intact cell

Pinched off portion of cell (secretion)

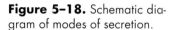

Figure 5–18. Schematic diagram of modes of secretion.

Cells of exocrine glands exhibit three different mechanisms for releasing their secretory products: **merocrine, apocrine,** and **holocrine** (Fig. 5–18). The release of the secretory product of **merocrine glands** (e.g., parotid gland) occurs via exocytosis, so neither cell membrane nor cytoplasm becomes a part of the secretion. Although many investigators question the existence of the apocrine mode of secretion, historically it was believed that in **apocrine glands** (e.g., lactating mammary gland), a small portion of the apical cytoplasm is released along with the secretory product. In **holocrine glands** (e.g., sebaceous gland), as a secretory cell matures, it dies and becomes the secretory product.

Unicellular Exocrine Glands

Unicellular exocrine glands, represented by isolated secretory cells in an epithelium, are the simplest form of exocrine gland. The primary example is **goblet cells,** which are dispersed individually in the epithelia lining the digestive tract and portions of the respiratory tract (Figs. 5–19, 5–20). The secretions released by these mucous glands protect the linings of these tracts. Goblet cells derive their name from their

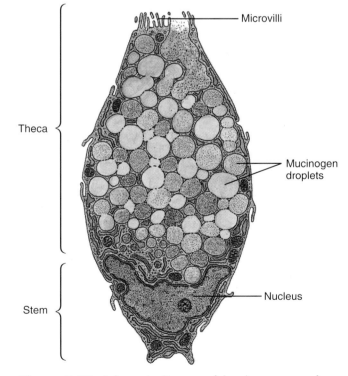

Microvilli

Theca

Mucinogen droplets

Nucleus

Stem

Figure 5–20. Schematic diagram of the ultrastructure of a goblet cell illustrating the tightly packed secretory granules of the theca. (From Lentz, T.L.: Cell Fine Structure. An Atlas of Drawings of Whole-Cell Structure. Philadelphia, W.B. Saunders Company, 1971.)

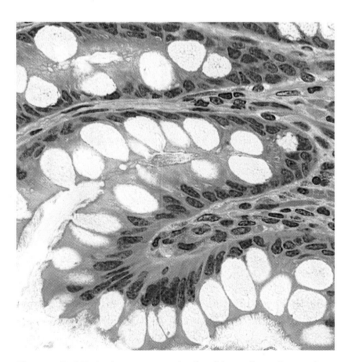

Figure 5-19. Light micrograph of goblet cells in the epithelial lining of the monkey ileum (× 540).

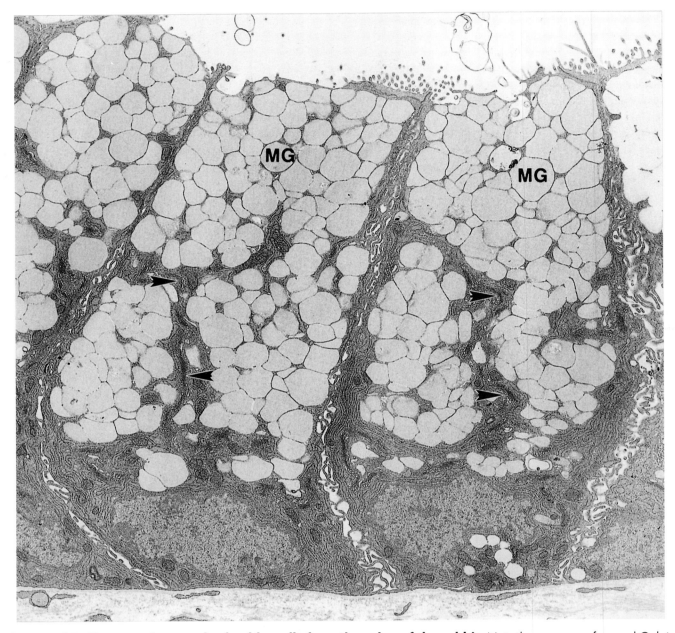

Figure 5–21. Electron micrograph of goblet cells from the colon of the rabbit. Note the presence of several Golgi complexes (*arrowheads*) and the numerous, compactly packed mucinogen granules (MG) that occupy much of the apical portion of the cells (× 11,170). (From Radwan, K.A., Oliver, M.G., and Specian, R.D.: Cytoarchitectural reorganization of rabbit colonic goblet cells during baseline secretion. Am. J. Anat. **198:**365–376, 1990.)

shape, that of a goblet (Fig. 5–21). Their thin basal region sits on the basal lamina, whereas their expanded apical portion, the **theca,** faces the lumen of the digestive tube or respiratory tract. The theca is filled with membrane-bound secretory droplets, which displace the cytoplasm to the cell's periphery and the nucleus toward its base. The process of mucinogen release is regulated and stimulated by chemical irritation and parasympathetic innervation, resulting in exocytosis of the entire secretory contents of the cell, thus lubricating and protecting the epithelial sheet.

Multicellular Exocrine Glands

Multicellular exocrine glands consist of clusters of secretory cells arranged in varying degrees of organization. These secretory cells do not act alone and independently but rather function as secretory organs. Multicellular glands may have a simple structure, exemplified by the glandular epithelium of the uterus and gastric mucosa, or a complex structure, composed of various types of secretory units and organized in a compound branching fashion.

Because of their structural arrangement, multicellular glands are subclassified according to the organization of their secretory and duct components, as well as according to the shape of their secretory units (Fig. 5–22).

Multicellular glands are classified as **simple** if their ducts do not branch and **compound** if their ducts branch. They are further categorized according to the morphology of their secretory units as **tubular, acinar, alveolar** (resembling a grape), or **tubuloalveolar.**

Larger multicellular glands are surrounded by a collagenous connective tissue **capsule,** which sends **septa**—strands of connective tissue—into the gland, subdividing it into smaller compartments known as **lobes** and **lobules.** Vascular elements, nerves, and ducts utilize the connective tissue septa to enter and leave the gland. Additionally, the connective tissue elements provide structural support for the gland (Fig. 5–23).

Acini of many multicellular exocrine glands such as sweat glands and major salivary glands possess **myoepithelial cells** that share the basal lamina of the acinar cells. Although myoepithelial cells are of epithelial origin, they possess some characteristics of smooth muscle cells, particularly contractility. These cells exhibit small nuclei and sparse fibrillar cytoplasm radiating out from the cell body, wrapping around the acini and some of the small ducts (Figs. 5–23, 5–24). Their contractions assist in expressing secretions from the acini and from some small ducts.

Endocrine Glands

Endocrine glands release their secretions, **hormones,** into blood or lymphatic vessels for distribution to target organs. The major endocrine glands of the body include the suprarenal (adrenal), pituitary, thyroid, parathyroid, and pineal glands, as well as the ovaries, placenta, and testes. The islets of Langerhans and the interstitial cells of Leydig are unusual, because they are composed of clusters of cells ensconced within the connective tissue stroma of other organs (the pancreas and the testes, respectively). Hormones secreted by endocrine glands include peptides, proteins, modified amino acids, steroids, and glycoproteins. Because of their complexity and important role in regulating bodily processes, the endocrine glands are covered in detail in Chapter 13.

The secretory cells of endocrine glands are organized either into cords of cells or into a follicular arrangement. In the **cord** type, the most common arrangement, cells form anastomosing cords around capillaries or blood sinusoids. The hormone to be secreted is stored intracellularly and is released upon the arrival of the proper signaling molecule or

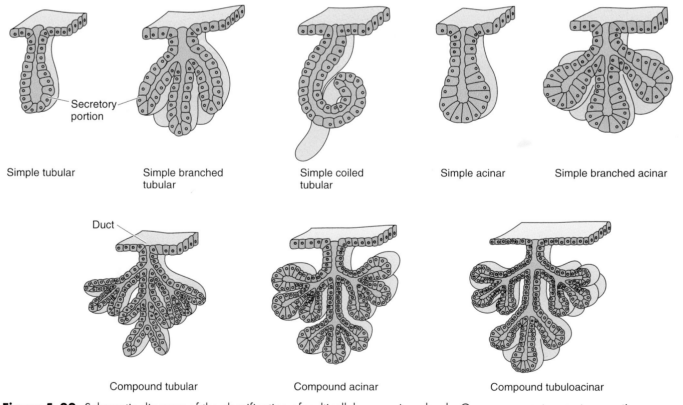

Figure 5–22. Schematic diagram of the classification of multicellular exocrine glands. Green represents secretory portion, lavender represents duct portion of gland.

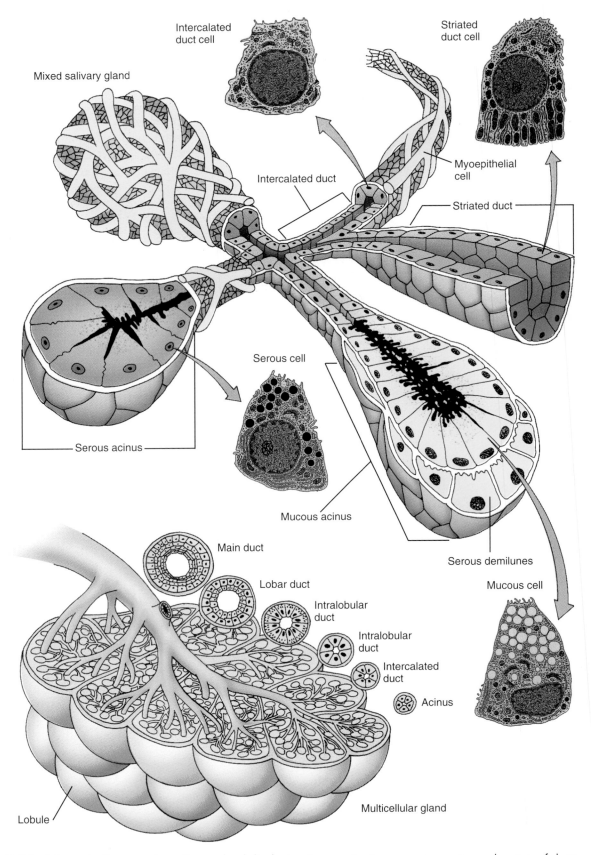

Figure 5–23. Schematic diagram of a salivary gland displaying its organization, secretory units, and system of ducts.

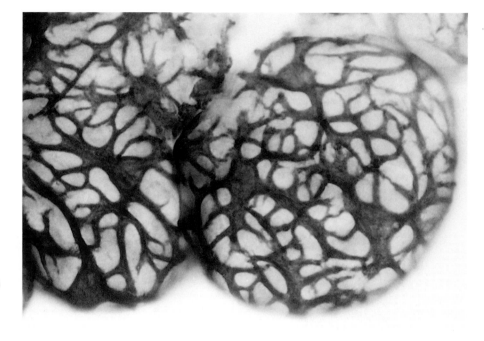

Figure 5–24. Light micrograph of myoepithelial cells immunostained for actin. Note that the myoepithelial cells surround the acini (× 700). (From Satoh, Y., Habara, Y., Kanno, T., and Ono, K.: Carbamylcholine-induced morphological changes and spatial dynamics of $[Ca^{2+}]_c$ in Harderian glands of guinea pigs: Calcium-dependent lipid secretion and contraction of myoepithelial cells. Cell. Tiss. Res. **274:**1–14, 1993. Copyright by Springer-Verlag.)

neural impulse. Examples of the cord type of endocrine gland include the suprarenal gland, anterior lobe of the pituitary gland, and parathyroid gland. In the **follicle** type of endocrine gland, secretory cells (**follicular cells**) form follicles that surround a cavity that receives and stores the secreted hormone. When a release signal is received, the stored hormone is resorbed by the follicular cells and released into the connective tissue to enter the blood capillaries. An example of the follicle type of endocrine gland is the thyroid gland.

It should be noted that some glands of the body are mixed—that is, the parenchyma contains both exocrine and endocrine secretory units. In these mixed glands (e.g., pancreas, ovary, and testes), the exocrine portion of the gland secretes its product into a duct, whereas the endocrine portion of the gland secretes its product into the bloodstream.

Diffuse Neuroendocrine System (DNES)

Widespread throughout the digestive tract and in the respiratory system are endocrine cells interspersed among other secretory cells. These cells, members of the **diffuse neuroendocrine system,** manufacture various paracrine and endocrine hormones. Because these cells are capable of taking up precursors of amines, as well decarboxylating amino acids, they are also called **APUD cells,** an acronym for **a**mine **p**recursor **u**ptake and **d**ecarboxylation. Because some of these cells stain with silver salts, they were also called **argentaffin** and **argyrophil cells.** Chapter 17 presents a more detailed description of these cells.

Connective Tissue

6

Connective tissues, as the name implies, form a continuum with epithelial tissue, muscle, and nervous tissue as well as other components of connective tissue to maintain a functionally integrated body. Most connective tissues originate from **mesoderm,** the middle germ layer of the embryonic tissue. From this layer, the multipotential cells of the embryo, the **mesenchyme,** develops. These mesenchymal cells migrate throughout the body, giving rise to the connective tissues and their cells, including those of bone, cartilage, tendons, capsules, blood and hemopoietic cells, and lymphoid cells (Fig. 6–1). Mature connective tissue is classified as **connective tissue proper,** the major subject of this chapter, or **specialized connective tissue** (i.e., cartilage, bone, and blood), which is detailed in Chapters 7 and 10.

Connective tissue is composed of **cells** and **extracellular matrix,** which consists of **ground substance** and **fibers** (Figs. 6–2, 6–3). The cells are the most important components in some connective tissues. For example, fibroblasts are the most important components of loose connective tissue; these cells manufacture and maintain the fibers and ground substance composing the extracellular matrix. In contrast, fibers are the most important components of tendons and ligaments. In still other connective tissues, the ground substance is most important because it is where certain specialized connective tissue cells carry out their functions. Thus, all three components are critical to the role of connective tissue in the body.

Functions of Connective Tissue

Although many functions are attributed to connective tissue, its primary functions include providing **structural support,** serving as a **medium of exchange,** aiding in the **defense** and **protection** of the body, and forming a site for **storage of fat.**

Bones, cartilage, and ligaments holding the bones together, as well as the tendons attaching muscles to bone, act as support. The connective tissue that forms the capsules encasing

the organs and the stroma forming the structural framework within the organs likewise have a support function.

Connective tissues also function as a **medium for exchange** of metabolic waste, nutrients, and oxygen between the blood and many of the cells of the body. The functions of **defense** and **protection** are carried out (1) by the body's phagocytic cells, which engulf and destroy cellular debris, foreign particles, and microorganisms; (2) by its immunocompetent cells, which produce antibodies against antigens; and (3) by certain cells that produce pharmacological substances that help in controlling inflammation. Connective tissues also help protect the body by forming a physical barrier to microorganism invasion and dissemination.

Extracellular Matrix

The extracellular matrix, composed of ground substance and fibers, resists both compressive and stretching forces. Although the components of the extracellular matrix are discussed in Chapter 4, their salient features are reviewed briefly here.

Ground Substance

Ground substance is a hydrated, amorphous material that is composed of **glycosaminoglycans,** long unbranched polymers of repeating disaccharides; **proteoglycans,** protein cores to which various glycosaminoglycans are covalently linked; and adhesive **glycoproteins,** large macromolecules responsible for fastening the various components of the extracellular matrix to each other and to integrins of the cell membrane (see Fig. 4–3).

Glycosaminoglycans are of two major types: sulfated, including keratan sulfate, heparan sulfate, heparin, chondroitin sulfates, and dermatan sulfate; and nonsulfated, including hyaluronic acid.

Proteoglycans are covalently linked to hyaluronic acid, forming huge macromolecules called **aggrecan aggregates,**

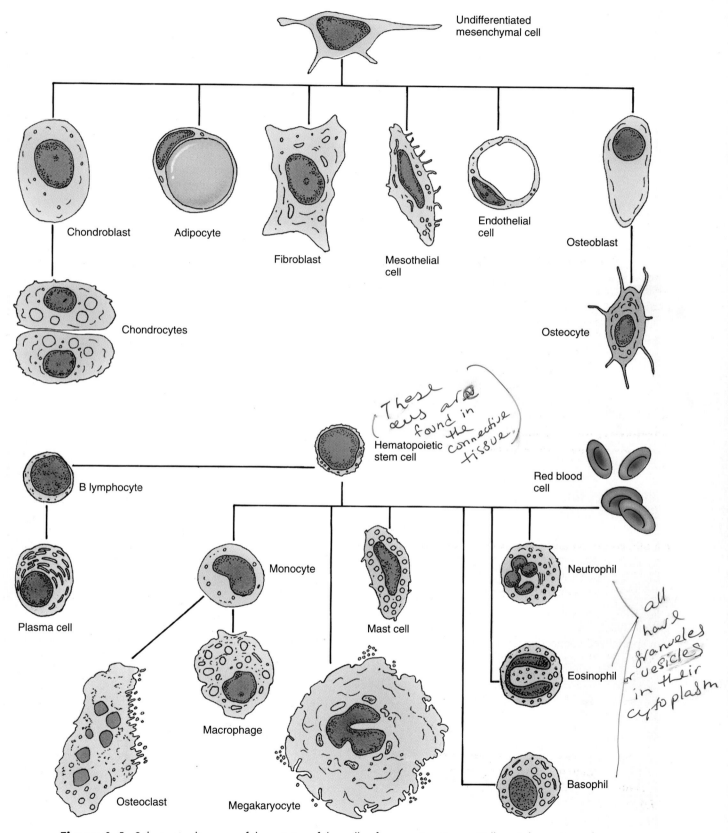

Figure 6-1. Schematic diagram of the origins of the cells of connective tissue. Cells not drawn to scale.

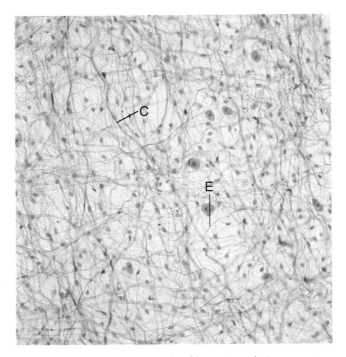

Figure 6–2. Light micrograph of loose (areolar) connective tissue displaying collagen (C) and elastic (E) fibers and some of the cell types common to loose connective tissue (× 132).

which are responsible for the gel state of the extracellular matrix.

Adhesive glycoproteins are of various types. Some are localized preferentially to the basal lamina, such as **laminin**, or to cartilage and bone, such as **chondronectin** and **osteonectin**, respectively. Still others are generally dispersed throughout the extracellular matrix, such as **fibronectin.**

Fibers

The **fibers** of the extracellular matrix are collagen (and reticular) and elastic fibers. **Collagen** fibers are inelastic and possess great tensile strength. Each fiber is composed of fine subunits, the **tropocollagen** molecule, composed of three α-chains wrapped around each other in a helical configuration. At least 15 different types of collagen fibers are known, which vary in the amino acid sequence of their α-chains. The most common amino acids of collagen are **glycine, proline, hydroxyproline,** and **hydroxylysine.** The six major collagen types are **type I** (in connective tissue proper, bone, dentin, and cementum), **type II** (in hyaline and elastic cartilages), **type III** (reticular fibers), **type IV** (lamina densa of the basal lamina), **type V** (associated with type I collagen and in the placenta), and **type VII** (attaching the basal lamina to the lamina reticularis). Most of the fiber types display a 67-nm periodicity in electron micrographs, which is due to the deposition of heavy metals in the **gap regions** of the fiber (see Fig. 4–5). Type IV collagen is not assembled into fibers, and thus does not possess a periodicity.

Elastic fibers are composed of **elastin** and **microfibrils.** These fibers are highly elastic and may be stretched up to 150% of their resting length without breaking. Their elasticity is due to the protein elastin, and their stability is due to the presence of microfibrils. Elastin is an amorphous material whose main amino acid components are **glycine** and **proline** as well as the unique amino acids **desmosine** and **isodesmosine.**

Cellular Components

The cells in connective tissues are grouped into two categories: **fixed cells** and **transient cells** (see Fig. 6–1).

Fixed cells are a resident population of cells that have developed and remain in place within the connective tissue, where they perform their functions. The fixed cells are a stable and long-lived population that include fibroblasts, adipose cells, mast cells, and pericytes. Some authors consider certain of the macrophages (e.g., Kupffer cells of the liver) to be fixed connective tissue cells.

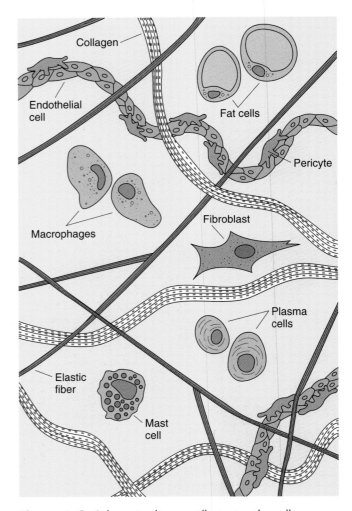

Figure 6–3. Schematic diagram illustrating the cell types and fiber types in loose connective tissue. Cells not drawn to scale.

Transient cells (free or wandering cells) originate mostly in the bone marrow and circulate in the bloodstream. Upon receiving the proper stimulus or signal, these cells leave the bloodstream and migrate into the connective tissue to perform their specific functions. Because most of these motile cells are usually short-lived, they must be replaced continually from a large population of stem cells. Transient cells include plasma cells, lymphocytes, neutrophils, eosinophils, basophils, monocytes, and some macrophages.

Fixed Connective Tissue Cells

Of the resident cells of connective tissue, fibroblasts are the most widely distributed and abundant. The four connective tissue cell types that are clearly fixed are described here; macrophages, which exhibit some fixed and some transient properties, are discussed later under the heading "Macrophages."

Fibroblasts

Fibroblasts, which synthesize the extracellular matrix of connective tissue, are derived from undifferentiated mesenchymal cells (see Fig. 6–1). Fibroblasts may occur in either an active state or a quiescent state. Some histologists differentiate between them, calling the quiescent cells **fibrocytes;** however, because the two states are temporary, the term fibroblast is used in this text.

Active fibroblasts often reside in close association with collagen bundles, where they lie parallel to the long axis of the fiber (Fig. 6–4). They are elongated, fusiform cells possessing pale-staining cytoplasm, which is often difficult to distinguish from collagen when stained with hematoxylin and eosin. The most obvious portion of the cell is the darker-stained, large, granular, ovoid nucleus containing a well-defined nucleolus. Electron microscopy reveals a prominent Golgi apparatus and abundant rough endoplasmic reticulum (RER), especially when the cell is actively manufacturing matrix, as in wound healing. Actin and α-actinin are localized at the periphery of the cell, and myosin is present throughout the cytoplasm.

Inactive fibroblasts are smaller and more ovoid, and they possess an acidophilic cytoplasm. Their nucleus is smaller, elongated, and more deeply stained. Electron microscopy reveals sparse amounts of RER but an abundance of free ribosomes.

Although considered to be fixed cells in the connective tissues, fibroblasts are capable of some movement. Fibroblasts seldom undergo cell division but may do so during wound healing. These cells, however, may differentiate into adipose cells, chondrocytes (during formation of fibrocartilage), and osteoblasts (under pathological conditions).

Myofibroblasts are modified fibroblasts that demonstrate characteristics similar to both fibroblasts and smooth muscle cells. Histologically, fibroblasts and myofibroblasts are not easily distinguished by routine light microscopy. However, electron microscopy reveals myofibroblasts to have bundles of actin filaments and dense bodies similar to those of smooth muscle cells. Additionally, the surface profile of the nucleus resembles that of a smooth muscle cell. Myofibroblasts differ from smooth muscle cells in that an external lamina (basal lamina) is absent. Myofibroblasts are abundant in areas undergoing wound healing; they also are found in the periodontal ligament, where they probably assist in tooth eruption.

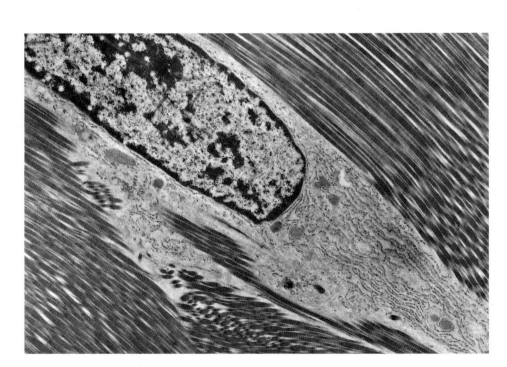

Figure 6–4. Electron micrograph displaying a portion of a fibroblast and the packed collagen fibers in rat tendon. Observe the heterochromatin in the nucleus and the rough endoplasmic reticulum (RER) in the cytoplasm. Banding in the collagen fibers may be observed also. (From Ralphs, J.R., Benjamin, M., and Thornett, A.: Cell and matrix biology of the suprapatella in the rat: A structural and immunocytochemical study of fibrocartilage in a tendon subject to compression. Anat. Rec. **231:**167–177, 1991. Copyright 1991. Reprinted by permission of John Wiley & Sons, Inc.)

Pericytes

Pericytes, derived from undifferentiated mesenchymal cells, partly surround the endothelial cells of capillaries and small venules (see Fig. 6–3). Technically, these perivascular cells are outside the connective tissue compartment because they are surrounded by their own basal lamina, which may be fused with that of the endothelial cells. Pericytes possess characteristics of smooth muscle cells and endothelial cells suggesting that, under certain conditions, they may differentiate into other cells. Pericytes are discussed more fully in Chapter 11.

Adipose cells

Fat cells, or **adipocytes,** also are derived from undifferentiated mesenchymal cells (Fig. 6–5), although some histolo-gists believe that fibroblasts may also give rise to adipose cells. Adipose cells are fully differentiated and do not undergo cell division. They function in the synthesis and storage of triglycerides. There are two types of fat cells, which constitute two types of adipose tissue. Cells with a single, large lipid droplet, called **unilocular fat cells,** form **white adipose tissue,** and cells with multiple, small lipid droplets, called **multilocular fat cells,** form **brown adipose tissue.** White fat is much more adundant than brown fat. As discussed later in this chapter, the distribution and histophysiology of the two types of fat tissue differ. Here we describe the histology of the adipocytes themselves.

Adipocytes of white fat are large spherical cells, up to 120 µm in diameter, that become polyhedral when crowded into adipose tissue (Fig. 6–6). Unilocular fat cells continually store fat in the form of a single droplet, which enlarges so much that the cytoplasm and nucleus are displaced peripher-

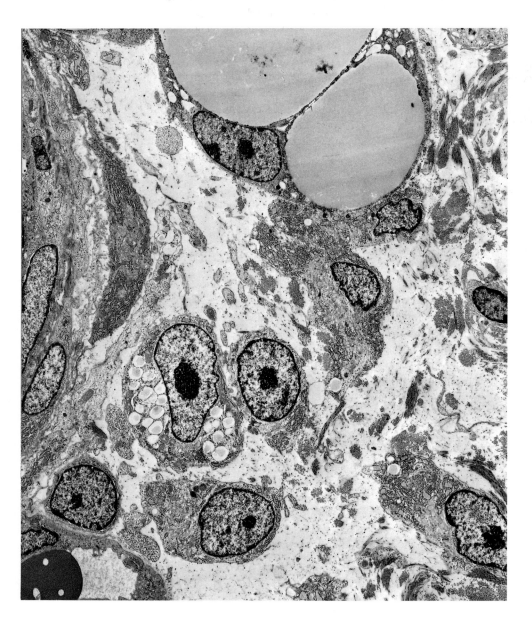

Figure 6–5. Electron micrograph of adipocytes in various stages of maturation in rat hypodermis. Observe the adipocyte at the top of the micrograph with its nucleus and cytoplasm crowded to the periphery by the fat droplet. (From Hausman, G.J., Campion, D.R., Richardson, R.L., and Martin, R.J.: Adipocyte development in the rat hypodermis. Am. J. Anat. **161:**85–100, 1981. Copyright 1991. Reprinted by permission of John Wiley & Sons, Inc.)

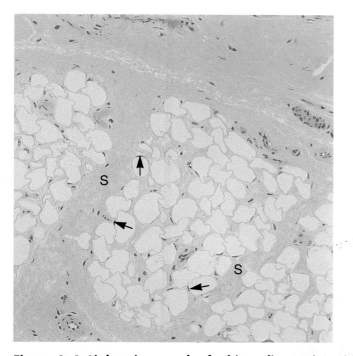

Figure 6–6. Light micrograph of white adipose tissue from monkey hypodermis (× 132). Observe that the lipid was extracted during tissue processing. Note how the cytoplasm and nuclei (*arrows*) are crowded to the periphery. Septa (S) divide the fat into lobules.

ally against the plasma membrane, thus giving these cells the "signet ring" profile when viewed by light microscopy. Electron micrographs reveal a small Golgi complex situated adjacent to the nucleus, only a few mitochondria, and sparse RER, but an abundance of free ribosomes. That the fat droplet is not bounded by a membrane is clear in electron micrographs but unclear in light micrographs. The external surfaces of the plasma membranes are enveloped by a basal lamina–like substance. Minute pinocytotic vesicles, whose function is unclear, have been noted on the surface of the plasma membrane. In fasting, the cell surface becomes irregular with pseudopod-like projections.

Multilocular adipocytes contrast with unilocular adipocytes in several ways. First, brown fat cells are smaller and more polygonal than white fat cells. Moreover, because these cells store fat in several small droplets rather than a single droplet, the spherical nucleus is not squeezed up against the plasma membrane. Multilocular fat cells contain many more mitochondria but fewer free ribosomes than unilocular fat cells (Fig. 6–7). Although brown fat cells lack RER, smooth ER is present.

STORAGE AND RELEASE OF FAT BY ADIPOSE CELLS. During digestion, fats are broken down in the duodenum by **pancreatic lipase** into **fatty acids** and **glycerol.** The intestinal epithelium absorbs these substances and reesterifies them in the smooth ER to **triglycerides,** which then are surrounded by proteins to form **chylomicrons.** Chylomicrons are released into the extracellular space at the basolateral membranes of the surface absorptive cells, enter the lacteals of the villus, and are carried by the lymph to the bloodstream. Additionally, very-low-density lipoprotein (VLDL), synthesized by the liver, and albumin-bound fatty acids are present in the bloodstream. Once in the capillaries of adipose tissue, very-low-density lipoprotein, fatty acids, and chylomicrons are exposed to **lipoprotein lipase** (manufactured by fat cells), which breaks them down into free fatty acids and glycerol (Fig. 6–8). The fatty acids enter the connective tissue and diffuse through the cell membranes of adipocytes. These cells then combine their own glycerol phosphate with the imported fatty acids to form triglycerides, which are added to the forming lipid droplets within the adipocytes until needed. It should be noted that adipose cells can convert glucose and amino acids into fatty acids when stimulated by insulin.

Norepinephrine is released from nerve endings of postganglionic sympathetic neurons in the vicinity of fat cells. Also, during strenuous exercise, **epinephrine** and **norepinephrine** are released from the suprarenal medulla. These two hormones bind to their respective receptors of the adipocyte plasmalemma, activating **adenylate cyclase** to form cyclic adenosine monophosphate (cAMP), a second messenger, resulting in activation of **hormone-sensitive lipase.** This enzyme cleaves triglycerides into fatty acids and glycerol, which are released into the bloodstream.

Fat cells are found throughout the body in loose connective tissue and concentrated along blood vessels. They may also accumulate into masses, forming adipose tissue.

Mast Cells

Mast cells, among the largest of the fixed cells of the connective tissue, are 20 to 30 μm in diameter, ovoid, and they possess a centrally placed, spherical nucleus (Fig. 6–9). Unlike the three types of fixed cells discussed earlier, mast cells probably derive from precursors in the bone marrow (see Fig. 6–1).

The presence of numerous granules in the cytoplasm is the identifying characteristic of mast cells (Fig. 6–10). These membrane-bounded granules range in size from 0.3 to 0.8 μm. Because these granules contain **heparin,** a sulfated glycosaminoglycan, they stain metachromatically with toluidine blue. Electron microscopic studies of the granules reveal differences in size and form and display variations in ultrastructure even within the same cell. Otherwise, the cytoplasm is unremarkable because it contains several mitochondria, a sparse number of RER profiles, and a relatively small Golgi complex.

In addition to heparin, mast cell granules also contain **histamine, neutral proteases, aryl sulfatase, eosinophil chemotactic factor (ECF),** and **neutrophil chemotactic**

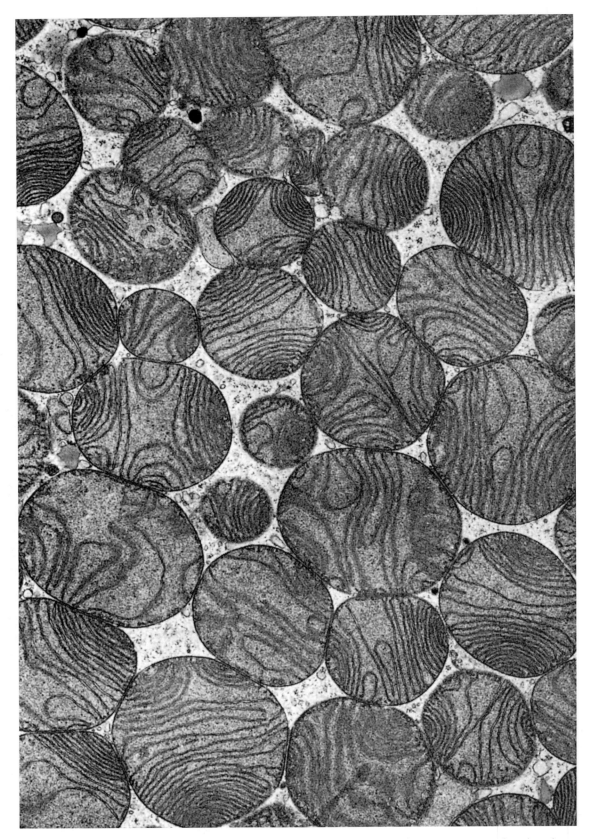

Figure 6-7. Multilocular tissues (brown fat) in the bat (× 16,000). Note the numerous mitochondria dispersed throughout the cell. (From Fawcett, D.W.: An Atlas of Fine Structure. The Cell. Philadelphia, W.B. Saunders Company, 1966.)

FAT CELL   CAPILLARY

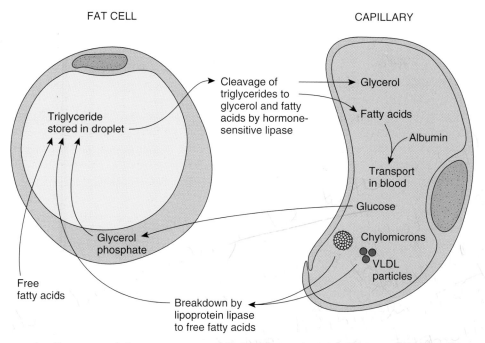

- Triglyceride stored in droplet
- Cleavage of triglycerides to glycerol and fatty acids by hormone-sensitive lipase
- Glycerol
- Fatty acids
- Albumin
- Transport in blood
- Glucose
- Glycerol phosphate
- Chylomicrons
- VLDL particles
- Free fatty acids
- Breakdown by lipoprotein lipase to free fatty acids

Figure 6–8. Schematic diagram of the transport of lipid between a capillary and an adipocyte. Lipids are transported in the bloodstream in the form of chylomicrons and very low-density lipoproteins (VLDL). The enzyme lipoprotein lipase, manufactured by the fat cell and transported to the capillary lumen, hydrolyzes the lipids to fatty acids and glycerol. Fatty acids diffuse into the connective tissue of the adipose tissue and into the lipocytes, where they are reesterified into triglycerides for storage. When required, triglycerides stored within the adipocyte are hydrolyzed by **hormone-sensitive lipase** into fatty acids and glycerol. These will then enter the connective tissue spaces of adipose tissue and from there into a capillary, where they will be bound to albumin and transported in the blood. Glucose from the capillary can be transported to adipocytes, which can manufacture lipids from carbohydrate sources.

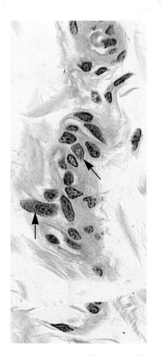

Figure 6–9. Light micrograph of mast cells (*arrows*) in monkey connective tissue. (× 540).

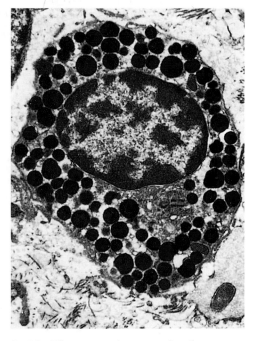

Figure 6–10. Electron micrograph of a mast cell in the rat (× 5500). Observe the dense granules filling the cytoplasm. (From Leeson, T.S., Leeson, C.R., and Paparo, A.A.: Text/Atlas of Histology. Philadelphia, W.B. Saunders Company, 1988.)

factor (NCF). Besides the substances found in the granules, mast cells also synthesize **leukotrienes** from membrane arachidonic acid precursors.

MAST CELL DEVELOPMENT AND DISTRIBUTION.

Because basophils and mast cells share some characteristics, it was once believed that mast cells were basophils that had left the bloodstream to perform their tasks in the connective tissues. It is now known that basophils and mast cells are different cells and have separate precursors (see Fig. 6–1). Mast cell precursors probably originate in the bone marrow, circulate in the blood for a short time, and then enter the connective tissues, where they differentiate into mast cells and acquire their characteristic cytoplasmic granules. These cells have a lifespan of less than a few months and occasionally undergo cell division.

Mast cells are located throughout the body in the connective tissue proper, where they are concentrated along small blood vessels. They also are present in the subepithelial connective tissue of the respiratory and digestive systems. Mast cells in connective tissue contain mostly heparin in their gran-

ules, whereas those located in the alimentary tract mucosa contain **chondroitin sulfate** instead of heparin. These cells are called **mucosal mast cells.** The reason for the existence of the two diverse populations of mast cells is not understood.

MAST CELL ACTIVATION AND DEGRANULATION.

Mast cells possess cell-surface Fc receptors for immunoglobulin E (IgE). They function in the immune system by initiating an inflammatory response known as the **immediate hypersensitivity reaction (anaphylactic reaction).** This response commonly is induced by foreign proteins (antigens) such as bee venom, pollen, and certain drugs.

1. The first exposure to any of these antigens elicits formation of IgE antibodies, which bind to the Fc receptors of the plasmalemma of mast cells, thereby **sensitizing** these cells.

2. On subsequent exposure to the *same* antigen, the antigen binds to the IgE on the mast cell surface, causing cross-linking of the bound IgE antibodies and clustering of the receptors (Fig. 6–11).

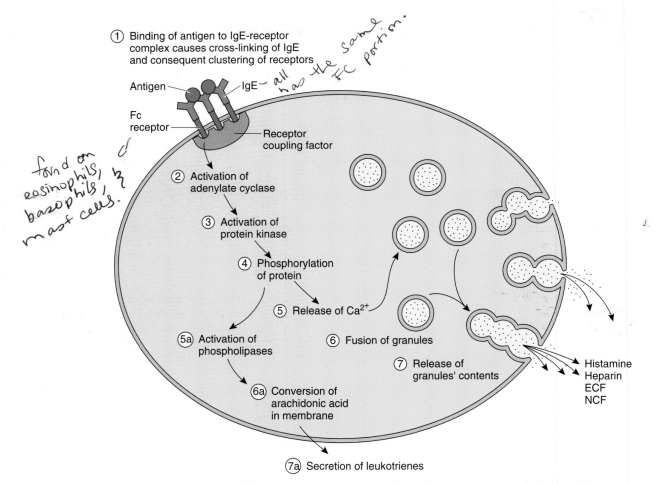

Figure 6–11. Schematic diagram illustrating the binding of antigens and cross-linking of IgE-receptor complexes on the mast cell plasma membrane. This event triggers a cascade that ultimately results in the synthesis and release of leukotrienes and prostaglandins, as well as degranulation, releasing histamine, heparin, eosinophil chemotactic factor (ECF), and neutrophil chemotactic factor (NCF).

3. Cross-linking and clustering activate membrane-bound **receptor coupling factors,** which, in turn, initiate at least two independent processes, the release of **primary** and **secondary mediators.**

4. The release of primary mediators is effected by activation of **adenylate cyclase,** the enzyme responsible for the conversion of adenosine triphosphate to cAMP.

5. This increase in cAMP activates release of Ca^{2+} from intracellular storage sites. The resulting increase in cytosolic Ca^{2+} causes the secretory granules to fuse with each other as well as with the cell membrane. These processes lead to **degranulation,** the release of the granule contents, namely histamine, heparin, proteases, aryl sulfatase, eosinophil chemotactic factor, and neutrophil chemotactic factor. These constitute primary mediators.

6. Cross-linking of the membrane-bound IgE also activates **phospholipase A$_2$,** which acts on membrane phospholipids to form **arachidonic acid.**

7. Arachidonic acid is converted into the secondary mediators **leukotrienes C$_4$ and D$_4$** and **prostaglandin D$_2$.** It is

important to note that these secondary mediators are *not* stored in the mast cell granules but are manufactured and immediately released.

Table 6–1 lists the sources and activity of the primary and secondary mediators released from mast cells.

The primary and secondary mediators released by mast cells during immediate hypersensitivity reactions initiate the inflammatory response, activate the body's defense system by attracting leukocytes to the site of inflammation, and modulate the degree of inflammation. The following sequence of events occurs during the inflammatory response:

1. **Histamine** causes vasodilation and increases vascular permeability of blood vessels in the vicinity. It also causes bronchiospasm and increases mucus production in the respiratory tract.

2. Complement components leak out of blood vessels and are cleaved by **neutral proteases** to form additional agents of inflammation.

Table 6–1. Primary and Secondary Mediators Released by Mast Cells

Substance	Type of Mediator	Source	Action
Histamine	Primary	Granule	Increases vascular permeability; vasodilation; smooth muscle contraction of bronchi; increases mucus production
Heparin	Primary	Granule	Anticoagulant (function in mast cells is not understood)
Chondroitin sulfate	Primary	Granule	Function not understood
Aryl sulfatase	Primary	Granule	Inactivates leukotriene C, thus limiting the inflammatory response
Neutral proteases	Primary	Granule	Protein cleavage to activate complement, increasing inflammatory response
Eosinophil chemotactic factor	Primary	Granule	Attracts eosinophils to site of inflammation
Neutrophil chemotactic factor	Primary	Granule	Attracts neutrophils to site of inflammation
Leukotrienes C$_4$ and D$_4$	Secondary	Membrane lipid	Vasodilator; increases vascular permeability; bronchial smooth muscle contractant
Prostaglandin D$_2$	Secondary	Membrane lipid	Causes contraction of bronchial smooth muscle; increases mucus secretion

3. **Eosinophil chemotactic factor** attracts eosinophils to the site of inflammation. These cells phagocytose antigen–antibody complexes; destroy any parasites present; and limit the inflammatory response.

4. **Neutrophil chemotactic factor** attracts neutrophils to the site of inflammation. These cells phagocytose and kill microorganisms, if present.

5. **Leukotrienes C_4 and D_4** increase vascular permeability and cause bronchiospasms. They are several thousand times more potent than histamine in their vasoactive effects.

6. **Prostaglandin D_2** causes bronchiospasm and increases mucus secretion by the bronchial mucosa.

Because degranulation of mast cells usually is a localized phenomenon, the typical inflammatory response is mild and site-specific. However, hyperallergic persons may experience systemic and severe immediate hypersensitivity reactions.

CLINICAL CORRELATIONS

Victims of **hay fever** attacks suffer from the effects of **histamine** being released by the mast cells of the nasal mucosa, causing localized edema from increased permeability of the small blood vessels. The swelling of the mucosa results in feeling "stuffed up" and hinders breathing.

Victims of **asthma** attacks suffer from difficulty in breathing as a result of bronchiospasm caused by **leukotrienes** released in the lungs.

Macrophages

As noted earlier, some macrophages behave as fixed cells and some as transient cells. Because macrophages are active phagocytes, they function in removing cellular debris and in protecting the body against foreign invaders.

Macrophages measure about 10 to 30 μm in diameter and are irregularly shaped cells (Fig. 6–12). The cell surface is uneven, varying from short, blunt projections to finger-like filopodia. More active macrophages have pleats and folds in their plasma membranes as a consequence of cell movement and phagocytosis. Their cytoplasm is basophilic and contains many small vacuoles and small dense granules. The eccentric nucleus is smaller and more darkly stained than that of fibroblasts, and it usually does not display nucleoli. The macrophage nucleus is somewhat distinctive in that it is ovoid and usually indented on one side, so that it resembles a kidney. Electron microscopic studies demonstrate a well-developed Golgi apparatus, a prominent RER, and an abundance of lysosomes, which appear as small, dense granules in light micrographs.

As young macrophages mature, they increase in size and there is a concomitant increase in RER profiles, Golgi complex, microtubules, lysosomes, microfilaments, and protein synthesis.

Macrophage Development and Distribution

Histologists once believed that macrophages were derived from precursor cells in the **reticuloendothelial system,** which included nonphagocytic cells such as reticulocytes. More recently, this classification has been replaced with the **mononuclear phagocyte system.** All members of the mononuclear phagocyte system arise from a common stem cell in the bone marrow, possess lysosomes, are capable of phagocytosis, and display Fc receptors and receptors for complement.

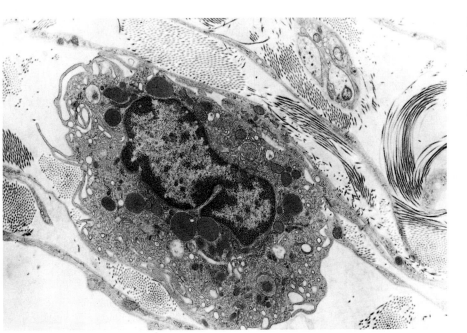

Figure 6–12. Electron micrograph of a macrophage in the rat epididymis. (From Flickinger, C.J., Herr, J.C., Sisak, J.R., and Howards, S.S.: Ultrastructure of epididymal interstitial reactions following vasectomy and vasovasostomy. Anat. Rec. **235**:61–73, 1993.)

Monocytes develop in the bone marrow and circulate in the blood. At the proper signal, they leave the bloodstream by migrating through the endothelium of capillaries or venules. In the connective tissue compartment they mature into macrophages, which normally have a lifespan of about 2 months.

Macrophages localized in certain regions of the body were given specific names before their origin was completely understood. Thus **Kupffer cells** of the liver, **dust cells** of the lung, **Langerhans cells** of the skin, **monocytes** of the blood, **macrophages** of the connective tissue, spleen, lymph nodes, thymus, and bone marrow are all members of the mononuclear phagocyte system and possess similar morphology and functions. Additionally, **osteoclasts** of bone and **microglia** of the brain, although morphologically different, also belong to the mononuclear phagocyte system.

Under chronic inflammatory conditions, macrophages congregate, greatly enlarge, and become polygonal-shaped **epithelioid cells.** When the particulate matter to be disposed of is excessively large, several to many macrophages may fuse to form a **foreign-body giant cell,** a giant multinucleated macrophage.

Macrophages residing in the connective tissues were previously called **fixed macrophages,** and those that developed as a result of an exogenous stimulus and migrated to the particular site were called **free macrophages.** These names have been replaced by the more descriptive **resident macrophages** and **elicited macrophages,** respectively.

Macrophage Function

Macrophages phagocytose senescent, damaged, and dead cells and cellular debris and digest the ingested material by action of hydrolytic enzymes in their lysosomes (see Chapter 2). Macrophages also assist in defense of the body by phagocytosing and destroying microorganisms. During the immune response, factors released by lymphocytes activate macrophages, increasing their phagocytic activity. **Activated macrophages** vary considerably in shape, possess microvilli and lamellipodia, and exhibit increased locomotion compared with unactivated macrophages. Macrophages also play a key role in presenting antigens to lymphocytes, as described in Chapter 12.

Transient Connective Tissue Cells

All the transient connective tissue cells are derived from precursors in the bone marrow (see Fig. 6–1). All of these cells are discussed in more detail in other chapters.

Plasma Cells

Although **plasma cells** are scattered throughout the connective tissues, they are found in greatest numbers in areas of chronic inflammation and where foreign substances or mi-

croorganisms have entered the tissues. These differentiated cells, which are derived from B lymphocytes that have interacted with antigen, produce and secrete antibodies (see Chapters 10 and 12). Plasma cells are large, ovoid cells, 20 µm in diameter, with an eccentrically placed nucleus with a relatively short lifespan of 2 to 3 weeks. Their cytoplasm is intensely basophilic as a result of a well-developed RER with closely spaced cisternae (Fig. 6–13). Only a few mitochondria are scattered between the profiles of RER. Electron micrographs also display a large juxtanuclear Golgi complex and a pair of centrioles (Figs. 6–14, 6–15). These structures are located in the pale-staining regions adjacent to the nucleus in light micrographs. The spherical nucleus possesses heterochromatin radiating out from the center, giving it a characteristic "clockface" or "spoked" appearance under the light microscope.

Leukocytes

Leukocytes are white blood cells that circulate in the bloodstream. However, they frequently migrate through the capillary walls to enter the connective tissues, especially during inflammation, when they carry out various functions.

Neutrophils phagocytose and digest bacteria in areas of acute inflammation, resulting in formation of **pus,** an accumulation of dead neutrophils and debris. **Eosinophils,** like neutrophils, are attracted to areas of inflammation by leukocyte chemotactic factors. Eosinophils combat parasites by

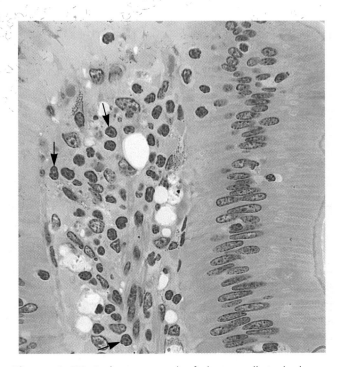

Figure 6–13. Light micrograph of plasma cells in the lamina propria of the monkey jejunum (× 540). Observe the "clockface" nucleus (*arrows*) and clear perinuclear zone.

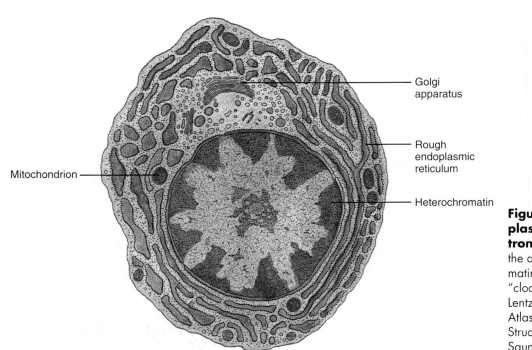

Figure 6–14. Drawing of a plasma cell from an electron micrograph. Note that the arrangement of heterochromatin gives the nucleus the "clockface" appearance. (From Lentz, T.L.: Cell Fine Structure. An Atlas of Drawings of Whole-Cell Structure. Philadelphia, W.B. Saunders Company, 1971.)

releasing cytotoxins. They also are attracted to sites of allergic inflammation, where they moderate the allergic reaction. **Lymphocytes** are present only in small numbers in most connective tissue, except at sites of chronic inflammation, where they are abundant. A more detailed discussion of leukocytes is presented in Chapter 10 and of lymphocytes in Chapter 12.

Classification of Connective Tissue

As noted earlier, connective tissue is classified into connective tissue proper, the major subject of this chapter, and specialized connective tissue, embracing cartilage, bone, and blood. The third recognized category of connective tissue is **embryonic connective tissue.** Table 6–2 summarizes the major classes of connective tissue and their subclasses.

Embryonic Connective Tissue

Embryonic connective tissue includes both mesenchymal tissue and mucous tissue. **Mesenchymal connective tissue** is present only in the embryo and consists of mesenchymal cells in a gel-like, amorphous ground substance containing scattered reticular fibers. **Mesenchymal cells** possess an oval nucleus exhibiting fine chromatin network and prominent nucleoli. The sparse, pale-staining cytoplasm extends small processes in several directions. Mitotic figures are frequently observed in mesenchymal cells because they give rise to most of the cells of loose connective tissue. It is generally believed that most if not all of the mesenchymal cells, once scattered throughout the embryo, are eventually depleted and do not exist as such in the adult. In adults,

pluripotential pericytes, which reside along capillaries, can differentiate into other cells of connective tissue.

Mucous tissue is a loose, amorphous connective tissue exhibiting a jelly-like matrix primarily composed of hyaluronic acid and sparsely populated with type I and type III collagen fibers and fibroblasts. This tissue—also known as **Wharton's jelly**—is found only in the umbilical cord and subdermal connective tissue of the embryo.

Connective Tissue Proper

The four recognized types of connective tissue proper differ in their histology, location, and functions.

Loose (Areolar) Connective Tissue

Loose connective tissue is also known as **areolar connective tissue;** this tissue fills in the spaces of the body just deep to the skin, lies below the mesothelial lining of the internal body cavity, is associated with the adventitia of blood vessels, and surrounds the parenchyma of glands. The loose connective tissue of mucous membranes (as in the alimentary canal) is called the **lamina propria.**

Loose connective tissue is characterized by abundant **ground substance** and tissue fluid (extracellular fluid) housing the fixed connective tissue cells: **fibroblasts, adipose cells, macrophages,** and **mast cells,** as well as some **undifferentiated cells.** Also scattered throughout the ground substance are loosely woven **collagen, reticular, and elastic fibers.** Coursing in this amorphous tissue are small nerve fibers, as well as blood vessels, which supply the cells with oxygen and nutrients.

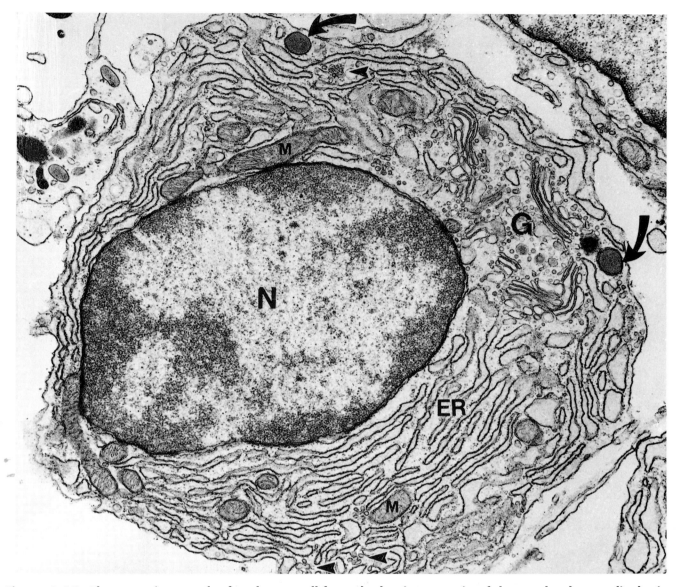

Figure 6–15. Electron micrograph of a plasma cell from the lamina propria of the rat duodenum displaying abundant rough endoplasmic reticulum and prominent Golgi complex (× 15,000). ER, Rough endoplasmic reticulum; G, Golgi apparatus; M, mitochondria; N, nucleus; arrowheads, small vesicles; arrows, dense granules. (From Rambourg, A., Clermont, Y., Hermo, L., and Chretien, M.: Formation of secretion granules in the Golgi apparatus of plasma cells in the rat. Am. J. Anat. **184:**52–61, 1988. Copyright 1988. Reprinted by permission of John Wiley & Sons, Inc.)

Because this tissue lies immediately beneath the thin epithelia of the digestive and respiratory tracts, it is where the body first attacks antigens, bacteria, and other foreign invaders. Therefore, loose connective tissue contains many transient cells responsible for inflammation, allergic reactions, and the immune response. These cells, which originally circulate in the bloodstream, are released from blood vessels in response to an inflammatory stimulus. Pharmacological agents released by mast cells increase the permeability of small vessels, so that excess plasma enters the loose connective tissue spaces, causing it to swell.

CLINICAL CORRELATIONS

Under normal circumstances tissue fluid returns back into the blood capillaries or enters lymph vessels to be returned to the blood. However, a potent and prolonged inflammatory response causes accumulation of excess tissue fluid within loose connective tissue beyond what can be returned via the capillaries and lymph vessels. This results in gross swelling, or **edema,** in the affected area. Edema can result from excessive release of histamine and leukotrienes C_4 and D_4, which all increase capillary permeability, as well as from obstructed venous or lymphatic vessels.

Table 6-2. Classification of Connective Tissues

A. Embryonic connective tissues
1. Mesenchymal connective tissue
2. Mucous connective tissue

B. Connective tissue proper
1. Loose (areolar) connective tissue
2. Dense connective tissue
   a. Dense irregular connective tissue
   b. Dense regular connective tissue
      (1) Collagenous
      (2) Elastic
3. Reticular tissue
4. Adipose tissue

C. Specialized connective tissue
1. Cartilage
2. Bone
3. Blood

Dense Connective Tissue

Dense connective tissue contains most of the same components found in loose connective tissue except that it has many more fibers and fewer cells. The orientation and the arrangements of the bundles of collagen fibers of this tissue make it resistant to stress. When the collagen fiber bundles are arranged randomly, the tissue is called **dense irregular connective tissue.** When fiber bundles of the tissue are arranged in parallel or organized fashion, the tissue is called **dense regular connective tissue,** which is divided into collagenous and elastic types.

Dense irregular connective tissue contains mostly coarse collagen fibers interwoven into a meshwork that resists stress from all directions (Fig. 6–16). The collagen bundles are packed so tightly that space is limited for ground substance and cells. Fine networks of elastic fibers are often scattered about the collagen bundles. Fibroblasts, the most abundant cells of this tissue, are located in the interstices between collagen bundles. Dense irregular connective tissue constitutes the dermis of skin, the sheaths of nerves, and the capsules of spleen, testes, ovary, kidney, and lymph nodes.

Dense regular collagenous connective tissue is composed of coarse collagen bundles densely packed and oriented into parallel cylinders or sheets that resist tensile forces (Fig. 6–17). Because of the tight packing of the collagen fibers, little space can be occupied by ground substance and cells. Thin, sheet-like fibroblasts are located between bundles of collagen with their long axis parallel to the bundles. Tendons, ligaments, and aponeuroses are examples of dense regular collagenous connective tissue.

Dense regular elastic connective tissue possesses coarse branching elastic fibers with only a few collagen fibers forming networks. Scattered throughout the interstitial spaces are fibroblasts. The elastic fibers are arranged parallel to each other and form either thin sheets or fenestrated membranes. The latter are found in large blood vessels, the ligamentum flava of the vertebral column, and the suspensory ligament of the penis.

Reticular Tissue

Type III collagen is the major fiber component of **reticular tissue.** The collagen fibers form mesh-like networks interspersed with fibroblasts and macrophages (Fig. 6–18). It is the fibroblasts that synthesize the type III collagen. Reticular tissue forms the architectural framework of liver sinusoids, adipose tissue, bone marrow, lymph nodes, spleen, smooth muscle, and the islets of Langerhans.

Adipose Tissue

Adipose tissue is classified into two types based on whether it is composed of unilocular or multilocular adipocytes. Other differences between the two types of adipose tissue include color, vascularity, and metabolic activity.

WHITE (UNILOCULAR) ADIPOSE TISSUE. Unilocular fat cells contain a single lipid droplet, giving the adipose tissue composed of these cells a white color. (If the diet is especially rich in foods containing carotenoids, such as carrots, this adipose tissue will have a yellow color.) White adipose tissue is heavily supplied with blood vessels, which

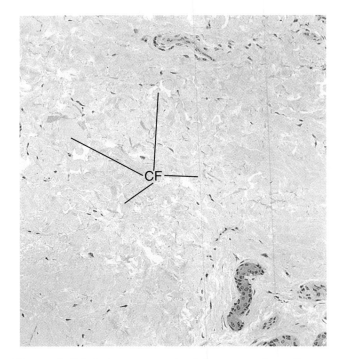

Figure 6-16. Light micrograph of dense irregular collagenous connective tissue from monkey skin (× 132). Observe the many bundles of collagen (CF) in random orientation.

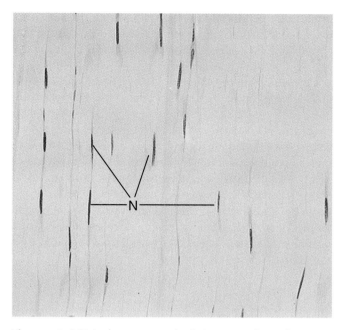

Figure 6–17. Light micrograph of dense regular collagenous connective tissue from monkey tendon (× 270). Note the ordered, parallel array of collagen bundles and the elongated nuclei (N) of the fibroblasts lying between collagen bundles.

form capillary networks throughout the tissue. The vessels gain access via connective tissue septa that partition the fat into lobules (see Fig. 6–6). The plasma membranes of the unilocular adipose cells contain receptors for several substances, including **insulin, growth hormone, norepinephrine,** and **glucocorticoids,** that facilitate the uptake and release of free fatty acids and glycerol.

Unilocular fat is the type present in the subcutaneous layers throughout the body. It also occurs in masses in characteristic sites influenced by sex and age. In men, fat is stored in the neck, in the shoulders, about the hips, and in the buttocks. As men age, the abdominal wall becomes an additional storage area. In women, fat is stored in the breasts, buttocks and hips, and lateral aspects of the thighs. Additionally, fat is stored in both sexes in the abdominal cavity about the omental apron and the mesenteries.

CLINICAL CORRELATIONS

Obesity increases the risks for many health problems, including those involving the cardiovascular system.

In adults, obesity develops in two different ways. **Hypertrophic obesity** results from the accumulation and storage of fat in unilocular fat cells, which may increase their size by as much as four times. **Hypercellular obesity,** as the name implies, results from an overabundance of adipocytes. This type of obesity usually is severe.

Although mature adipocytes do not divide, their precur-

sors proliferate in early postnatal life. There is substantial evidence that overfeeding newborn infants for a few weeks may actually increase the number of adipocyte precursors, leading to an increase in the number of adipocytes and setting the stage for hypercellular obesity in the adult. Overweight infants are at least three times more apt to exhibit obesity as adults than are infants of average weight.

BROWN (MULTILOCULAR) ADIPOSE TISSUE. Brown adipose tissue is composed of multilocular fat cells, which store fat in multiple droplets. This tissue may appear tan to reddish brown because of its extensive vascularity and the chytochromes present in its abundant mitochondria (see Fig. 6–7).

Multilocular adipose tissue has a lobular organization and vascular supply similar to those of a gland. Brown fat tissue is very vascular because the vessels are located near the adipocytes. Unmyelinated nerve fibers enter the tissue with the axons ending on the blood vessels as well as on fat cells, whereas in white fat tissue, the neurons end only on the blood vessels.

Although it has long been known that multilocular fat is found in many mammal species, especially those that hibernate, and in the infants of most mammals, it was unclear whether it existed in adult humans. In the newborn human, brown fat is located in the neck region and in the interscapular region. As humans mature, the fat droplets in brown fat cells coalesce and form into one droplet (similar to white fat

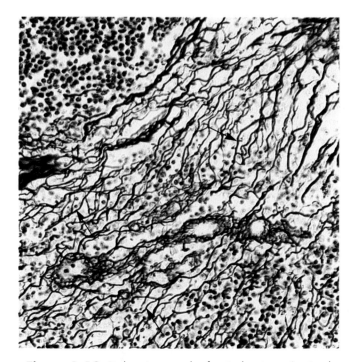

Figure 6–18. Light micrograph of reticular tissue (stained with silver) displaying the networks of reticular fibers (× 270). Many lymphoid cells are interspersed between the reticular fibers (*arrows*).

cells), and the cells become more like those in unilocular fat tissue. Thus, although adults appear to contain only unilocular fat, the evidence is that they also possess brown fat. This can be demonstrated in some of the wasting diseases of the elderly in which multilocular fat tissue forms again and in the same areas as in the newborn.

Brown adipose tissue (brown fat) is associated with body-heat production due to the large number of mitochondria in the multilocular adipocytes composing this tissue. These cells can oxidize fatty acids at up to 20 times the rate of white fat, increasing body-heat production threefold in cold environments. Sensory receptors in the skin send signals to the temperature-regulating center of the brain, which results in sympathetic nerve impulses being relayed directly to the brown fat cells. The neurotransmitter norepinephrine activates the enzyme that cleaves triglycerides into fatty acids and glycerol, initiating heat production by fatty-acid oxidation in the mitochondria. **Thermogenin,** a transmembrane protein located on the inner membrane of mitochondria, permits backflow of protons instead of utilizing them for synthesis of adenosine triphosphate; as a result of uncoupling oxidation from phosphorylation, the proton flow generates energy that is dispersed as heat.

Histogenesis of Adipose Tissue

It is believed that adipose cells are derived from undifferentiated mesenchymal cells, as previously stated, although the actual stem cell, **lipoblast** or **preadipocyte,** has not been identified. However, recent in vitro studies have shown that cells exhibiting adipose-like qualities differ from those displaying fibroblast-like qualities.

The most predominant view is that adipose tissue develops via two separate processes. **Primary fat formation** occurs early in fetal life wherein groups of **epithelioid precursor cells** are distributed at certain locations in the developing fetus; in these tissues, lipid droplets begin to accumulate in the form of brown adipose tissue. Near the end of fetal life, other **fusiform precursor cells** differentiate in many areas of the connective tissues within the fetus and begin to accumulate lipids that coalesce into the single droplet in each cell, thus forming unilocular fat cells found in adults. The latter process has been named **secondary fat formation.**

CLINICAL CORRELATIONS

Tumors of the adipose tissues may be benign or malignant. **Lipomas** are common benign tumors of adipocytes, whereas **liposarcomas** are malignant tumors of adipocytes. The latter form most commonly in the leg and in retroperitoneal tissues, though they may form anywhere in the body. The tumor cells may resemble unilocular adipocytes or they may resemble multilocular adipocytes, another indication that adult humans do indeed possess the two kinds of adipose tissue.

Cartilage and Bone

7

Cartilage and bone are both specialized connective tissues. Cartilage possesses a firm pliable matrix that resists mechanical stresses. Bone matrix, on the other hand, is one of the hardest tissues of the body, and it too resists stresses placed upon it. Both of these connective tissues possess cells that are specialized to secrete the matrix in which the cells become trapped. Although cartilage and bone have many varied functions, some of their functions are similar and related. Both are involved in supporting the body, because they are intimately associated in the skeletal system. Most of the long bones of the body are formed first in the embryo as cartilage, which forms a template that is later replaced by bone; this is referred to as **endochondral bone formation.** This system begins early in the fetus and continues after birth, with more and more of the cartilage being replaced by bone until the person has attained full growth in the skeletal system. Most of the flat bones are formed within preexisting membranous sheaths; this method of osteogenesis is known as **intramembranous bone formation.**

Cartilage

Cartilage possesses cells called **chondrocytes,** which occupy small cavities called **lacunae** within the **extracellular matrix** they secreted. The substance of cartilage is neither vascularized nor supplied with nerves or lymphatic vessels; however, the cells receive their nourishment from blood vessels of surrounding connective tissues by diffusion through the matrix. The extracellular matrix is composed of **glycosaminoglycans** and **proteoglycans,** which are intimately associated with the collagen and elastic fibers embedded in the matrix. The flexibility and resiliency of cartilage to compression permit it to function as a shock absorber, whereas its smooth surface permits almost friction-free movement of the joints of the body as it covers the articulating surfaces of the bones.

There are three types of cartilage based on the fibers present in the matrix (Fig. 7–1). **Hyaline cartilage,** containing type II collagen in its matrix, is the most abundant cartilage in the body and serves many functions. **Elastic cartilage** contains type II collagen and abundant elastic fibers scattered throughout its matrix, giving it more pliability. **Fibrocartilage** possesses dense, coarse type I collagen fibers in its matrix, allowing it to withstand strong tensile forces (Table 7–1).

The perichondrium is a connective tissue sheath covering that lies over most cartilage. It has an outer fibrous layer and inner cellular layer, whose cells secrete cartilage matrix. The perichondrium is vascular, and its vessels supply nutrients to the cells of cartilage. In areas where the cartilage has no perichondrium—for example, the articular surfaces of the bones forming a joint—the cartilage cells receive their nourishment from the synovial fluid that bathes the joint surfaces.

Hyaline Cartilage

Hyaline cartilage, a bluish-gray, semitranslucent, pliable substance, is the most common cartilage of the body. It is located in the nose and larynx, on the ventral ends of the ribs where they articulate with the sternum, and in the tracheal rings and bronchi. Hyaline cartilage is also located on the articulating surfaces of the moveable joints of the body. This cartilage forms the cartilage template of many of the bones during embryonic development and constitutes the epiphyseal plates of growing bones.

Histogenesis and Growth of Hyaline Cartilage

Where cartilage is to form, individual mesenchymal cells retract their processes, round up, and congregate in dense masses called **chondrification centers.** These cells differentiate into **chondroblasts** and commence secreting a matrix around themselves. As this process continues, the chondroblasts become entrapped in their own matrix in small individual compartments called **lacunae.**

HYALINE CARTILAGE

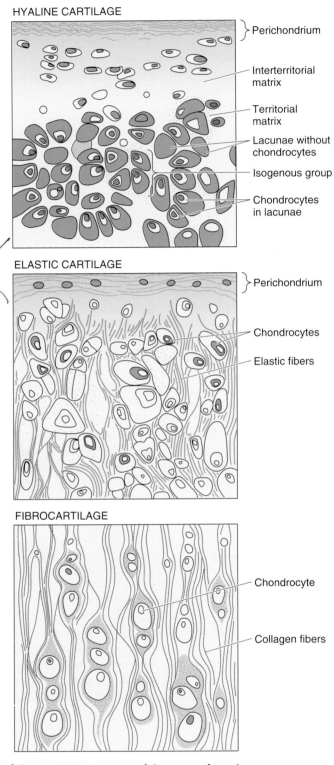

Perichondrium

Interterritorial matrix

Territorial matrix

Lacunae without chondrocytes

Isogenous group

Chondrocytes in lacunae

ELASTIC CARTILAGE

Perichondrium

Chondrocytes

Elastic fibers

FIBROCARTILAGE

Chondrocyte

Collagen fibers

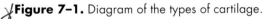

Figure 7–1. Diagram of the types of cartilage.

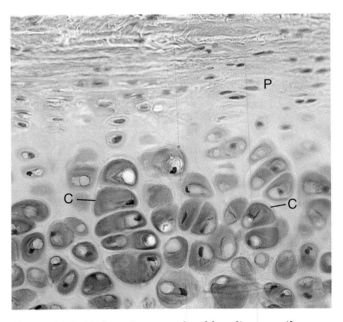

Figure 7–2. Light micrograph of hyaline cartilage (× 270). Observe the large ovoid chondrocytes (C) trapped in their lacunae. Directly above them are the elongated chondroblasts, and at the very top is the perichondrium (P) and the underlying chondrogenic cell layer.

represent one, two, or more cell divisions from an original chondrocyte (see Fig. 7–1). As the cells of an isogenous group manufacture matrix, they are pushed away from each other, forming separate lacunae and thus enlarging the cartilage from within. This type of growth is called **interstitial growth.**

Mesenchymal cells at the periphery of cartilage development differentiate to form fibroblasts. These cells manufacture a dense irregular collagenous connective tissue, the **perichondrium,** responsible for the growth and maintenance of the cartilage. The perichondrium has two layers, an **outer fibrous layer** composed of type I collagen, fibroblasts, and blood vessels, and an **inner cellular layer** composed mostly of **chondrogenic cells.** The chondrogenic cells undergo division and differentiate into chondroblasts, which begin to elaborate matrix. In this way cartilage also grows by adding to its periphery, a process called **appositional growth.**

Interstitial growth occurs only in the early phase of hyaline cartilage formation. However, articular cartilage, which lacks a perichondrium, grows only by interstitial growth. This type also occurs in the **epiphyseal plates** of long bones, where the lacunae are arranged in a longitudinal orientation parallel to the long axis of the bone; therefore, the interstitial growth serves to lengthen the bone. The cartilage in the remainder of the body grows mostly by apposition, a controlled process that may continue during the life of the cartilage.

Chondroblasts surrounded by matrix are referred to as **chondrocytes** (Fig. 7–2). These cells are still capable of cell division, forming a cluster of two to four or more cells in a lacuna. These groups are known as **isogenous groups** and

Table 7–1. Cartilage Types, Characteristics, and Locations

Type of Cartilage	Identifying Characteristics	Perichondrium	Location
Hyaline	Type II collagen, basophilic matrix, chondrocytes usually arranged in groups	Perichondrium present in most places. *Exceptions:* Articular cartilages and epiphyses	Articular ends of long bones, nose, larynx, trachea, bronchi, ventral ends of ribs
Elastic	Type II collagen, elastic fibers	Perichondrium present	Pinna of ear, walls of auditory canal, auditory tube, epiglottis, cuneiform cartilage of larynx
Fibrocartilage	Type I collagen, acidophilic matrix, chondrocytes arranged in parallel rows between bundles of collagen, always associated with dense regular collagenous connective tissue or hyaline cartilage	Perichondrium absent	Intervertebral disks, articular disks, pubic symphysis, insertion of some tendons

Cartilage Cells

Three types of cells are associated with cartilage: chondrogenic cells, chondroblasts, and chondrocytes (see Fig. 7–2).

Chondrogenic cells are spindle-shaped, narrow cells that are derived from mesenchymal cells. They possess an ovoid nucleus with one or two nucleoli. Their cytoplasm is sparse, and electron micrographs of chondrogenic cells display a small Golgi apparatus, a few mitochondria, some profiles of rough endoplasmic reticulum (RER), and an abundance of free ribosomes. These cells can differentiate into chondroblasts as well as into osteoprogenitor cells.

Chondroblasts are derived from two sources: mesenchymal cells within the center of chondrification and **chondrogenic cells** of the inner cellular layer of the perichondrium (as in appositional growth). Chondroblasts are plump, basophilic cells that display the organelles required for protein synthesis. Electron micrographs of these cells demonstrate a rich network of RER, a well-developed Golgi complex, numerous mitochondria, and an abundance of secretory vesicles.

Chondrocytes are chondroblasts that are surrounded by matrix. Those near the periphery are ovoid, whereas those deeper in the cartilage are more rounded, with a diameter of 10 to 30 µm. It should be noted that histological processing creates artifactual shrinkage and distortion of the cells. They display a large nucleus with a prominent nucleolus and the usual organelles of protein-secreting cells. Young chondrocytes possess a pale-staining cytoplasm with many mitochondria, an elaborate RER, a well-developed Golgi

apparatus, and glycogen. Older chondrocytes, which are relatively quiescent, display a greatly reduced complement of organelles, with an abundance of free ribosomes. Thus, these cells can resume active protein synthesis if they revert back to chondroblasts.

Matrix of Hyaline Cartilage

The semitranslucent blue-gray matrix of hyaline cartilage contains up to 40% of its dry weight in collagen. Additionally it contains proteoglycans, glycoproteins, and extracellular fluid. Because the refractive index of the collagen fibrils and the ground substance is nearly the same, the matrix appears to be an amorphous, homogeneous mass with the light microscope. The matrix of hyaline cartilage primarily contains **type II collagen,** but types IX, X, and XI and other minor collagens are also present in small quantities. Type II collagen does not form large bundles, although the bundle thickness increases with distance from the lacunae. Fiber orientation appears to be related to the stresses placed on the cartilage. For example, in articular cartilage, the fibers near the surface are oriented parallel to the surface, whereas deeper fibers seem to be oriented in curved columns.

The matrix is subdivided into two regions: the **territorial matrix** around each lacuna and the **interterritorial matrix.** The **territorial matrix,** a 50 µm wide band, is poor in collagen and rich in chondroitin sulfate, which contributes to its basophilic and intense staining with periodic acid-Schiff (PAS) reagent. The bulk of the matrix is interterritorial matrix, which is richer in type II collagen and poorer in proteoglycans than the territorial matrix.

A small region of the matrix, 1 to 3 μm thick, immediately surrounding the lacuna, and known as the **pericellular capsule** was recently identified. It displays a fine meshwork of collagen fibers embedded in a basal lamina-like substance. These fibers may represent some of the other minor collagens present in hyaline cartilage; some research suggests that the pericellular capsule may protect chondrocytes from mechanical stresses.

Cartilage matrix is rich in **aggrecans,** large proteoglycans molecules composed of protein cores to which glycosaminoglycan molecules (chondroitin-4-sulfate, chondroitin-6-sulfate, and the heparan sulfate) are covalently linked (see Fig. 4–3). As many as 100 to 200 aggrecans molecules are linked noncovalently to hyaluronic acid, forming huge aggrecan composites that can be 3 to 4 μm long. The abundant negative charges associated with these exceedingly large proteoglycan molecules attract cations, predominantly Na^+ ions, which in turn attract water molecules. In this way the cartilage matrix becomes hydrated to such an extent that up to 80% of the wet weight of cartilage is water, resisting forces of compression.

Not only do hydrated proteoglycans fill the interstices among the collagen fiber bundles, but their glycosaminoglycan sidechains also form electrostatic bonds with the collagen. Thus the ground substance and fibers of the matrix form a cross-linked molecular framework that resists tensile forces.

Cartilage matrix also contains the adhesive glycoprotein **chondronectin.** This large molecule, similar to fibronectin, has binding sites for type II collagen, chondroitin-4 and chondroitin-6 sulfates, hyaluronic acid, and integrins (transmembrane proteins) of chondroblasts and chondrocytes. Chondronectin thus assists these cells in maintaining their contact with fibrous and amorphous components of the matrix.

Histophysiology of Cartilage

The smoothness of hyaline cartilage and its ability to resist forces of both compression and tension are essential to its function at the articular surfaces of joints. Because cartilage is avascular, nutrients and oxygen must diffuse through the water of hydration present in the matrix. The inefficiency of such a system necessitates a limit on the width of cartilage. There is a constant turnover in the proteoglycans of cartilage that changes with age. Hormones and vitamins also exert influence over the growth, development, and function of cartilage. Many of these substances also affect skeletal formation and growth (Table 7–2).

Table 7–2. Effects of Hormones and Vitamins on Hyaline Cartilage

Hormones	Effects on Cartilage
Thyroxine, testosterone, and somatotropin (via somatomedin)	Stimulate cartilage growth and matrix formation
Cortisone, hydrocortisone, and estradiol	Inhibit cartilage growth and matrix formation
Vitamins	
Hypovitaminosis A	Reduces width of epiphyseal plates
Hypervitaminosis A	Accelerates ossification of epiphyseal plates
Hypovitaminosis C	Inhibits matrix synthesis and deforms architecture of epiphyseal plate; leads to scurvy
Absence of vitamin D resulting in deficiency in absorption of calcium and phosphorus	Proliferation of chondrocytes is normal but matrix does not become calcified properly; results in rickets

CLINICAL CORRELATIONS

Hyaline cartilage degenerates when the chondrocytes hypertrophy and die and the matrix begins to calcify. This process is a normal and integral part of endochondral bone formation. However, it is also a natural process of aging, often resulting in less mobility and pain in the joints.

Cartilage regeneration is usually poor except in children. Chondrogenic cells from the perichondrium enter the defect and form new cartilage. If the defect is large, the cells will form dense connective tissue to repair the scar.

Elastic Cartilage

Elastic cartilage is located in the pinna of the ear, the external and internal auditory tubes, the epiglottis, and the larynx (cuneiform cartilage). Because of the presence of elastic fibers, elastic cartilage is somewhat yellow and is more opaque than hyaline cartilage in the fresh state.

In most respects, elastic cartilage is identical to hyaline cartilage and is often associated with it. The outer fibrous layer of the perichondrium is rich in elastic fibers. The matrix of elastic cartilage possesses abundant fine-to-course branching elastic fibers interposed with type II collagen fiber bundles, giving it much more flexibility than the matrix of hyaline cartilage (Fig. 7–3). The chondrocytes of elastic cartilage are more abundant and larger than those of hyaline

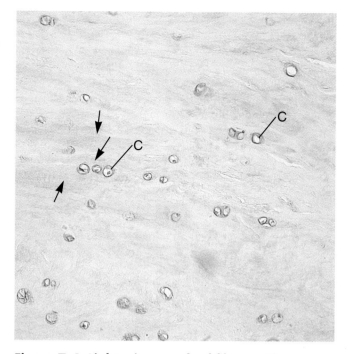

Figure 7–4. Light micrograph of fibrocartilage (×132). Note alignment of the chondrocytes (C) in rows interspersed with thick bundles of collagen fibers (*arrows*).

cartilage. The matrix is not as ample as in hyaline cartilage, and the elastic fiber bundles of the territorial matrix are larger and coarser than those of the interterritorial matrix.

Fibrocartilage

Fibrocartilage is found in intervertebral disks, in pubic symphysis, in articular disks, and attached to bone. It is associated with hyaline cartilage and with dense connective tissue, which it resembles. Unlike the other two types of cartilage, fibrocartilage does not possess a perichondrium, displays a scant amount of matrix (rich in chondroitin sulfate and dermatan sulfate), and exhibits bundles of type I collagen, which stain acidophilic (Fig. 7–4). Chondrocytes are often aligned in alternating parallel rows with the thick, coarse bundles of collagen, which parallel the tensile forces attendant on this tissue.

Chondrocytes of fibrocartilage usually arise from fibroblasts that begin to manufacture proteoglycans. As the ground substance surrounds the fibroblast, the cell becomes incarcerated in its own matrix and differentiates into a chondrocyte.

Intervertebral disks represent an example of the organization of fibrocartilage. They are interposed between the hyaline cartilage coverings of the articular surface of successive vertebrae. Each disk contains a gelatinous center, called the **nucleus pulposus,** which is composed of cells derived from the notochord, lying within a hyaluronic acid–rich matrix.

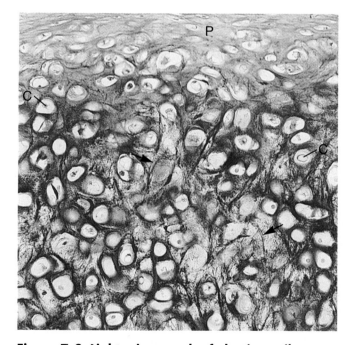

Figure 7–3. Light micrograph of elastic cartilage (×132). Observe the perichondrium (P) and the chondrocytes (C) in their lacunae (shrunken from the walls because of processing), some of which contain more than one cell, evidence of interstitial growth. Note the elastic fibers (*arrows*) scattered throughout.

These cells disappear by the 20th year of life. Much of the nucleus pulposus is surrounded by the **annulus fibrosus,** layers of fibrocartilage whose type I collagen fibers run vertically between the hyaline cartilages of the two vertebrae. The fibers of adjacent lamellae are oriented obliquely to each other, providing support to the gelatinous nucleus pulposus. The annulus fibrosus provides resistance against tensile forces, whereas the nucleus pulposus resists forces of compression.

CLINICAL CORRELATIONS

A **ruptured disk** refers to a tear or break in the laminae of the annulus fibrosus, through which the gel-like nucleus pulposus extrudes. This condition occurs more often on the posterior portions of the disks, particularly in the lumbar portion of the back where the disk may dislocate, or slip. A **"slipped disk"** leads to severe, intense pain in the lower back and extremities from the displaced disk compressing the lower spinal nerves.

Bone

Bone is a specialized connective tissue whose extracellular matrix is calcified, incarcerating the cells that secreted it. Although bone is one of the hardest substances of the body, it is a dynamic tissue that constantly changes shape in relation to the stresses placed on it. For example, pressures applied to bone lead to its resorption, whereas tension applied to it results in development of new bone.

Bone is the primary structural framework for support and protection of the organs of the body, including the brain and spinal cord and the structures within the thoracic cavity, namely the lungs and heart. The bones also serve as levers for the muscles attached to them, thereby multiplying the force of the muscles to attain movement. Bone is a reservoir for several minerals of the body—for example, it stores about 99% of the body's calcium. Bone contains a central cavity, the **marrow cavity,** which houses the **bone marrow,** a hemopoietic organ.

Bone is covered on its external surface, except at synovial articulations, with a **periosteum,** which consists of an outer layer of dense fibrous connective tissue and an inner cellular layer containing osteoprogenitor (osteogenic) cells. The central cavity of a bone is lined with **endosteum,** a specialized thin connective tissue composed of a monolayer of **osteoprogenitor cells** and **osteoblasts.**

Bone is composed of cells lying in an extracellular matrix that has become calcified. The calcified matrix is composed of fibers and ground substance. The fibers constituting bone are primarily type I collagen. The ground substance is rich in proteoglycans with chondroitin sulfate and keratan sulfate sidechains. Additionally glycoproteins, such as osteonectin, osteocalcin, osteopontin, and bone sialoprotein, are also present.

The cells of bone include **osteogenic cells,** which differentiate into **osteoblasts.** Osteoblasts are responsible for secreting the matrix. Once these cells are surrounded by matrix, they become quiescent and are known as osteocytes. The spaces osteocytes occupy are known as lacunae (Fig. 7–5). **Osteoclasts,** multinucleated giant cells derived from fused bone marrow precursors, are responsible for bone resorption and remodeling.

Because bone is such a hard tissue there are two methods employed to prepare it for study. **Decalcified sections** can be prepared by decalcifying the bone in an acid solution to remove the calcium salts. The tissue can then be embedded, sectioned, and routinely stained for study. **Ground sections,** the other method of preparing bone sections for study, involve sawing the bone into thin slices, followed by grinding the sections with abrasives between glass plates. When the section is sufficiently thin for study with light microscope, it is mounted for study. Each system has disadvantages: in decalcified sections, osteocytes are distorted from the decalcifying acid bath; in ground sections, the cells are destroyed, and the lacunae and canaliculi are filled in with bone debris.

Bone Matrix

Bone matrix has inorganic and organic constituents.

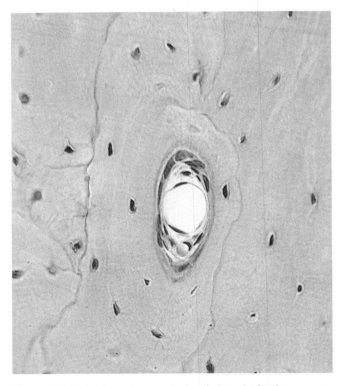

Figure 7–5. Light micrograph of decalcified compact bone (× 540). Osteocytes may be observed in lacunae. Also note the osteon and the cementing lines.

Inorganic Component

The **inorganic portion** of bone, which constitutes about 65% of its dry weight, is composed mainly of calcium and phosphorus, along with other components including bicarbonate, citrate, magnesium, sodium, and potassium. Calcium and phosphorus exist primarily in the form of **hydroxyapatite crystals** [$Ca_{10}(PO_4)_6(OH)_2$], but calcium phosphate is also present in an amorphous form. Hydroxyapatite crystals (40 nm in length by 25 nm in width and 1.5 to 3 nm in thickness) are arranged in an ordered fashion along the type I collagen fibers; they are deposited into the gap regions of the collagen but also are present along the overlap region. The free surface of the crystals is surrounded by amorphous ground substance. The surface ions of the crystals attract H_2O and form a **hydration shell,** which permits ion exchange with the extracellular fluid.

Bone is one of the hardest and strongest substances in the body. Its hardness and strength are due to the association of hydroxyapatite crystals with collagen. If bone is decalcified (i.e., all of the mineral is removed from the bone), it still retains its original shape but becomes so flexible that it can be bent like a piece of tough rubber. If the organic component is extracted from bone, the mineralized skeleton still retains its original shape, but it becomes extremely brittle and can be fractured with ease.

Organic Component

The **organic component** of bone matrix, constituting approximately 35% of the dry weight of bone, includes fibers that are almost exclusively type I collagen.

Collagen, most of which is type I, makes up about 90% of the organic component of bone. It is formed in large (50 to 70 nm in diameter) bundles displaying the typical 67-nm periodicity. Type I collagen in bone is highly cross-linked, preventing it from being easily extracted.

The fact that bone matrix stains with PAS reagent and displays slight metachromasia indicates the presence of sulfated glycosaminoglycans—namely, chondroitin sulfate and keratan sulfate. These form small proteoglycan molecules, with short protein cores to which the glycosaminoglycans are covalently bound. The proteoglycans are covalently bound, via link proteins, to hyaluronic acid, forming **aggrecan composites.** The abundance of collagen, however, causes the matrix to be acidophilic.

Several glycoproteins also are present in the bone matrix. These appear to be restricted to bone, including **osteocalcin,** which binds to hydroxyapatite, and **osteopontin,** which also binds to hydroxyapatite but has additional binding sites for other components as well as for integrins present on osteoblasts and osteoclasts. Vitamin D stimulates the synthesis of these glycoproteins. **Bone sialoprotein,** another matrix protein, has binding sites for matrix components and integrins of osteoblasts and osteocytes, suggesting its involvement in the adherence of these cells to bone matrix.

Cells of Bone

Osteoprogenitor Cells

Osteoprogenitor cells are located in the inner cellular layer of the periosteum, lining haversian canals, and in the endosteum (see Fig. 7–5). These cells, derived from embryonic mesenchyme, can undergo mitotic division and have the potential of differentiating into osteoblasts. Moreover, under certain conditions of low oxygen tension, these cells may differentiate into chondrogenic cells. Osteoprogenitor cells are spindle-shaped and possesses a pale-staining oval nucleus; their scant pale-staining cytoplasm displays sparse RER and a poorly developed Golgi apparatus but an abundance of free ribosomes. These cells are most active during the period of intense bone growth.

Osteoblasts

Osteoblasts, derived from osteoprogenitor cells, are responsible for the synthesis of the organic components of the bone matrix, including collagen, proteoglycans, and glycoproteins. Osteoblasts are located on the surface of the bone in a sheet-like arrangement of cuboidal-to-columnar cells (Fig. 7–6). When actively secreting matrix, they exhibit a basophilic cytoplasm.

The organelles of osteoblasts are polarized so that the nucleus is located away from the region of secretory activity, which houses secretory granules believed to contain matrix

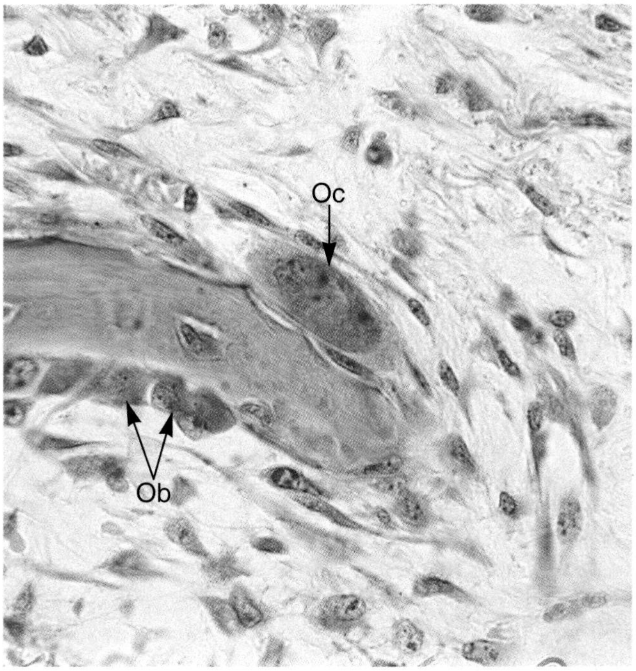

Figure 7–6. Light micrograph of intramembranous ossification (× 540). Osteoblasts (Ob) line the bony spicule where they are secreting osteoid onto the bone. Osteoclasts (Oc) may be observed housed in Howship's lacunae.

precursors. The contents of these vesicles stain pink with PAS reagent.

Electron micrographs exhibit abundant RER, a well-developed Golgi complex (Fig. 7–7A), and numerous secretory vesicles containing flocculent material that accounts for the PAS-staining pink vacuoles observed in the light microscope. Osteoblasts extend processes that contact neighboring osteoblasts and form **gap junctions.**

CLINICAL CORRELATIONS

During active bone formation, osteoblasts secrete high levels of alkaline phosphatase, which elevates the levels of this enzyme in the blood. Thus the clinician can monitor bone formation by measuring the blood alkaline phosphatase level.

A clear zone is observed between osteoblasts and bone; this represents the **osteoid,** the uncalcified bone matrix. During calcification, calcium salts are deposited in the osteoid, but osteoblasts that remain on the bone surface are always separated from calcified bone by an osteoid. As the secreted matrix accumulates, each osteoblast becomes surrounded by the matrix; once this occurs, the cell is referred to as an osteocyte, and the space it occupies is known as a **lacuna.**

Surface osteoblasts that cease to form matrix revert to a quiescent state and are called **bone-lining cells.** Although these cells appear to be similar to osteoprogenitor cells, they most likely are incapable of dividing but can be reactivated to the secreting form with the proper stimulus. These quiescent osteoblasts are also separated from the calcified bone by a thin layer of bone matrix.

Osteoblasts have **parathyroid hormone receptors** on their cell membranes. When parathyroid hormone binds to these receptors, it stimulates osteoblasts to secrete **osteoclast-stimulating factor,** which activates osteoclasts to resorb bone. Osteoblasts also secrete enzymes responsible for removing osteoid, so that osteolclasts can contact the bone.

Osteocytes

Osteocytes are mature bone cells, derived from osteoblasts, that are housed in **lacunae** within the calcified bony matrix (see Figs. 7–5, 7–7B). Radiating out in all directions from the lacuna are narrow, tunnel-like spaces called **canaliculi,** which house cytoplasmic processes of the osteocyte. These processes contact similar processes of neighboring osteocytes, forming **gap junctions** through which ions and small molecules can move between the cells. The canaliculi also contain nutrients and metabolites, which nourish the osteocytes.

Osteocytes conform to the shape of their lacunae. Their nucleus is flattened, and their cytoplasm is poor in or-

ganelles, displaying scant RER and a greatly reduced Golgi apparatus. Though osteocytes appear to be inactive cells, they secrete substances necessary for bone maintenance.

Osteoclasts

The precursor of the **osteoclast** originates in the bone marrow. Osteoclasts have receptors for osteoclast-stimulating factor and for calcitonin. These cells are responsible for resorbing bone.

MORPHOLOGY OF OSTEOCLASTS. Osteoclasts are large, motile, multinucleated cells 150 μm in diameter; they contain up to 50 nuclei, and have an acidophilic cytoplasm (see Fig. 7–6). Until recently, osteoclasts were thought to be derived from the fusion of many blood-derived monocytes, but the newest evidence shows that they have a bone-marrow precursor in common with monocytes, the **granulocyte-macrophage progenitor cell (GM-CSF).** In the presence of bone, these osteoclast precursors fuse to produce the multinucleated osteoclast in response to a factor (or factors) released by osteoblasts (or osteocytes).

Osteoclasts occupy shallow depressions, called **Howship's lacunae,** which identify regions of bone resorption. An osteoclast active in bone resorption may be subdivided into four morphologically recognizable regions: the basal zone, ruffled border, clear zone, and vesicular zone.

The **basal zone,** located the farthest from Howship's lacuna, houses most of the organelles, including the multiple nuclei and their associated Golgi complexes and centrioles. Mitochondria, RER, and polysomes are distributed throughout the cell but are more numerous near the ruffled border.

The **ruffled border** is that portion of the cell that is directly involved in the resorption of bone. Its finger-like processes are active and dynamic, changing their configuration continually as they project into the resorption compartment, known as the **subosteoclastic compartment.** The cytoplasmic aspect of the ruffled border plasmalemma displays a regularly spaced, bristle-like coat that increases the thickness of the plasma membrane of this region.

The **clear zone** is the region of the cell that immediately surrounds the periphery of the ruffled border. It is organelle-free but contains many actin microfilaments, which appear to function in helping integrins of the clear-zone plasmalemma maintain contact with the bony periphery of Howship's lacuna. The cytoplasm in this region is so closely applied to the bone that it is called the **sealing zone** of the **subosteoclastic compartment.**

The **vesicular zone** of the osteoclast consists of numerous endocytotic and exocytotic vesicles that ferry lysosomal enzymes into the subosteoclastic compartment and the products of bone degradation into the cell (Fig. 7–8). The vesicular zone is between the basal zone and the ruffled border.

By isolating the subosteoclastic compartment from the surrounding region, the clear zone delimits a microenviron-

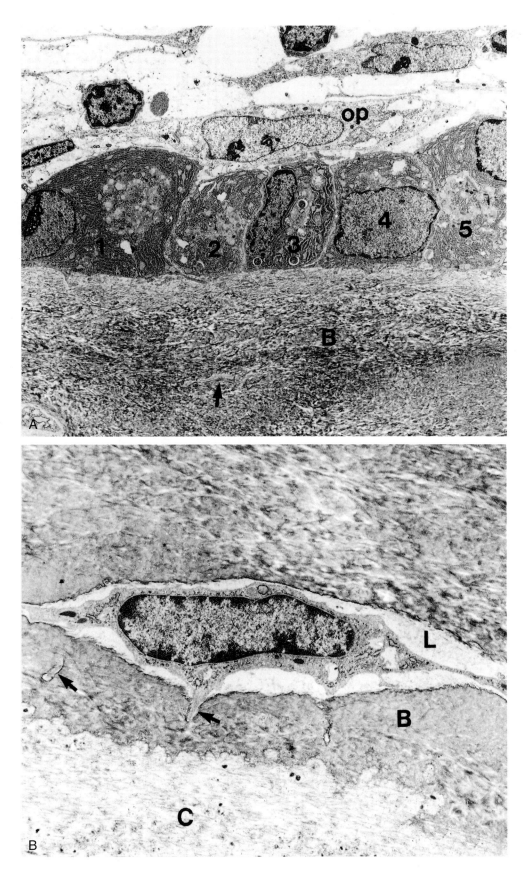

Figure 7–7. Electron micrograph of bone-forming cells. A, Observe the five osteoblasts (numbered 1 to 5) lined up on the surface of bone (B) displaying abundant rough endoplasmic reticulum. The arrow indicates the process of an osteocyte in a canaliculus. The cell with the elongated nucleus lying above the osteoblasts is an osteoprogenitor cell (op). (× 2900.) **B,** Note the osteocyte in its lacuna (L) with its processes extending into canaliculi. B, bone; C, cartilage. (× 1200.) (From Marks, S.C. Jr., and Popoff, S.N.: Bone cell biology: The regulation of development, structure, and function in the skeleton. Am. J. Anat. **183:**1–44, 1988. Copyright © 1988. Reprinted by permission of John Wiley & Sons, Inc.)

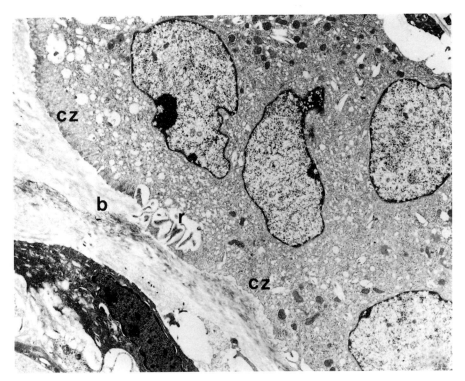

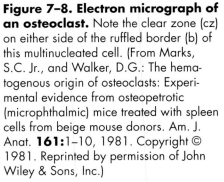

Figure 7–8. Electron micrograph of an osteoclast. Note the clear zone (cz) on either side of the ruffled border (b) of this multinucleated cell. (From Marks, S.C. Jr., and Walker, D.G.: The hematogenous origin of osteoclasts: Experimental evidence from osteopetrotic (microphthalmic) mice treated with spleen cells from beige mouse donors. Am. J. Anat. **161:**1–10, 1981. Copyright © 1981. Reprinted by permission of John Wiley & Sons, Inc.)

ment whose contents may be modulated by cellular activities. The formation of the ruffled border increases the surface area of the plasmalemma in the region of bone resorption, enhancing the resorptive process.

MECHANISM OF BONE RESORPTION. Within osteoclasts, the enzyme **carbonic anhydrase** catalyzes the intracellular formation of carbonic acid (H_2CO_3) from carbon dioxide and water. Carbonic acid is unstable and dissociates within the cells into H^+ ions and bicarbonate ions, HCO_3^-. The bicarbonate ions, accompanied by Na^+ ions, cross the plasmalemma and enter nearby capillaries. Proton pumps in the plasmalemma of the ruffled border of the osteoclasts actively transport H^+ ions into the subosteoclastic compartment, reducing the pH of the microenvironment (Cl^- ions follow passively). The inorganic component of the matrix is dissolved as the environment becomes acidic; the liberated minerals enter the osteoclast cytoplasm to be delivered to nearby capillaries.

Lysosomal hydrolases and **collagenase,** which are secreted by osteoclasts into the subosteoclastic compartment, degrade the organic components of the decalcified bone matrix. The degradation products are endocytosed by the osteoclasts and further broken down into amino acids, monosaccharides, and disaccharides, which then are released into nearby capillaries.

HORMONAL CONTROL OF BONE RESORPTION. The bone-resorbing activity of osteoclasts is regulated by two hormones: parathyroid hormone and calcitonin, produced by the parathyroid and thyroid gland, respectively.

Bone Structure

Bones are classified according to their shape: **long bones,** which display a shaft located between two heads (e.g., tibia); **short bones,** which have more or less the same width and length (e.g., carpal bones of the wrist); **flat bones,** which are flat, thin, and plate-like (e.g., bones forming the brain case of the skull); and **irregular bones,** which have an irregular shape that does not fit into the other classes (e.g., sphenoid and ethmoid bones within the skull). **Sesamoid bones,** another type of bone, develop within tendons, where they increase the mechanical advantage for the muscle (e.g., patella) across a joint.

Gross Observation of Bone

Gross observations of the femur (a long bone) cut in longitudinal section reveal two different types of bone structure. The very dense bone on the outside surface is **compact bone,** whereas the porous portion lining the marrow cavity is **cancellous** or **spongy bone** (Fig. 7–9). Closer observation of the spongy bone reveals branching bony **trabeculae** and **spicules** jutting out from the internal surface of the compact bone into the marrow cavity. There are no haversian systems in spongy bone, but there are irregular arrangements of lamellae. These contain lacunae housing osteocytes that are nourished by diffusion from the marrow cavity, which is

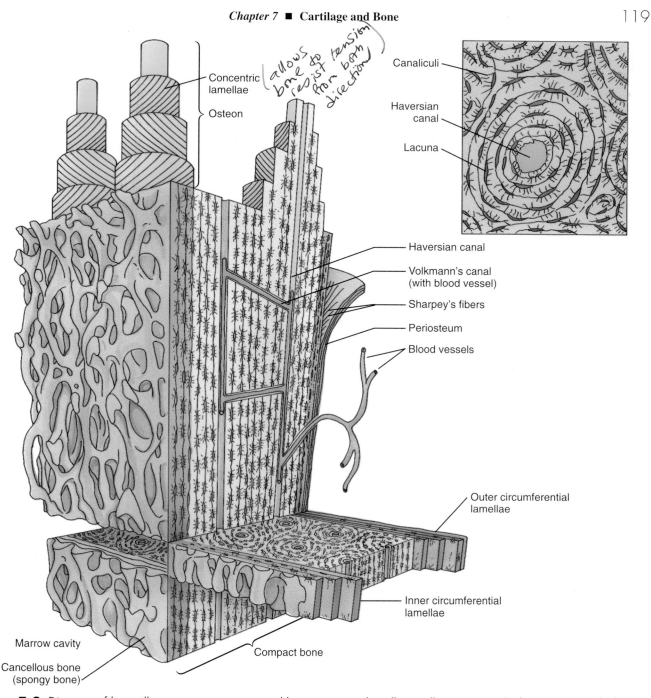

Figure 7–9. Diagram of bone illustrating compact cortical bone, osteons, lamellae, Volkmann's canals, haversian canals, lacunae, canaliculi, and spongy bone.

filled with bone marrow. Bone marrow exists as two types: **red bone marrow,** where blood cells are forming, and **yellow bone marrow,** composed mostly of fat.

The shaft of the bone is called the **diaphysis,** and the articular ends are called the **epiphyses** (singular form: *epiphysis*). In a person who is still growing, the diaphysis is separated from each epiphysis by the **epiphyseal plate** of cartilage. The articular end of the bone is enlarged and sculpted to articulate with its bony counterpart of the joint.

The surface of the articulating end is covered with only a thin layer of compact bone overlying spongy bone. On top of this is the highly polished articular hyaline cartilage, which reduces friction as it moves against the articular cartilage of the bony counterpart of the joint. The area of transition between the epiphyseal plate and the diaphysis is called the **metaphysis,** where columns of spongy bone are located. It is from the epiphyseal plate and the metaphysis that bone grows in length.

The diaphysis is covered by a **periosteum** except where tendons and muscles insert into the bone. Also, there is no periosteum on the surfaces of bone covered by articular cartilage. Periosteum is also absent from sesamoid bones (e.g., patella), which are formed within tendons and function to increase the mechanical advantage across a joint. The periosteum is a noncalcified, dense, irregular, collagenous connective tissue covering the bone on its external surface and inserting into it via **Sharpey's fibers** (see Fig. 7–9). Periosteum is composed of two layers, an **outer fibrous layer,** whose primary function is to distribute vascular and nerve supply to bone, and an **inner cellular layer,** possessing osteoprogenitor cells.

The flat bones of the skull develop by a different method than most of the long bones of the body. The inner and outer surfaces of the calvaria (skull cap) possess two relatively thick layers of compact bone called the **inner** and **outer tables,** which surround the spongy bone (**diploë**) sandwiched between them. The outer table possesses a periosteum, the **pericranium;** internally the inner table is lined with **dura mater,** which serves as a periosteum for the inner table and as a protective covering for the brain.

Bone Types Based on Microscopic Observations

Microscopic observations reveal two types of bone: **primary bone,** known also as **immature** or **woven bone;** and **secondary bones,** known also as **mature** or **lamellar bone.**

Primary bone is an immature form of bone in that it is the first bone to form during fetal development and during bone repair. It has abundant osteocytes and irregular bundles of collagen, which are later replaced and organized as secondary bone except in certain areas (e.g., at sutures of the calvaria, insertions sites of tendons, and alveoli of teeth). The mineral content of primary bone is also much less than that of secondary bone.

Secondary bone is mature bone composed of parallel or concentric lamellae, 3 to 7 μm thick. Osteocytes in their lacunae are dispersed at regular intervals between, or occasionally within, lamellae. Canaliculi, housing osteocytic processes, connect neighboring lacunae with each other, forming a network of intercommunicating channels that facilitate the flow of nutrients, hormones, and waste products to and from osteocytes. Additionally, osteocytic processes within these canaliculi contact similar processes of neighboring osteocytes and form gap junctions, permitting these cells to communicate with each other.

Because the matrix of secondary bone is more calcified, it is stronger than primary bone. Additionally, the collagen fibers of secondary bone are arranged so that they parallel each other within a given lamella.

Lamellar Systems of Compact Bone

Compact bone is composed of lamellae arranged in four lamellar systems that are especially evident in the diaphyses of long bones. These lamellar systems are: outer circumferential lamellae, inner circumferential lamellae, haversian canal systems (osteons), and interstitial lamellae.

OUTER AND INNER CIRCUMFERENTIAL LAMELLAE. The **outer circumferential lamellae** are just deep to the periosteum, forming the outermost region of the diaphysis, and contain Sharpey's fibers anchoring the periosteum to the bone (see Fig. 7–9).

The **inner circumferential lamellae,** analogous to but not as extensive as outer circumferential lamellae, completely encircle the marrow cavity. Trabeculae of spongy bone extend from the inner circumferential lamellae into the marrow cavity, interrupting the endosteal lining of the inner circumferential lamellae.

HAVERSIAN CANAL SYSTEM (OSTEON) AND INTERSTITIAL LAMELLAE. The bulk of compact bone is composed of an abundance of **haversian canal systems (osteons);** each system is composed of cylinders of lamellae, concentrically arranged around a vascular space known as the **haversian canal** (see Figs. 7–9, 7–10). Frequently the osteons bifurcate along their considerable length. Each osteon is bounded by a thin **cementing line,** composed mostly

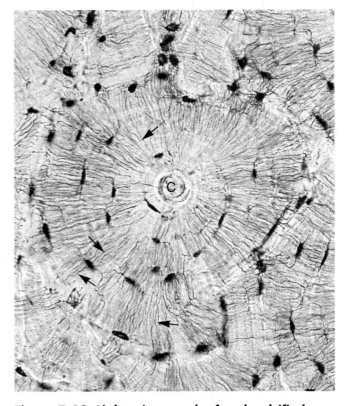

Figure 7–10. Light micrograph of undecalcified ground bone (× **270**). Observe the haversian system containing the haversian canal (C) and concentric lamellae with lacunae with their canaliculi (*arrows*).

of calcified ground substance with a scant amount of collagen fibers (see Fig. 7–5).

Collagen fiber bundles are parallel to each other within a lamella but are oriented almost perpendicular to those of adjacent lamellae. This arrangement is possible because the collagen fibers follow a helical arrangement around the haversian canal within each lamella but are pitched differently in adjacent lamellae.

Each haversian canal, lined by a layer of osteoblasts and osteoprogenitor cells, houses a neurovascular bundle with its associated connective tissue. Haversian canals of adjacent osteons are connected to each other by **Volkmann canals** (Figs. 7–9, 7–11). These vascular spaces are oriented oblique to or perpendicular to haversian canals.

The diameter of haversian canals varies from approximately 20 to about 100 μm. During the formation of osteons, the lamella closest to the cementing line is the first one to be formed. As additional lamellae are added to the system, the diameter of the haversian canal is reduced, and the thickness of the osteon wall increases. Because nutrients from blood vessels of the haversian canal must traverse canaliculi to reach osteocytes, an inefficient process, most osteons possess only 4 to 20 lamellae.

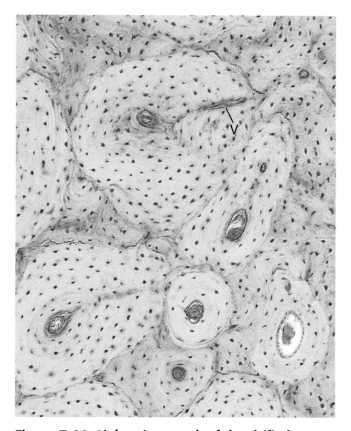

Figure 7–11. Light micrograph of decalcified compact bone (× 132). Several osteons are displayed with their concentric lamellae. A Volkmann's canal (V) is also displayed.

As bone is being remodeled, osteoclasts resorb osteons and osteoblasts replace them. Remnants of osteons remain as irregular arcs of lamellar fragments, known as **interstitial lamellae,** surrounded by osteons. Similar to osteons, interstitial lamellae are also surrounded by cementing lines.

Histogenesis of Bone

Bone formation during embryonic development may occur in two ways: **intramembranous bone formation** and **endochondral bone formation.** The bone that is formed by either of the two methods is identical histologically. The first bone formed is primary bone, which is later resorbed and replaced by secondary bone. Secondary bone continues to be resorbed throughout life, although at a slower rate.

Intramembranous Bone Formation

Most flat bones are formed by **intramembranous bone formation.** This process occurs in a richly vascularized mesenchymal tissue, whose cells contact each other via long processes.

Mesenchymal cells differentiate into **osteoblasts** that secrete **bone matrix,** forming a network of **spicules** and **trabeculae** whose surfaces are populated by these cells (Figs. 7–12, 7–13). This region of initial osteogenesis is known as the **primary ossification center.** The collagen fibers of these developing spicules and trabeculae are randomly oriented as expected in primary bone. Calcification quickly follows osteoid formation, and osteoblasts trapped in their matrices become osteocytes. The processes of these osteocytes are also surrounded by forming bone, establishing a system of canaliculi. Continuous mitotic activity of mesenchymal cells provides a supply of undifferentiated **osteoprogenitor cells,** which form osteoblasts.

As the sponge-like network of trabeculae is established, the vascular connective tissue in their interstices is transformed into bone marrow. The addition of trabeculae to the periphery increases the size of the forming bone. Larger bones, such as the occipital bone of the base of the skull, have several ossification centers, which fuse with each other to form a single bone. The fontanelles ("soft spots") on the frontal and parietal bones of a newborn infant represent ossification centers that are not fused prenatally.

Regions of the mesenchymal tissues that remain uncalcified differentiate into the periosteum and endosteum of developing bone. Moreover, the spongy bone deep to the periosteum and the periosteal layer of the dura mater of flat bones are transformed into compact bone, forming the **inner** and **outer tables** with the intervening diploë.

Endochondral Bone Formation

Most of the long and short bones of the body develop by **endochondral bone formation.** This type of bone formation

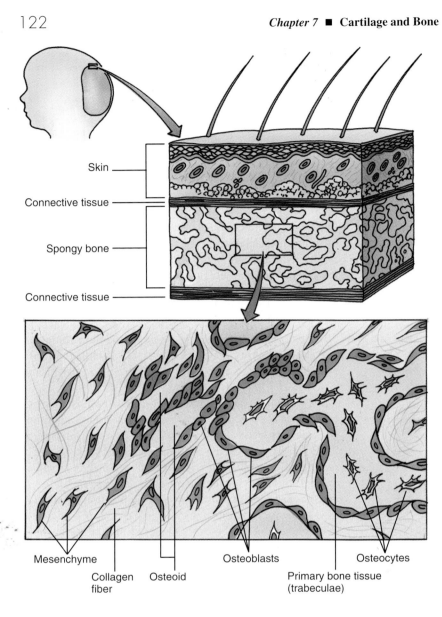

Skin

Connective tissue

Spongy bone

Connective tissue

Mesenchyme

Collagen fiber   Osteoid

Osteoblasts

Primary bone tissue (trabeculae)

Osteocytes

Figure 7–12. Diagram of intramembranous bone formation.

occurs in two steps: (1) a miniature hyaline cartilage model is formed; and (2) the cartilage model continues to grow and serves as a structural scaffold for bone development, is resorbed, and is replaced by bone. Table 7–3 summarizes the events in endochondral bone formation, and Figure 7–14 illustrates the process.

EVENTS IN ENDOCHONDRAL BONE FORMATION

- In the region where bone is to grow within the embryo, a **hyaline cartilage model of that bone is developed.** This event begins in exactly the same way that hyaline cartilage at any location would be developed, as discussed earlier. For a period this model grows, both appositionally and interstitially. Eventually the chondrocytes in the center of the cartilage model hypertrophy, accumulate glycogen in their cytoplasm, and become vacuolated (Fig. 7–15). Hypertrophy of the chondrocytes results in enlargement of

their lacunae and reduction in the intervening cartilage matrix septa, which become calcified.

PRIMARY CENTER OF OSSIFICATION

- Concurrently the perichondrium at the **midriff of the diaphysis of cartilage becomes vascularized** (Fig. 7–16). When this happens, chondrogenic cells become osteoprogenitor cells forming osteoblasts, and the overlying perichondrium becomes a periosteum.
- The newly formed **osteoblasts secrete bone matrix, forming the subperiosteal bone collar** on the surface of the cartilage template by intramembranous bone formation.
- The bone collar prevents the diffusion of nutrients to the hypertrophied chondrocytes within the core of the cartilage model, causing them to die. This process is responsible for the presence of empty, confluent lacunae forming

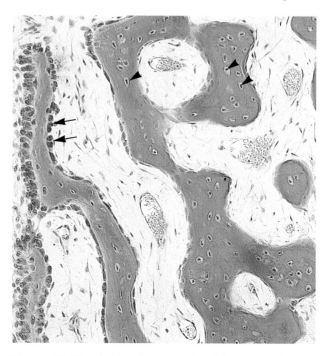

Figure 7–13. Light micrograph of intramembranous ossification (× 132). Trabeculae of bone are being formed by osteoblasts lining their surface (*arrows*). Observe osteocytes trapped in lacunae (*arrowheads*) and that primitive osteons are beginning to form.

large concavities—the future marrow cavity—in the center of the cartilage model.

- Holes etched in the bone collar by osteoclasts permit an osteogenic or **periosteal bud,** composed of osteoprogenitor cells, hemopoietic cells, and blood vessels, to enter the concavities within the cartilage model (see Fig. 7–14).
- Osteoprogenitor cells divide to form osteoblasts. These newly formed cells elaborate bone matrix on the surface of the calcified cartilage. The bone matrix becomes calcified to form a **calcified cartilage/calcified bone complex.** This complex can be appreciated in routinely stained histological sections because calcified cartilage stains basophilic, whereas calcified bone stains acidophilic.
- As the subperiosteal bone becomes thicker and grows in each direction from the midriff of the diaphysis toward the epiphyses, osteoclasts begin resorbing the calcified cartilage/calcified bone complex enlarging the marrow cavity. As this process continues, the cartilage of the diaphysis is replaced by bone, except for the **epiphyseal plates,** which are responsible for the continued growth of the bone for 18 to 20 years.

SECONDARY CENTERS OF OSSIFICATION. Secondary centers of ossification begin to form at the epiphysis at each end of the bone by a process similar to that in the diaphysis, except that a bone collar is not formed.

Rather, osteoprogenitor cells invade the cartilage of the epiphysis, differentiate into osteoblasts, and begin secreting matrix on the cartilage scaffold (see Fig. 7–14). These events take place and progress much as they do in the diaphysis, and eventually the cartilage of the epiphysis is replaced with bone, except at the articular surface and at the epiphyseal plate. The articular surface of the bone remains cartilaginous throughout life. The process at the epiphyseal plate, which controls bone length, is described in the next section.

These events are a dynamic continuum that is completed over a number of years as bone growth and development progresses toward the growing epiphyses at each end of the bone (see Table 7-3). At the same time the bone is constantly being remodeled to meet the changing needs placed on it.

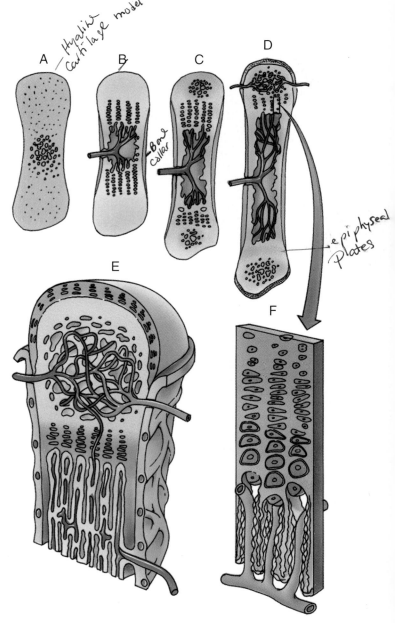

Figure 7–14. Diagram of endochondral bone formation.

Table 7-3. Events in Endochondral Bone Formation

Event	Description
Hyaline cartilage model formed	Miniature hyaline cartilage model formed in region of developing embryo where bone is to develop. Some chondrocytes mature, hypertrophy, and die. Cartilage matrix becomes calcified.
Primary Center of Ossification	
Endochondrium at the midriff of diaphysis becomes vascularized	Vascularization of endochondrium [*Perichondrium*] changes it to periosteum. Chondrogenic cells become osteoprogenitor cells.
Osteoblasts secrete matrix, forming subperiosteal bone collar	The subperiosteal bone collar is formed of primary bone (intramembranous bone formation).
Chondrocytes within the diaphysis core hypertrophy, die, and degenerate	Presence of periosteum and bone collar prevents diffusion of nutrients to chondrocytes. Their degeneration leaves lacunae, opening large spaces in septa of cartilage.
Osteoclasts etch holes in subperiosteal bone collar, permitting entrance of osteogenic bud	Holes permit osteoprogenitor cells and capillaries to invade cartilage model, now calcified, and begin laying down bone matrix.
Formation of calcified cartilage/calcified bone complex	Bone matrix laid down on septa of calcified cartilage forms this complex. Histologically: calcified cartilage stains blue, calcified bone stains red.
Osteoclasts begin resorbing the calcified cartilage/calcified bone complex	Destruction of the calcified cartilage/calcified bone complex enlarges the marrow cavity.
Subperiosteal bone collar thickens, begins growing toward epiphyses	This event, over a number of years, completely replaces diaphyseal cartilage with bone.
Secondary Center of Ossification	
Ossification begins at epiphysis	Begins in same way as primary center except there is no bone collar. Osteoblasts lay down bone matrix on calcified cartilage scaffold.
Growth of bone at epiphyseal plate	Cartilaginous articular surface of bone remains. Epiphyseal plate persists—growth added at epiphyseal end of plate. Bone added at diaphyseal end of plate.
Epiphysis and diaphysis become continuous	At end of bone growth, cartilage of epiphyseal plate ceases proliferation. Bone development continues to unite the diaphysis and epiphysis.

[handwritten margin note: *bone collar formed*]

[handwritten margin note: *no bone collar formed*]

BONE GROWTH IN LENGTH. The continued lengthening of bone depends on the **epiphyseal plate,** whose chondrocytes proliferate and participate in the process of endochondral bone formation. Proliferation occurs at the epiphyseal aspect, and replacement by bone takes place at the diaphyseal side of the plate. Histologically, the epiphyseal plate is divided into five recognizable zones. These zones, beginning at the epiphyseal side, are:

Zone of reserve cartilage—chondrocytes randomly distributed throughout the matrix are mitotically active.

Zone of proliferation—chondrocytes, rapidly proliferating, form rows of isogenous cells that parallel the direction of bone growth.

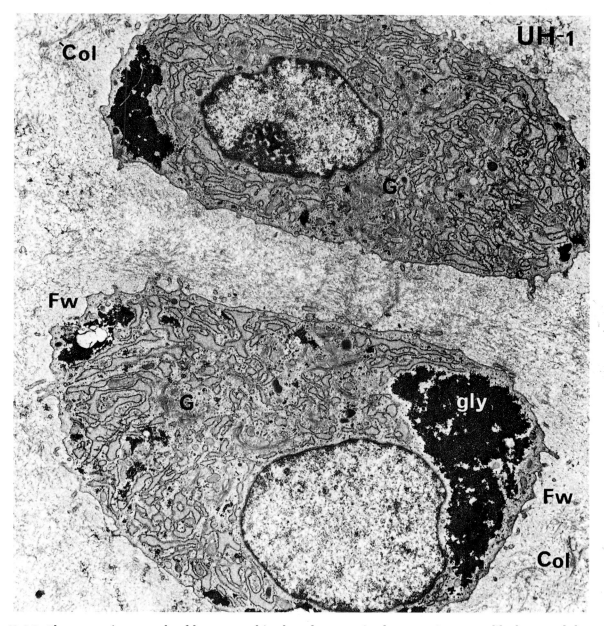

Figure 7–15. Electron micrograph of hypertrophic chondrocytes in the growing mandibular condyle (× 10,750). Observe the abundant rough endoplasmic reticulum and developing Golgi apparatus (G). Note also glycogen (gly) deposits in one end of the cells, a characteristic of these cells shortly before death. Col, collagen fibers; Fw, territorial matrix. (From Marchi, F., Luder, H.U., and Leblond, C.P.: Changes in cells' secretory organelles and extracellular matrix during endochondral ossification in the mandibular condyle of the growing rat. Am. J. Anat. **190:**41–73, 1991. Copyright © 1991. Reprinted by permission of John Wiley & Sons, Inc.)

Zone of maturation and hypertrophy—chondrocytes mature, hypertrophy, and accumulate glycogen in their cytoplasm (see Fig. 7–15). The matrix between their lacunae narrows with a corresponding growth of lacunae.

Zone of calcification—lacunae become confluent, hypertrophied chondrocytes die, and cartilage matrix becomes calcified.

Zone of ossification—osteoprogenitor cells invade the area and differentiate into osteoblasts, which elaborate matrix that becomes calcified on the surface of calcified

cartilage. This is followed by resorption of the calcified cartilage/calcified bone complex.

As long as the rate of mitotic activity in the zone of proliferation equals the rate of resorption in the zone of ossification, the epiphyseal plate remains the same width, and the bone continues to grow longer. At about the 20th year of age, the rate of mitosis decreases in the zone of proliferation, and the zone of ossification overtakes the zones of proliferation and cartilage reserve. The cartilage of the epiphyseal plate becomes replaced by a plate of calcified

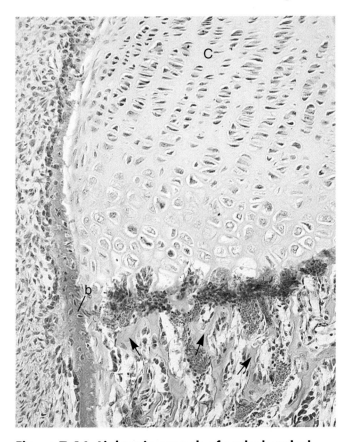

Figure 7–16. Light micrograph of endochondral bone formation (× 14). The upper half of the photograph demonstrates cartilage (C) containing chondrocytes that mature, hypertrophy, and calcify at the interface; the lower half of the photograph shows where calcified cartilage/bone complex (*arrows*) is being resorbed and bone (b) is being formed.

cartilage/calcified bone complex, which becomes resorbed by osteoclastic activity, and the marrow cavity of the diaphysis becomes confluent with the bone marrow cavity of the epiphysis. Once the epiphyseal plate is resorbed, growth in length is no longer possible.

BONE GROWTH IN WIDTH. The events just described detail how bone lengthening is accomplished by the proliferation and interstitial growth of cartilage, which eventually is replaced by bone. Growth of the diaphysis in girth, however, takes place by appositional growth. The osteogenic layer of cells of the periosteum proliferate and differentiate into osteoblasts that begin elaborating bone matrix on the subperiosteal bone surface. This process occurs continuously throughout the total period of bone growth and development, so that in a mature long bone the shaft is built via subperiosteal intramembranous bone formation. It is worth remembering that during bone growth and development, bone resorption is as important as bone deposition. Formation of bone on the outside of the shaft must be accompanied

by osteoclastic activity internally so that the marrow space can be enlarged.

Calcification of Bone

Calcification begins when there are deposits of calcium phosphate on the collagen fibrils. Exactly how this occurs is still unclear, though it is known to be stimulated by certain proteoglycans and the Ca^{2+}-binding glycoprotein **osteonectin.** One theory, **heterogeneous nucleation,** is that collagen fibers in the matrix are nucleation sites for the metastable calcium and phosphate solution, and the solution begins to crystalize into the gap region of the collagen. Once this region has "nucleated," the calcification proceeds.

The most common theory of calcification is based on the presence of matrix vesicles within the osteoid. Osteoblasts release these small, membrane-bounded matrix vesicles, 100 to 200 nm in diameter, which contain a high concentration of Ca^{2+} and PO_4^{3-} ions, cyclic AMP, ATP, ATPase, alkaline phosphatase, pyrophosphatase, calcium-binding proteins, and phosphoserine. The matrix vesicle membrane possesses numerous calcium pumps, which transport Ca^{2+} ions into the vesicle. As the concentration of ions within the vesicle increases, crystallization occurs and the growing calcium hydroxyapatite crystal pierces the membrane, bursting the matrix vesicle and releasing its contents.

Alkaline phosphatase cleaves pyrophosphate groups from the macromolecules of the matrix. The liberated pyrophosphate molecules are inhibitors of calcification, but they are cleaved by the enzyme pyrophosphatase into PO_4^{3-} ions, increasing the concentration of this ion in the microenvironment.

The calcium hydroxyapatite crystals released from the matrix vesicles act as **nidi of crystallization.** The high concentration of ions in their vicinity, along with the presence of calcification factors and calcium-binding proteins, fosters the calcification of the matrix. As crystals are deposited into the gap regions on the surface of collagen molecules, water is resorbed from the matrix.

Mineralization occurs around numerous closely spaced nidi of crystallization; as it progresses, these centers enlarge and fuse with each other. In this fashion an increasingly larger region of the matrix is dehydrated and calcified.

Bone Remodeling

In young persons, bone development exceeds bone resorption because new haversian systems are being developed much faster than old ones are being resorbed. Later, as an adult, when the epiphyseal plates close and bone growth has been attained, new bone development is balanced with bone resorption.

Growing bones largely retain the general architectural shape from the beginning of bone development in the fetus to the end of bone growth in the adult. This is accomplished by **surface remodeling,** a process involving bone deposition under certain regions of the periosteum, with concomitant bone resorption under other regions of the periosteum. Similarly, bone is being deposited in certain regions of the endosteal surface, whereas in other regions it is being resorbed. The bones of the calvarium are being reshaped in a similar way to accommodate the growing brain; however, how this process is regulated is unclear.

The internal structure of adult bone is continually being remodeled as new bone is being formed and dead and dying bone is being resorbed. This is related to the fact that (1) haversian systems are continually being replaced and (2) bone must be resorbed from one area and added to another to meet changing stresses placed on it (e.g., weight, posture, fractures). As haversian systems are resorbed, their osteocytes die; additionally, osteoclasts are recruited to the area to resorb the bone matrix, forming **absorption cavities.** Continual osteoclastic activity increases the diameter and length of these cavities, which are invaded by blood vessels. At this point, bone resorption ceases and osteoblasts deposit new concentric lamellae around the blood vessels, forming new haversian systems. Although primary bone is remodeled in this fashion, which strengthens the bone by ordered collagen alignment about the haversian system, remodeling continues throughout life as resorption is replaced by deposition and the formation of new haversian systems. The interstitial lamellae observed in adult bone are remnants of remodeled haversian systems.

Bone Repair

A bone fracture causes damage and destruction to the bone matrix, death of cells, tears in the periosteum and endosteum, and possible displacement of the ends of the broken bone (fragments). Blood vessels are severed near the break, and localized hemorrhaging fills in the zone of the break, resulting in blood clot formation at the site of injury. Soon the blood supply is shut down in a retrograde fashion from the injury site back to regions of anastomosing vessels, which can reestablish a new circulation route. This results in a widening zone of injury, on either side of the original break, as a lack of a blood supply to many haversian systems causes the zone of dead and dying osteocytes to increase appreciably. Because bone marrow and the periosteum are highly vascularized, the initial injury site in either of these two areas does not grow significantly, nor is there a notable increase in dead and dying cells much beyond the original injury site. Wherever the bone's haversian systems are without a blood supply, osteocytes become pyknotic and undergo lysis, leaving empty lacunae.

The blood clot filling the site of the fracture is invaded by small capillaries and fibroblasts from the surrounding connective tissue, forming **granulation tissue.** A similar event occurs in the marrow cavities as a clot forms that is soon invaded by osteogenic cells of the endosteum and multipoten-

tial cells of the bone marrow, eventually forming an **internal callus** of bony trabeculae within 1 week or so (Fig. 7–17). Within 48 hours post injury, osteogenic cells build up because of increased mitotic activity of the osteogenic layer of the periosteum and endosteum and from undifferentiated cells of the bone marrow. The deepest layer of proliferating osteogenic cells of the periosteum (those closest to the bone), which are in the vicinity of capillaries, differentiate into osteoblasts and begin elaborating a collar of bone, cementing it to the dead bone about the injury site.

Although the capillaries are growing, their rate of proliferation is much slower than that of the osteogenic cells; thus, the osteogenic cells in the middle of the proliferating

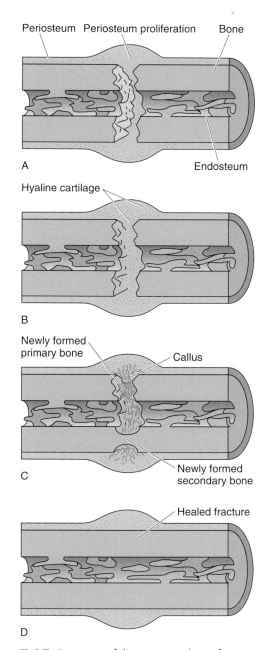

Figure 7–17. Diagram of the events in bone fracture repair.

mass are now without a profuse capillary bed. This results in lowered oxygen tension, and these cells become chondrogenic cells, giving rise to chondroblasts that form cartilage in the outer parts of the collar. The outermost layer of the proliferating osteogenic cells (those adjacent to the fibrous layer of the periosteum), having some capillaries in their midst, continue to proliferate as osteogenic cells. Thus, the collar exhibits three zones that blend together: a layer of new bone cemented to the bone of the fragment, an intermediate layer of cartilage, and a proliferating osteogenic surface layer. In the meantime, the collars formed on the ends of each fragment fuse into one collar, known as the **external callus,** thus rendering union of the fragments. Continued growth of the external collar is derived mainly from the proliferation of osteogenic cells and to some degree from interstitial growth of the cartilage in its intermediate zone.

The cartilage matrix adjacent to the new bone formed in the deepest region of the collar becomes calcified and is eventually replaced with cancellous bone. Ultimately, all of the cartilage is replaced with primary bone by endochondral bone formation.

Once the fragments of bone are united by bridging with cancellous bone, it is necessary to remodel the injury site by replacing the primary bone with secondary bone and resolving the callus.

The first bone elaborated against injured bone develops by intermembranous bone formation, and the new trabeculae become firmly cemented to the injured or dead bone. Matrices of dead bone, located in the empty spaces between newly developing bony trabeculae, are resorbed, and the spaces are filled in by new bone. Eventually all of the dead bone is resorbed and replaced by new bone formed by the osteoblasts that invade the region. These events are concurrent, resulting in repair of the fracture with cancellous bone surrounded by a bony callus.

Through the events of remodeling, the primary bone of intermembranous bone formation is replaced with secondary bone, further reinforcing the mended fracture zone, and at the same time the callus is resorbed. It appears that the healing and remodeling processes at the fracture site are in direct response to the stresses placed on it; eventually, the repaired zone is restored to its original shape and strength. It is interesting that bone repair involves cartilage formation and both intramembranous and endochondral bone formation.

CLINICAL CORRELATIONS

If segments of bone are lost or damaged so severely that they have to be removed, a **"bony union"** is not possible; that is, the process of bone repair cannot occur because a bony callus will not form. In cases of this sort, a bone graft is required. Since the 1970s, bone banks have become available, supplying viable bone for grafting purposes. The bone fragments are harvested and frozen to preserve their osteogenic potential and are then utilized as transplants by orthopedic surgeons. **Autographs** are the most successful, as the transplant recipient is also the donor. **Homographs** are from different individuals of the same species and may be rejected because of immunological response. **Heterographs,** grafts from different species, are least successful, although it has been shown that calf bone loses some of its antigenicity after being refrigerated, making it a worthy bone graft when necessary.

Histophysiology of Bone

Bone supports soft tissues of the body and protects the central nervous system and hemopoietic tissue. It also provides for attachment of the tendons of muscle that use the bone as levers to increase the mechanical advantage needed for locomotion. Just as important, bone serves as a reservoir of calcium and phosphate essential for maintaining adequate levels of these elements in the blood and other tissues of the body.

Maintenance of Blood Calcium Levels

Calcium is vital for the activity of many enzymes and also functions in membrane permeability, cell adhesion, blood coagulation, and muscle contraction, among other bodily processes. To fulfill all of the necessary functional requirements for which calcium is responsible, a tightly controlled blood plasma concentration of 9 to 11 mg per 100 ml must be maintained.

Because 99% of the calcium in the body is stored in bone as hydroxyapatite crystals, the remaining 1% must be available for mobilization from the bone on short notice. Indeed there is a constant turnover between the calcium ions in bone and in blood. The calcium ions retrieved from bone to maintain blood calcium levels come from new and young osteons, where mineralization is incomplete. Because bone remodeling is constant, new osteons are always forming where labile calcium ions are available for this purpose. It seems that older osteons are more heavily mineralized; because of this, their calcium ions are less available.

Hormonal Effects

Osteoclastic activity is necessary for maintaining a constant supply of calcium ions for the body. Parenchymal cells of the parathyroid gland are sensitive to the blood calcium level; when it falls below normal, **parathyroid hormone** is secreted. As discussed earlier, this hormone activates receptors on osteoblasts, suppressing matrix formation and initiating manufacture and secretion of **osteoclast-stimulating factor** by the osteoblasts. This factor induces quiescent osteoclasts into activity, leading in bone resorption and the release of calcium ions.

Parafollicular cells of the thyroid gland also monitor calcium ion levels in the plasma. When the calcium ion level becomes elevated, these cells secrete **calcitonin,** a polypeptide hormone, that activates receptors on osteoclasts, inhibiting them from resorbing bone.

The growth hormone **somatotropin,** secreted by cells in the anterior lobe of the pituitary gland, influences bone development via somatomedins, especially stimulating growth of the epiphyseal plates. Children deficient in this hormone exhibit dwarfism, whereas persons who produce an excess of somatotropin in their growing years display **pituitary gigantism.**

CLINICAL CORRELATIONS

Acromegaly occurs in adults who produce an excess of somatotropin, causing an abnormal increase in bone deposition without normal bone resorption. This condition creates thickening of the bones, especially those about the face, in addition to soft-tissue disfiguring.

Skeletal maturation also is influenced by hormones produced in the male and female gonads. Closure of the epiphyseal plates is normally rather stable and constant and is related to sexual maturation. For example, precocious sexual maturation will stunt skeletal development because the epiphyseal plates are stimulated to close too early. In other persons whose sexual maturation is retarded, however, skeletal growth continues beyond normal because the epiphyseal plates do not close.

CLINICAL CORRELATIONS

Osteoporosis affects some women over the age of 40 and many postmenopausal women not on estrogen therapy. Osteoporosis is related to decreasing bone mass, which be-

comes more serious as estrogen secretion drops appreciably after menopause. Binding of estrogen to specific receptors on osteoblasts activate the cells to manufacture and secrete bone matrix. With diminished secretion of estrogen, osteoclastic activity is greater than bone deposition, potentially reducing bone mass to the point at which it cannot withstand stresses and breaks easily. Estrogen therapy may reduce or eliminate this condition.

Nutritional Effects

Normal bone growth is sensitive and dependent on several nutritional factors. Unless a person's intake of protein, minerals, and vitamins is sufficient, the amino acids essential for collagen synthesis by osteoblasts will be lacking, thus reducing collagen formation. Insufficient intake of calcium or phosphorus leads to poorly calcified bone, which is subject to fracture. A deficiency of vitamin D prevents calcium absorption from the intestines, causing rickets in children. Vitamins A and C also are necessary for proper skeletal development (Table 7–4).

CLINICAL CORRELATIONS

Rickets is a disease in children who are deficient in vitamin D. Without vitamin D the intestinal mucosa is unable to absorb calcium even though there may be an adequate intake in the diet. This results in disturbances in ossification of the epiphyseal cartilages and disorientation of the cells at the metaphysis, giving rise to poorly calcified bone matrix. Children with rickets display deformed bones, particularly in the legs, simply because the bones cannot bear the weight.

Osteomalacia is adult rickets resulting from prolonged

Table 7–4. Vitamins and Their Effects on Skeletal Development

Vitamin	Effects on Skeletal Development
Vitamin A deficiency	Inhibits proper bone formation as coordination of osteoblast and osteoclast activities fail. Failure of resorption and remodeling of cranial vault to accommodate the brain with serious damage to the central nervous system.
Hypervitaminosis A	Erosion of cartilage columns without increases of cells in proliferation zone. Epiphyseal plates may become obliterated ceasing growth prematurely.
Vitamin C deficiency	Mesenchymal tissue affected as connective tissue is unable to produce and maintain extracellular matrix. Deficient production of collagen and bone matrix result in retarded growth and delayed healing.
Vitamin D deficiency	Ossification of epiphyseal cartilages disturbed. Cells become disordered at metaphysis, leading to poorly calcified bones, which become deformed by weight-bearing. In children—rickets. In adults—osteomalacia.

deficiency of vitamin D. When this occurs, the newly formed bone in the process of remodeling fails to calcify properly. This condition may become severe during pregnancy because the fetus requires calcium that needs to be supplied by the mother.

Scurvy is a condition resulting from a deficiency of vitamin C. One effect is deficient collagen production, causing a reduction in formation of bone matrix and bone development. Healing is also delayed.

Joints

Bones articulate or come into close proximity with one another at **joints,** which are classified according to the degree of movement available between the bones of the joint. Those that are closely bound together with only a minimum of movement between them are called **synarthroses;** joints in which the bones are free to articulate over a fairly wide range of motion are classified as **diarthroses.**

There are three types of **synarthroses joints,** based on the tissue making up the union. These include **synostosis,** in which there is little if any movement and joint-uniting tissue is bone (e.g., skull bones of adults); **synchondrosis,** in which there is little movement and joint-uniting tissue is hyaline cartilage (e.g., joint of first rib and sternum); and **syndesmosis,** again in which there is little movement and bones are joined by dense connective tissue (e.g., pubic symphysis).

Most of the joints of the extremities are **diarthroses** (Fig. 7–18). The bones making up these joints are covered by persistent **hyaline cartilage,** referred to as the articular cartilage. Usually ligaments maintain the contact between the bones of the joint, which is sealed by the **joint capsule.** The **capsule** is composed of an outer **fibrous layer** of dense connective tissue, which is continuous with the periosteum of the bones, and an inner cellular **synovial layer,** which covers all nonarticular surfaces. Some prefer to call this a **synovial membrane.**

Two kinds of cells are located in the synovial layer. **Type A cells** are macrophages displaying a well-developed Golgi

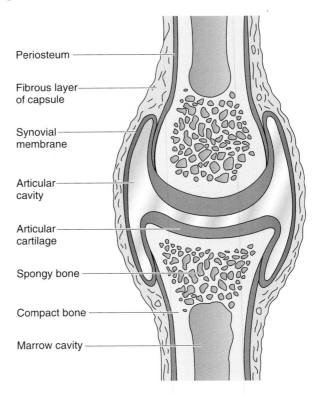

Figure 7-18. Drawing of the anatomy of a diarthroidal joint.

apparatus and many lysosomes but only a small amount of RER. These phagocytic cells are responsible for removing debris from the joint space. **Type B cells** resemble fibroblasts, exhibiting a well-developed RER; these cells are thought to secrete the **synovial fluid.** This fluid contains a high concentration of **hyaluronic acid** and the glycoprotein **lubricin** combined with filtrate of plasma. In addition to supplying nutrients and oxygen to the chondrocytes of the articular cartilage, this fluid has a high content of hyaluronic acid and lubricin that permits it to function as a lubricant for the joint. Moreover, macrophages in the synovial fluid act to phagocytose debris in the joint space.

Muscle

8

Although many cells of multicellular organisms have limited contractile abilities, it is the capability of muscle cells, specialized for contraction, that permits animals to move. Organisms harness the contraction of muscle cells and the arrangement of the extracellular components of muscle to permit locomotion, constriction, pumping, and other propulsive movements.

Cells of muscle are elongated and are called **striated** or **smooth** muscle, depending on the respective presence or absence of a regularly repeated arrangement of myofibrillar contractile proteins, the myofilaments. Striated muscle cells display characteristic alternations of light and dark crossbands, which are absent in smooth muscle (Fig. 8–1). There are two types of striated muscle: **skeletal,** accounting for most of the voluntary muscle mass of the body, and involuntary **cardiac** muscle, limited almost exclusively to the heart. **Smooth muscle** is located in the walls of blood vessels and the viscera, as well as in the dermis of the skin.

Unique terms are often used in describing the components of muscle cells. Thus muscle cell membrane is referred to as **sarcolemma;** the cytoplasm, as **sarcoplasm;** the smooth endoplasmic reticulum, as **sarcoplasmic reticulum;** and occasionally, the mitochondria, as **sarcosomes.** Because they are much longer than they are wide, muscle cells frequently are called **muscle fibers;** unlike collagen fibers, however, they are **living** entities.

All three muscle types are derived from mesoderm. Cardiac muscle originates in splanchnopleuric mesoderm, most smooth muscle is derived from splanchnic and somatic mesoderm, and most skeletal muscles originate from somatic mesoderm.

Skeletal Muscle

Several hundred **myoblasts,** precursors of skeletal muscle fibers, line up end to end, fusing with one another to form long cells known as **myotubes.** These newly formed myotubes manufacture cytoplasmic constituents as well as contractile elements, called **myofibrils.** Myofibrils are composed of specific arrays of **myofilaments,** the proteins responsible for the contractile capability of the cell.

Muscle fibers are arranged parallel to each other, with their intervening intercellular spaces housing parallel arrays of **continuous capillaries.** Each skeletal muscle fiber is long, cylindrical, multinucleated, and striated. The diameter of the fibers vary, ranging from 10 to 100 μm, although hypertrophied fibers may exceed the latter figure. The relative strength of a muscle fiber directly depends on its diameter, whereas the strength of the entire muscle is a function of the number and thickness of its component fibers.

Skeletal muscle is pink to red because of its rich vascular supply as well as the presence of **myoglobin pigments,**

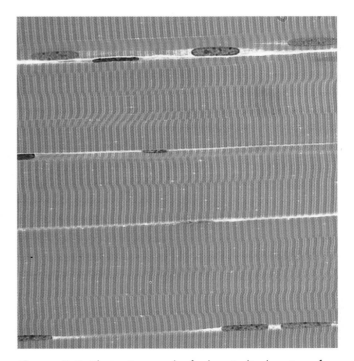

Figure 8–1. Photomicrograph of a longitudinal section of skeletal muscle (× 540).

131

oxygen-transporting proteins that resemble, but are smaller than, hemoglobin. Depending on the quantity of myoglobin, number of mitochondria, concentration of various enzymes, and rate of contraction, the muscle fiber may be classified as **red, white,** or **intermediate** (Table 8–1).

Usually, a gross muscle (e.g., biceps) will contain all three types of muscle fibers (red, white, and intermediate) in relatively constant proportions characteristic of that particular muscle. In chickens, for instance, the thigh muscles are predominantly red, whereas breast muscles are predominantly white. The innervation of the muscle fiber appears to be the factor that determines fiber type. If the innervation is experimentally switched, the fiber will accommodate itself to the new nerve supply.

Investments

The entire muscle is surrounded by **epimysium,** a dense irregular collagenous connective tissue. **Perimysium,** a less dense collagenous connective tissue, derived from epimysium, surrounds bundles **(fascicles)** of muscle fibers, and **endomysium,** composed of reticular fibers and an **external lamina** (basal lamina), surrounds each muscle cell (Fig. 8–2).

Because these connective tissue elements are interconnected, contractile forces exerted by individual muscle cells are transferred to them. Tendons and aponeuroses, which connect muscle to bone and other tissues, are continuous with the connective tissue encasements of muscle and, therefore, act in harnessing the contractile forces for motion.

Light Microscopy of Skeletal Muscle Fibers

Skeletal muscle fibers are multinucleated cells, with their nuclei peripherally located just beneath the cell membrane (Fig. 8–3). Each cell is surrounded by endomysium, whose fine reticular fibers intermingle with those of neighboring muscle cells. Small **satellite cells,** which possess a single nucleus and act as regenerative cells, are located in shallow depressions on the muscle cell's surface, sharing the muscle fiber's external lamina. The chromatin network of the satellite cell nucleus is denser and more coarse than that of the muscle fiber.

Much of the skeletal muscle cell is composed of longitudinal arrays of cylinder-shaped **myofibrils,** each 1 to 2 μm in diameter (Fig. 8–4). They extend the entire length of the cell and are aligned precisely with their neighbors. This strictly ordered parallel arrangement of the myofibrils is responsible for the cross-striations of light and dark banding that is characteristic of skeletal muscle viewed in longitudinal section (see Fig. 8–1).

The dark bands are known as **A bands** (anisotropic with polarized light) and the light bands as **I bands** (isotropic with polarized light). The center of each A band is occupied by a pale area, the **H band,** which is bisected by a thin **M line.** Each I band is bisected by a thin dark line, the **Z disk (Z line).** The region of the myofibril between two successive Z disks, known as a **sarcomere,** is 2.5 μm in length and is considered to be the contractile unit of skeletal muscle fibers (Figs. 8–4, 8–5).

During muscle contraction the various transverse bands behave characteristically. The I band becomes narrower, the H band is extinguished, and the Z disks move closer together (approaching the interface between the A and I bands), but the width of the A bands remains unaltered.

Fine Structure of Skeletal Muscle Fibers

Electron microscopy has helped reveal the functional and morphological significance of skeletal muscle cross-striations and other structural components.

T Tubules and Sarcoplasmic Reticulum

The fine structure of the sarcolemma is similar to that of other cell membranes. However, a distinguishing feature of this membrane is that it is continued within the skeletal muscle fiber as numerous **T tubules (transverse tubules),** long, tubular invaginations that intertwine among the myofibrils (see Fig. 8–5).

T tubules pass transversely across the fiber and lie specifically in the plane of the junction of the A and I bands in mammalian skeletal muscle. These tubules branch and anastomose but usually remain in a single plane; hence each sarcomere possesses two sets of T tubules, one at each interface of the A and I bands. Thus, T tubules extend deep into the

Table 8–1. Types of Skeletal Muscle Fibers

Type	Myoglobin	Mitochondria	Enzymes	Contraction
Red	Rich	Numerous	Rich in oxidative, weak ATPase	Slow but repetitive; not easily fatigued
White	Poor	Poor	Poor in oxidative, rich in phosphorylases and ATPase	Fast but easily fatigued
Intermediate	Intermediate	Intermediate	Intermediate	Intermediate

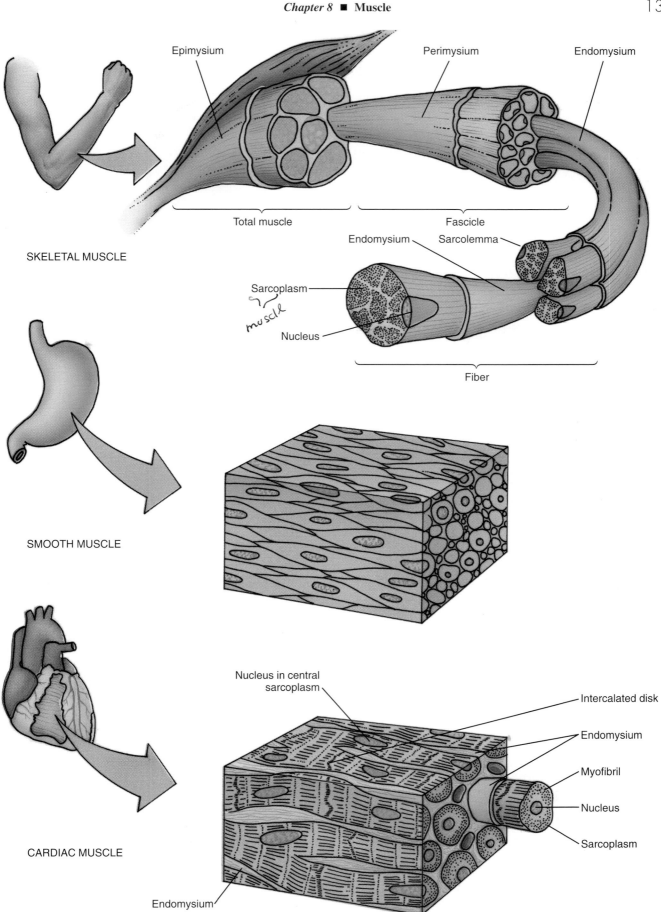

Figure 8–2. Diagram of the three types of muscle. *Top,* Skeletal muscle; *center,* smooth muscle; *bottom,* cardiac muscle.

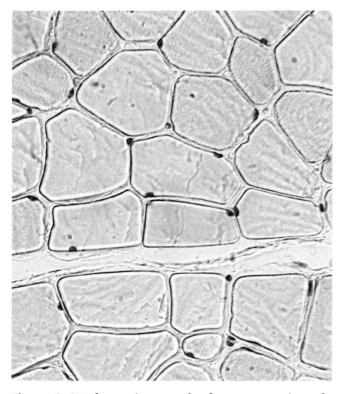

Figure 8–3. Photomicrograph of a cross-section of skeletal muscle (× 540). Note the peripheral location of the nuclei.

interior of the fiber and facilitate the conduction of waves of depolarization along the sarcolemma (Figs. 8–6, 8–7).

Associated with this system of T tubules is the **sarcoplasmic reticulum,** which is maintained in close register with the A and I bands as well as with the T tubules. The sarcoplasmic reticulum, which stores intracellular calcium, forms a meshwork around each myofibril and displays dilated **terminal cisternae** at each A–I junction. Thus two of these cisternae are always in close apposition to a T tubule, forming a **triad** in which a T tubule is flanked by two cisternae. This arrangement permits a wave of depolarization to spread, almost instantaneously, from the surface of the sarcolemma throughout the cell, reaching the terminal cisternae, which have voltage-gated Ca²⁺-release channels **(junctional feet)** in their membrane.

The sarcoplasmic reticulum regulates muscle contraction by controlled sequestering (leading to relaxation) and release (leading to contraction) of Ca^{2+} ions within the sarcoplasm. The trigger for the calcium release is the wave of depolarization transmitted by T tubules, which causes opening of the calcium-release channels of the terminal cisternae, resulting in release of calcium into the cytosol in the vicinity of the myofibrils.

Myofibrils are held in register with each other by the intermediate filaments **desmin** and **vimentin,** which secure the periphery of the Z disks of neighboring myofibrils to

each other. These bundles of myofibrils are attached to the cytoplasmic aspect of the sarcolemma by various proteins, including **dystrophin,** a protein that binds to actin.

Deep to the sarcolemma, and interspersed between and among myofibrils, are numerous elongated mitochondria with many highly interdigitating cristae. The mitochondria may either parallel the longitudinal axis of the myofibril or wrap around the myofibril. Moreover, numerous mitochondria are located just deep to the sarcoplasm.

Structural Organization of Myofibrils

Electron microscopy reveals the same banding as noted by light microscopy, but it also demonstrates the presence of parallel, interdigitating thick and thin rod-like **myofilaments.** The **thick filaments** (15 nm in diameter and 1.5 μm long) are composed of **myosin,** whereas the **thin filaments** (7 nm in diameter and 1.0 μm long) are composed primarily of **actin.**

Thin filaments originate at the Z disk and project toward the center of the two adjacent sarcomeres, thus pointing in opposite directions. Hence, a single sarcomere will have two groups of parallel arrays of thin filaments, each attached to one Z disk, with all the filaments in each group pointing toward the middle of the sarcomere (Fig. 8–8). Thick filaments also form parallel arrays, interdigitating with the thin filaments in a specific fashion.

In a relaxed skeletal muscle fiber, the thick filaments do not extend the entire length of the sarcomere, nor do the thin filaments projecting from the two Z disks of the sarcomere meet in the midline. Therefore, there are regions of each sarcomere, on either side of each Z disk, where only thin filaments are present. These adjacent portions of two successive sarcomeres correspond to the I band seen by light microscopy. The region of each sarcomere that encompasses the entire length of the thick filaments is the A band. The zone in the middle of the A band, which is devoid of thin filaments, is the H band. As noted earlier, the H band is bisected by the M line, which consists of **myomesin, C protein,** and other as yet poorly characterized proteins that interconnect thick filaments to maintain their specific lattice arrangement.

During contraction, individual thick and thin filaments do not shorten; instead, the two Z disks are brought closer together as the thin filaments slide past the thick filaments **(sliding filament theory).** Thus, when contraction occurs, the motion of the thin filaments toward the center of the sarcomere creates a greater overlap between the two groups of filaments, effectively reducing the width of the I and H bands without influencing the width of the A band.

The arrangement of the thick and thin filaments bears a specific and constant relationship. In mammalian skeletal muscle each thick filament is surrounded equidistantly by six thin filaments. Cross-sections through the region of overlapping thin and thick filaments display a hexagonal pattern,

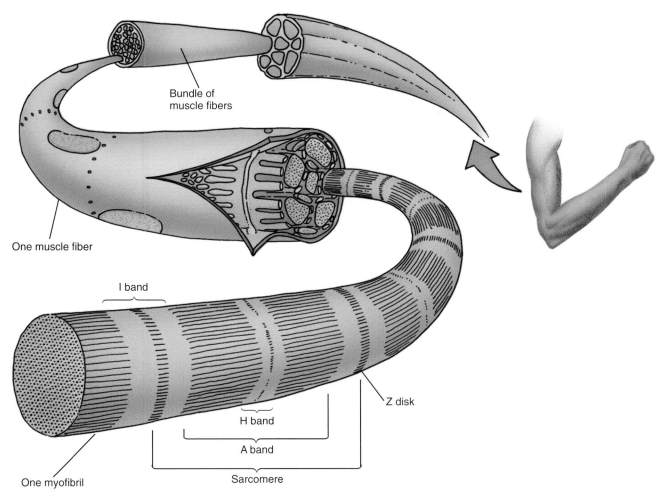

Figure 8–4. Diagram of the organization of myofibrils and sarcomeres within a skeletal muscle cell.

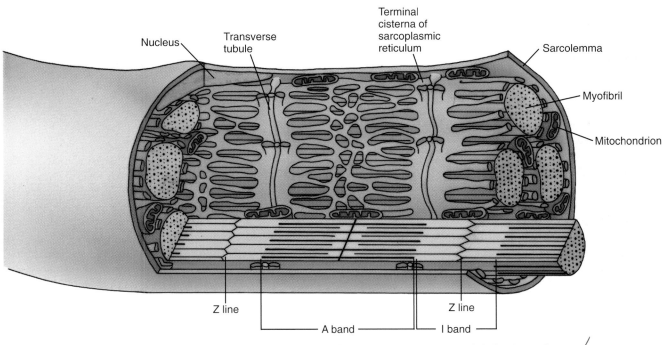

Figure 8–5. Diagram of the organization of triads and sarcomeres of skeletal muscle.

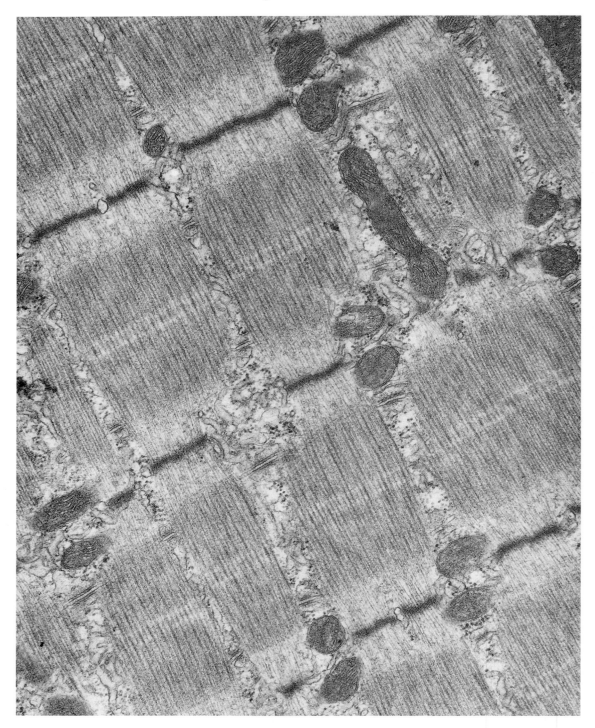

Figure 8–6. Electron micrograph of longitudinal section of rat skeletal muscle (× 28,800). (Courtesy of Dr. J. Strum.)

with thin filaments for the apices of each hexagon, the center of which is occupied by a thick filament (see Fig. 8–8; Fig. 8–9). Thick filaments are separated from each other by a distance of 40 to 50 nm, whereas the distance between thick and thin filaments is only 15 to 20 nm.

The structural organization of myofibrils is maintained largely by three proteins: titin, α-actinin, and nebulin. Thick filaments are positioned precisely within the sarcomere with

the assistance of **titin,** a large, linear, elastic protein. A titin molecule extends from each half of a thick filament to the adjacent Z disk, thus anchoring the filament between the two Z disks of each sarcomere. Thin filaments are held in register by the rod-shaped protein **α-actinin,** a component of the Z disk that can bind thin filaments in parallel arrays. In addition, two molecules of **nebulin**—a long, nonelastic protein—are wrapped around the entire length of each thin

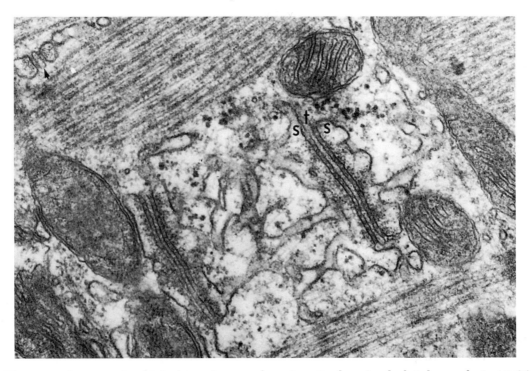

Figure 8–7. Electron micrograph of triads and sarcoplasmic reticulum in skeletal muscle (× 64,000). t, T tubule; s, terminal cisternae of the sarcoplasmic reticulum; (arrow), cross-section of T tubule flanked by terminal cisternae. (From Leeson, T.S., Leeson, C.R., and Papparo, A.A.: Text/Atlas of Histology. Philadelphia, W.B. Saunders Company, 1988.)

filament, further anchoring it in the Z disk and ensuring the maintenance of the specific array (see Fig. 8–8). Table 8–2 summarizes the structure and function of the proteins that make up myofilaments and keep them correctly positioned within myofibrils.

Thick Filaments

Every thick filament consists of 200 to 300 myosin molecules. Each **myosin** molecule (150 nm long; 2 to 3 nm in diameter) is composed of two identical **heavy chains** and two pairs of **light chains.** The heavy chains resemble two golf clubs, whose rod-like polypeptide chains are wrapped around each other in an α-helix. The heavy chains can be cleaved by trypsin into a rod-like tail, **light meromyosin,** and a globular head, **heavy meromyosin.** The former functions in the proper assembly of the molecules into the bipolar thick filament. Heavy meromyosin is cleaved by papain into two globular (S_1) moieties and a short, helical, rod-like segment (S_2) (see Fig. 8–8). The S_1 subfragment binds **adenosine triphosphate (ATP)** and functions in the formation of cross-bridges between thick and thin myofilaments. Light chains (not to be confused with light meromyosin) are of two types, and one of each is associated with each S_1 subfragment of the myosin molecule. So—for each heavy chain there are two light chains, and a myosin molecule is composed of two heavy chains and four light chains.

Myosin molecules are closely packed in a specific fashion in the thick filament. They are lined up in a parallel but staggered manner, spaced at regular intervals, lying head to tail, so that the middle of each thick filament is composed solely of tail regions, whereas the two ends of the thick filament consist of both heads and tails. The spatial orientation of the myosin molecules permits the heavy meromyosin portion to project from the thick filament at a 60-degree angle relative to neighboring heavy meromyosin, so that the head regions are always in register with the thin filaments.

Thin Filament

The major component of each thin filament is **F-actin,** a polymer of globular **G-actin** units. Although G-actin molecules are globular, they all polymerize in the same spatial orientation, imparting to the filament a distinct polarity. The **plus end** of each filament is bound to the Z disk by α-actinin; the **minus end** extends toward the center of the sarcomere. Each G-actin molecule also contains an **active site** where the head region (S_1 subfragment) of myosin binds. Two chains of F-actin are wound around each other in a tight helix (36-nm periodicity) like two strands of pearls (see Fig. 8–8).

Running along the length of the F-actin double-stranded helix are two shallow grooves. Pencil-shaped **tropomyosin molecules,** about 40 nm long, polymerize to form head-to-tail filaments that occupy the shallow grooves in the actin filaments. Bound tropomyosin masks the active sites on the actin molecules by partially overlapping them.

active sites on the actin filament, so that myosin heads can bind.

Muscle Contraction and Relaxation

Contraction effectively reduces the resting length of the muscle fiber by an amount that is equal to the sum of all shortenings that occur in all sarcomeres of that particular muscle cell. The process of contraction, usually triggered by neural impulses, obeys the **"all-or-none law"** in that a single muscle fiber will either contract or not contract as a result of stimulation. The strength of contraction of a gross anatomical muscle, such as the biceps, is a function of the number of muscle fibers that undergo contraction. The stimulus is transferred at the neuromuscular junction. During muscle contraction the thin filaments slide past the thick filaments, as proposed by Huxley's sliding filament theory.

The following sequence of events leads to contraction in skeletal muscle:

1. Impulse, generated along the sarcolemma, is transmitted into the interior of the fiber via the T tubules, where it is conveyed to the terminal cisternae of the sarcoplasmic reticulum (see Fig. 8–5).

2. Calcium ions leave the terminal cisternae through voltage-gated **calcium-release channels,** enter the cytosol, and bind to the TnC subunit of troponin, altering its conformation.

3. Conformational change in troponin shifts the position of tropomyosin deeper into the groove, unmasking the active site (myosin-binding site) on the actin molecule.

4. ATP present on the S_1 fragment of myosin is hydrolyzed, but both adenosine diphosphate (ADP) and inorganic phosphate (P_i) remain attached to the S_1 fragment, and the complex binds to the active site on actin (Fig. 8–10).

5. P_i is released, resulting not only in an increased bond strength between the actin and myosin but also in a conformational alteration of the S_1 fragment.

6. ADP is also released, and the thin filament is dragged toward the center of the sarcomere ("power stroke").

7. A new ATP molecule binds to the S_1 fragment, which causes the release of the bond between actin and myosin.

The attachment and release cycles must be repeated numerous times for contraction to be completed. Each attachment and release requires ATP for the conversion of chemical energy into motion.

CLINICAL CORRELATIONS

Rigor mortis occurs subsequent to death because the lack of ATP prevents the dissociation of actin and myosin.

As long as cytosolic calcium concentration remains high enough, actin filaments will remain in the active state and

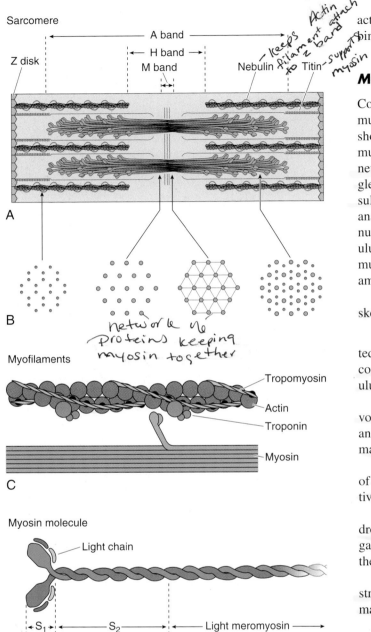

Sarcomere

A band

H band

M band

Z disk

Nebulin   Titin

(handwritten annotations: "Keeps Actin filament attach to Z band", "Titin – support myosin")

A

B

(handwritten: "network up Proteins keeping myosin together")

Myofilaments

Tropomyosin

Actin

Troponin

Myosin

C

Myosin molecule

Light chain

S_1 S_2 Light meromyosin

D   Heavy meromyosin

Figure 8–8. Diagram of a sarcomere and its components. A, Sarcomere; **B,** cross-sectional profiles of sarcomere at indicated regions; **C,** thick and thin filaments; **D,** myosin molecule.

Approximately 25 to 30 nm from the beginning of each tropomyosin molecule is a single **troponin molecule,** composed of three globular polypeptides, TnT, TnC, and TnI. The **TnT** subunit binds the entire troponin molecule to tropomyosin; **TnC** has a great affinity for calcium; and **TnI** binds to actin, preventing the interaction between actin and myosin. Binding of calcium by **TnC** induces a conformational shift in tropomyosin, exposing the previously blocked

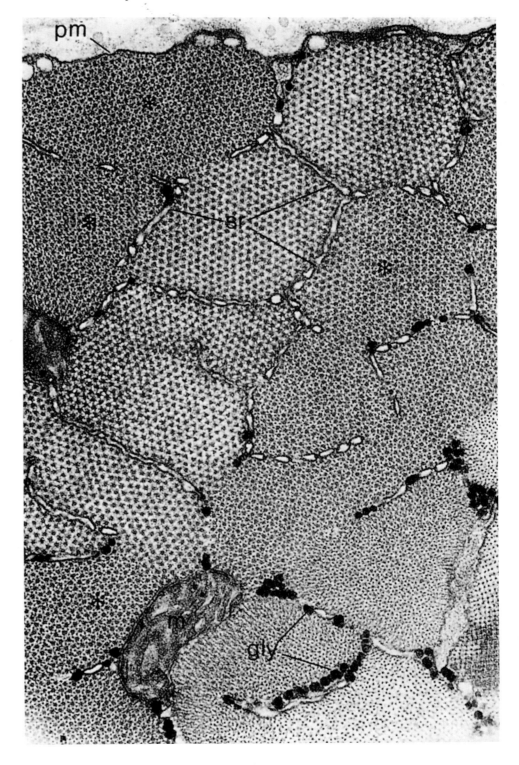

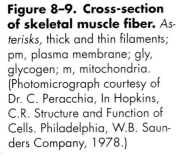

Figure 8–9. Cross-section of skeletal muscle fiber. *Asterisks,* thick and thin filaments; pm, plasma membrane; gly, glycogen; m, mitochondria. (Photomicrograph courtesy of Dr. C. Peracchia, In Hopkins, C.R. Structure and Function of Cells. Philadelphia, W.B. Saunders Company, 1978.)

contraction cycles will continue. However, once the stimulating impulses cease, muscle relaxation occurs, involving a reversal of the steps that led to contraction. First, calcium pumps in the membrane of the sarcoplasmic reticulum actively drive Ca^{2+} back into the terminal cisternae, where the Ca^{2+} ions are bound by the protein **calsequestrin.** The reduced levels of Ca^{2+} in the cytosol cause TnC to lose its bound Ca^{2+}; tropomyosin then reverts to the position in which it masks the active site of actin, preventing the interaction of actin and myosin.

Energy Sources for Muscle Contraction

Because the process of muscle contraction consumes a great deal of energy, skeletal muscle cells maintain a high concentration of the energy-rich compounds ATP and creatine

Table 8–2. Proteins Associated With Skeletal Muscle

Protein	Molecular Weight	No. of Subunits and Their Molecular Weight	Function
Myosin	510 kDa	2 heavy chains, 222 kDa each 2 pairs light chains, 18 kDa and 22 kDa	Major protein of thick filament; its interaction with actin hydrolyzes ATP and produces contraction
Myomesin	185 kDa	None	Cross-links adjacent thick filaments at M line
Titin	2500 kDa	None	Forms an elastic lattice that anchors thick filaments to Z disks
C protein	140 kDa	None	Binds to thick filaments at the M line
G-Actin	42 kDa	None	Polymerizes to form thin filaments of F-actin; interaction of G-actin with myosin assists in hydrolyzing ATP, resulting in contraction
Tropomyosin	64 kDa	2 chains 32 kDa each	Occupies grooves of the thin filaments
Troponin	78 kDa	TnC, 18 kDa TnT, 30 kDa TnI, 30 kDa	Binds calcium; binds to tropomyosin; binds to actin, thus inhibiting actin–myosin interaction
α-Actinin	190 kDa	2 units, each 95 kDa	Anchors plus ends of thin filaments to Z disk
Nebulin	600 kDa	None	Z-disk protein that may assist α-actinin anchor thin filaments to Z disk

phosphate. ATP is manufactured via oxidative phosphorylation within the abundant mitochondria of muscle cells during periods of inactivity or low activity. Lipid droplets and glycogen, which abound in the sarcoplasm, also are readily converted into energy sources. During prolonged periods of muscle contraction, the ADP generated is rephosphorylated by two means: anaerobic **glycolysis,** leading to accumulation of lactic acid, and transfer of high-energy phosphate from creatine phosphate catalyzed by **phosphocreatine kinase.**

Myotendinous Junctions

The connective tissue elements of the muscle fiber are continuous with the tendon to which the muscle is attached. At the myotendinous junctions, the cells become tapered and highly fluted. Collagen fibers of the tendon penetrate deep into these infoldings and probably become continuous with

the reticular fibers of the endomysium. Within the cell, the myofilaments are anchored to the internal aspect of the sarcolemma, so that the force of contraction is transmitted to the collagen fibers of the tendon.

Innervation of Skeletal Muscle

Each skeletal muscle receives at least two types of nerve fibers, namely motor and sensory. The motor nerve functions in eliciting contraction, whereas the sensory fibers pass to muscle spindles (discussed later). Additionally, autonomic fibers supply the vascular elements of skeletal muscle. The specificity of motor innervation is a function of the muscle innervated. If the muscle acts fastidiously, as do some muscles of the eye, a single motor neuron may be responsible for as few as 5 to 10 skeletal muscle fibers, whereas a muscle located in the abdominal wall may have as

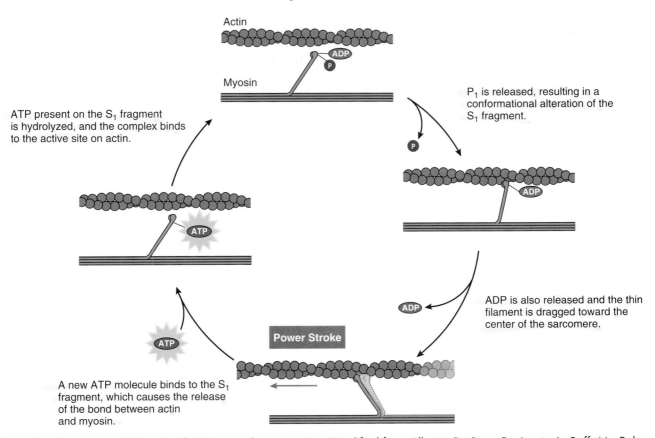

Actin

Myosin

ATP present on the S₁ fragment is hydrolyzed, and the complex binds to the active site on actin.

P₁ is released, resulting in a conformational alteration of the S₁ fragment.

ADP is also released and the thin filament is dragged toward the center of the sarcomere.

Power Stroke

A new ATP molecule binds to the S₁ fragment, which causes the release of the bond between actin and myosin.

Figure 8–10. Diagram of the role of ATP in muscle contraction. (Modified from Alberts, B., Bray, D., Lewis, J., Raff, M., Roberts, K., and Watson, J.D.: Molecular Biology of the Cell. New York, Garland Publishing, 1994.)

many a 1000 fibers under the control of a single motor neuron. Each motor neuron and the muscle fibers it controls form a **motor unit.** The muscle fibers of a motor unit contract in unison and follow the "all-or-none law" of muscle contraction.

Impulse Transmission at the Myoneural Junctions

Motor fibers are **myelinated axons of α-motor neurons,** which pass in the connective tissue of the muscle. The axon arborizes, eventually losing its myelin sheath (but not its Schwann cells). The terminal of each arborized twig becomes dilated and overlies the **motor end plate** of individual muscle fibers. Each of these muscle-nerve junctions, known as a **myoneural junction,** is composed of an axon terminal, synaptic cleft, and the muscle cell membrane (Figs. 8–11, 8–12, 8–13).

The muscle cell membrane (**postsynaptic membrane**) is modified, forming the **primary synaptic cleft,** a trough-like structure occupied by the **axon terminal.** Opening into the primary synaptic clefts are numerous **secondary synaptic clefts (junctional folds),** a further modification of the sarcolemma. Both the primary synaptic cleft and the junctional folds are lined by a basal lamina-like **external lamina.** The

sarcoplasm in the vicinity of the secondary synaptic cleft is rich in glycogen, nuclei, ribosomes, and mitochondria.

The axon terminal, covered by Schwann cells, houses mitochondria, smooth endoplasmic reticulum, and as many as 300,000 **synaptic vesicles** (each 40 to 50 nm in diameter) containing the neurotransmitter **acetylcholine.** The function of the myoneural junction is to transmit a stimulus from the nerve fiber to the muscle cell.

Stimulus transmission across a synaptic cleft involves the following sequence of events (Fig. 8–14):

1. A stimulus, traveling along the axon, depolarizes the membrane of the axon terminal, thus opening **voltage-gated calcium channels.**

2. The influx of calcium into the axon terminal results in the fusion of synaptic vesicles with the axon terminal's membrane (**presynaptic membrane**) and subsequent release of acetylcholine (along with proteoglycans and ATP) into the primary synaptic cleft. Fusion occurs along specific regions of the presynaptic membrane known as **active sites.**

3. The neurotransmitter acetylcholine (ligand) is liberated in large quantities, known as **quanta** (= 10 to 20 thousand molecules), from the nerve terminal.

4. Acetylcholine then diffuses across the synaptic cleft and binds to postsynaptic **acetylcholine receptors** in the

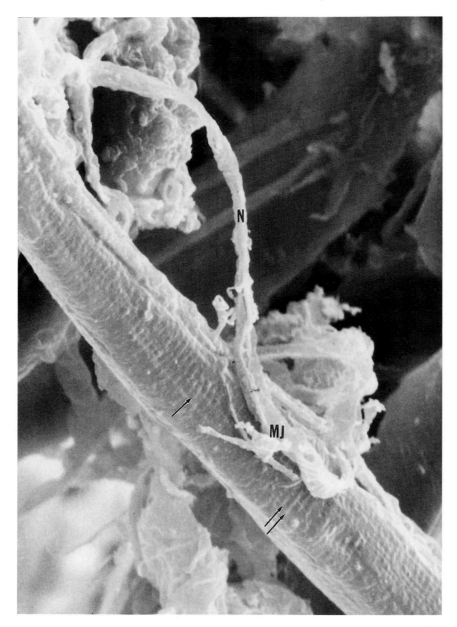

Figure 8–11. Scanning electron micrograph of a myoneural junction from the tongue of a cat (× 2610).
MJ, myoneural junction; N, nerve fiber; *arrows*, striations. (Courtesy of Dr. L. Litke.)

muscle cell membrane. These receptors, located in the vicinity of the presynaptic active sites, are ligand-gated ion channels, which open when acetylcholine binds. The resulting ion influx leads to **depolarization** of the sarcolemma and generation of an **action potential** (see Chapter 9 for further discussion).

5. The impulse generated spreads quickly throughout the muscle fiber via the system of T tubules, initiating muscle contraction.

To prevent a single stimulus from eliciting multiple responses, **acetylcholinesterase,** an enzyme located in the external lamina lining the primary and secondary synaptic clefts, degrades acetylcholine into acetate and choline, thus permitting the reestablishment of the resting potential.

Degradation is so rapid that all of the released acetylcholine is cleaved within a few hundred milliseconds.

Choline is transported back into the axon terminal by a sodium-choline symport protein, powered by the sodium concentration gradient. Within the axon terminal the acetylcholine is synthesized from activated acetate (produced in mitochondria) and the recycled choline, a reaction catalyzed by **choline acetyl transferase.** The newly formed acetylcholine is transported, utilizing an antiport system powered by a proton concentration gradient, into forming synaptic vesicles.

In addition to recycling of choline, the synaptic vesicle membrane also is recycled to conserve the surface area of the presynaptic membrane. This membrane recycling is accomplished by the formation of **clathrin-coated vesicles.**

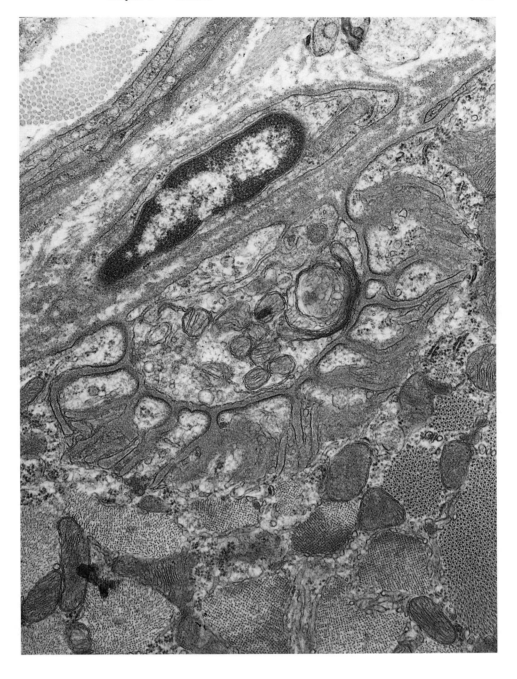

Figure 8-12. Electron micrograph of a mouse myoneural junction. (From Feczko, J.D., and Klueber, K.M.: Cytoarchitecture of muscle in a genetic model of murine diabetes. Am. J. Anat. **182:**224–240, 1988. Copyright © 1988. Reprinted by permission of John Wiley & Sons, Inc.)

CLINICAL CORRELATIONS

Botulism is usually caused by ingestion of improperly preserved canned foods. The toxin, produced by the microbe **Clostridium botulinum,** interferes with the release of acetylcholine, with resultant muscle paralysis and, if untreated, death.

Myasthenia gravis is an autoimmune disease in which autoantibodies attach to acetylcholine receptors, blocking their availability to acetylcholine. Receptors thus inactivated are endocytosed and replaced by new receptors, which are also inactivated by the autoantibodies. Thus the number of locations for the initiation of muscle depolar-

ization is reduced and the skeletal muscles will weaken gradually. The condition results in pulmonary infections, respiratory compromise, and subsequent death. Certain **neurotoxins,** such as bungarotoxin of some poisonous snakes, also bind to acetylcholine receptors, causing paralysis and eventual death due to respiratory compromise.

Muscle Spindles

When muscle is stretched it normally undergoes reflex contraction, known as the **stretch reflex.** This protective response, preventing the tearing of muscle fibers, is initiated by the **muscle spindle,** an encapsulated sensory receptor lo-

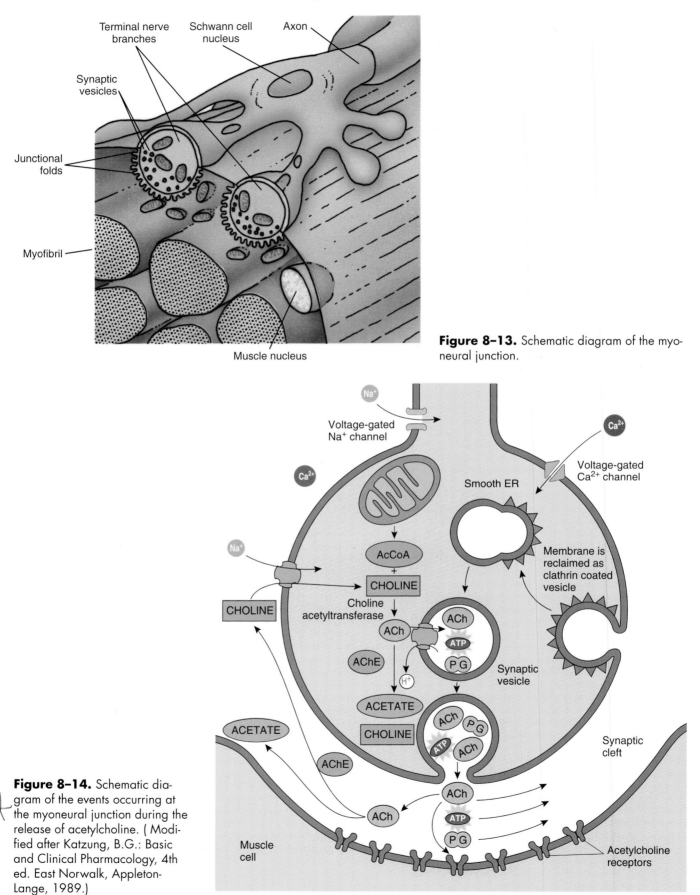

Figure 8–13. Schematic diagram of the myoneural junction.

Figure 8–14. Schematic diagram of the events occurring at the myoneural junction during the release of acetylcholine. (Modified after Katzung, B.G.: Basic and Clinical Pharmacology, 4th ed. East Norwalk, Appleton-Lange, 1989.)

cated among the muscle cells (Fig. 8–15). Each muscle spindle is composed of 8 to 10 elongated, narrow, very small, modified muscle cells called **intrafusal fibers,** surrounded by the fluid-containing **periaxial space,** which, in turn, is enclosed by the capsule. The connective tissue elements of the capsule are continuous with the collagen fibers of the perimysium and endomysium.

Intrafusal fibers are of two types: **nuclear bag fibers** and the more numerous, thinner **nuclear chain fibers.** The nuclei of both types of fibers occupy the center of the cell: their myofibrils are located on either side of the nuclear region, limiting contraction to the poles of these spindle-shaped cells. The nuclei in the nuclear bag fibers are aggregated, whereas they are aligned in a single row in nuclear chain fibers. The skeletal muscle fibers surrounding the muscle spindle are unremarkable and are called **extrafusal fibers.**

Large, sensory nerve fibers form **annulospiral** or **primary nerve endings** (type Ia, *rapidly adapting*), which wrap spirally around the nuclear regions of both types of intrafusal fibers. On either side of these nerve endings, **flowerspray** or **secondary nerve endings** (type IIa, *slowly adapting*) also wrap around the nuclear region. Additionally, slowly conducting axons of small **γ-efferent (motor) neurons** terminate on motor endplates on the myofibrillar aspects of the intrafusal fibers. The extrafusal fibers receive their normal nerve fibers, large, rapidly conducting axons of **α-efferent (motor) neurons.**

When a muscle is stretched, the annulospiral and flowerspray nerve endings become distorted and stimulated, relaying information to the α-motor neurons that supply the extrafusal fibers (i.e., the muscle cells), resulting in muscle contraction. The flower-spray nerve endings respond to the **duration,** whereas annulospiral nerve endings respond to the **rate,** of stretching. The sensitivity of the muscle spindle

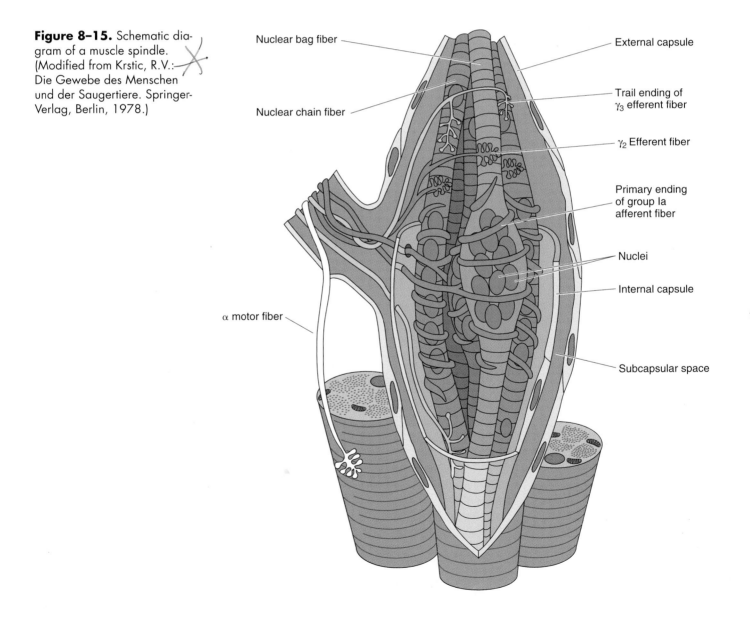

Figure 8–15. Schematic diagram of a muscle spindle. (Modified from Krstic, R.V.: Die Gewebe des Menschen und der Saugertiere. Springer-Verlag, Berlin, 1978.)

Nuclear bag fiber

Nuclear chain fiber

α motor fiber

External capsule

Trail ending of γ₃ efferent fiber

γ₂ Efferent fiber

Primary ending of group Ia afferent fiber

Nuclei

Internal capsule

Subcapsular space

is increased if the γ-efferent neurons stimulate the contractile regions of the intrafusal fibers, because this causes a stretching of their nuclear regions.

CLINICAL CORRELATIONS

The **simple reflex arc,** such as the knee jerk, is an example of the function of muscle spindles. Tapping on the patellar tendon results in a sudden stretching of the muscle (and of the muscle spindles). The annulospiral and flower-spray nerve endings are stimulated, relaying the stimulus to the α-motor neurons of the spinal cord, resulting in muscle contraction.

Golgi Tendon Organs (Neurotendinous Spindles)

When a muscle undergoes strenuous contraction it may place undue stress on its tendons. To protect the tendon, **Golgi tendon organs** provide an inhibitory feedback to the α-motor neuron of the muscle, resulting in relaxation of the contracting tendon's muscle. Thus, the function of Golgi tendon organs, also called **neurotendinous spindles,** is opposite that of muscle spindles. These two sensory organs act in concert to integrate spinal reflex systems.

Golgi tendon organs are composed of encapsulated, thin intrafusal collagen fibers that receive the nerve endings of type-Ib sensory neurons. The nerve endings become stimulated upon excessive stretching of the intrafusal collagen fibers.

CLINICAL CORRELATIONS

The ability of a person to touch his/her nose in absolute darkness is due to the integrative activities of muscle spindles and, possibly, Golgi tendon organs. These structures provide feedback not only on the amount of tension placed on the muscle and tendon but also on their position in three-dimensional space.

Cardiac Muscle

Heart muscle, another form of striated muscle, is found only in the heart and in pulmonary veins where they join the heart. Cardiac muscle is derived from a strictly defined mass of splanchnic mesenchyme, the **myoepicardial mantle,** whose cells give rise to the epicardium and **myocardium.**

The adult myocardium consists of an anastomosing network of branching cardiac muscle cells arranged in layers **(laminae).** Laminae are separated from each other by slender connective tissue sheets that convey blood vessels, nerves, and the conducting system of the heart. Capillaries, derived from these branches, invade the intercellular connective tissue, forming a rich, dense network of capillary beds surrounding every cardiac muscle cell.

Heart muscle differs from skeletal and smooth muscles in

that it possesses an **inherent rhythmicity** as well as the ability to **contract spontaneously.** A system of modified cardiac muscle cells has been adapted to ensure the coordination of its contractile actions. This specialized system as well as the associated autonomic nerve supply is discussed in Chapter 11 on the circulatory system.

Cardiac Muscle Cells

The resting lengths of individual cardiac muscle cells vary, but on the average they are 15 μm in diameter and 80 μm long. Each cell possesses a single, large, oval, centrally placed nucleus, though occasionally two nuclei are present (Figs. 8–16, 8–17).

Intercalated Disks

Cardiac muscle cells form highly specialized end-to-end junctions, referred to as **intercalated disks** (see Fig. 8–16; Figs. 8–18, 8–19, 8–20). The cell membranes involved in these junctions approximate each other, so that in most areas they are separated by a space of less than 15 to 20 nm.

Intercalated disks have **transverse portions,** where fasciae adherentes and desmosomes abound, as well as **lateral portions** rich in gap junctions (see Figs. 8–18, 8–20). On the cytoplasmic aspect of the sarcolemma of the intercalated disks, **thin myofilaments** attach to the fasciae adherentes, which are thus analogous to Z disks. Gap junctions, which function in permitting rapid flow of information from one

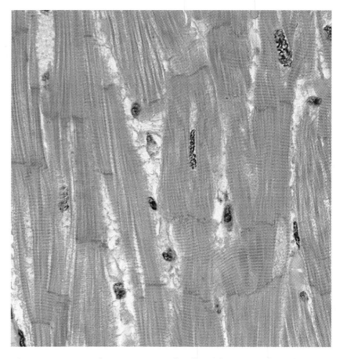

Figure 8–16. Photomicrograph of cardiac muscle in longitudinal section (× 540).

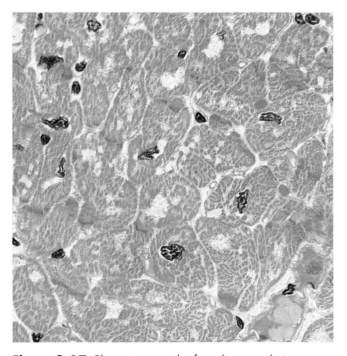

Figure 8-17. Photomicrograph of cardiac muscle in cross-section.

cell to the next, also form in regions where cells lying side by side come in close contact with each other.

Organelles

The bandings of cardiac muscle fibers are identical with those of skeletal muscle, including alternating I and A bands. Each sarcomere possesses the same substructure as its skeletal muscle counterpart; therefore, the mode and mechanism of contraction are virtually identical in the two striated muscles. Two major differences should be noted, however—one in the membranous system and the other in the Ca^{2+} supply of cardiac muscle.

The sarcoplasmic reticulum of cardiac muscle does not form terminal cisternae as in skeletal muscle; instead, small terminals of sarcoplasmic reticulum approximate the **T tubules.** These structures do not normally form a triad as in skeletal muscle; rather the association is usually limited to two partners, resulting in a **diad.** Unlike in skeletal muscle, the diads are located in the vicinity of the Z line. The T tubules of cardiac muscle cells are almost two and a half times the diameter of those in skeletal muscle and are lined by an **external lamina.** The significance of these differences may be attributed to the faster contraction rate of skeletal muscle in contrast with that of cardiac muscle. The second major difference is that Ca^{2+} *must be actively transported* into the cardiac muscle cell from the extracellular fluid compartment.

Almost half of the volume of the cardiac muscle cell is occupied by mitochondria, attesting to its great energy consumption. Glycogen to a certain extent, but mostly triglycerides (about 60% during basal rate), form the energy supply of the heart. Because the oxygen requirement of cardiac muscle cells is high, they contain an abundant supply of myoglobin.

Atrial muscle cells are somewhat smaller than those of the ventricles. These cells also house granules (especially in the right atrium) containing **atrial natriuretic peptide,**

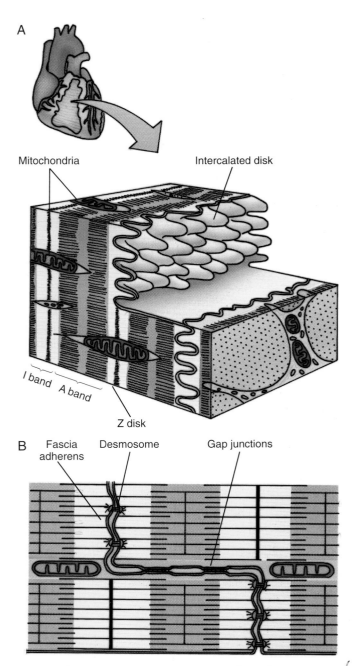

Figure 8-18. Schematic diagram of cardiac muscle. A, Three-dimensional view of the intercalated disk. **B,** Two-dimensional view of the intercated disk, displaying adhering and communicating junctions.

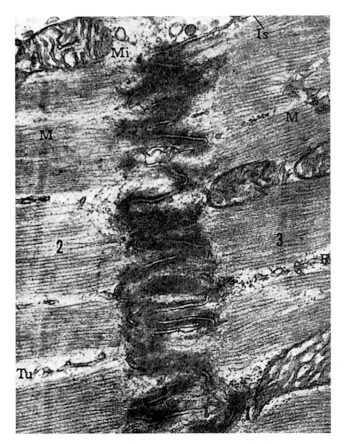

Figure 8–19. Electron micrograph of an intercalated disk from a steer heart (× 31,000). Mi, mitochondrion; Tu, sarcoplasmic reticulum; Ri, ribosomes; M, M-line; Is, intercellular space; 2 and 3 denote the two cells, one on either side of the intercalated disk. (From Rhodin, J.A.G.: An Atlas of Ultrastructure. Philadelphia, W.B. Saunders Company, 1963.)

which function to lower blood pressure (Fig. 8–21). This peptide acts by decreasing the capabilities of renal tubules to resorb (conserve) sodium and water.

CLINICAL CORRELATIONS

During cardiac hypertrophy there is no increase in myocardial fiber number; instead, heart muscle cells become longer and larger in diameter. Damage to the heart does not result in regeneration of muscle tissue; instead, the dead muscle cells are replaced by fibrous connective tissue.

Lack of Ca^{2+} in the extracellular compartment results in cessation of cardiac muscle contraction within 1 minute, whereas skeletal muscle fibers can continue to contract for several hours.

Although a small percentage of energy production may be achieved by anaerobic metabolism (up to 10% during hypoxia), total anaerobic conditions cannot sustain ventricular contraction.

Smooth Muscle

The cells of the third type of muscle exhibit no striations; therefore, they are referred to as **smooth muscle.** Additionally, smooth muscle cells do not possess a system of T tubules. Smooth muscle is found in the walls of hollow viscera (e.g., the gastrointestinal, some of the reproductive, and the urinary tracts), walls of blood vessels, larger ducts of compound glands, respiratory passages, and small bundles within the dermis of skin. Smooth muscle is not under voluntary control; instead, it is regulated by the autonomic nervous system, hormones (such as bradykinins), and local physiological conditions. Hence, smooth muscle is also referred to as **involuntary muscle.**

In addition to its contractile functions, some smooth muscle is capable of exogenous **protein synthesis.** Among the

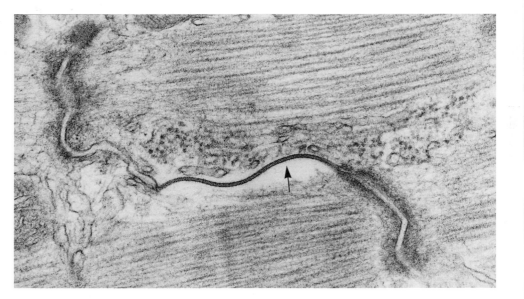

Figure 8–20. Intercalated disk from the atrium of a mouse heart (×61,500). The arrow points to gap junctions. (From Forbes, M.S., and Sperelakis, N.: Intercalated disks of mammalian heart: A review of structure and function. Tissue Cell **17:**605, 1985.)

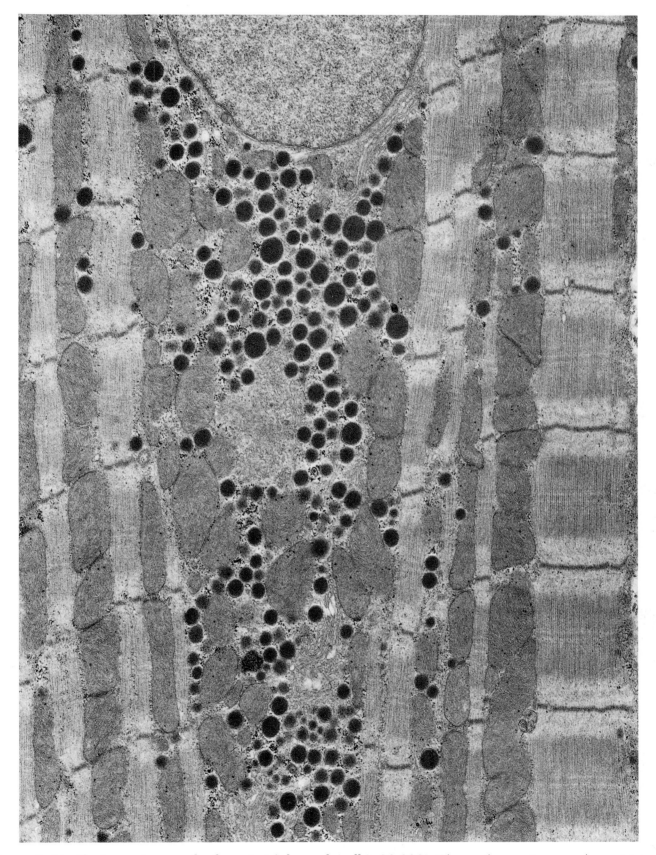

Figure 8–21. Electron micrograph of a rat atrial muscle cell (× 23,000). Observe the secretory granules containing atrial natriuretic peptide. (Courtesy of Dr. Stephen C. Pang.)

substances manufactured by smooth muscle cells for extracellular utilization are collagen, elastin, glycosaminoglycans, proteoglycans, and growth factors.

Light Microscopy of Smooth Muscle Fibers

Smooth muscle fibers are **fusiform,** elongated cells, whose average length is about 0.2 mm with a diameter of 5 to 6 μm. The cells taper at either end, whereas the central portion contains an oval-shaped nucleus, housing two or more nucleoli (see Fig. 8–2; Figs. 8–22, 8–23). During muscle shortening the nucleus assumes a characteristic **cork-screw appearance,** due to the method of smooth muscle contraction (Fig. 8–24).

Each smooth muscle cell is surrounded by an **external lamina,** which invariably separates the sarcolemma of contiguous muscle cells (Fig. 8–25). Embedded in the external lamina are numerous **reticular fibers,** which appear to envelop individual smooth muscle cells and function in harnessing the force of contraction.

Under hematoxylin and eosin staining, the cytoplasm of smooth muscle fibers appears unremarkable; however, iron hematoxylin stain demonstrates the presence of **dense bodies** adhering to the cytoplasmic aspect of the cell membrane. In addition to dense bodies, thin longitudinal striations may

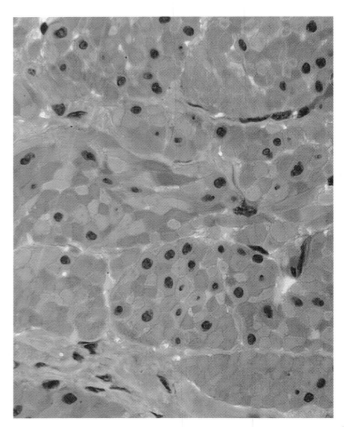

Figure 8–23. Photomicrograph of smooth muscle in cross-section (× 540).

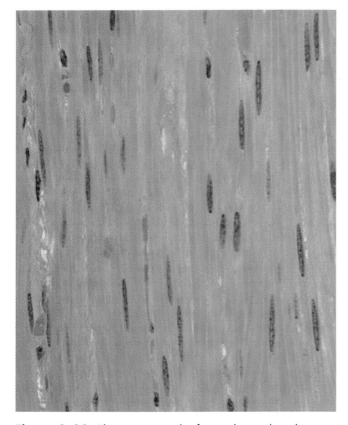

Figure 8–22. Photomicrograph of smooth muscle in longitudinal section (× 540).

be evident in the sarcoplasm of smooth muscle cells, representing clumped associations of **myofilaments.**

Smooth muscle cells usually form sheets of various thicknesses, although they may also occur as individual cells. When they form sheets, the cells are arranged such that they form a continuous network in which their tapered portions fit almost precisely into existing spaces between the expanded regions of neighboring smooth muscle cells (see Fig. 8–2). In cross-section, outlines of various diameters may be noted, some containing nuclei, some not (see Fig. 8–23). Cross-sections without nuclei represent the tapered ends of smooth muscle cells as they interdigitate with the other smooth muscle fibers.

Sheets of smooth muscle cells are frequently arranged in two layers, perpendicular to each other, as in the digestive and urinary systems. This arrangement permits waves of peristalsis.

Fine Structure of Smooth Muscle

The perinuclear cytoplasm of smooth muscle cells, especially the regions adjacent the two poles of the nucleus, contains numerous mitochondria, Golgi apparatus, rough and smooth endoplasmic reticulum, and inclusions such as glycogen (see Fig. 8–25). Additionally, an extensive array of

cytoplasmic aspect of the smooth muscle sarcolemma and are believed to resemble Z disks in function. The force of contraction is relayed, through the association of myofilaments with dense bodies, to the intermediate filaments, which act to twist and shorten the cell along its longitudinal axis.

Lying just beneath the cell membrane are structures that may be associated with the sparse sarcoplasmic reticulum, known as **caveolae (sarcolemmal vesicles).** These vesicles may function in the release and sequestering of calcium ions.

Control of Smooth Muscle Contraction

Although the regulation of contraction in smooth muscle depends on Ca²⁺, the control mechanism differs from that encountered in striated muscle, because smooth muscle thin filaments are devoid of troponin. Additionally, not only do myosin molecules assume a different configuration in that their actin-binding site is masked by their light meromyosin moiety (Fig. 8–26), but their light chains are different from those of striated muscle.

Contraction of smooth muscle fibers proceeds as follows:

1. Calcium ions, released from caveolae, bind to **calmodulin** (a regulatory protein ubiquitous in living organisms), thereby altering its conformation. The Ca²⁺-calmodulin complex then activates **myosin light-chain kinase.**
2. Myosin light-chain kinase phosphorylates one of the myosin light chains, which permits the unfolding of the light meromyosin moiety to form the typical "golf club"–shaped myosin molecule (see Fig. 8–26).
3. The phosphorylated light chain unmasks the myosin's actin binding site, permitting the interaction between actin and the S₁ fragment of myosin, resulting in contraction.

Because phosphorylation occurs slowly, the process of smooth muscle contraction takes longer than does contraction of skeletal and cardiac muscles. Interestingly, ATP hydrolysis occurs more slowly in smooth muscle than in striated muscles. Thus smooth muscle contraction is not only *prolonged* but also requires *less energy.*

Decrease in the sarcoplasmic calcium level results in the dissociation of the **calmodulin–calcium complex,** causing inactivation of **myosin light-chain kinase.** The subsequent dephosphorylation of myosin light chains brings about *masking* of the myosin's actin binding site and the subsequent *relaxation* of the muscle.

Innervation of Smooth Muscle

Neuromuscular junctions in smooth muscle are not as specifically organized as those of skeletal muscle. The synapses may vary from 15 to 100 nm in width. The neural component of the synapse is the **en passant** type, which occurs as axonal swellings that contain **synaptic vesicles,**

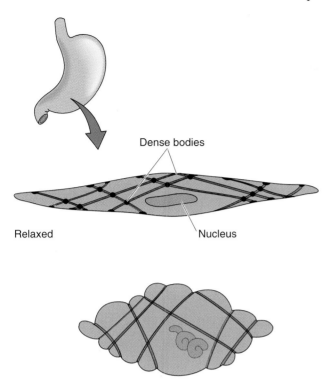

Figure 8–24. Schematic diagram of a relaxed and contracted smooth muscle cell.

interweaving **thin** (7-nm) and **thick** (15-nm) filaments are present. The thin filaments are composed of actin (with its associated tropomyosin but with the notable **absence of troponin),** whereas the thick filaments are composed of myosin.

Myofilaments of smooth muscle are not arranged in the paracrystalline fashion of striated muscle, nor is the organization of the thick filaments the same. Instead, the myosin molecules are lined up so that the **heavy meromyosin heads** (S₁) project from the thick filaments throughout the length of the filament with the two ends lacking heavy meromyosin. The middle of the filament, unlike in striated muscle, also possesses heavy meromyosin, making available a larger surface area for the interaction of actin with myosin and permitting **contractions of long duration.**

The **all-or-none law** of striated muscle contraction does *not* apply to smooth muscle. The entire cell or only a portion of the cell may contract at a given instant, even though the method of contraction probably follows the "sliding filament theory" of contraction.

The contractile forces are harnessed, intracellularly, by an additional system of intermediate filaments, **vimentin** and **desmin** in *vascular* smooth muscle, and **desmin** (only) in *nonvascular* smooth muscle. These intermediate filaments as well as thin filaments insert into **dense bodies,** formed of **α-actinin** and other Z disk–associated proteins. Dense bodies may be located in the cytoplasm or associated with the

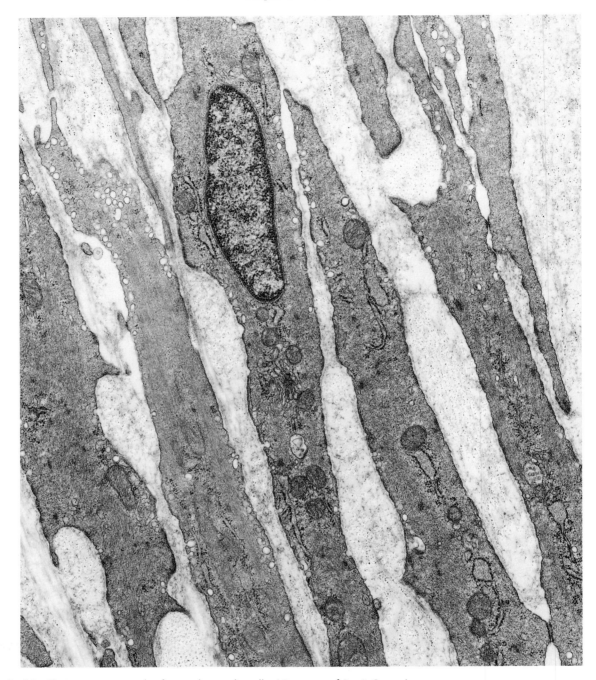

Figure 8–25. Electron micrograph of smooth muscle cells. (Courtesy of Dr. J. Strum.)

housing either **norepinephrine** for sympathetic or **acetylcholine** for parasympathetic innervation.

In certain cases every smooth muscle cell receives individual innervation, as in the iris of the eye and vas deferens of the male reproductive tract. Smooth muscle innervated in this fashion is referred to as **multiunit type.**

Other smooth muscle cells, such as those of the gastrointestinal tract and uterus, do not possess individual innervation; rather, only a few muscle cells are equipped with neuromuscular junctions. In these muscles, referred to as **vis-** **ceral smooth muscles,** impulse transmission occurs via **nexus** (gap junctions) located between neighboring smooth muscle cells. Visceral smooth muscle may also be regulated by humoral or microenvironmental factors, such as oxytocin in the uterus or stretching of the muscle fibers in the intestines.

Still other smooth muscles of the body are of an **intermediate type,** in which a certain percentage (30% to 60%) of the cells receive individual innervation.

Table 8–3 summarizes the similarities and differences among the three types of muscle.

Table 8–3. Comparison of the Three Types of Muscle

Features	Skeletal	Cardiac	Smooth
Sarcomeres	Yes	Yes	No
Nuclei	Multinucleated; peripherally located	One (or two); centrally located	One; centrally located
Sarcoplasmic reticulum	Well-developed with terminal cisterns	Poorly defined; some small terminals	Some smooth endoplasmic reticulum (but not involved in calcium storage)
T tubules	Yes; small, involved in triad formation	Yes; large, involved in diad formation	None
Cell junctions	None	Intercalated disks	Nexus (gap junctions)
Contraction	Voluntary; "all or none"	Involuntary; rhythmic and spontaneous	Involuntary; slow and forceful; not "all or none"
Calcium control	Calsequestrin in terminal cisternae	Calcium from extracellular sources	Caveolae
Calcium binding	Troponin C	Troponin C	Calmodulin
Regeneration	Yes, via satellite cells	None	Yes
Mitosis	No	No	Yes
Nerve fibers	Somatic motor	Autonomic	Autonomic
Connective tissue	Epimysium, perimysium and endomysium	Connective tissue sheaths and endomysium	Connective tissue sheaths and endomysium
Distinctive features	Long; cylinder-shaped; many peripheral nuclei	Branched cells; intercalated disks; single nucleus	Fusiform cells with no striations; one nucleus

Regeneration of Muscle

Although **skeletal muscle** cells do not have the capability of mitotic activity, the tissue can regenerate because of the presence of satellite cells. These cells may undergo mitotic activity, resulting in **hyperplasia,** subsequent to muscle injury. Under certain other conditions, such as "muscle building," satellite cells may fuse with existing muscle cells, thus increasing muscle mass during skeletal muscle **hypertrophy.**

Cardiac muscle is incapable of regeneration. Subsequent to damage, such as myocardial infarct, **fibroblasts** invade the damaged region, undergo cell division, and form fibrous connective tissue (scar tissue) to repair the damage.

Smooth muscle cells retain their mitotic capability to form more smooth muscle cells. This ability is especially evident in the pregnant uterus, where the muscular wall becomes thicker both by hypertrophy of individual cells and by hyperplasia derived from mitotic activity of the smooth muscle cells. Small defects, subsequent to injury, may result in formation of new smooth muscle cells. These new cells may be derived via mitotic activity of existing smooth muscle cells, as in the gastrointestinal and urinary tracts, or from

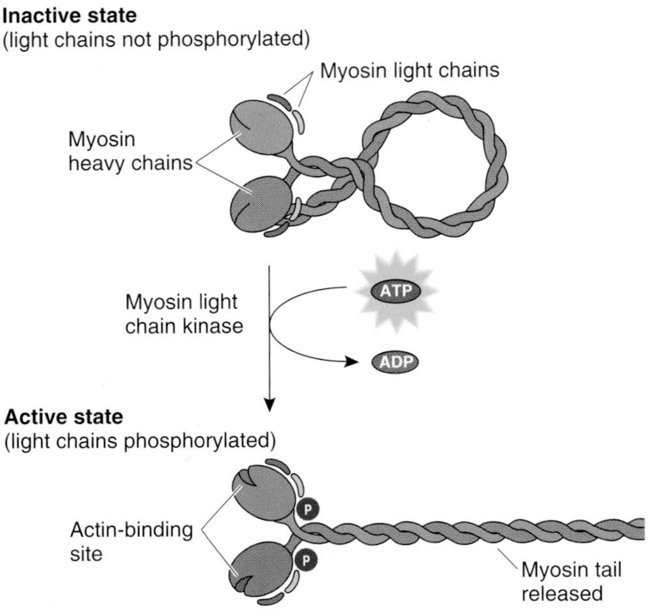

Inactive state
(light chains not phosphorylated)

Myosin light chains

Myosin
heavy chains

Myosin light
chain kinase

ATP

ADP

Active state
(light chains phosphorylated)

Actin-binding
site

P

P

Myosin tail
released

Figure 8–26. Schematic diagram of activation of a myosin molecule of smooth muscle. (Modified from Alberts, B., Bray, D., Lewis, J., Raff, M., Roberts, K., and Watson, J.D.: Molecular Biology of the Cell. New York, Garland Publishing, 1994. Copyright Cell Press.)

differentiation of relatively undifferentiated **pericytes** accompanying some blood vessels.

Myoepithelial Cells and Myofibroblasts

Certain cells associated with glandular secretory units possess contractile capabilities. These **myoepithelial cells** are modified to assist in the delivery of the secretory products into the ducts of the gland. Myoepithelial cells are flattened in morphology and possess long processes, which wrap around the glandular units (see Figs. 5–23, 5–24). Myoepithelial cells contain both actin and myosin. Mechanisms and control of contraction resemble, but are not identical to, that occurring in smooth muscle.

In lactating mammary glands myoepithelial cells contract upon the release of **oxytocin,** whereas in the lacrimal gland they contract because of the action of **acetylcholine.**

Myofibroblasts resemble fibroblasts but have abundant actin and myosin. They can contract and are especially prominent in **wound contraction** and in tooth eruption.

Nervous Tissue

9

Nervous tissue, comprising perhaps as many as a trillion neurons with multitudes of interconnections, forms the complex system of neuronal communication within the body. Certain **receptors,** elaborated on the terminals of the neurons, are specialized for receiving different types of stimuli (e.g., mechanical, chemical, thermal) and transducing them into nerve impulses that may eventually be conducted to nerve centers. These impulses are then transferred to other neurons for processing and transmission to higher centers for perceiving sensations or for initiating motor responses.

To accomplish these functions, the nervous system is organized anatomically into the **central nervous system (CNS),** which includes the brain and spinal cord, and the **peripheral nervous system (PNS).** The latter, which lies outside the CNS, includes cranial nerves, emanating from the brain; spinal nerves, emanating from the spinal cord; and their associated ganglia.

Functionally, the nervous system is divided into a **sensory (afferent) component,** which receives and transmits impulses to the CNS for processing, and a **motor (efferent) component,** which originates in the CNS and transmits impulses to effector organs throughout the body. The motor component is further subdivided into the somatic system and the autonomic system. In the **somatic system,** impulses originating in the CNS are transmitted directly, via a single neuron, to skeletal muscles. In the **autonomic system,** by contrast, impulses from the CNS first are transmitted to an autonomic **ganglion** via one neuron; a second neuron originating in the autonomic ganglion then transmits the impulses to smooth muscles, cardiac muscles, or glands.

In addition to neurons, nervous tissue contains numerous other cells, collectively called **neuroglial cells,** which do not receive or transmit impulses. These cells support neurons.

Development of Nervous Tissue

As the notochord develops early in embryonic life, it induces the ectoderm to form **neuroepithelium,** which thickens and forms the **neural plate.** As the margins of this plate continue to thicken, the plate buckles, forming a **neural groove** whose edges continue to grow toward each other until they come together, forming the **neural tube.** The rostral (anterior) end of this structure develops into the brain; the remaining (caudal) portion of the neural tube develops into the spinal cord. Additionally, the neural tube gives rise to the neuroglia, ependyma, neurons, and choroid plexus.

A small mass of cells at the lateral margins of the neural plate, which does not become incorporated into the neural plate complex, forms the **neural crest cells.** This group of cells begins to migrate away from the developing neural plate early in development. These cells eventually form many structures, including the following:

- Most of the sensory components of the peripheral nervous system
- Sensory neurons of cranial and spinal sensory ganglia (dorsal root ganglia)
- Autonomic ganglia and the postganglionic autonomic neurons originating in them
- Much of the mesenchyme of the anterior head and neck
- Melanocytes of the skin and oral mucosa
- Odontoblasts (cells responsible for production of dentin)
- Chromaffin cells of the adrenal medulla
- Cells of the arachnoid and pia mater
- Satellite cells of peripheral ganglia
- Schwann cells

CLINICAL CORRELATIONS

Abnormal organogenesis of the CNS results in various types of congenital malformations. **Spina bifida** is a defective closure of the spinal column. In severe cases the spinal cord and meninges may protrude through the unfused areas. **Spina bifida anterior** is a defective closure of the vertebrae. In severe cases there may be defective development of the viscera of the thorax and abdomen.

Anencephaly is failure of the developmental anterior

neuropore to close with a poorly formed brain and an absent cranial vault. It is usually not compatible with life.

Epilepsy results from abnormal migration of cortical cells, which disrupts normal interneuronal functioning.

Hirschsprung disease, also known as **congenital megacolon,** is caused by failure of the neural crest cells to invade the wall of the gut. As a result the wall lacks **Auerbach plexus,** the parasympathetic system innervating the distal end of the colon, leading to dilatation and hypertrophy of the colon.

Cells

The cells of the nervous system may be subdivided into two categories: **Neurons,** responsible for the receptive, integrative, and motor functions of the nervous system and **neuroglial cells,** responsible for supporting and protecting neurons.

Neurons

The cells responsible for the reception and transmission of nerve impulses to and from the CNS are the **neurons.** These cells, ranging in diameter from 5 to 150 μm, are among both the smallest and the largest cells in the body. Most neurons are composed of three distinct parts: a cell body, multiple dendrites, and a single axon.

Structure and Function of Neurons

The **cell body** of a neuron, also known as the **perikaryon** or **soma,** is the central portion of the cell where the nucleus and perinuclear cytoplasm are contained. Generally, neurons in the CNS are polygonal (Fig. 9–1) with concave surfaces between the many cell processes, whereas neurons in the dorsal root ganglion (a sensory ganglion of the PNS) have a round cell body from which only one process exits (Fig. 9–2). Cell bodies present different sizes and shapes that are characteristic for their type and location, recognizable by the neurohistologist. These different morphologies are described later when the various regions of the nervous system are discussed.

Projecting from the cell body are the **dendrites,** processes specialized for receiving stimuli from sensory cells, axons, and other neurons (Fig. 9–3). Often the dendrites are multibranched and the terminals are arborized so that they can receive multiple stimuli from many other neurons simultaneously. The nerve impulses received by the dendrites are then transmitted toward the soma.

On the opposite side of the cell body from the dendrites is the **axon,** a single process of varying diameter and up to 100 cm in length. The axon conducts the impulse away from the soma to other neurons, muscles, or glands. The axon may also receive stimuli from other neurons, thus modifying its behavior. As with dendrites, the terminals of the axon are arborized. These axon terminals, known as **end bulbs (termi-**

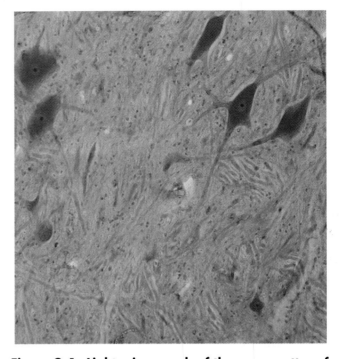

Figure 9–1. Light micrograph of the gray matter of the spinal cord (× 270). Observe the multipolar neuron cell bodies and their processes.

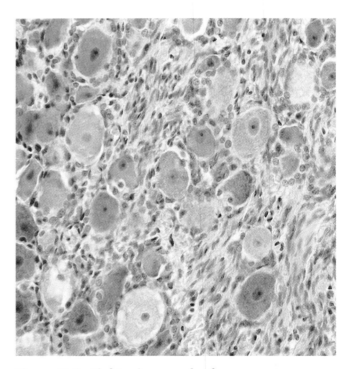

Figure 9–2. Light micrograph of a sensory ganglion (× 270). Observe the large neuronal cell bodies with singular nucleoli.

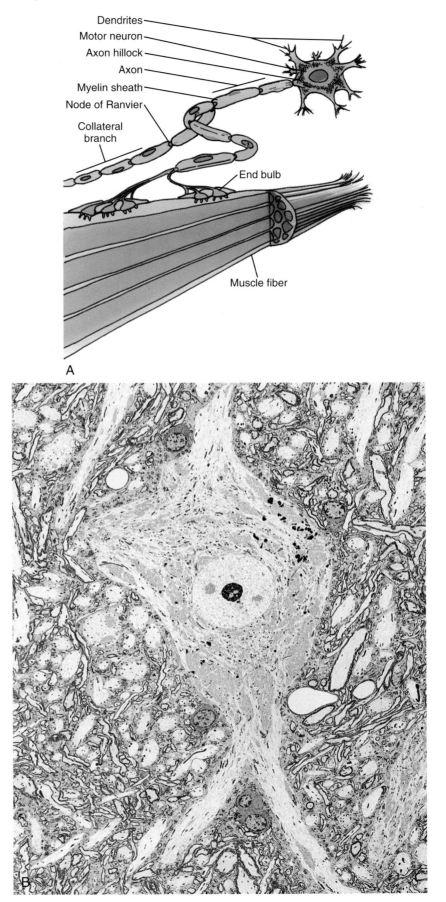

Dendrites
Motor neuron
Axon hillock
Axon
Myelin sheath
Node of Ranvier
Collateral branch

End bulb

Muscle fiber

A

B

Figure 9–3. Motor neuron. A, Diagram of a typical motor neuron. **B,** Electron micrograph of a ventral horn neuron with several of its dendrites (× 1410). (From Ling, E.A., Wen, C.Y., Shieh, J.Y., Yick, T.Y., and Leong, S.K.: Neuroglial response to neuron injury: A study using intraneural injection of *Ricinus communis* agglutinin-60. J. Anat. **164:**201–213, 1989. Reprinted with the permission of Cambridge University Press.)

nal boutons), come close to another cell and form a **synapse,** the region where the impulse can be transmitted to the receiving cell.

Neurons can be classified according to their shape and the arrangement of their processes (Fig. 9–4). The prevalence and typical location of the various neuron types are discussed later.

NEURONAL CELL BODY. The cell body (soma, perikaryon) is the region of the neuron containing the large pale-staining nucleus and perinuclear cytoplasm (Fig. 9–5). The remainder of the neuron's cytoplasm is located in the processes originating from the cell body. The **nucleus** is large, usually spherical to ovoid, and centrally located. It contains finely dispersed chromatin, indicative of a rich synthetic activity, although smaller neurons may present some condensed, inactive heterochromatin. A well-defined nucleolus is also common.

The **cytoplasm** of the cell body has abundant rough endoplasmic reticulum (RER) with many cisternae in parallel arrays, a characteristic especially prominent in large motor neurons. Polyribosomes are also scattered throughout the cytoplasm. When these cisternae and polyribosomes are stained with basic dyes, they appear as clumps of basophilic material called **Nissl bodies,** which are visible with the light microscope. RER is also present in the dendritic region of the neuron but only as scattered short or branching cisternae. Rough endoplasmic reticulum is absent at the **axon hillock,** the region on the cell body where the axon arises; however, smooth endoplasmic reticulum (SER) is present in the axon.

Although Nissl bodies in each type of neuron have a characteristic size, shape, and form, no pattern has been observed. Generally, small neurons display small granular Nissl bodies, but not all large neurons display larger Nissl bodies. It is suggested that these differences may be related to changing physiological and pathological conditions within the neuron.

Most neurons have abundant SER throughout the cell body; this extends into the dendrites and the axon, forming **hypolemmal cisternae** directly beneath the plasmalemma. These cisternae are continuous with the RER in the cell body and weave between the Nissl bodies on their way into the dendrites and axon. Although it is unclear how they

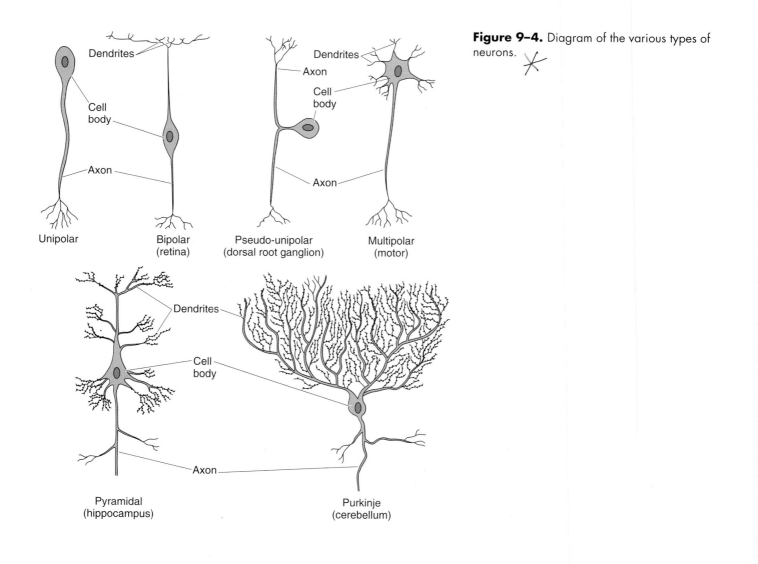

Figure 9–4. Diagram of the various types of neurons.

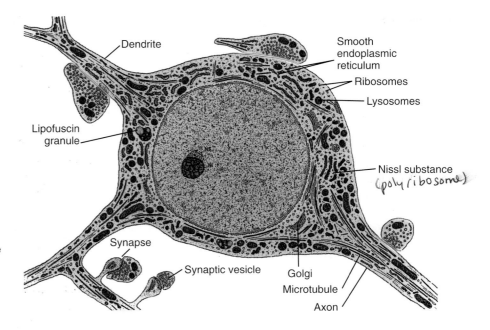

Figure 9-5. Diagram of the ultrastructure of a neuronal cell body. (From Lentz, T.L.: Cell Fine Structure. An Atlas of Drawings of Whole-Cell Structure. Philadelphia, W.B. Saunders Company, 1971.)

function, it is known that hypolemmal cisternae sequester calcium and contain protein. These cisternae may serve as a conduit for distributing protein throughout the cell. Some theorize that transport and synaptic vesicles bud from these cisternae, but much of this is still unclear.

A prominent juxtanuclear **Golgi complex** is present, composed of several closely associated cisternae exhibiting a dilated periphery, characteristic of protein-secreting cells. The Golgi complex is also thought to be responsible for the packaging of neurotransmitter substances or the enzymes essential for their production in the axon.

Numerous **mitochondria** are scattered throughout the cytoplasm of the soma, dendrites, and axon, but they are most abundant at the axon terminals. Generally, the mitochondria in neurons are more slender than those in other cells and, occasionally, their cristae are oriented longitudinally rather than transversely. It has been shown that neuronal mitochondria are constantly moving along microtubules in the cytoplasm.

Most adult neurons display only one **centriole** associated with a basal body of a cilium; it possesses the 9+0 arrangement of microtubules (see Chapter 2 concerning microtubule structure). The centriole is thought to be a vestigial structure in neurons.

Inclusions. Dark brown to black **melanin granules** are found in neurons in certain regions of the CNS (e.g., substantia nigra, locus ceruleus, dorsal motor nucleus of the vagus, and the spinal cord) and in the sympathetic ganglia of the PNS. The function of these granules in these various locations is unknown.

Lipofuscin, an irregularly shaped pigment granule, is more prevalent in the neuronal cytoplasm of older persons and is thought to be the remnants of lysosomal enzymatic activity. These granules increase with advancing age and may even crowd the organelles and nucleus to one side in the cell, possibly affecting cellular function. Iron-containing pigments also may be observed in certain neurons of the CNS and may accumulate with age.

Lipid droplets sometimes are observed in the neuronal cytoplasm and may be the result of faulty metabolism, or they may be energy reserves. **Secretory granules** are observed in neurosecretory cells; many of them contain signaling molecules.

Cytoskeletal Components. When prepared by silver impregnation for visualization by light microscopy, the neuronal cytoskeleton exhibits **neurofibrils** (up to 2 μm in diameter) coursing through the cytoplasm of the soma and extending into the processes. Electron microscopic studies reveal three different filamentous structures: microtubules (24 nm in diameter), neurofilaments (intermediate filaments 10 nm in diameter), and microfilaments (6 nm in diameter). It has been suggested that the neurofibrils observed in light microscopy represent clumped bundles of neurofilaments, an observation supported by the fact that neurofilaments are stained by silver nitrate. Microfilaments (actin filaments) are associated with the plasma membrane. The **microtubules** in neurons are identical to those in other cells except that MAP-2 (**microtubule-associated protein**) is found in the cytoplasm of the cell body and dendrite, whereas MAP-3 is present only in the axon.

DENDRITES. Dendrites are the sensory (afferent) terminals of the neuron. In some neurons, however, the cell body and the proximal end of the axon may also serve in a sensory capacity. Most neurons possess multiple dendrites, each of which arise from the cell body, usually as a single short trunk that ramifies several times into smaller and smaller branches, tapering to the terminals. The dendrite branching pattern is characteristic of each kind of neuron. The base of the dendrite arises from the cell body and contains the usual complement of organelles except for Golgi complexes (see Fig. 9–5). Farther away from the base, toward the distal end of the dendrite, many of the organelles become sparse or are absent. In the dendrites of most neurons, neurofilaments are reduced to small bundles or single filaments, which may be cross-linked to microtubules. Mitochondria, however, are abundant in dendrites. The branching of dendrites, resulting in numerous synaptic terminals, permits a neuron to receive and integrate multiple impulses so that the electrical potential of the cell membrane eventually exceeds the threshold. **Spines** located on the surfaces of some dendrites may be related to sensory selectivity and control. These spines diminish with age and poor nutrition, and they exhibit structural changes in persons with trisomy 13 and trisomy 21 (Down's syndrome). Dendrites sometimes transmit impulses to other dendrites.

AXONS. The **axon** arises from the cell body at the axon hillock as a single thin process extending longer distances from the cell body than the dendrite. In some instances axons of motor neurons may be 1 m or more in length. Axon thickness is directly related to conduction velocity, so that velocity increases as axon diameter increases. Although axon thickness varies, it is constant for a particular type of neuron. Recent evidence indicates that the relative abundance of neurofilaments in axons may be responsible for regulating axon diameter. Some axons possess **collateral branches,** which arise at right angles from the axonal trunk (see Fig. 9–2). As the axon terminates, it may ramify, forming many small **axon terminals.**

That portion of the axon from its origin to the beginning of the myelin sheath is called the **initial segment.** Deep to the **axolemma** (plasmalemma) of the initial segment is a thin, electron-dense layer whose function is not known but resembles that located at the nodes of Ranvier.

The axoplasm contains short profiles of SER and remarkably long, thin mitochondria and many microtubules. These microtubules are grouped in small bundles at the origin of the axon and in its initial segment, but distally, they become arranged as uniformly spaced, single microtubules interspersed with neurofilaments.

In the region of the axon hillock and the initial segment of the axon, also referred to as the **spike trigger zone,** action potentials give rise to nerve impulses, one of the functions of axons (see later discussion). This region also is the site for synapses of inhibitory afferents with the axon.

The plasmalemma of certain neuroglial cells form a **myelin sheath** around some axons in both the CNS and the PNS, referred to as **myelinated axons** (Figs. 9–6, 9–7). The process of myelination is described in detail later. Axons lacking myelin sheaths are called **unmyelinated axons** (Fig.

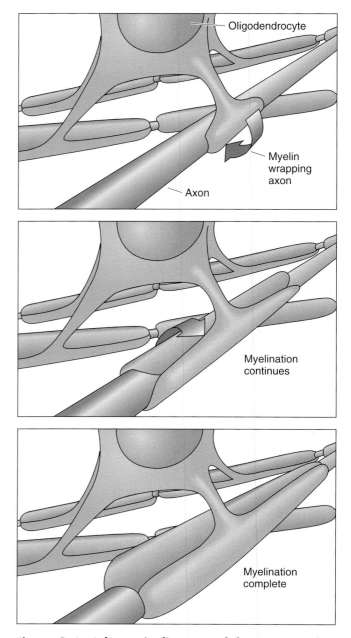

Figure 9–6. Schematic diagram of the process of myelination in the central nervous system. Note that unlike Schwann cells of the peripheral nervous system, each oligodendroglion is capable of myelinating several axons.

9–8). Nerve impulses are conducted much faster along myelinated axons than along unmyelinated axons. In the fresh state the myelin sheath imparts a white, glistening appearance to the axon. The presence of myelin permits the subdivision of the CNS into **white matter** and **gray matter.**

In addition to impulse conduction, another important function of the axon is **axonal transport** of materials between the soma and the axon terminals. In **anterograde transport,** the direction is from the cell body to the axon terminal; in **retrograde transport,** the direction is from the

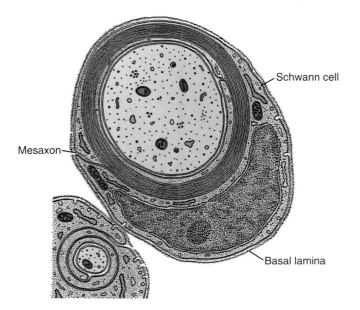

Figure 9–7. Diagram of the fine structure of a myelinated nerve fiber and its Schwann cell. (From Lentz, T.L.: Cell Fine Structure. An Atlas of Drawings of Whole-Cell Structure. Philadelphia, W.B. Saunders Company, 1971.)

axon terminal to the cell body. Axonal transport is crucial to **trophic relationships** between neurons and muscles or glands. If these relationships are interrupted, the target cells will atrophy.

Axonal transport occurs at three velocities: fast, intermediate, and slow. The most rapid transport (up to 400 mm/day) takes place in anterograde transport of organelles, which move more rapidly in the cytosol. In retrograde transport, the fastest speed is less than one half that observed in anterograde transport, with the slowest being only about 0.2 mm/day. Axonal transport speeds between these two extremes are considered intermediate.

Anterograde transport is utilized in the translocation of organelles and vesicles, as well as of macromolecules, such as actin, myosin, and clathrin, and some of the enzymes necessary for neurotransmitter synthesis at the axon terminals. Items returned to the cell body from the axon in retrograde transport include protein building blocks of neurofilaments, subunits of microtubules, and soluble enzymes. Additionally, small molecules and proteins destined for degradation are transported to endolysosomes of the soma.

Axonal transport not only distributes materials for nerve conduction and neurotransmitter synthesis but also serves to provide and ensure general maintenance of the axon. Viruses (e.g., herpes simplex and rabies virus) can utilize axonal transport to enter and spread from one neuron to another between the cell body and the nerve ending.

Since the 1970s much has been learned about the nature and functioning of the neuron by studying the mechanism of axonal retrograde transport, using the enzyme **horseradish peroxidase.** When this enzyme is injected into the axon ter-

minal, it can be detected later by histochemical techniques that mark its pathway to the cell body. In studying anterograde axonal transport, researchers inject radiolabeled amino acids into the cell body and then later determine the radioactivity at the axon terminals using autoradiography.

Microtubules are important to fast anterograde transport, because they exhibit a polarity with their plus-ends directed toward the axon terminal. **Tubulin dimers,** reaching the axoplasm via anterograde transport, are assembled onto the microtubules at their plus-ends and depolymerized at the minus-ends. The mechanism for anterograde transport involves **kinesin,** a microtubule-associated protein, because one end attaches to a vesicle and the other end interacts in a cyclic fashion with a microtubule, thus permitting the kinesin to transport the vesicle at a speed of about 3 µm/second. **Dynein,** another microtubule-associated protein, is responsible for moving vesicles along the microtubules in retrograde transport.

CLINICAL CORRELATIONS

Although **neurological tumors** account for about 50% of the intracranial tumors, those of neurons of the CNS are rare. Most intracranial tumors originate from neuroglial

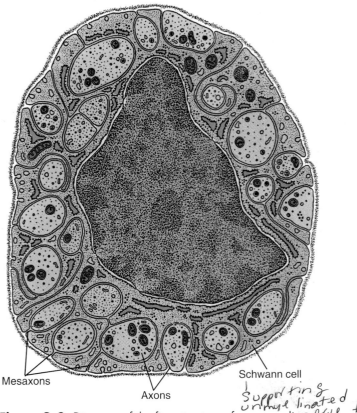

Figure 9–8. Diagram of the fine structure of an unmyelinated nerve fiber. (From Lentz, T.L.: Cell Fine Structure. An Atlas of Drawings of Whole-Cell Structure. Philadelphia, W.B. Saunders Company, 1971.)

cells (e.g., **benign oligodendrogliomas** and fatal **malignant astrocytomas**). Tumors that arise from cells of connective tissue associated with nervous tissue (e.g., **benign fibroma** or **malignant sarcoma**) are connective tissue tumors and are not related to the nervous system. Tumors of neurons in the PNS may be extremely malignant (e.g., **neuroblastoma** in the suprarenal gland, which attacks mostly infants and young children).

Classification of Neurons

As noted already, neurons are commonly classified morphologically into four major types according to their shape and arrangement of their processes (see Fig. 9–4):

- **Unipolar neurons** possess a single process and are rare in vertebrates except in early embryonic development.
- **Bipolar neurons** possess two processes emanating from the soma, a single dendrite and a single axon. Bipolar neurons are located in the vestibular and cochlear ganglia and in the olfactory epithelium of the nasal cavity.
- **Pseudounipolar neurons** possess only one process emanating from the cell body, but this process branches later into a peripheral and a central branch. The central branch enters the CNS, and the peripheral branch proceeds to its destination in the body. Each of the branches are morphologically axonal and can propagate nerve impulses, although the very distal aspect of the peripheral branch arborizes and displays small dendritic ends, indicating its receptor function. Pseudounipolar neurons develop from embryonic bipolar neurons whose processes migrate around the cell body during development and eventually fuse into a single process. During impulse transmission, the impulse passes from the dendritic (receiving) end of the peripheral process to the central process without involving the cell body. Pseudounipolar neurons are present in the dorsal root ganglia and in some of the cranial nerve ganglia. Recently, neuroanatomists have begun calling pseudounipolar neurons "unipolar neurons."
- **Multipolar neurons** are the most common type of neurons. They possess various arrangements of multiple dendrites emanating from the soma and a single axon. They are present throughout the nervous system, and most of them are motor neurons. Some multipolar neurons are named according to their morphology (e.g., pyramidal cells) or after the scientist who described them (e.g., Purkinje cells).

Neurons also are classified into three general groups according to their function:

- **Sensory (afferent) neurons** receive sensory input at their dendritic terminals and conduct impulses to the CNS for processing. Those located in the periphery of the body monitor changes in the environment, and those within the body monitor the internal environment.

- **Motor (efferent) neurons** originate in the CNS and conduct their impulses to muscles, glands, and other neurons.
- **Interneurons,** which are located completely in the CNS, function as interconnectors or integrators that establish networks of neuronal circuits between sensory and motor neurons and other interneurons. With evolution the number of neurons in the human nervous system has increased enormously, but the greatest increase has involved the interneurons that are responsible for the complex functioning of the body.

Neuroglial Cells

Cells whose function is the metabolic and mechanical support and protection of neurons collectively form the **neuroglia** (Fig. 9–9). There may be as many as 10 times more neuroglial cells than neurons in the nervous system. Although neuroglial cells form gap junctions with other neuroglial cells, they do not react to or propagate nerve impulses. Neuroglial cells that reside exclusively in the CNS include astrocytes, oligodendrocytes, microglia, and ependymal cells. Schwann cells, although located in the PNS, are now also considered to be neuroglial cells.

Astrocytes

Astrocytes are the largest of the neuroglial cells and exist as two distinct types: protoplasmic astrocytes in the gray matter of the CNS and fibrous astrocytes present mostly in the white matter of the CNS. It is difficult to distinguish between the two types of astrocytes in light micrographs.

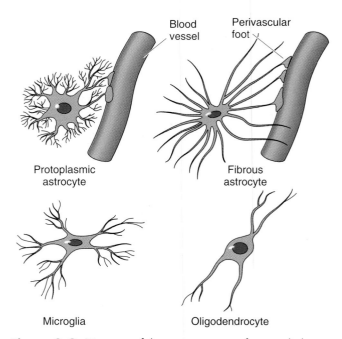

Figure 9–9. Diagram of the various types of neuroglial cells.

Some researchers have suggested that they may be the same cells functioning in different environments. Electron micrographs display distinct cytoplasmic bundles of 8- to 11-nm intermediate filaments composed of **glial fibrillar acidic protein,** which is unique to astrocytes.

Protoplasmic astrocytes are stellate-shaped cells displaying abundant cytoplasm, a large nucleus, and many short branching processes (Fig. 9–10). The tips of some processes end as **pedicles (vascular feet)** that come into contact with blood vessels. Other astrocytes lie adjacent to

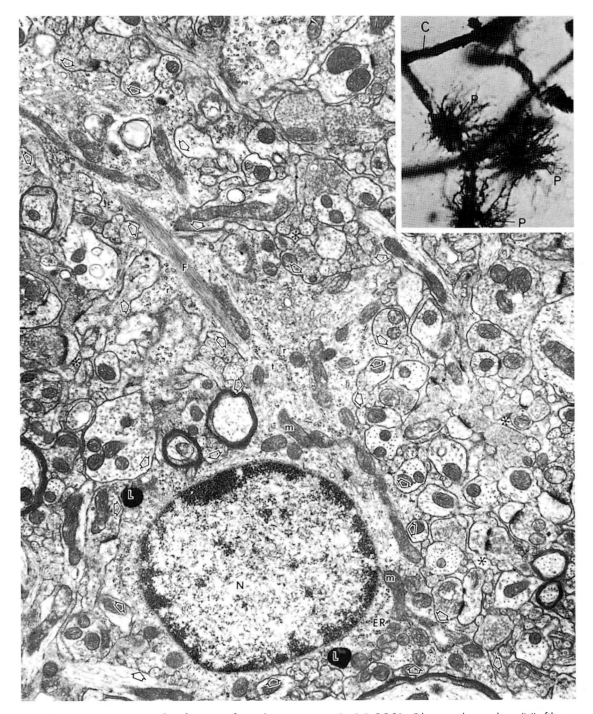

Figure 9–10. Electron micrograph of protoplasmic astrocyte (× 14,000). Observe the nucleus (N), filaments (F), mitochondria (m), microtubules (t), free ribosomes (r), and granular reticulum (ER). Two lysosomes (l) are also identified in the cytoplasm, processes of neuroglia (*). Note the irregular cell boundary indicated by arrowheads. (From Peters, A., Palay, S.L., and Webster, H.F.: The Fine Structure of the Nervous System. Philadelphia, W.B. Saunders Company, 1976.) **Inset,** Light micrograph of three highly branched protoplasmic astrocytes (P) surrounding capillaries (C). (From Leeson, T.S., Leeson, C.R., and Paparo, A.A.: Text/Atlas of Histology. Philadelphia, W.B. Saunders Company, 1988.)

blood vessels with their cell body apposed to the vessel wall. Still other protoplasmic astrocytes near the brain or spinal-cord surface exhibit pedicle-tipped processes that contact the pia mater, forming the **pia-glial membrane.** Some smaller protoplasmic astrocytes located adjacent to neuronal cell bodies are a form of satellite cells.

Fibrous astrocytes possess a euchromatic cytoplasm containing only a few organelles, free ribosomes, and glycogen (Fig. 9–11). The processes of these cells are long and mostly unbranched. These processes are closely associated with the pia mater and blood vessels but are separated from these structures by their own basal lamina.

Astrocytes function in scavenging ions and remnants of neuronal metabolism, such as K^+ ions, glutamate, and α-aminobutyric acid, accumulated in the microenvironment of the neurons. They also contribute to energy metabolism within the cerebral cortex by releasing glucose from their stored glycogen when induced by the neurotransmitters norepinephrine and vasoactive intestinal peptide (VIP). Astrocytes located at the periphery of the CNS form a continuous layer over the blood vessels and may assist in maintaining the **blood–brain barrier.** Astrocytes are also recruited to damaged areas of the CNS, where they form cellular scar tissue.

Oligodendrocytes

Oligodendrocytes resemble astrocytes, but they are smaller and contain fewer processes with sparse branching. The darkest-staining neuroglial cells, oligodendrocytes, are located in both the gray and the white matter of the CNS. Their dense cytoplasm contains a relatively small nucleus, abundant RER, many free ribosomes and mitochondria, and a conspicuous Golgi complex (Fig. 9–12). Microtubules also are present, especially in the perinuclear zone and in the processes.

Interfascicular oligodendrocytes, located in rows beside bundles of axons, are responsible for manufacturing and maintaining **myelin** about the axons of the CNS, serv-

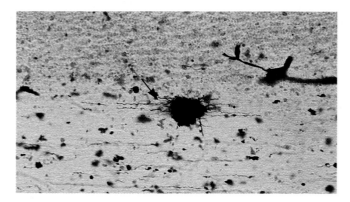

Figure 9–11. Light micrograph of a fibrous astrocyte (*arrow*) in the human cerebellum (× 132).

ing to insulate them (see Fig. 9–6). In producing myelin, oligodendrocytes function similarly to the Schwann cells of the PNS, except that a single oligodendrocyte may wrap several axons with segments of myelin, whereas a single Schwann cell wraps only one axon with myelin. Schwann cells also differ from interfascicular oligodendrocytes in the following ways: Schwann cells possess a basal lamina and retain some cytoplasm within the intracellular domains of the myelin lamellae; in addition, connective tissue invests the myelin sheaths and their surrounding Schwann cells.

Satellite oligodendrocytes are closely applied to cell bodies of neurons; their function is not clear.

Microglial Cells

Scattered throughout the CNS, **microglial cells** are small, dark-staining cells that faintly resemble oligodendrocytes. These cells exhibit scant cytoplasm, an oval to triangular nucleus, and irregular short processes. Spines also adorn the cell body and processes. These cells function as phagocytes in clearing debris and damaged structures in the CNS. Unlike the other neuroglial cells, which are derived embryologically from the neural tube, microglial cells originate in the bone marrow and are part of the mononuclear phagocytic cell population.

Ependymal Cells

Ependymal cells are the low columnar to cuboidal epithelial cells lining the ventricles of the brain and central canal of the spinal cord. They are derived from embryonic neuroepithelium of the developing nervous system. Their cytoplasm contains abundant mitochondria and bundles of intermediate filaments. In some regions these cells are ciliated, which facilitates the movement of cerebrospinal fluid. Processes emanating from the cell body reach the surface of the brain in the embryo, but in the adult they are reduced, ending on nearby cells.

Where the neural tissue is thin, ependymal cells form an **internal limiting membrane** lining the ventricle and an **external limiting membrane,** beneath the pia, formed by thin fused pedicles. Modifications of some of the ependymal cells in the ventricles of the brain participate in the formation of the **choroid plexus,** responsible for secreting **cerebrospinal fluid (CSF). Tanycytes,** a specialized type of ependymal cell, extend processes into the hypothalamus, where they terminate near blood vessels and neurosecretory cells. It is thought that tanycytes transport CSF to these neurosecretory cells.

Schwann Cells

Unlike other neuroglial cells, **Schwann cells** are located in the PNS, where they envelop axons. They can form two types of coverings over these axons: myelinated and non-

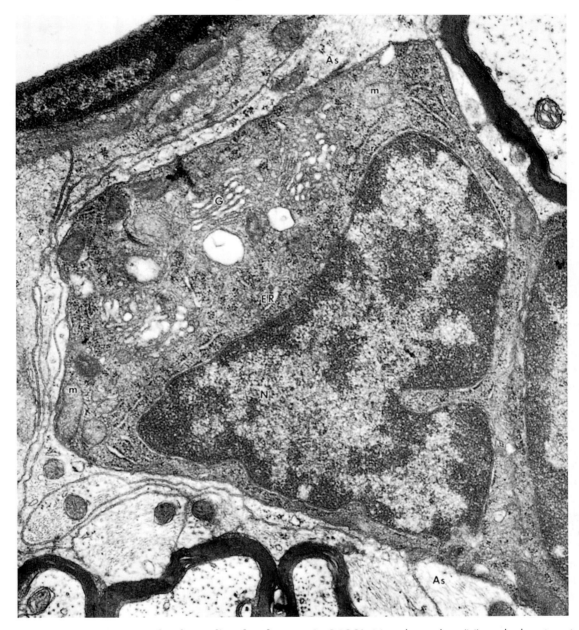

Figure 9–12. Electron micrograph of an oligodendrocyte (× 3600). Note the nucleus (N), endoplasmic reticulum (ER), Golgi apparatus (G), and mitochondria (m). Processes of fibrous astrocytes (As) contact the oligodendrocyte. (From Leeson, T.S., Leeson, C.R., and Paparo, A.A.: Text/Atlas of Histology. Philadelphia, W.B. Saunders Company, 1988.)

myelinated. Axons that have myelin wrapped around them are referred to as myelinated nerves.

Schwann cells are flattened cells whose cytoplasm contains a flattened nucleus, a small Golgi apparatus, and a few mitochondria. Electron microscopy has revealed that myelin is the plasmalemma of the Schwann cell organized into a sheath that is wrapped several times around the axon. At regular intervals along the length of the axon, interruptions occur in the myelin sheath, called **nodes of Ranvier,** exposing the axon (Fig. 9–13). The nodes of Ranvier indicate an interface between the myelin sheaths of two different Schwann cells located along the axon.

The outer portion of Schwann cells is covered by a basal lamina that dips into the nodes of Ranvier, covering the overlapped areas of the myelin sheath lamellae of adjacent Schwann cells. Thus each Schwann cell is covered by a basal lamina, as is the axon at the node of Ranvier. It is important to note that after nerve injury, the regenerating nerve is guided by the basal lamina to its location.

Areas of the axon covered by concentric lamellae of myelin and the single Schwann cell that produced the myelin are called **internodal segments,** which range in length from 200 to 1000 μm. Light microscopy has revealed several cone-shaped oblique clefts in the myelin sheath

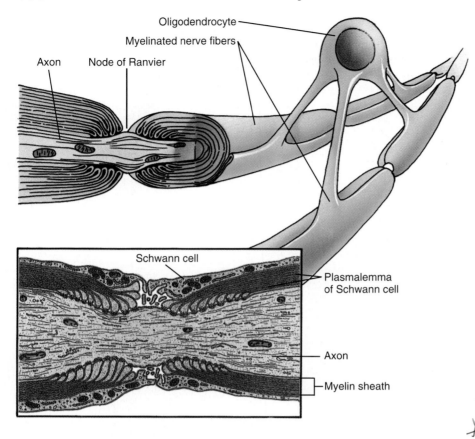

Oligodendrocyte

Myelinated nerve fibers

Axon   Node of Ranvier

Schwann cell

Plasmalemma
of Schwann cell

Axon

Myelin sheath

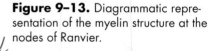

Figure 9-13. Diagrammatic representation of the myelin structure at the nodes of Ranvier.

of each internodal segment called **clefts (incisures) of Schmidt-Lantermann.** These clefts, viewed by the electron microscope, were demonstrated to be Schwann cell cytoplasm trapped within the lamellae of myelin. As the membrane spirals around the axon, it produces a series of alternating wide, dense lines with narrower, less-dense lines occurring at 12-nm intervals. The wider line (3 nm in width) is known as the **major dense line.** It represents the fused cytoplasmic surfaces of the Schwann cell plasma membrane. The narrower **intraperiod line** represents the apposing outer leaflets of the Schwann cell plasma membrane. High-resolution electron microscopy has revealed a small gap within the intraperiod line between each spiraled layer of the myelin sheath called the **intraperiod gap.** This gap is thought to provide access for small molecules to reach the axon. The region of the intraperiod line that is in intimate contact with the axon is known as the **internal mesaxon,** whereas its outermost aspect, in contact with the body of the Schwann cell, is the **external mesaxon** (see Figs. 9–7, 9–14).

The mechanism of **myelination,** the process whereby the Schwann cell (or oligodendrocyte) concentrically wraps its membrane around the axon to form the myelin sheath, is unclear. It is believed to begin as a Schwann cell envelops an axon and somehow wraps its membrane around the axon. The wrapping may continue for more than 50 turns. During this process the cytoplasm is squeezed back into the body of the Schwann cell, bringing the cytoplasmic surfaces of the

membranes in contact with each other, thus forming the major dense line that spirals through the myelin sheath. It is important to note that a single Schwann cell can myelinate only one internode of a single axon (and only in the PNS), whereas oligodendroglia cells can myelinate an internode of several axons (and only in the CNS).

Nerves are not myelinated simultaneously during development. Indeed, the onset and completion of myelination varies considerably in different areas of the nervous system. This variation seems to be correlated with function. For example, motor nerves are nearly completely myelinated at birth, whereas sensory roots are not myelinated for several months thereafter. Some CNS nerve tracts and commissural axons are not fully myelinated for several years after birth.

Some axons in the PNS are not wrapped with the many layers of myelin typical of myelinated axons. These unmyelinated axons are surrounded by a single layer of Schwann cell plasma membrane and cytoplasm of the Schwann cell (see Fig. 9–8). Although a single Schwann cell can myelinate only one axon, several unmyelinated axons may be enveloped by a single Schwann cell.

CLINICAL CORRELATIONS

Multiple sclerosis (MS), a relatively common disease affecting myelin, is 1.5 times more common in females

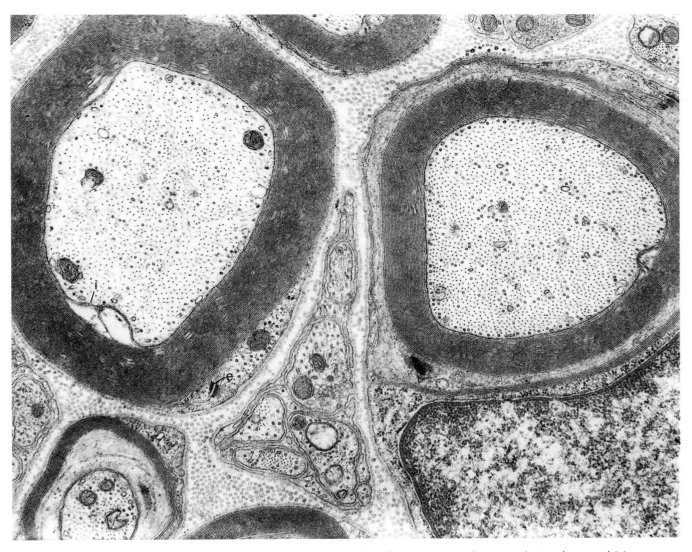

Figure 9–14. Electron micrograph of a myelinated peripheral nerve. Note the internal (i) and external (e) mesaxons as well as the Schwann cell cytoplasm and nucleus. (From Jennes, L., Traurig, H.H., and Conn, P.M.: Atlas of the Human Brain. Philadelphia, Lippincott-Raven, 1995.)

than in males. It usually occurs between 15 and 45 years of age and is characterized by its principal pathology of demyelination in the CNS (optic nerve, cerebellum, and white matter of the cerebrum, spinal cord, and cranial and spinal nerves). The disease is distinguished by episodes of random, multifocal inflammation, edema, and subsequent demyelination of axons in the CNS, followed by periods of remission that may last for several months to decades. Each episode may further jeopardize the patient's vitality. Any single episode of demyelination may deteriorate, become malignant, and lead to death in a matter of months. Because this demyelination is thought to result from an autoimmune disease (as a possible aftermath of an infectious agent), immunosuppression with corticosteroids is the most common therapy for multiple sclerosis, although it is believed that the antiinflammatory activity of the therapy is most beneficial.

Radiation therapy can lead to demyelination of the brain or spinal cord when these structures are in the radiation field during therapy. Also, toxic agents such as those used in **chemotherapy** for cancer may lead to demyelination, resulting in neurological problems.

Generation and Conduction of Nerve Impulses

Nerve impulses are electrical signals that are generated in the spike trigger zone of a neuron as the result of **membrane depolarization** and conducted along the axon to the axon terminal. Transmission of impulses from the terminals of a neuron to another neuron, muscle cell, or gland occurs at synapses (see next section).

Neurons and other cells are electrically **polarized** with a **resting potential** of about –70 mV (the inside is less positive than the outside) across the plasma membrane. This potential arises because of the difference of ion concentration inside and outside the cell. In mammalian cells the concentration of K+ ions is much higher inside the cell than outside the cell, whereas the concentration of Na+ and Cl− ions is much higher outside cells than inside (Fig. 9–15). **K+ leak channels** in the plasmalemma permit a relatively free flow of K+ ions out of a cell down its concentration gradient. Because there are few open Na+ and Cl− channels in a resting cell, more K+ ions leave the cell than Na+ and Cl− ions enter; thus, a small net positive charge accumulates on the outside of the plasma membrane. Although the maintenance of the resting potential depends primarily on K+ leak channels, **Na+-K+ pumps** in the plasma membrane assist by actively pumping Na+ ions out of the cell and K+ ions into the cell. For every three Na+ ions pumped out, two K+ ions enter the cell.

In most cells the potential across the plasma membrane is generally constant. However, in neurons and muscle cells, the membrane potential can undergo controlled changes, making these cells capable of conducting an electrical signal. Stimulation of a neuron causes opening of voltage-gated Na+ channels in a small region of the membrane, leading to an influx of Na+ into the cell at that site (Fig. 9–16). Eventually the overabundance of Na+ ions inside the cell causes a reversal of the resting potential (i.e., the inside becomes positive relative to the outside), and the membrane is said to be **depolarized.** This results in the Na+ channels closing for 1 to 2 msec, which is known as the **refractory period,** when the closed channels are inactive and cannot

open. During this period, **voltage-gated K+ channels** open, permitting an efflux of K+ ions into the extracellular fluid that eventually restores the resting membrane potential; however, there may be a brief period of hyperpolarization. Once the resting potential is restored, the voltage-gated K+ channels close and the refractory period ends.

The cycle of membrane depolarization, hyperpolarization, and return to the resting membrane potential is called the **action potential,** an all-or-none response that can occur at rates of 1000 impulses/second. The membrane depolarization that occurs by opening of voltage-gated Na+ channels at one point on an axon spreads passively for a short distance and triggers opening of adjacent channels, resulting in the generation of another action potential. In this way, the wave of depolarization, or impulse, is conducted along the axon. *In vivo,* an impulse is conducted only in one direction, from the site of initial depolarization to the axon terminal. The inactivation of closed Na+ channels during the refractory periods prevents retrograde propagation of the depolarization wave.

Synapses and the Transmission of the Nerve Impulse

Synapses are the sites where nerve impulses are transmitted from a presynaptic cell (a neuron) to a postsynaptic cell (another neuron, muscle cell, or gland cell). Synapses thus permit neurons to communicate with each other and with effector cells. Impulse transmission at synapses can occur electrically or chemically.

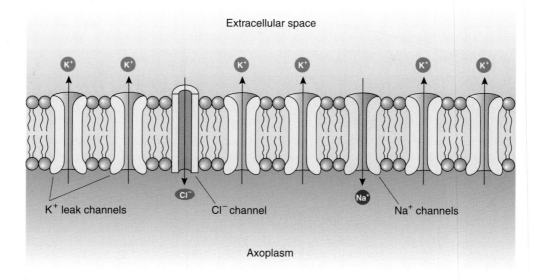

Figure 9–15. Schematic diagram of the establishment of the resting potential in a typical neuron. Observe that the K+ leak channels outnumber the Na+ and Cl− channels; consequently, more K+ can leave the cell than Na+ or Cl− can enter. Because there are more positive ions outside than inside the cell, the outside is more positive than the inside, establishing a potential difference across the membrane. Note that ion channels and ion pumps not directly responsible for the establishment of resting membrane potential are not shown.

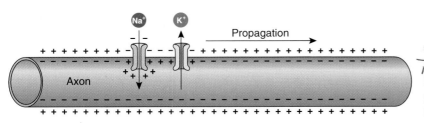

Figure 9–16. Schematic diagram of the propagation of the action potential (see text for explanation).

Although **electrical synapses** are uncommon in mammals, they are present in the brainstem, retina, and cerebral cortex. Electrical synapses are usually represented by gap junctions that permit free movement of ions from one cell to another. When this occurs between neurons, there is a flow of current. Impulse transmission is much faster across electrical synapses than across chemical synapses.

Chemical synapses are the most common mode of communication between two nerve cells. The **presynaptic membrane** releases one or more **neurotransmitters** into the **synaptic cleft** a small (20- to 30-nm) gap, located between the presynaptic membrane of the first cell and the **postsynaptic membrane** of the second cell (Fig. 9–17). The neurotransmitter diffuses across the synaptic cleft to gated ion-channel **receptors** on the postsynaptic membrane. Binding of the neurotransmitter to these receptors initiates the opening of ion channels that permits the passage of certain ions, altering the permeability of the postsynaptic membrane and reversing its membrane potential. It is important to realize that neurotransmitters do not effect the reaction events at the postsynaptic membrane; they only activate the response.

When the stimulus at a synapse results in depolarization of the postsynaptic membrane to a threshold value that initiates an action potential, it is called an **excitatory postsynaptic potential.** A stimulus at the synapse that results in maintaining a membrane potential or increasing its hyperpolarization is called an **inhibitory postsynaptic potential.**

Various types of synaptic contacts between neurons have been observed. The following are the most common (see Figs. 9–17, 9–18):

- **Axodendritic synapse**—between an axon and a dendrite
- **Axosomatic synapse**—between an axon and a soma
- **Axoaxonic synapse**—between two axons
- **Dendrodendritic synapse**—between two dendrites

Synaptic Morphology

Terminals of axons vary according to the type of synaptic contact. Often the axon forms a bulbous expansion at its terminal end called **boutons terminaux.** Other forms of synaptic contacts in axons are derived from swellings along the axon called **boutons en passage,** where each bouton may serve as a synaptic site.

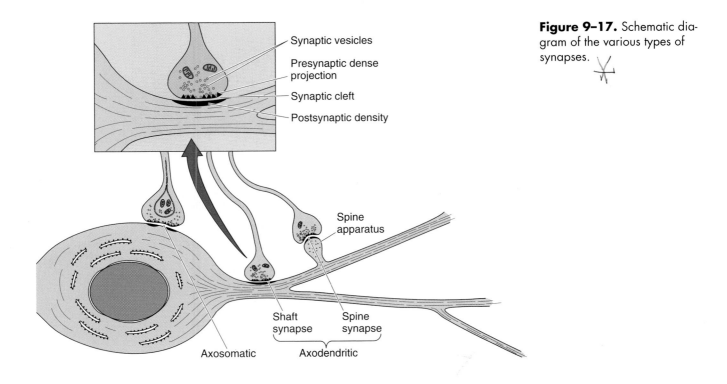

Synaptic vesicles

Presynaptic dense projection

Synaptic cleft

Postsynaptic density

Spine apparatus

Shaft synapse

Spine synapse

Axosomatic

Axodendritic

Figure 9–17. Schematic diagram of the various types of synapses.

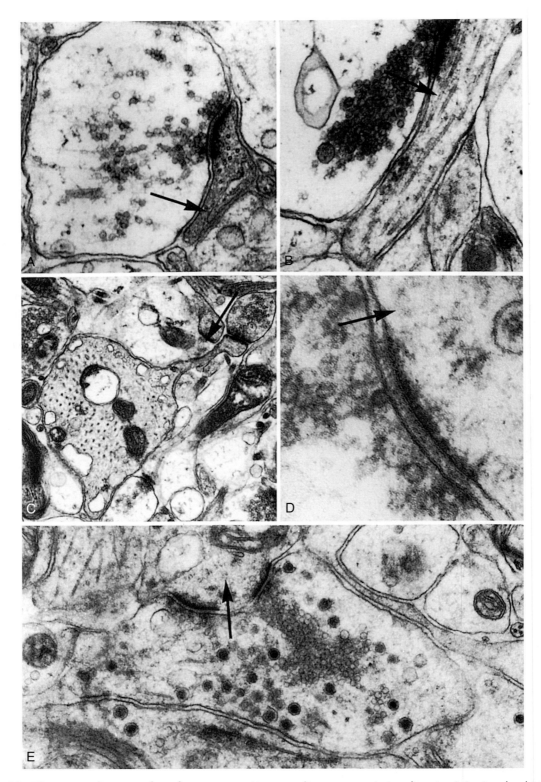

Figure 9–18. Electron micrographs of synapses. (Arrow indicates transmission direction.) **A,** Axodendritic synapse. Presynaptic vesicles are located to the left (× 45,000). **B,** Axodendritic synapse. Note neurotubules in dendrite (× 52,000). **C,** Dendrite in cross-section. Note the synapse (× 22,500). **D,** Axodendritic synapse. Note presynaptic vesicle fusing with the axolemma (× 98,000). **E,** Axon terminal with clear synaptic vesicles and dense-cored vesicles (× 37,000). (From Leeson, T.S., Leeson, C.R., and Paparo, A.A.: Text/Atlas of Histology. Philadelphia, W.B. Saunders Company, 1988.)

The cytoplasm at the **presynaptic membrane** contains mitochondria, a few elements of smooth endoplasmic reticulum, and an abundance of synaptic vesicles, assembled around the presynaptic membrane (Fig. 9–19). **Synaptic vesicles** are spherical structures (40 to 60 nm in diameter) filled with neurotransmitter substance that was manufactured and packaged, usually, near the axon terminal. Peptide neurotransmitters, however, are manufactured and packaged in the cell body and transported to the axon terminal via anterograde transport. Enzymes located in the axoplasm protect neurotransmitters from degradation.

Also located on the cytoplasmic side of the presynaptic membrane are conically shaped densities that project from the membrane into the cytoplasm; these appear to be associated with many of the synaptic vesicles, forming the **active site** of the synapse. Those synaptic vesicles associated with

the active site are released at stimulation. Additional synaptic vesicles, forming a reserve pool, adhere to actin microfilaments. **Synapsin-I,** a small protein that forms a complex with the vesicle surface, appears to assist in the clustering of synaptic vesicles held in reserve. When synapsin-I is phosphorylated, these synaptic vesicles become free to move to the active zone in preparation for release of the neurotransmitter; dephosphorylation of synapsin-I reverses the process. **Synapsin-II** and another small protein **(rab3a)** control association of the vesicles with actin microfilaments. Docking of the synaptic vesicles with the presynaptic membrane is under control of two additional proteins: **synaptotagmin** and **synaptophysin.** When an action potential reaches the presynaptic membrane, it initiates opening of the **voltage-gated Ca^{2+} channels,** permitting Ca^{2+} ions to enter. This Ca^{2+} influx causes synaptic vesicles to fuse with

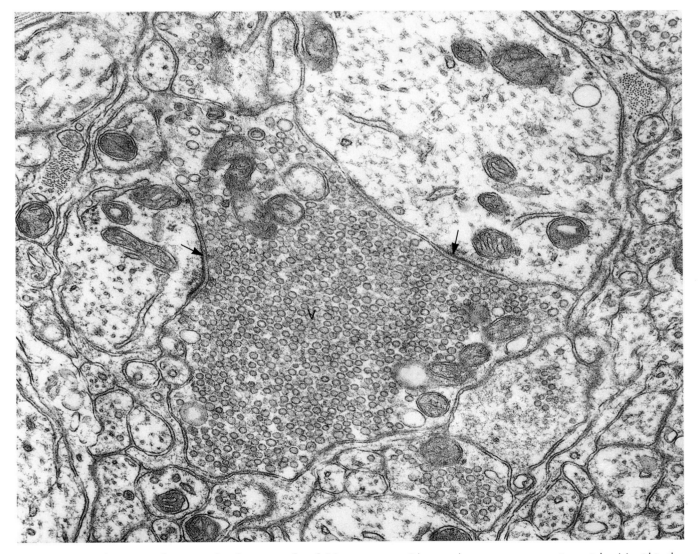

Figure 9–19. Electron micrograph of an axodendritic synapse. Observe the numerous synaptic vesicles (v) within the axon terminal synapsing with dendrites. Also note the synaptic clefts at these sites (*arrows*). (From Jennes, L., Traurig, H.H., and Conn, P.M.: Atlas of the Human Brain. Philadelphia, Lippincott-Raven, 1995.)

the presynaptic membrane, emptying neurotransmitter into the synaptic cleft via exocytosis. Excess membrane is recaptured via **clathrin-mediated endocytosis.** The formed vesicle fuses with the SER, where new membrane is continuously recycled.

The **postsynaptic membrane,** a thickened portion of the plasma membrane of the postsynaptic cell, contains neurotransmitter receptors, and the cytoplasmic area contains some dense material. Coupling of the neurotransmitter with the receptors in the plasmalemma initiates an action potential (an excitatory response) or hyperpolarization (an inhibitory response) of the postsynaptic membrane.

It is interesting to note that the relative thickness and densities of the presynaptic and postsynaptic membranes coupled with the width of the synaptic cleft generally correlate with the nature of the response. A thick postganglionic density and a 30-nm synaptic cleft is called an **asymmetric** synapse, which usually is the site of **excitatory responses.** A thin postsynaptic density and a 20-nm synaptic cleft is called a **symmetric synapse,** which usually is the site of **inhibitory responses.**

Neurotransmitters

Cells of the nervous system communicate mostly by the release of signaling molecules. The released molecules contact receptor molecules protruding from the plasmalemma of the target cell, eliciting a response from the target cell. These signaling molecules were called **neurotransmitters.** However, these signaling molecules may act on two types of receptors: (1) those directly associated with ion channels and (2) those associated with G proteins or receptor kinases, which activate a second messenger. Therefore, signaling molecules that act as first messenger systems—that is, they act on receptors directly associated with ion channels—are referred to as **neurotransmitters.** Signaling molecules that invoke the second messenger system are referred to as **neuromodulators** or **neurohormones.** Because neurotransmitters act directly, the entire process is fast, lasting usually less than 1 msec. Events utilizing neuromodulators are much slower and may last as long as a few minutes.

There are perhaps 100 known neurotransmitters (and neuromodulators) represented by the following three groups: small molecule transmitters, neuropeptides, and gases.

Small molecule transmitters are of three major types: *acetylcholine* (the only one in this group that is not an amino acid derivative); the *amino acids* glutamate, aspartate, glycine, and γ-amino butyrate (GABA); and the *biogenic amines* (monoamines) serotonin and the three catecholamines: dopamine, norepinephrine (noradrenalin), and epinephrine (adrenalin).

Neuropeptides, many of which are neuromodulators, form a large group. They include the opioid peptides enkephalins and endorphins; the gastrointestinal peptides, produced by cells of the diffuse neuroendocrine system—

substance P, neurotensin, and vasoactive intestinal peptide; the hypothalamic releasing hormones, such as thyrotropin-releasing hormone and somatostatin; and hormones stored in and released from the neurohypophysis (antidiurrhetic hormone and oxytocin).

Recently, certain **gases** have been shown to act as neuromodulators. These are NO (nitric oxide) and CO (carbon monoxide).

The most common neurotransmitters are listed in Table 9–1.

CLINICAL CORRELATIONS

Huntington's chorea (HC) is a hereditary condition with an onset at about the third or fourth decade of life, beginning as flicking of the joints that progresses to severe distortions, dementia, and motor dysfunction. The condition is thought to be related to loss of cells producing **GABA,** an inhibitory neurotransmitter. Without it, outbursts are uncontrolled. The dementia associated with HC is thought to be related to subsequent loss of acetylcholine-secreting cells.

Parkinson's disease, a crippling disease related to the absence of **dopamine** in certain regions of the brain, is characterized by muscular rigidity, constant tremor, bradykinesia (slow movement), and finally a mask-like face with difficult voluntary movement. Because dopamine cannot cross the blood–brain barrier, therapy is administered as L-dopa, which relieves the problem, although the neurons in the affected area continue to die. Recent efforts to transplant fetal adrenal gland tissue have provided only transient relief.

Several principles appear to describe the functioning of neurotransmitters. First, a specific neurotransmitter may elicit different actions under varied circumstances. Second, the nature of the postsynaptic receptors determines the effect of a neurotransmitter on postsynaptic cells. Synaptic communication commonly involves multiple neurotransmitters. Additionally, there is mounting evidence for **volume transmission** as a method of communication between brain cells. According to this concept, chemical and electric "neurotransmitters," believed to exist in the intercellular fluid-filled spaces between brain cells, activate groups or fields of cells that contain appropriate receptors, rather than individual cells. Whereas synaptic communication is fast-acting, volume transmission is thought to be slow and may be related to such conditions as autonomic function, alertness, awareness, changes in brain patterns during sleep, sensitivity to pain, and moods.

Peripheral Nerves

Peripheral nerves are bundles of nerve fibers (axons) surrounded by several investments of connective tissue sheaths

Table 9–1. Common Neurotransmitters and Functions Their Receptors Elicit

Neurotransmitter	Compound Group	Function
Acetylcholine	Non–amino acid derived small molecule transmitter	Myoneural junctions; all parasympathetic synapses; and preganglionic sympathetic synapses
Norepinephrine	Small molecule transmitter; biogenic amine; catecholamine	Postganglionic sympathetic synapses (except for eccrine sweat glands)
Glutamic acid	Small molecule transmitter; amino acid	Presynaptic sensory and cortex: most common excitatory neurotransmitter of CNS
γ-Aminobutyric acid (GABA)	Small molecule transmitter; amino acid	Most common inhibitory neurotransmitter of the CNS
Dopamine	Small molecule transmitter; biogenic amine; catecholamine	Basal ganglia of CNS; inhibitory
Serotonin	Small molecule transmitter; biogenic amine	Inhibits pain; mood control; sleep
Glycine	Small molecule transmitter; amino acid	Spinal cord; inhibitory
Endorphins	Neuropeptide; opioid peptide	Analgesic; inhibit pain transmission?
Enkephalins	Neuropeptide; opioid peptide	Analgesic; inhibit pain transmission?

CNS, central nervous system.

(Figs. 9–20, 9–21, 9–22). These bundles **(fascicles)** may be observed with the unaided eye; those that are myelinated appear white because of the presence of myelin. Each bundle of nerve fibers, regardless of size, contains both sensory and motor components.

Connective Tissue Investments

The **epineurium** is the outermost layer of the three connective tissue investments covering a nerve (see Fig. 9–22). The epineurium is composed of dense irregular fibrous connective tissue containing some thick elastic fibers that completely ensheathes the nerve. Collagen fibers within the sheath are aligned and oriented to prevent damage by overstretching of the nerve bundle. The epineurium is thickest where it is continuous with the dura covering the CNS at the spinal cord or brain where the spinal or cranial nerves originate, respectively. It becomes progressively thinner as the nerves branch into smaller nerve components, and eventually it becomes absent.

The **perineurium,** the middle layer of connective tissue investments, covers each bundle of nerve fibers within the nerve. The perineurium is composed of dense connective tissue but is thinner than epineurium. Its inner surface is lined by several layers of epithelioid cells joined by zonulae occludentes and surrounded by a basal lamina that isolates the neural environment. Between the layers of epithelioid cells are sparse collagen fibers oriented longitudinally and intertwined with a few elastic fibers. The thickness of the perineurium is progressively reduced to a sheet of flattened cells.

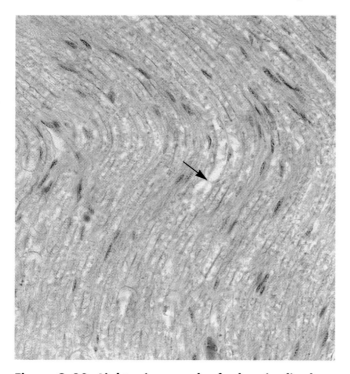

Figure 9-20. Light micrograph of a longitudinal section of a peripheral nerve (× 270). Myelin and nodes of Ranvier (*arrow*) may be observed as well as the lightly stained oval nuclei of Schwann cells.

The **endoneurium,** the innermost layer of the three connective tissue investments of a nerve, surrounds each axon. It is a loose connective tissue composed of a thin layer of reticular fibers (produced by the underlying Schwann cells), scattered fibroblasts, fixed macrophages, capillaries, and perivascular mast cells in extracellular fluid, and it is in contact with the basal lamina of the Schwann cells. Thus the endoneurium is housed in a completely isolated compartment from the perineurium and Schwann cells, an important factor in regulating the microenvironment of the nerve fiber. Near the distal terminus of the axon, the endoneurium is reduced to a few reticular fibers surrounding the basal lamina of the Schwann cells of the axon.

Functional Classification of Nerves

Nerve fibers are segregated functionally into sensory **(afferent)** fibers and motor **(efferent)** fibers. Sensory nerve fibers carry sensory input from the cutaneous areas of the body and from the viscera back to the CNS for processing. Motor nerve fibers originate in the CNS and carry motor impulses to the effector organs. The sensory roots and motor roots of the spinal cord unite to form a mixed peripheral nerve, the **spinal nerve,** which carries both sensory and motor fibers.

Conduction Velocity

The conduction velocity of peripheral nerve fibers depends on the extent of their myelination. In myelinated nerves, ions can cross the axonal plasma membrane, initiating depolarization, only at the nodes of Ranvier, for two reasons: One, voltage-gated Na^+ ion channels of the axon plasmalemma are clustered mostly at the nodes of Ranvier; and two, the myelin sheath covering the internodes prevents the outward movement of the excess Na^+ ions in the axoplasm associated with the action potential. The excess positive ions can diffuse through the axoplasm to the next node, triggering depolarization there. In this way, the action potential "jumps" from node to node, a process called **saltatory conduction.**

As noted earlier, unmyelinated fibers lack a thick myelin sheath and nodes of Ranvier. These fibers are surrounded by a single layer of Schwann cell plasma membrane and cytoplasm, which provides little insulation. Moreover, voltage-gated Na^+ ion channels are distributed along the entire length of the axon plasma membrane. Therefore, impulse propagation in unmyelinated fibers occurs by **continuous conduction,** which is slower and requires more energy than the saltatory conduction occurring in myelinated fibers.

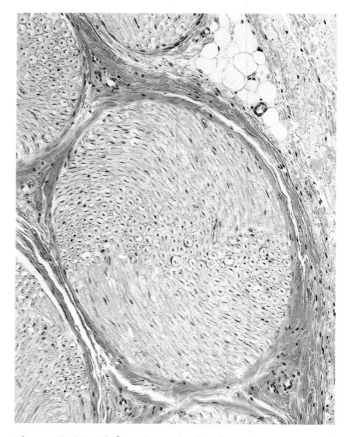

Figure 9-21. Light micrograph of a cross-section of a peripheral nerve (× 132). Observe the axons and the perineurium surrounding the fascicle.

vides motor impulses to the skeletal muscles, whereas the **autonomic nervous system** provides motor impulses to the smooth muscles of the viscera, cardiac muscle of the heart, and secretory cells of the exocrine and endocrine glands, thus functioning in maintaining homeostasis.

Somatic Nervous System

The skeletal muscles receive motor nerve impulses conducted to them by spinal and select cranial nerves of the somatic nervous system. The cell bodies of these nerve fibers originate in the CNS. The cranial nerves containing **somatic efferent components** are III, IV, VI, and XII (excluding those nerves supplying muscles of branchiomeric origin). Most of the 31 pairs of spinal nerves contain somatic efferent components to skeletal muscles.

Cell bodies of neurons of the somatic nervous system in the cranial nerves originate in motor nuclei of the cranial nerves embedded within the brain or in the ventral horn of the spinal cord. These neurons are multipolar, and their axons leave the brain or spinal cord and travel to the skeletal muscle by the cranial nerves or spinal nerves (Fig. 9–23). They synapse with the skeletal muscle at the motor endplate (see Chapter 8).

Autonomic Nervous System

The **autonomic (involuntary, visceral) nervous system** is generally defined as a motor system, although agreement on this point is not universal. Nevertheless, it shall be regarded as a motor system in this discussion. The autonomic nervous system controls the viscera of the body by supplying the **general visceral efferent (visceral motor)** component to smooth muscle, cardiac muscle, and glands. In contrast with the somatic system, in which one neuron, originating in the

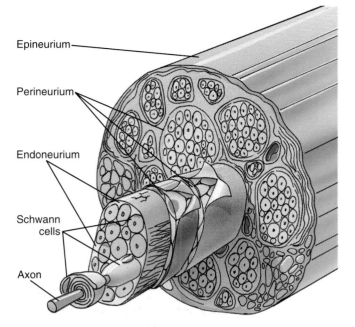

Figure 9–22. Diagram of the structure of a nerve bundle.

Epineurium
Perineurium
Endoneurium
Schwann cells
Axon

As shown in Table 9–2, peripheral nerve fibers are classified into three major groups based on their conduction velocity. In thin unmyelinated fibers, the conduction velocity ranges from about 0.5 to 2 m/sec, whereas in heavily myelinated fibers it ranges from 15 up to 120 m/sec.

Somatic and Autonomic Nervous System

The motor component of the nervous system is divided functionally into the somatic nervous system and the autonomic nervous system. The **somatic nervous system** pro-

Table 9–2. Classification of Peripheral Nerve Fibers			
Fiber Group	**Diameter**	**Conduction Velocity**	**Function**
Type-A fibers—heavily myelinated	1–20 μm	15–120 m/sec	**(High-velocity fibers)** Acute pain, temperature, touch, pressure, proprioception, somatic efferent fibers
Type-B fibers—less heavily myelinated	1–3 μm	3–15 m/sec	**(Moderate-velocity fibers)** Visceral afferents, preganglionic autonomics
Type-C fibers—unmyelinated	0.5–1.5 μm	0.5–2 m/sec	**(Slow-velocity fibers)** Postganglionic autonomics, chronic pain

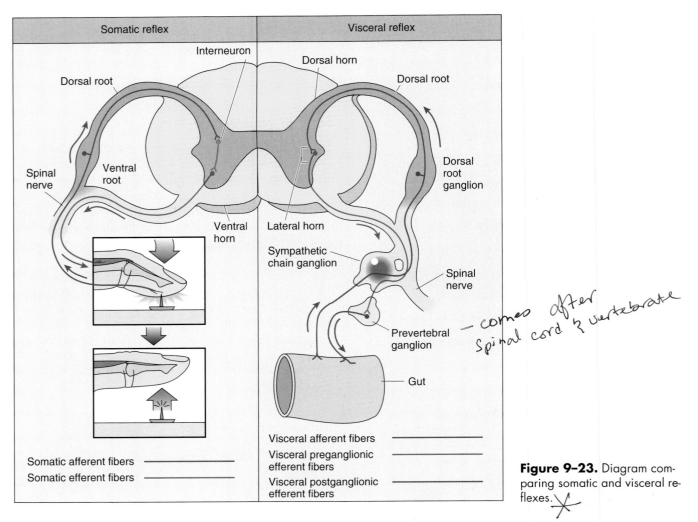

| Somatic reflex | Visceral reflex |

Interneuron
Dorsal horn
Dorsal root
Dorsal root
Dorsal root ganglion
Spinal nerve
Ventral root
Spinal nerve
Ventral horn
Lateral horn
Sympathetic chain ganglion
Prevertebral ganglion
— comes after
Spinal cord & vertebrate
Gut

Somatic afferent fibers ——————
Somatic efferent fibers ——————

Visceral afferent fibers ——————
Visceral preganglionic efferent fibers ——————
Visceral postganglionic efferent fibers ——————

Figure 9–23. Diagram comparing somatic and visceral reflexes.

CNS, acts directly on the effector organ, the autonomic nervous system possesses two neurons between the CNS and the effector organ. In addition, synapses between postganglionic fibers and effector organs differ in the two systems. In contrast with the somatic system, the autonomic system has postganglionic synapses that branch out and the neurotransmitter diffuses out for some distance to the effector cells, thus contributing to more prolonged and widespread effects than occur in the somatic system. Smooth muscle cells stimulated by neurotransmitter activate adjacent smooth muscle cells to contract by relaying the information via gap junctions.

Cell bodies of the first neurons in the autonomic chain are located in the CNS, and their axons are usually myelinated, whereas cell bodies of the second neurons are located in autonomic ganglia, which lie outside the CNS, and their axons are usually unmyelinated, although they are always enveloped by Schwann cells. It is in these ganglia that axons of the **preganglionic fibers** (first neurons) synapse with the multipolar **postganglionic fibers** (second neurons), whose axons subsequently exit the ganglia to reach the effector or-

gans (smooth muscle, cardiac muscle, and glands). It is important to remember that preganglionic fibers synapse only once and only with cell bodies of postganglionic fibers.

Acetylcholine is the neurotransmitter at all synapses between preganglionic and postganglionic fibers and between parasympathetic postganglionic endings and effector organs. **Norepinephrine** is the neurotransmitter at synapses between postganglionic sympathetic fibers and effector organs. Generally, preganglionic fibers of the sympathetic system are short, whereas the postganglionic fibers are long. In contrast, preganglionic parasympathetic fibers are long, whereas postganglionic fibers are short.

The autonomic nervous system is subdivided into two functionally different divisions, the sympathetic and the parasympathetic systems (Fig. 9–24). The **sympathetic system** generally prepares the body for action by increasing respiration, blood pressure, heart rate, and blood flow to the skeletal muscles, dilating pupils of the eye, and generally slowing down visceral function. The **parasympathetic system,** on the other hand, tends to be functionally antagonistic to the sympathetic system by decreasing respiration, blood

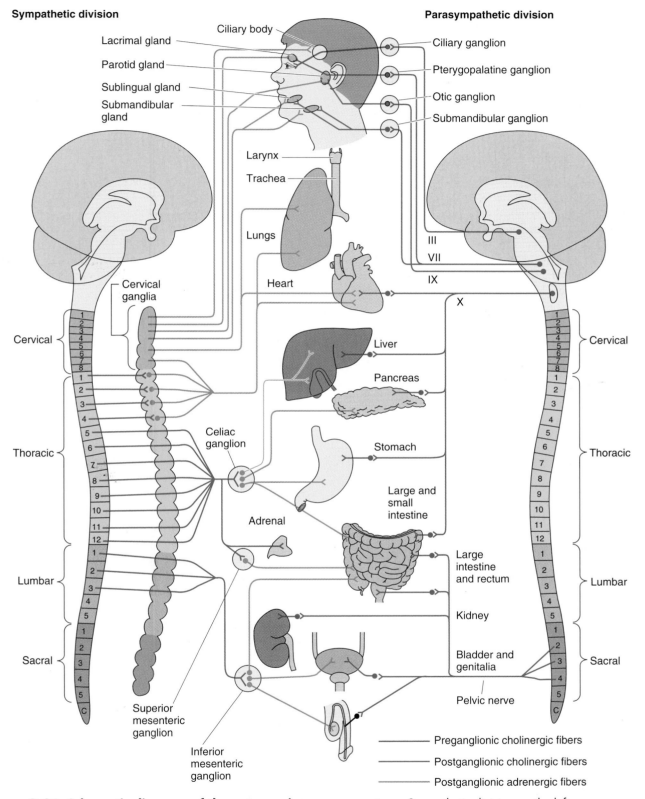

Figure 9–24. Schematic diagram of the autonomic nervous system. Sympathetic division on the left; parasympathetic division on the right.

pressure, heart rate, and generally reducing blood flow to skeletal muscles, constricting the pupils and generally increasing the actions and functions of the visceral system. Thus the parasympathetic system brings about homeostasis, whereas the sympathetic system prepares the body for "fight or flight." Because the visceral components of the body receive innervation from both divisions of the autonomic system, these two systems are balanced in health.

Sympathetic System

The **sympathetic system** originates in the spinal cord from segments of the thoracic spinal cord and upper lumbar spinal cord (T_1 to L_2). Thus the sympathetic system is sometimes called the **thoracolumbar outflow** (see Fig. 9–24). Cell bodies of preganglionic neurons are small spindle-shaped cells that originate in the lateral horn of the spinal cord; their axons exit the cord via the ventral roots to join the spinal nerve. After a short distance the fibers leave the peripheral nerve, via white rami communicates, to enter one of the paravertebral chain ganglia. Typically, the preganglionic neuron will synapse on a cell body of one of the multipolar postganglionic neurons residing in the ganglion associated with that spinal cord segment, or it may ascend or descend in the sympathetic trunk to synapse on a cell in another of the chain ganglia. Certain of the preganglionic fibers do not synapse in the chain ganglia, however, but pass through to enter the abdominal cavity as splanchnic nerves. Here they seek collateral ganglia located along the abdominal aorta for synapsing on cell bodies of postganglionic fibers residing there.

Axons of postganglionic neurons housed in the chain ganglia exit the ganglia, via gray rami communicantes, to reenter the peripheral nerve for distribution to effector organs in the periphery (i.e., sweat glands, blood vessels, dilator pupillae muscles, cardiac muscle, bronchial tree, salivary glands, and arrector pili muscles).

Axons of postganglionic neurons housed in the collateral ganglia exit the ganglia and accompany the myriad blood vessels to the viscera, where they synapse on the effector organs (i.e., blood vessels and the smooth muscles and glands of the viscera).

Parasympathetic System

The **parasympathetic system** originates in the brain and the sacral segments of the spinal cord (S_2 to S_4); thus the parasympathetic system is called the **craniosacral outflow** (see Fig. 9–24). Cell bodies of **preganglionic parasympathetic neurons** originating in the brain lie in the **visceromotor nuclei** of the four cranial nerves that carry visceral motor components (III, VII, IX, and X). Axons of the preganglionic parasympathetic fibers of cranial nerves III, VII, and IX seek **parasympathetic (terminal) ganglia** located outside the brain case, where they synapse on cell bodies of

postganglionic parasympathetic fibers housed in the ganglia. Axons of these nerves are usually delivered by cranial nerve V to the effector organs they serve, including salivary glands, ciliary muscle, sphincter pupillae muscles, and mucous glands.

Axons of **preganglionic parasympathetic fibers** in cranial nerve X travel to the thorax and abdomen before synapsing in the terminal ganglia within the respective viscera. Axons of postganglionic parasympathetic nerves synapse on the glands, smooth muscles, and cardiac muscle.

Cell bodies of preganglionic parasympathetic nerves originating in segments of the sacral spinal cord are located in the lateral segment of the ventral horn and leave via the ventral root with the sacral nerves. From here the axons project to terminal ganglia (**Meissner's** and **Auerbach's plexuses**) in the walls of the lower gastrointestinal tract, where they synapse on cell bodies of postganglionic parasympathetic neurons. Axons of postganglionic neurons synapse on the effector organs in the viscera of the lower abdominal wall and the pelvis.

Ganglia

Ganglia are aggregations of cell bodies of neurons located outside the CNS. There are two types, **sensory ganglia** and **autonomic ganglia.**

Sensory Ganglia

Sensory ganglia are associated with cranial nerves V, VII, IX, and X and with each of the spinal nerves originating from the spinal cord. Sensory ganglia of the cranial nerves present as a swelling of the nerve either inside the cranial vault or at its exit. They are usually identified with a specific name that relates to the nerve. Sensory ganglia of the spinal nerves are called **dorsal root ganglia.** Sensory ganglia house pseudounipolar cell bodies of the sensory nerves enveloped by cuboidal **capsule cells.** These are then surrounded by a connective tissue capsule composed of **satellite cells** and collagen. The endoneurium of each axon becomes continuous with the connective tissue surrounding the ganglia. Peripheral processes of the nerves possess specialized receptors at their terminals to transduce various types of stimuli from the internal and external environments. Central processes pass from the ganglion unsynapsed to the brain within the cranial nerves or to the spinal cord within the spinal nerves, where they will terminate on other neurons for processing.

Autonomic Ganglia

By definition, nerve cell bodies of **autonomic ganglia** are motor in function because they cause smooth or cardiac muscle contraction or glandular secretion. In the sympathetic system **preganglionic sympathetic fibers** synapse on postganglionic sympathetic cell bodies in the sympathetic ganglia located in either the **sympathetic chain ganglia,** adjacent to the spinal cord, or the **collateral ganglia** along the abdominal aorta in the abdomen. **Postganglionic sympathetic nerves** originating in these ganglia are then distributed, for the most part, by peripheral nerves that they join after exiting the ganglia. They then terminate in the effector organs that they innervate.

In the parasympathetic system, **preganglionic parasympathetic fibers** originate in one of two places: in certain cranial nerves or in certain segments of the sacral spinal cord. These fibers synapse on postganglionic cell bodies (Fig. 9–25) located in **terminal ganglia.** Preganglionic parasympathetic fibers originating in the nuclei of the cranial nerves conducting parasympathetic fibers synapse in one of the four **terminal ganglia** located in the head (except those of cranial nerve X). Terminal ganglia associated with cranial nerve X and preganglionic fibers from the sacral spinal cord are located in the walls of the viscera.

Postganglionic parasympathetic nerves originating in the terminal ganglia within the head exit the ganglia and usually join the trigeminal nerve (V) to be distributed to the effector organs. Those postganglionic parasympathetic nerves originating in the ganglia located in the walls of the

viscera pass directly to the effector organs located within the viscera.

Central Nervous System (CNS)

The **central nervous system,** the brain and the spinal cord, consists of white matter and gray matter without intervening connective tissue elements; therefore, the CNS has the consistency of a semifirm gel. **White matter** is composed mostly of myelinated nerve fibers, along with some unmyelinated fibers and neuroglial cells; its white color results from the abundance of myelin surrounding the axons. **Gray matter** consists of aggregations of neuronal cell bodies, dendrites, and unmyelinated portions of axons, as well as neuroglial cells; the absence of myelin causes these regions to have a gray color. Axons, dendrites, and neuroglia processes form an intertangled network of neural tissue called the **neuropil** (Fig. 9–26). In certain regions, aggregations of gray matter completely surrounded by white matter are called **nuclei.**

Gray matter in the brain is located at the periphery (**cortex**) of the cerebrum and cerebellum and forms the deeper basal ganglia, whereas the white matter lies deep to the cortex and surrounds the basal ganglia. The reverse is true in the spinal cord: white matter is located in the periphery of

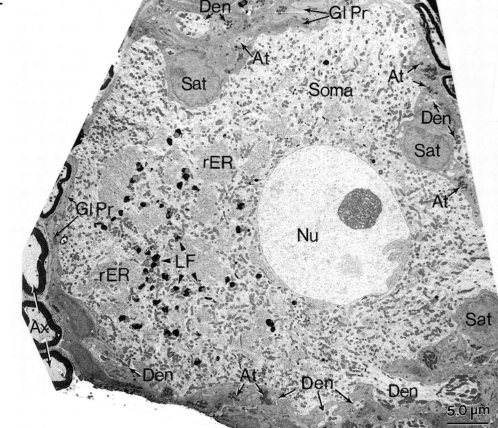

Figure 9–25. Electron micrograph of the ciliary ganglion. At, axon terminal; Ax, axon; Den, dendrite; LF, lipofuscin granules; Nu, nucleus; rER, rough endoplasmic reticulum; Sat, satellite cells. (From May, P.J., and Warren, S.: Ultrastructure of the macaque ciliary ganglion. J. Neurocytol. **22:**1073–1095, 1993.)

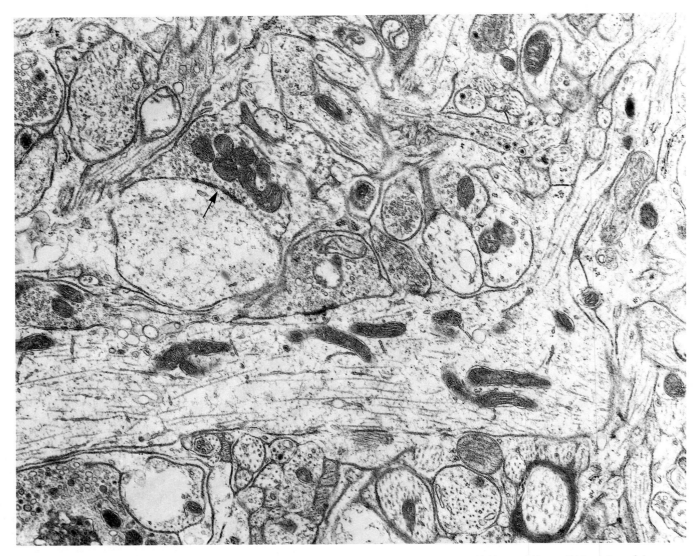

Figure 9–26. Electron micrograph of axodendritic synapses. (From Jennes, L., Traurig, H.H., and Conn, P.M.: Atlas of the Human Brain. Philadelphia, Lippincott-Raven, 1995.)

the spinal cord, whereas gray matter lies deep in the spinal cord, where it forms the shape of an **H** in cross-section. A small **central canal,** lined by **ependymal cells** and representing the lumen of the original neural tube, lies in the center of the cross-bar of the H. The upper vertical bars of the H represent the **dorsal horns** of the spinal cord, which receive central processes of the sensory neurons whose cell bodies lie in the **dorsal root ganglion.** Cell bodies of interneurons are also located in the dorsal horns. Cell bodies of **interneurons (internuncial neurons** or **intercalated neurons)** originate in the CNS and are entirely confined there, where they form networks of communication for integration between sensory and motor neurons. Interneurons constitute the vast majority of the neurons of the body. The lower vertical bars of the H represent the **ventral horns** of the spinal cord, which house cell bodies of large multipolar motor neurons, whose axons exit the spinal cord via the ventral roots.

Meninges

The three connective tissue coverings of the brain and spinal cord are the **meninges.** The outermost layer of the meninges is the **dura mater,** the intermediate layer is the **arachnoid,** and the innermost intimate layer of the meninges is the **pia mater** (Fig. 9–27).

Dura Mater

The **dura mater** covering the brain is a dense, collagenous connective tissue composed of two layers that are closely apposed in the adult. **Periosteal dura,** the outer layer, is composed of osteoprogenitor cells, fibroblasts, and organized bundles of collagen fibers that are loosely attached to the inner surface of the skull except at the sutures and base of the skull, where the attachment is firm. Periosteal dura, as the name implies, serves as the periosteum of the inner sur-

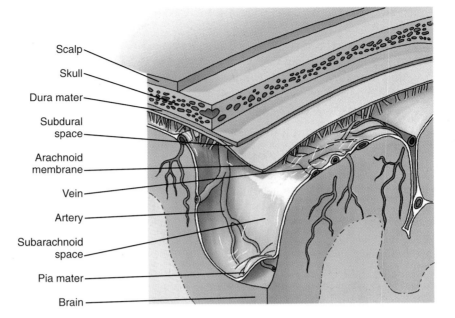

Scalp
Skull
Dura mater
Subdural
space
Arachnoid
membrane
Vein
Artery
Subarachnoid
space
Pia mater
Brain

Figure 9–27. Diagram of the skull and the layers of the meninges covering the brain.

face of the skull, and as such it is well-vascularized. The inner layer of the dura, **meningeal dura,** is composed of fibroblasts displaying darkly staining cytoplasm, elongated processes, ovoid nuclei, and sheet-like layers of fine collagen fibers. This layer also contains small blood vessels. A layer of cells, internal to the meningeal layer, called the **border cell layer** is composed of flattened fibroblasts exhibiting long processes that are occasionally attached to each other by desmosomes and gap junctions. Collagen fibers are lacking in this layer, but in their place an extracellular, amorphous, flocculent material (thought to be a proteoglycan) surrounds the fibroblasts and extends into the interface between this layer and the meningeal dural layer.

Spinal dura does not adhere to the walls of the vertebral canal; rather, it forms a continuous tube from the foramen magnum to the second segment of the sacrum and is pierced by the spinal nerves. The **epidural space,** the space between the dura and the bony walls of the vertebral canal, is filled with epidural fat and a venous plexus.

Arachnoid

The **arachnoid** layer of the meninges is avascular, although blood vessels course through it. This intermediate layer of the meninges consists of fibroblasts, collagen, and some elastic fibers. The fibroblasts form gap junctions and desmosomes with each other. The arachnoid is composed of two regions, a flat, sheet-like membrane, in contact with the dura, and a deeper, gossamer-like region composed of loosely arranged **arachnoid trabecular cells** (modified fibroblasts), along with a few collagen fibers, that form trabeculae that contact the underlying pia mater. These arachnoid trabeculae span the **subarachnoid space,** the

space between the sheet-like portion of the arachnoid and the pia. The arachnoid trabecular cells have long processes that attach to each other via desmosomes and communicate with one another by gap junctions.

The interface between the dura and arachnoid, the **subdural space,** is considered to be a "potential space," because it appears only as the aftermath of injury resulting in subdural hemorrhage, when blood forces these two layers apart.

Blood vessels from the dura pierce the arachnoid on their way to the vascular pia mater. However, they are isolated both from the arachnoid and the subarachnoid space by a close investment of arachnoid-derived modified fibroblasts. In certain regions the arachnoid extends through the dura to form **arachnoid villi,** which protrude into the spaces connected to the lumina of the dural venous sinuses. These specialized regions of the arachnoid function in transporting CSF from the subarachnoid space into the venous system. In later life, the villi enlarge and become sites for calcium deposits.

The interface between the arachnoid and pial layers is difficult to distinguish; therefore, the two are often called the **pia-arachnoid,** with both surfaces being covered by a thin layer of squamous epithelioid cells composed of modified fibroblasts.

Pia Mater

The **pia mater** is the innermost layer of the meninges and is intimately associated with the brain tissue, following closely all of its contours. It is composed of a thin layer of flattened, modified fibroblasts that resemble arachnoid trabecular cells. Blood vessels, abundant in this layer, are surrounded by pial cells interspersed with macrophages, mast cells, and lymphocytes. Fine collagenous and elastic fibers lie between the pia and neural tissue. The pia is completely separated from the underlying neural tissue by neuroglial cells. Blood vessels penetrate the neural tissues and are covered by pia until they form the **continuous capillaries** characteristic of the CNS. Endfeet of astrocytes, rather than pia, cover capillaries within the neural tissue.

Blood–Brain Barrier

A highly selective barrier, known as the **blood–brain barrier,** exists between specific bloodborne substances and the neural tissue of the CNS. This barrier is established by the endothelial cells lining the **continuous capillaries** that course through the CNS. These endothelial cells form fasciae occludentes with one another, retarding the flow of materials between cells. Additionally, these endothelial cells have relatively few pinocytotic vesicles, and vesicular traffic is almost completely restricted to **receptor-mediated transport.** Macromolecules injected into the vascular system cannot enter the intercellular spaces of the CNS; conversely, macromolecules injected into the intercellular spaces of the CNS cannot enter the capillary lumen. Certain substances, however, such as O_2, H_2O, CO_2, and other small lipid-soluble materials, including some drugs, can easily penetrate the blood–brain barrier. Molecules, such as glucose, amino acids, certain vitamins, and nucleosides, are transferred across the blood–brain barrier by specific carrier proteins, many via facilitated diffusion. Ions are also transported across the blood–brain barrier through ion channels via active transport. The energy requirement for this process is satisfied by the presence of large numbers of mitochondria within the endothelial cell cytoplasm.

Capillaries of the CNS are invested by well-defined basal laminae, which in turn are almost completely surrounded by the endfeet of numerous astrocytes, collectively called the **perivascular glia limitans.** It is believed that these astrocytes help convey metabolites from blood vessel to neurons. Additionally, astrocytes remove excess K^+ ions and neurotransmitters from the neuron's environment, thus maintaining the neurochemical balance of the CNS's extracellular milieu.

CLINICAL CORRELATIONS

Because the blood–brain barrier is so selective, antibiotics, some therapeutic drugs, and certain neurotransmitters (e.g., dopamine) cannot pass the barrier. Perfusion of a hypertonic solution of **mannitol** transiently opens the tight junctions of the capillary endothelial cells for administration of therapeutic drugs. Therapeutic drugs can also be bound to antibodies developed against **transferrin receptors** in the endothelial cells of the capillaries, which permits their transport across the blood–brain barrier and into the CNS.

In some diseases of the CNS (e.g., stroke, infection, tumors), the integrity of the blood–brain barrier is compromised, resulting in the accumulation of toxins and extraneous metabolites in the extracellular environment.

Choroid Plexus

Folds of pia mater housing an abundance of fenestrated capillaries and invested by the simple cuboidal (ependymal) lining extend into the third, fourth, and lateral ventricles of the brain, forming the **choroid plexus** (Fig. 9–28). The choroid plexus produces **cerebrospinal fluid,** which fills the ventricles of the brain and central canal of the spinal cord. The CSF bathes the CNS as it circulates through the subarachnoid space. Although more than half of the CSF is produced by the choroid plexus, there is evidence that parenchyma in several other regions of the brain produces a substantial amount of CSF, which diffuses through the ependymal lining to enter the ventricles.

Cerebrospinal Fluid (CSF)

Cerebrospinal fluid is produced by the choroid plexus at the rate of about 14 to 36 ml/hour, replacing its total volume about four to five times daily. CSF circulates through the ventricles of the brain, the subarachnoid space, the perivascular space, and the central canal of the spinal cord. CSF is low in protein but rich in sodium, potassium, and chloride ions. It is clear and has a low density. It is about 90% water and ions; however, it may contain a few desquamated cells and occasional lymphocytes. CSF is important to the meta-

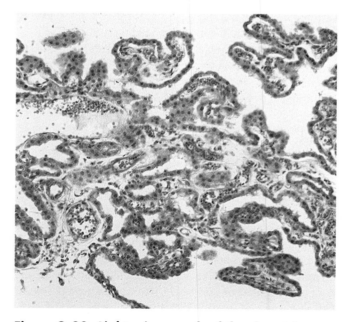

Figure 9–28. Light micrograph of the choroid plexus (× 270). Observe capillaries and the simple cuboidal epithelium of the choroid plexus.

Chapter 9 ■ Nervous Tissue
183

bolic activity of the CNS because brain metabolites diffuse into the CSF as it passes through the subarachnoid space. It also serves as a liquid cushion for protection of the CNS. CSF is able to flow by diffusion and is reabsorbed through the thin cells of the arachnoid villi in the superior sagittal venous sinus where the CSF is returned to the bloodstream.

CLINICAL CORRELATIONS

Because CSF is constantly being produced by the choroid plexus, any decrease in absorption of the fluid by the arachnoid villi or blockage within the ventricles of the brain will cause swelling in the brain tissue. This condition, called **hydrocephalus,** leads to enlargement of the head in the fetus and neonate, impaired mental and muscular function, and death if left untreated.

BLOOD–CSF BARRIER. The chemical stability of the CSF is maintained by the **blood–CSF barrier,** composed of zonulae occludentes between the cells of the simple cuboidal epithelium. These tight junctions impede the movement of substances between cells, compelling them to take the transcellular route. The production of CSF thus depends on facilitated and active transport across the simple cuboidal epithelium, resulting in differences in the composition of CSF and plasma (Table 9–3).

Cerebral Cortex

The gray matter at the periphery of the cerebral hemispheres is folded into many **gyri** and **sulci** called the **cerebral cortex.** This portion of the brain is responsible for learning, memory, information analysis, initiation of motor response, and integration of sensory signals.

The cerebral cortex is divided into six layers composed of neuronal cells that exhibit a morphology unique to that particular layer. The most superficial layer lies just deep to the pia; the sixth layer is the deepest layer of the cortex, bordered by white matter of the cerebrum. The six layers and their components are as follows:

1. **Molecular layer** is composed mostly of nerve terminals originating in other areas of the brain, **horizontal cells,** and neuroglia.
2. **External granular layer** contains mostly **granule (stellate) cells** and neuroglial cells.
3. **External pyramidal layer** contains neuroglial cells and large **pyramidal cells,** which become increasingly larger from the external to the internal border of this layer.
4. **Internal granular layer** is a thin layer and is characterized by closely arranged, small **granule (stellate) cells, pyramidal cells,** and neuroglia. This layer has the greatest cell density of the cerebral cortex.
5. **Internal pyramidal layer** contains the largest **pyramidal cells** and neuroglia. This layer has the lowest cell density of the cerebral cortex.
6. **Multiform layer** consists of various multiform cells called **Martinotti cells** and neuroglia.

Cerebellar Cortex

The layer of gray matter located in the periphery of the cerebellum is called the **cerebellar cortex.** This portion of the brain is responsible for maintaining balance and equilibrium, muscle tone, and coordination of skeletal muscles (Fig. 9–29). Histologically, the cerebellar cortex is divided into three layers: the molecular layer, lying directly below the pia; the Purkinje cell layer; and the deepest, the granule cell layer.

Table 9–3. Comparison Between Serum and Cerebrospinal Fluid

Constituent	Serum	Cerebrospinal Fluid
White blood cells	0	0–5 cells/ml
Protein	60–80 g/L	Negligible
Glucose	4.0–5.5 mMol/L	2.1–4.0 mMol/L
Na^+	135–150 mMol/L	135–150 mMol/L
K^+	4.0–5.1 mMol/L	2.8–3.2 mMol/L
Cl^-	100–105 mMol/L	115–130 mMol/L
Ca^{2+}	2.1–2.5 mMol/L	1.0–1.4 mMol/L
Mg^{2+}	0.7–1.0 mMol/L	0.8–1.3 mMol/L
pH	7.4	7.3

The **molecular layer** contains superficially located stellate cells, dendrites of Purkinje cells, basket cells, and unmyelinated axons from the granular layer. The **Purkinje cell layer** contains the large, flask-shaped **Purkinje cells,** which are present only in the cerebellum (see Fig. 9–4). Their arborized dendrites project into the molecular layer, and their myelinated axons project into the granular layer. Each Purkinje cell receives hundreds of thousands of excitatory and inhibitory synapses that it must integrate to form the proper response. The Purkinje cell is the only cell of the cerebellar cortex that sends information to the outside, and it is always an **inhibitory output** using GABA as the neurotransmitter. The **granular layer** consists of small granule cells and **glomeruli (cerebellar islands).** Glomeruli are regions of the cerebellar cortex where synapses are taking place between axons entering the cerebellum and the granule cells.

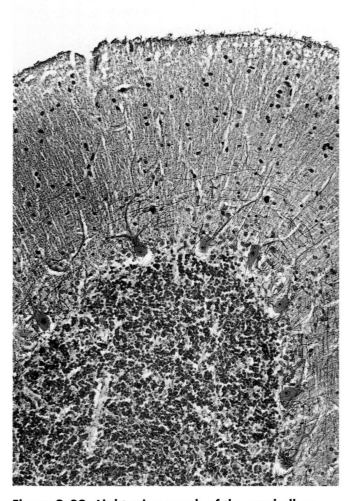

Figure 9–29. Light micrograph of the cerebellum showing its layers (× 132). Especially note the prominent Purkinje cells.

Nerve Regeneration

When a traumatic event destroys neurons they are not replaced because neurons cannot proliferate; therefore, the damage to the central nervous system is permanent. However, if a peripheral nerve fiber is injured or transected, the neuron attempts to repair the damage, regenerate the process, and restore function by initiating a series of structural and metabolic events, collectively called the **axon reaction.** The reaction to the trauma is characteristically localized in three regions of the neuron: at the site of damage, **local changes;** distal to the site of damage, **anterograde changes;** and proximal to the site of damage, **retrograde changes.** Some of the changes occur simultaneously, whereas others may occur weeks or months apart. The following description of nerve regeneration assumes that the cut ends remain near each other; otherwise, regeneration is unsuccessful (Fig. 9–30).

Local Reaction

- The severed ends of the axon retract away from each other, and the cut membrane of each stump fuses to cover the open end, preventing loss of axoplasm. Each severed end begins to expand as material delivered by axoplasmic flow accumulates. Macrophages invade the damaged area and phagocytose the debris.

Anterograde Reaction

- The axon terminal becomes hypertrophied and degenerates within a week; as a result, contact with the postsynaptic membrane is terminated. Schwann cells proliferate and phagocytose the remnants of the axon terminal, and the newly formed Schwann cells occupy the synaptic space.
- The distal portion of the axon undergoes **wallerian degeneration,** whereby the axon disintegrates and Schwann cells proliferate and phagocytose the remnants of the axon and the myelin sheath. The connective tissue covering of the nerve is unaltered, and the space it encloses becomes filled with Schwann cells, which will direct the regenerating axon to its postsynaptic cell.

Retrograde Reaction

- The perikaryon of the damaged neuron becomes hypertrophied, its Nissl bodies disperse, and its nucleus is displaced. These events are called **chromatolysis,** and the soma is actively producing free ribosomes, synthesizing proteins and various macromolecules, including RNA. The process of chromatolysis may last several months.
- During this time the proximal axon stump and surrounding myelin sheath degenerate as far proximally as the nearest collateral axon. Then several "sprouts" of axon emerge from the proximal axon stump, enter the connective tissue sheath, and are guided by the Schwann cells

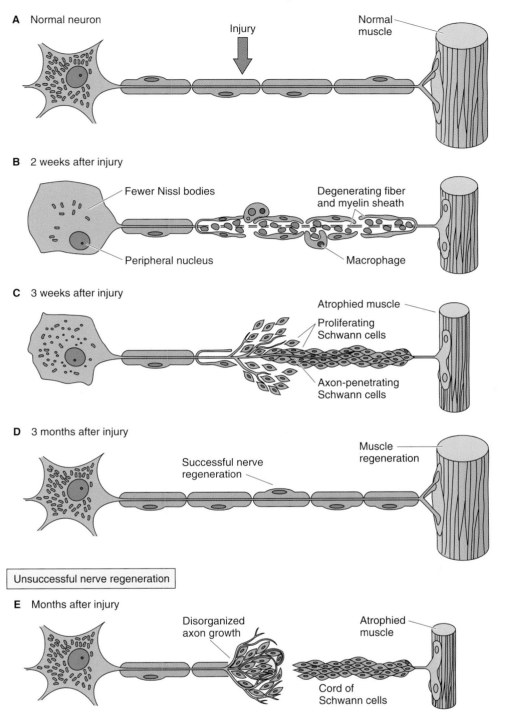

A Normal neuron

Injury

Normal muscle

B 2 weeks after injury

Fewer Nissl bodies

Degenerating fiber and myelin sheath

Peripheral nucleus

Macrophage

C 3 weeks after injury

Atrophied muscle

Proliferating Schwann cells

Axon-penetrating Schwann cells

D 3 months after injury

Muscle regeneration

Successful nerve regeneration

Unsuccessful nerve regeneration

E Months after injury

Disorganized axon growth

Atrophied muscle

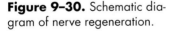

Cord of Schwann cells

Figure 9–30. Schematic diagram of nerve regeneration.

to their target cell. The sprout that reaches the target cell first forms a synapse, whereas the other sprouts degenerate. The process of regeneration proceeds at about 3 to 4 mm/day.

The nerve cell has a **trophic influence** on the cells it contacts. If the neuron dies, not only does its target cell atrophy and degenerate, but other cells targeting that particular neuron also atrophy and degenerate. This process, called **transneuronal degeneration,** may thus be anterograde or retrograde.

Regeneration in the CNS is much less likely than in the PNS, because connective tissue sheaths are absent in the CNS. Injured cells within the CNS are phagocytosed by special macrophages, known as **microglia,** and the space liberated by the phagocytosis is occupied by proliferation of glial cells, which form a cell mass called **glial scars.** It is believed that these glial cell masses hinder the process of repair. Thus, generally, neuronal damage within the CNS is irreparable.

Blood and Hemopoiesis

10

Blood is a bright to dark red, viscous, slightly alkaline fluid (pH 7.4) that accounts for approximately 7% of body weight. The total volume of blood of an average adult is about 5 L, and it circulates throughout the body within the confines of the blood vessels of the circulatory system. Blood is a specialized connective tissue composed of formed elements—**red blood cells (RBCs; erythrocytes), white blood cells (leukocytes),** and **platelets**—suspended in a fluid component, the extracellular matrix, known as **plasma** (Figs. 10–1, 10–2).

Because blood circulates throughout the body, it is an ideal vehicle for the transport of materials. The primary functions of blood include conveying nutrients from the gastrointestinal system to all of the cells of the body and subsequently delivering the waste products of these cells to specific organs for elimination. Numerous other metabolites, cellular products (such as hormones and other signaling molecules), and electrolytes are also ferried by the bloodstream to their final destinations. Oxygen is carried by the hemoglobin within erythrocytes from the lungs for distribution to the cells of the organism, and CO_2 is conveyed both by hemoglobin and by the fluid component of plasma (as HCO_3^- and in its free form) for elimination by the lungs. Additionally, blood functions in regulating body temperature and maintaining the acid/base and osmotic balance of the body fluids. Finally, blood acts as a pathway for migration of white blood cells between various connective tissue compartments of the body.

The fluid state of blood necessitates the presence of a protective mechanism, **coagulation,** to staunch its flow in case of damage to the vascular tree. The process of coagulation is mediated by platelets and bloodborne solutes that transform the blood from a sol to a gel state.

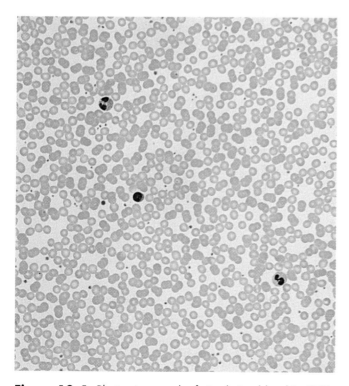

Figure 10–1. Photomicrograph of circulating blood (× 270).

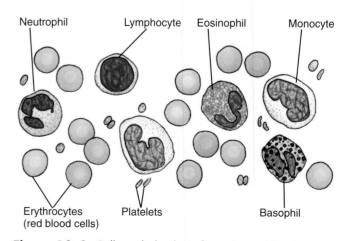

Figure 10–2. Cells and platelets of circulating blood.

When blood is removed from the body and placed in a test tube, clotting occurs unless the tube is coated by an anticoagulant such as heparin. Upon centrifugation, the formed elements settle to the bottom of the tube as a red precipitate (44%) covered by a thin translucent layer, the **buffy coat** (1%), and the fluid plasma remains on top as the supernatant (55%). The red precipitate is composed of red blood cells, the buffy coat consists of white blood cells and platelets, and the combined formed elements are called the **hematocrit.**

The finite lifespan of blood cells requires their constant renewal to maintain a steady circulating population. This process of blood cell formation from established blood cell precursors is called **hemopoiesis.**

Light microscopic examination of circulating blood cells is performed by evenly smearing a drop of blood on a glass slide, air-drying the preparation, and staining it with mixtures of dyes specifically designed to demonstrate distinctive characteristics of the cells. The current methods are derived from the technique developed in the late 19th century by Romanovsky, who used a mixture of methylene blue and eosin. Most laboratories now use either Wright's or Giemsa's modifications of the original procedure, and identification of blood cells is based on the colors produced by these stains. Methylene blue stains acidic cellular components blue, and eosin stains alkaline components pink. Still other components are colored a reddish-blue by binding to **azures,** substances formed when methylene blue is oxidized.

Plasma

Plasma is a yellowish fluid in which cells, platelets, organic compounds, and electrolytes are suspended, dissolved, or both. During coagulation some of the organic and inorganic components leave the plasma to become integrated into the clot. The remaining fluid, which differs from plasma, is straw-colored and is called **serum.**

The major component of plasma is water, constituting about 90% of its volume. Proteins compose 9%, and inorganic salts, ions, nitrogenous compounds, nutrients, and gases constitute the remaining 1%. The types, origins, and functions of the blood proteins are listed in Table 10–1.

The fluid component of blood leaves the capillaries and small venules to enter the connective tissue spaces as **tissue fluid,** which thus has a similar composition of electrolytes and small molecules as plasma. However, the concentration of proteins in tissue fluid is much lower than that in plasma, because it is difficult even for small proteins, such as albumin, to traverse the endothelial lining of a capillary. In fact, albumin is chiefly responsible for the establishment of blood's **colloid osmotic pressure,** the force that maintains normal blood and interstitial fluid volumes.

Table 10–1. Proteins of Plasma

Protein	Size	Source	Function
Albumin	60,000–69,000 Da	Liver	Maintains colloid osmotic pressure and transports certain insoluble metabolites
Globulins α- and β-Globulins	80,000–1 × 10⁶ Da	Liver	Transport metal ions, protein-bound lipids, and lipid-soluble vitamins
γ-Globulin		Plasma cells	Antibodies of immune defense
Clotting proteins (e.g., prothrombin, fibrinogen, accelerator globulin)	Varied	Liver	Formation of fibrin threads
Complement proteins C1 through C9	Varied	Liver	Destruction of microorganisms and initiation of inflammation
Plasma lipoproteins Chylomicrons	100–500 μm	Intestinal epithelial cells	Transport of triglycerides to liver
Very low-density lipoprotein (VLDL)	25–70 nm	Liver	Transport of triglycerides from liver to body cells
Low-density lipoprotein (LDL)	3 × 10⁶ Da	Liver	Transport of cholesterol from liver to body cells

Formed Elements

Erythrocytes

Each **erythrocyte (red blood cell)** resembles a biconcave-shaped disk, 7.5 μm in diameter, 2.0 μm thick at its widest region, and less than 1 μm thick at its center (Figs. 10–3, 10–4). This shape provides the cell with a large surface area relative to its volume, thus enhancing its capability for the exchange of gases. Although erythrocyte precursor cells within the bone marrow are nucleated, they expel not only their nuclei but all of their organelles as they achieve matu-

rity and enter circulation. Thus, mature erythrocytes are anucleate. When stained with Giemsa or Wright stains, erythrocytes have a salmon-pink color.

Although erythrocytes possess no organelles, they do have soluble enzymes in their cytosol. Within the erythrocyte, the enzyme **carbonic anhydrase** facilitates the formation of carbonic acid from CO_2 and water. This acid dissociates to form bicarbonate (HCO_3^-) and H^+. It is as bicarbonate that most of the carbon dioxide is ferried to the lungs for exhalation. The ability of bicarbonate to cross the erythrocyte cell membrane is mediated by the integral mem-

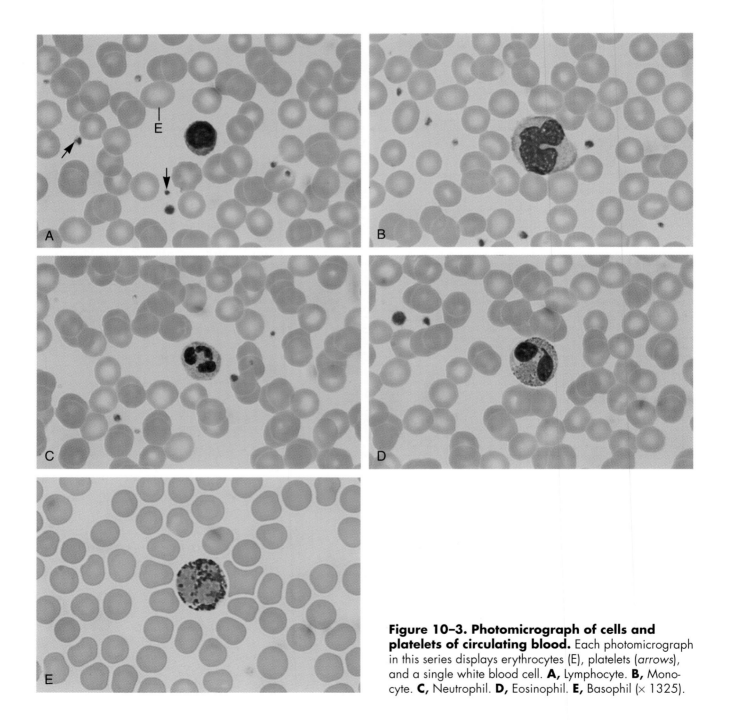

Figure 10–3. Photomicrograph of cells and platelets of circulating blood. Each photomicrograph in this series displays erythrocytes (E), platelets (*arrows*), and a single white blood cell. **A,** Lymphocyte. **B,** Monocyte. **C,** Neutrophil. **D,** Eosinophil. **E,** Basophil (× 1325).

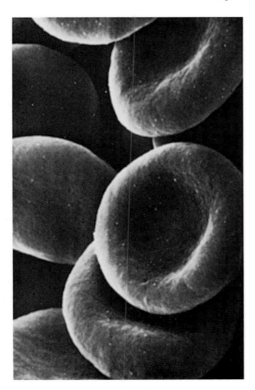

Figure 10–4. Scanning electron micrograph of circulating red blood cells (× 5850). (From Leeson, T.S., Leeson, C.R., and Paparo, A.A.: Text/Atlas of Histology. Philadelphia, W.B Saunders Company, 1988.)

brane protein, **band 3,** a coupled anion transporter that exchanges intracellular bicarbonate for extracellular Cl^-. Additional enzymes include those of the glycolytic pathway and those responsible for the monophosphate shunt. The former does not require the presence of oxygen, and is the chief method whereby the erythrocyte produces adenosine triphosphate (ATP), necessary for its energy requirement.

Males have more erythrocytes per unit volume of blood than do females (5×10^6 vs. 4.5×10^6 per mm^3), and members of both sexes living at higher altitudes have correspondingly more red blood cells than do those living at lower altitudes.

Human erythrocytes have an average lifespan of 120 days; once they reach that age, they display on their surface a group of oligosaccharides. Red blood cells bearing these sugar groups are destroyed by macrophages of the spleen, bone marrow, and liver.

Hemoglobin

Red blood cells are packed with **hemoglobin,** a large tetrameric protein (MW 68,000) composed of four polypeptide chains, each of which is covalently bound to an iron-containing **heme.** It is hemoglobin that provides the *unstained* cell with its pale-yellow color. The globin moiety of hemoglobin releases CO_2, and the iron binds to O_2 in regions of high oxygen concentration, as in the lung. However, in oxygen-poor regions, as in tissues, hemoglobin releases O_2 and binds CO_2. This property of hemoglobin makes it ideal for the conveyance of respiratory gases. Hemoglobin carrying O_2 is known as **oxyhemoglobin,** and hemoglobin carrying CO_2 is called **carbaminohemoglobin.** Hypoxic tissues release 2,3-diphosphoglyceride, a carbohydrate that facilitates the release of oxygen from the erythrocyte.

CLINICAL CORRELATIONS

Carbon monoxide has a much greater affinity for the heme portion of hemoglobin compared with oxygen. Persons trapped in areas of poor ventilation with a running gasoline-powered engine or in a building on fire frequently succumb to CO poisoning. Many such victims, when fair-skinned, instead of being cyanotic (having a bluish pallor), present with healthy-looking, cherry-red skin due to the color of the CO-hemoglobin complex.

Based on the amino acid sequences, there are four normal, human polypeptide chains of hemoglobin, designated α, β, γ, and δ. The principal hemoglobin of the fetus, **fetal hemoglobin (HbF),** composed of two α- and two γ-chains, is replaced shortly after birth by adult hemoglobin (HbA). There are two types of normal adult hemoglobins, HbA_1 ($\alpha_2\beta_2$) and the much rarer form, HbA_2 ($\alpha_2\delta_2$). In the adult, approximately 96% of the hemoglobin is HbA_1, 2% is HbA_2, and the remaining 2% is HbF.

CLINICAL CORRELATIONS

Several hereditary diseases result from defects in the genes encoding the hemoglobin polypeptide chains. Diseases referred to as **thalassemia** are marked by decreased synthesis of one or more hemoglobin chains. In β-thalassemia, synthesis of the β-chains is impaired. In the homozygous form of this disease, which is most prevalent among persons of Mediterranean descent, HbA is missing and high levels of HbF persist after birth.

Sickle cell anemia is the result of a point mutation at a single locus of the β-chain (valine is incorporated into the sequence instead of glutamate), forming the abnormal hemoglobin HbS. When the oxygen tension is reduced (e.g., during strenuous exercise), HbS changes shape, producing abnormal-shaped (crescent-shaped) erythrocytes that are less pliant, more fragile, and more prone to hemolysis than normal cells. Sickle cell anemia is prevalent in the black population, especially in persons whose ancestors lived in regions of Africa where malaria is endemic. In the United States, about 1 of 600 newborn African-American babies is stricken with this condition.

Erythrocyte Cell Membrane

The red blood cell plasma membrane, a typical lipid bilayer, is composed of about 50% protein, 40% lipids, and 10% carbohydrates. The majority of the proteins are integral proteins, mostly glycophorins, ion channels, and the anion transporter, **band 3 protein,** which also acts as an anchoring site for **ankyrin** (Fig. 10–5). Ankyrin assists in affixing the cytoskeleton, a hexagonal lattice composed chiefly of **spectrin tetramers, actin,** and **band 4.1,** to the cytoplasmic aspect of the plasmalemma, as detailed in Chapter 2. This subplasmalemmal cytoskeleton helps maintain the biconcave disk shape of the erythrocyte.

CLINICAL CORRELATIONS

Defects in the cytoskeletal components of erythrocytes result in various conditions marked by abnormally shaped cells. **Hereditary spherocytosis,** for instance, is caused by synthesis of an abnormal spectrin that exhibits defective binding to band 4.1 protein. Red blood cells of persons afflicted with this condition are more fragile and transport less oxygen than do normal erythrocytes. Moreover, these spherocytes are preferentially destroyed in the spleen, leading to **anemia.**

The extracellular surface of the red blood cell plasmalemma possesses specific inherited carbohydrate chains that act as antigens and thus determine the blood group of an individual for the purposes of blood transfusion. The most notable of these are the **A** and **B antigens,** which determine the four primary blood groups, **A, B, AB,** and **O** (Table 10–2). Persons who lack the A or B antigen, or both of them, have antibodies against the missing antigen(s) in their blood; if they are transfused with blood containing the missing antigen(s), the donor erythrocytes are attacked by the recipient's serum antibodies and are eventually lysed.

An important blood group is the **Rh** group, so named because it was first identified in rhesus monkeys. This complex group comprises more than two dozen antigens, although many are relatively rare. Three of the Rh antigens (C, D, and E) are so common in the human population that the erythrocytes of 85% of Americans possess one of these antigens on their surface and are thus said to be **Rh+.**

CLINICAL CORRELATIONS

When an Rh⁻ pregnant woman delivers her first Rh+ baby, enough of the baby's blood is likely to enter her circulation to induce the formation of anti-Rh antibodies. During a subsequent pregnancy with an Rh+ fetus, these antibodies will attack the erythrocytes of the fetus, causing **erythroblastosis fetalis,** a condition that may be fatal to the newborn. Prenatal and postnatal transfusions of the fetus are necessary to prevent brain damage and death of the newborn unless the mother was treated with anti-Rh agglutinins (RhoGAM) before or shortly after the birth of the first Rh+ baby.

Leukocytes

The number of **leukocytes** (white blood cells) is much smaller than that of red blood cells; in fact, in a normal adult there are only between 6500 and 10,000 white blood cells per mm³ of blood. Unlike erythrocytes, leukocytes do not function within the bloodstream but use it as a means of traveling from one region of the body to another. When they reach their destination, they leave the bloodstream by migrating between the endothelial cells of the blood vessels **(diapedesis),** enter the connective tissue spaces, and perform their function. Within the bloodstream, as well as in smears, leukocytes are round, but in connective tissue, they are pleomorphic. They generally defend the body against foreign substances.

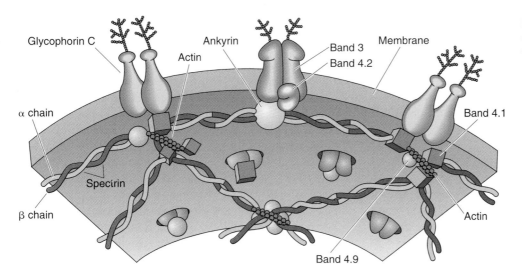

Figure 10–5. Diagram of the cytoskeleton and integral proteins of the erythrocyte cell membrane.

Glycophorin C • Ankyrin • Actin • Band 3 • Band 4.2 • Membrane • α chain • Spectrin • β chain • Band 4.1 • Actin • Band 4.9

(handwritten notes in margins)

has lipo or polysaccarides of gram negative bacteria that recognize

★ I person is given wrong blood, body will mount a massive Immune response, because it has memory cells w/ Antigens against. against gram negative bacteria.

Table 10-2. ABO Blood Group System

Blood Group	Antigens Present	Miscellaneous
A	Antigen A	
B	Antigen B	
AB	Antigens A and B	Universal acceptor
O	Neither antigens A nor B	Universal donor

White blood cells are classified into two groups: **granulocytes,** which possess **specific granules** in their cytoplasm, and **agranulocytes,** which lack specific granules. Both granulocytes and agranulocytes possess nonspecific **(azurophilic)** granules, which have been demonstrated to be **lysosomes.** There are three types of granulocytes—neutrophils, eosinophils, and basophils—differentiated according to the color of their staining reaction with Romanovsky-type stains. There are two types of agranulocytes, namely lymphocytes and monocytes. The differential leukocyte count and various properties of the leukocytes are detailed in Table 10–3.

Neutrophils

Polymorphonuclear leukocytes (polys, neutrophils) are the most numerous of the white blood cells, comprising 60% to 70% of the total leukocyte population. In blood smears, neutrophils are 9 to 12 μm in diameter and have a multilobed nucleus (see Figs. 10–2, 10–3). The lobes, connected to each other by slender chromatin threads, increase in number with the age of the cell. In females, the nucleus presents a characteristic small appendage, the "drumstick," which contains the condensed, inactive second X chromosome. It is also called the Barr body or sex chromosome but is not always evident in every cell. Neutrophils are among the first cells to appear in acute bacterial infections.

Neutrophil Granules

Three types of granules are present in the cytoplasm of neutrophils: small, specific granules (0.1 μm in diameter); larger azurophilic granules (0.5 μm in diameter); and the newly discovered tertiary granules. **Specific granules** contain various enzymes and pharmacological agents that aid the neutrophil in performing its antimicrobial functions (see Table 10–3). In electron micrographs these granules appear somewhat oblong (Fig. 10–6). **Azurophilic granules** are lysosomes, containing acid hydrolases, myeloperoxidase, the antibacterial agent lysozyme, bactericidal permeability increasing (BPI) protein, cathepsin G, elastase, and nonspecific collagenase. **Tertiary granules** contain gelatinase and cathepsins, as well as glycoproteins that are inserted into the plasmalemma.

Neutrophil Functions

Neutrophils interact with chemotactic agents to migrate to sites invaded by microorganisms. Once there, they destroy the microorganisms by phagocytosis and release of hydrolytic enzymes (and respiratory burst). Additionally, by manufacturing and releasing leukotrienes, neutrophils assist in the initiation of the inflammatory process. The sequence of events is as follows:

1. The binding of neutrophil chemotactic agents to the neutrophil's plasmalemma facilitates the release of the contents of tertiary granules into the extracellular matrix.

2. Gelatinase degrades the basal lamina, facilitating neutrophil migration. Glycoproteins that become inserted in the cell membrane aid the process of phagocytosis.

3. The contents of the specific granules are also released into the extracellular matrix, where they attack the invading microorganisms and aid neutrophil migration.

4. Microorganisms, phagocytosed by neutrophils, become enclosed in **phagosomes** (Fig. 10–7A, B). Enzymes and pharmacological agents of the azurophilic granules are usually released into the lumina of these intracellular vacuoles, where they destroy the ingested microorganisms. Because of their phagocytic functions, neutrophils are also known as **microphages** to distinguish them from the larger phagocytic cells, the **macrophages.**

5. Bacteria are killed not only by the action of enzymes but also by the formation of reactive oxygen compounds within the phagosomes of neutrophils. These are **superoxide** (O_2^-), formed by the action of NADPH oxidase on O_2 in a respiratory burst; **hydrogen peroxide,** formed by the action of superoxide dismutase on superoxide; and **hypochlorous acid** (HOCP), formed by the interaction of myeloperoxidase (MPO) and chloride ions with hydrogen peroxide (Fig. 10–7C, D).

6. Occasionally, the contents of the azurophilic granules are released into the extracellular matrix, causing tissue damage.

7. Once neutrophils perform their function of killing microorganisms they also die, resulting in the formation of **pus,** the accumulation of dead leukocytes, bacteria, and tissue fluid.

8. Not only do neutrophils destroy bacteria, they also synthesize **leukotrienes** from arachidonic acids in their cell

Table 10–3. Leukocytes

Features	Granulocytes			Agranulocytes	
	Neutrophils	**Eosinophils**	**Basophils**	**Lymphocytes**	**Monocytes**
Number/mm³ % of WBC	3500–7000 60–70%	150–400 2–4%	50–100 < 1%	1500–2500 20–25%	200–800 3–8%
Diameter (μm) (section) (smear)	8–9 9–12	9–11 10–14	7–8 8–10	7–8 8–10	10–12 12–15
Nucleus	3–4 lobes	2 lobes (sausage-shaped)	S-shaped	Round	Kidney-shaped
Specific granules	0.1 μm, light pink*	1–1.5 μm, dark pink*	0.5 μm, blue/black*	None	None
Contents of specific granules	Type IV collagenase, phospholipase A₂, lactoferrin, lysozyme, phagocytin, alkaline phosphatase	Aryl sulfatase, histaminase, β-glucuronidase, acid phosphatase, phospholipase, major basic protein, eosinophil cationic protein, neurotoxin, ribonuclease, cathepsin, peroxidase	Histamine, heparin, eosinophil chemotactic factor, neutrophil chemotactic factor, peroxidase	None	None
Surface markers	Fc receptors, platelet-activating factor receptor, leukotriene B₄ receptor, leukocyte cell adhesion molecule-1	IgE receptors, eosinophil chemotactic factor receptor	IgE receptors	*T cells:* T-cell receptors, CD molecules, IL receptors; *B cells:* surface immunoglobulins	Class II HLA, Fc receptors
Lifespan	< 1 week	< 2 weeks	1–2 years (in murines)	Few months to several years	Few days in blood, several months in connective tissue
Function	Phagocytosis and destruction of bacteria	Phagocytosis of antigen–antibody complex; destruction of parasites	Similar to mast cells to mediate inflammatory responses	*T cells:* cell-mediated immune response; *B cells:* humorally mediated immune response	Differentiate into macrophage: phagocytosis, presentation of antigens

*Using Romanovsky-type stains (or their modifications).

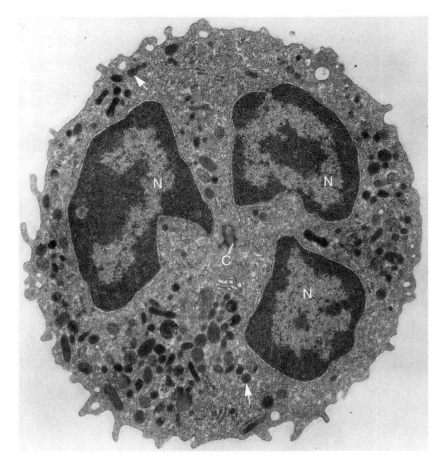

Figure 10-6. Electron micrograph of a human neutrophil. Note the three lobes of the nucleus (N), the presence of granules (*arrows*) throughout the cytoplasm, and the centrally located centriole (C). (From Zucker-Franklin, D., et al. [eds.]: Atlas of Blood Cells, vol. 1. Milan, Edi Ermes, 1981.)

membranes. These newly formed leukotrienes aid the initiation of the inflammatory process.

CLINICAL CORRELATIONS

Children with hereditary deficiency of NADPH oxidase are subject to persistent bacterial infections, because their neutrophils cannot form a respiratory burst response to the bacterial challenge. Their neutrophils cannot generate superoxide, hydrogen peroxide, or hypochlorous acid during phagocytosis of bacteria.

Eosinophils

Eosinophils constitute less than 4% of the total white blood cell population. They are round cells in suspension and in blood smears, but they may be pleomorphic during their migration through connective tissue. Eosinophils are 10 to 14 μm in diameter (in blood smears) and possess a sausage-shaped, bilobed nucleus in which the two lobes are connected by a thin chromatin strand and nuclear envelope (see Figs. 10–2, 10–3). Electron micrographs display a small, centrally located Golgi apparatus, a limited amount of rough endoplasmic reticulum (RER), and only a few mitochondria, usually in the vicinity of the centrioles near the cytocenter.

Eosinophil Granules

Eosinophils possess specific granules and azurophilic granules. Specific granules are oblong (1.0 to 1.5 μm in length and < 1.0 μm in width) and stain deep pink with Giemsa and Wright stains. Electron micrographs display that specific granules have a crystal-like, electron-dense center, the **internum,** surrounded by a less electron-dense **externum** (Fig. 10–8). The internum contains **major basic protein, eosinophilic cationic protein,** and **eosinophil-derived neurotoxin,** the first two of which are highly efficacious agents in combating parasites. The externum also contains the enzymes listed in Table 10–3.

The nonspecific azurophilic granules are lysosomes (0.5 μm in diameter) containing hydrolytic enzymes similar to those found in neutrophils. These function both in the destruction of parasitic worms and in the hydrolysis of antigen-antibody complexes internalized by eosinophils.

Eosinophil Functions

1. The binding of histamine, leukotrienes, and eosinophil chemotactic factor (released by mast cells, basophils, and neutrophils) to eosinophil plasmalemma receptors results in the migration of eosinophils to the site of allergic reaction, inflammatory reaction, or parasitic worm invasion.

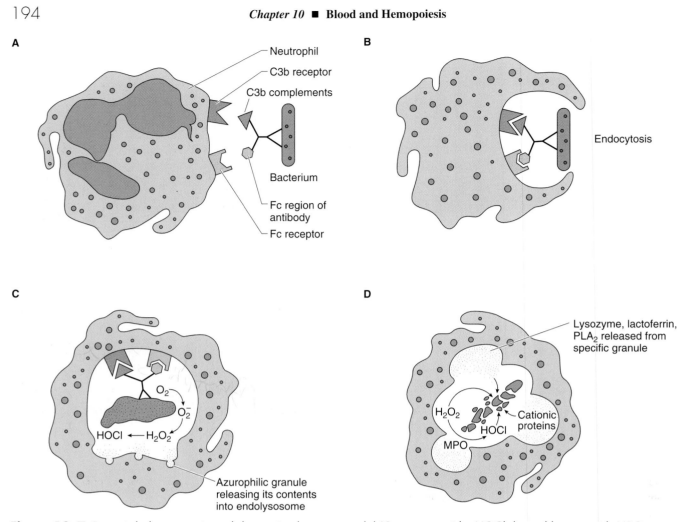

Figure 10–7. Bacterial phagocytosis and destruction by a neutrophil (O_2^-, superoxide; HOCl, hypochlorous acid; MPO, myeloperoxidase).

2. Eosinophils degranulate their major basic protein or eosinophil cationic protein on the surface of the parasitic worms, killing them by forming pores in their pellicles, thus facilitating access of agents such as **superoxides** and **hydrogen peroxide** to the parasite; or they release substances that inactivate the pharmacological initiators of the inflammatory response, such as **histamine** and **leukotriene C;** or they engulf antigen–antibody complexes.

3. Internalized antigen–antibody complexes pass into the **endosomal** compartment for eventual degradation.

CLINICAL CORRELATIONS

Connective tissue cells in the vicinity of antigen–antibody complexes release the pharmacological agents histamine and interleukin-5, causing increased formation and release of eosinophils from the bone marrow. On the contrary, elevation of blood corticosteroid levels depresses the number of eosinophils in circulation.

Basophils

Basophils constitute fewer than 1% of the total leukocyte population. They are round cells in suspension but may be pleomorphic during migration through connective tissue. Basophils are 8 to 10 μm in diameter (in blood smears) and possess an S-shaped nucleus, which is frequently masked by the large specific granules present in the cytoplasm (see Figs. 10–2, 10–3). In electron micrographs, the small Golgi apparatus, few mitochondria, extensive RER, and occasional glycogen deposits are clearly evident. Basophils possess several surface receptors on their plasmalemma, including **IgE receptors.**

Basophil Granules

The **specific granules** of basophils stain dark blue to black with Giemsa and Wright stains. They are approximately 0.5 μm in diameter and frequently press against the periphery of the cell, creating the basophil's characteristic "roughened

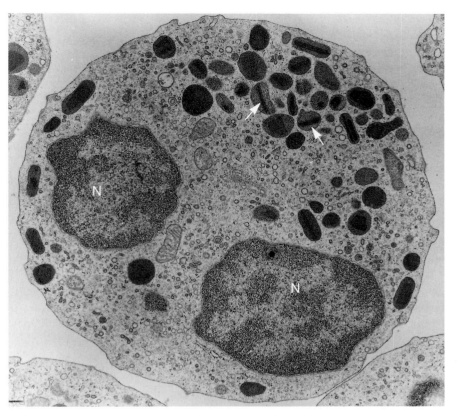

Figure 10–8. Electron micrograph of a human eosinophil. Note the electron-dense internum (*arrows*) of the eosinophilic granules and the two lobes of the nucleus (N). (From Zucker-Franklin, D.: *In* Stollerman, G.H., et al. [eds.]: Advances in Internal Medicine, vol. 19. Chicago, Year Book, 1974.)

perimeter." The granules contain heparin, histamine, eosinophil chemotactic factor, neutrophil chemotactic factor, and peroxidase, as detailed in Table 10–3. The nonspecific **azurophilic granules** are lysosomes, which contain enzymes similar to those of neutrophils.

Basophil Functions

In response to the presence of some antigens in certain individuals, plasma cells manufacture and release a particular class of immunoglobulin, IgE. The Fc portions of the IgE molecules become attached to the Fc receptors of basophils and mast cells without any apparent effect. However, the next time the same antigens enter the body, they bind to the IgE molecules on the surface of these cells. It should be understood that although mast cells and basophils appear to possess similar functions, they are different cells, although possibly arising from the same precursor.

Although the following sequence of steps occurs in both mast cells and basophils, the basophil will be utilized for descriptive purposes.

1. Binding of antigens to the IgE molecules on the surface of a basophil causes the cell to release the contents of its specific granules into the extracellular space.

2. Additionally, phospholipases act on certain phospholipids of the basophil plasmalemma to form **arachidonic acids.** Arachidonic acids are metabolized to produce

leukotrienes C$_4$, D$_4$, and E$_4$ (previously known as slow-reacting substance of anaphylaxis, or **SRS-A).**

3. The release of histamine causes vasodilation, smooth muscle contraction (in the bronchial tree), and leakiness of blood vessels.

4. Leukotrienes have similar effects, but these actions are slower and more persistent than those associated with histamine. Additionally, leukotrienes activate leukocytes, causing them to migrate to the site of antigenic challenge.

CLINICAL CORRELATIONS

In certain allergic persons, second exposure to the same allergen may result in an intense generalized response. A large number of basophils (and mast cells) degranulate, resulting in widespread vasodilation and sweeping reduction in blood volume (due to vessel leakiness). Thus the victim goes into circulatory shock. Additionally, the smooth muscles of the bronchial tree constrict, causing respiratory insufficiency. The combined effect is a life-threatening condition known as **anaphylactic shock.**

Monocytes

Monocytes are the largest of the circulating blood cells, 12 to 15 μm in diameter in blood smears, and constitute 3% to 8% of the leukocyte population. They have a large, acentric, kidney-shaped nucleus that frequently has a "moth-eaten," soap-bubbly appearance and whose lobe-like extensions seem to overlap one another. The chromatin network is coarse but not overly dense, and typically two nucleoli are present, although they are not always evident in smears. The cytoplasm is bluish-gray and has numerous azurophilic granules (lysosomes) and occasional vacuole-like spaces (see Figs. 10–2, 10–3).

Electron micrographs display both heterochromatin and euchromatin in the nucleus as well as two nucleoli. The Golgi apparatus is usually near the indentation of the kidney-shaped nucleus. The cytoplasm contains deposits of glycogen granules, a few profiles of RER, some mitochondria, free ribosomes, and numerous lysosomes. The periphery of the cell displays microtubules, microfilaments, pinocytotic vesicles, and filopodia.

Monocytes stay in circulation for only a few days; they then migrate through the endothelium of venules and capillaries into the connective tissue, where they differentiate into **macrophages.**

Function of Macrophages

1. Macrophages are avid phagocytes, and as members of the **mononuclear phagocyte system,** they phagocytose and destroy dead and defunct cells (such as senescent erythrocytes), as well as antigens and foreign particulate matter (such as bacteria). The destruction occurs within the phagosomes both via enzymatic digestion and through the formation of superoxide, hydrogen peroxide, and hypochlorous acid.

2. They produce cytokines that activate the inflammatory response as well as the proliferation and maturation of other cells.

3. Certain macrophages, known as **antigen-presenting cells,** phagocytose antigens and present their most antigenic portions, the **epitopes,** in conjunction with the integral proteins, **class II human leukocyte antigen** (class II HLA) to immunocompetent cells.

4. In response to large foreign particulate matter, macrophages fuse with one another, forming **foreign-body giant cells** that are large enough to phagocytose the foreign particle.

Lymphocytes

Lymphocytes make up 20% to 25% of the total circulating leukocyte population. They are round cells in blood smears, but they may be pleomorphic as they migrate through connective tissue. Lymphocytes are somewhat larger than erythrocytes, 8 to 10 μm in diameter (in blood smears), and have a slightly indented, round nucleus that occupies most of the cell. The nucleus is dense, with a lot of heterochromatin, and it is acentrically located. The peripherally situated cytoplasm stains a light blue and contains a few azurophilic granules. On the basis of size, lymphocytes may

be described as small, medium (12 to 15 μm in diameter), or large (15 to 18 μm), although the latter two are much less numerous (see Figs. 10–2, 10–3).

Electron micrographs of lymphocytes display a scant amount of peripheral cytoplasm housing a few mitochondria, a small Golgi apparatus, and a few profiles of RER. Additionally, a small number of lysosomes, representing azurophilic granules 0.5 μm in diameter, and an abundant supply of ribosomes are also evident (Fig. 10–9).

Although lymphocytes are discussed in greater detail in Chapter 12, an introduction to their properties and functions follows.

Types of Lymphocytes

Lymphocytes can be subdivided into three functional categories, namely **B lymphocytes (B cells), T lymphocytes (T cells),** and **null cells.** Although morphologically they are indistinct, they may be distinguished immunocytochemically by the differences in their surface markers (see Table 10–3). Approximately 80% of the circulating lymphocytes are T cells, about 15% are B cells, and the remainder are null cells. Their lifespans also differ widely: some T cells may live for years, whereas some B cells may die in a few months.

Functions of B and T Cells

Lymphocytes have no function in the bloodstream, but in the connective tissue these cells are responsible for the proper functioning of the immune system. In order to be immunologically competent, they migrate to specific body compartments to mature and to express specific surface markers and receptors. B cells enter as-yet unidentified regions of the **bone marrow,** whereas T cells migrate to the cortex of the **thymus.** Once they have become immunologically competent, they leave their respective sites of maturation, enter the lymphoid system, and undergo mitosis, forming a **clone** of identical cells. All members of a particular clone can recognize and respond to the same antigen.

After stimulation by a specific antigen, both B and T cells proliferate and differentiate into two subpopulations, **memory cells** and **effector cells.** Memory cells do not participate in the immune response but remain as part of the clone with an "immunological memory," ready to mount a response against a subsequent exposure to a particular antigen or foreign substance.

Effector Cells

B cells are responsible for the **humorally mediated immune system;** that is, they differentiate into **plasma cells,** which produce **antibodies** against **antigens.** T cells are responsible for the **cellularly mediated immune system.** Some T cells differentiate into **cytotoxic T cells (CTL; T**

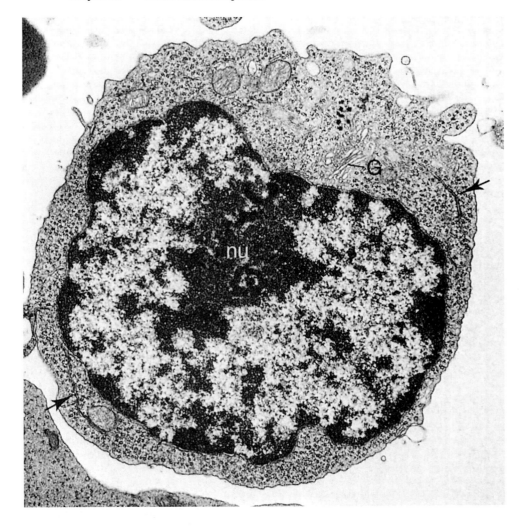

Figure 10–9. Electron micrograph of a lymphocyte (× 18,000). G, Golgi apparatus; nu, nucleus; arrows point to the rough endoplasmic reticulum. (From Hopkins, C.R.: Structure and Function of Cells. Philadelphia, W.B. Saunders Company, 1978.)

killer cells), which physically contact and kill **foreign** or **virally altered cells.** Additionally, certain T cells are responsible for the initiation and development (**T helper cells**) or for the suppression (**T suppressor cells**) of most humorally and cellularly mediated immune responses. They do this by releasing signaling molecules known as **cytokines (lymphokines)** that elicit specific responses from other cells of the immune system (detailed in Chapter 12).

Null Cells

Null cells are composed of two distinct populations, circulating **stem cells,** which give rise to all of the formed elements of blood, and **NK cells (natural killer cells).** These NK cells can kill some foreign and virally altered cells without the influence of the thymus or T cells.

Platelets

Platelets (thromboplastids) are small, disk-shaped, nonnucleated cell fragments derived from **megakaryocytes** in the bone marrow. Platelets are about 2 to 4 μm in diameter

(in blood smears) (see Figs. 10–2, 10–3); in light micrographs, they display a peripheral clear region, the **hyalomere,** and a central darker region, the **granulomere.** The platelet plasmalemma has numerous receptor molecules as well as a relatively thick (15 to 20 nm) glycocalyx. There are between 250,000 and 400,000 platelets per mm³ of blood with a lifespan of less than 14 days.

Platelet Tubules and Granules

Electron micrographs of platelets display 10 to 15 microtubules arranged parallel to each other and forming a ring within the hyalomere. The microtubules assist platelets in maintaining their diskoid morphology. Associated with this bundle of microtubules are actin and myosin monomers, which can rapidly assemble to form a contractile apparatus. Additionally, two tubular systems are present in the hyalomere, the **surface-opening (connecting)** and the **dense tubular systems** (Figs. 10–10, 10–11).

The ultrastructure of the granulomere displays the presence of a small number of mitochondria, glycogen deposits, peroxisomes, and three types of granules: **α-granules,**

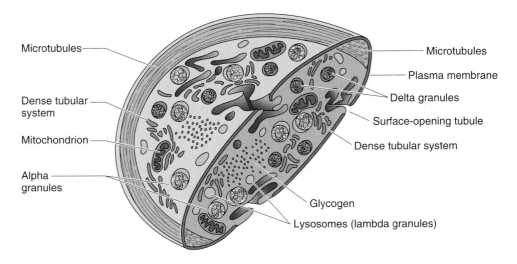

Microtubules

Dense tubular system

Mitochondrion

Alpha granules

Microtubules

Plasma membrane

Delta granules

Surface-opening tubule

Dense tubular system

Glycogen

Lysosomes (lambda granules)

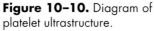

Figure 10–10. Diagram of platelet ultrastructure.

δ-granules, and λ-granules (lysosomes). The tubules and granules, as well as their contents and functions, are listed in Table 10–4. The granulomere also houses a system of enzymes that permits platelets to catabolize glycogen, consume oxygen, and generate ATP.

Platelet Function

Platelets function in limiting hemorrhage to the endothelial lining of the blood vessel in case of injury. If the endothelial lining is disrupted and platelets contact the subendothelial collagen, they become **activated,** release the contents of their granules, adhere to the damaged region of the vessel wall **(platelet adhesion),** and adhere to each other **(platelet aggregation).** Interactions of tissue factors, plasma-borne factors, and platelet-derived factors form a blood clot (Fig. 10–12). Although the mechanism of platelet aggregation, adhesion, and blood clotting is beyond the scope of histology, some of its salient features follow.

1. Normally the intact endothelium produces **prostacyclins** and NO_2, which inhibit platelet aggregation. It also blocks coagulation by the presence of **thrombomodulin** and **heparin-like molecule** on its luminal plasmalemma. These two membrane-associated molecules inactivate specific coagulation factors.

2. Injured endothelial cells release **von Willebrand factor** and **tissue thromboplastin** and cease the production and expression of the inhibitors of coagulation and platelet aggregation. They also release **endothelin,** a powerful vasoconstrictor that reduces the loss of blood.

3. Platelets avidly adhere to subendothelial collagen, especially in the presence of von Willebrand factor, release the contents of their granules, and adhere to one another. These three events are collectively called **platelet activation.**

4. The release of some of their granular contents, especially **adenosine diphosphate (ADP)** and **thrombospondin,** makes platelets "sticky," causing circulating platelets to adhere to the collagen-bound platelets and to degranulate.

5. Arachidonic acid, formed in the activated platelet plasmalemma, is converted to **thromboxane A_2,** a potent vasoconstrictor and platelet activator.

6. The aggregated platelets act as a plug, blocking hemorrhage. Additionally, they express **platelet factor 3** on their plasmalemma, providing the necessary phospholipid surface for the proper assembly of the coagulation factors (especially of **thrombin).**

7. As part of the complex cascade of reactions involving the various **coagulation factors,** tissue thromboplastin and platelet thromboplastin both act on circulating **prothrombin,** converting it into **thrombin.** Thrombin is an enzyme that facilitates platelet aggregation. It also converts, in the presence of Ca^{2+}, **fibrinogen** to **fibrin.**

8. The fibrin monomers thus produced polymerize and form a **reticulum of clot,** entangling additional platelets, erythrocytes, and leukocytes into a stable, gelatinous **blood clot (thrombus).** The erythrocytes facilitate platelet activation, whereas neutrophils and endothelial cells limit both platelet activation and thrombus size.

9. Approximately 1 hour after clot formation, actin and myosin monomers form thin and thick filaments, which interact by utilizing ATP as their energy source. This results in clot contraction to about half its previous size, pulling the edges of the vessel closer together, minimizing blood loss.

10. When the vessel is repaired, the endothelial cells release **plasminogen activators,** which convert circulating plasminogen to **plasmin,** the enzyme that initiates lysis of the thrombus. The hydrolytic enzymes of λ-granules assist in this process.

CLINICAL CORRELATIONS

In **thromboembolism,** the most common type of embolism, clots break free and circulate in the bloodstream

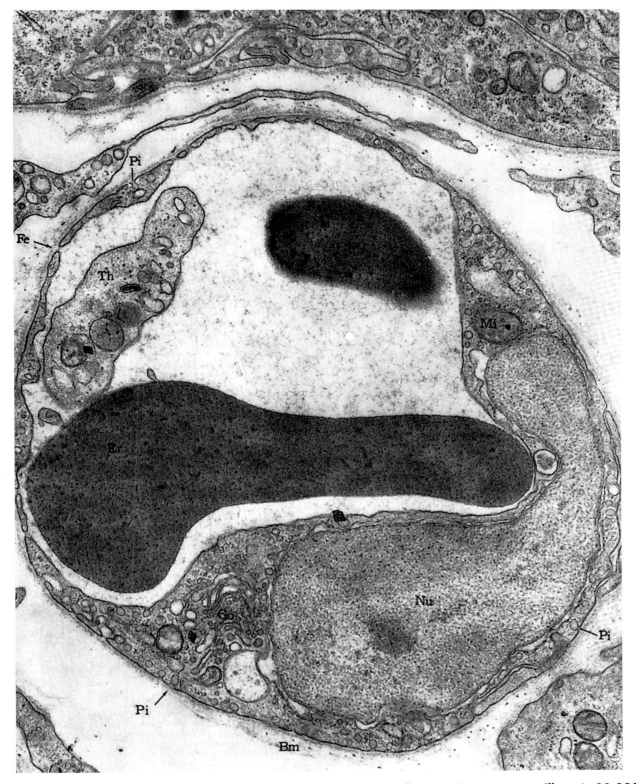

Figure 10–11. Electron micrograph of a platelet and erythrocyte in the gastric mucosa capillary (× 30,000).
Th, platelet; Er, erythrocyte; Nu, nucleus of the capillary; Fe, fenestra; Go, Golgi apparatus; Pi, pinocytotic vesicles; Bm, basal lamina. (From Rhodin, J.A.G.: An Atlas of Ultrastructure. Philadelphia, W.B. Saunders Company, 1963.)

Table 10–4. Platelet Tubules and Granules

Structure (Size)	Location	Contents	Function
Surface-opening tubule system	Hyalomere		Expedites rapid uptake and release of molecules from activated platelets
Dense tubular system	Hyalomere		Probably sequesters calcium ions to prevent platelet "stickiness"
α-Granules (300–500 nm)	Granulomere	Fibrinogen, platelet-derived growth factor, platelet thromboplastin, thrombospondin, coagulation factors	Contained factors facilitate vessel repair, platelet aggregation, and coagulation of blood
δ-Granules (dense bodies) (250–300 nm)	Granulomere	Calcium, ADP, ATP, serotonin, histamine, pyrophosphatase	Contained factors facilitate platelet aggregation and adhesion, as well as vasoconstriction
λ-Granules (lysosomes) (200–250 nm)	Granulomere	Hydrolytic enzymes	Contained enzymes aid clot resorption

ADP, adenosine diphosphate; ATP, adenosine triphosphate.

until they reach a vessel whose lumen is too small to accommodate the clot. If the clot is large enough to occlude the bifurcation of the pulmonary artery (**saddle embolus),** it can result in sudden, unexpected death. If a clot obstructs branches of the coronary artery, a **myocardial infarct** may occur.

Several types of coagulation disorders that result in excessive bleeding are known. The disorder may be acquired (as in vitamin K deficiency), hereditary (as in hemophilia), or due to low levels of blood platelets (thrombocytopenia). **Vitamin K** is required by the liver as a cofactor in the synthesis of the **clotting factors VII, IX,** and **X,** and **prothrombin.** The absence or reduced levels of these factors result in partial or complete dysfunction of the clotting process.

The most common type of **hemophilia** is due to factor VIII deficiency (**classic hemophilia),** a recessive hereditary trait transmitted by mothers to their male children. Because it is carried on the X chromosomes, female children would not be affected unless both parents had deficient X chromosomes. Affected persons are prone to bleeding subsequent to trauma, usually occurring from damage to larger vessels.

Thrombocytopenia is a condition in which the blood level of platelets is decreased. The condition becomes serious when the platelet level is below $50,000/mm^3$. Bleeding is common in persons suffering from this condition, but the bleeding is generalized and occurs from small vessels, resulting in purplish splotches on the skin. This condition is believed to be an **autoimmune disease,** in which antibodies are formed to one's own platelets and these antibodies destroy the platelets.

Bone Marrow

The medullary cavity of long bones and the interstices between trabeculae of spongy bones house the soft, gelatinous, highly vascular and cellular tissue known as **marrow.** It is isolated from bone by the endosteum (composed of osteogenic cells, osteoblasts, and occasional osteoclasts). Bone marrow constitutes almost 5% of the total body weight. It is responsible for the formation of blood cells (**hemopoiesis)** and their delivery into the circulatory system, and it performs this function from the fifth month of prenatal life until the person dies. Bone marrow also provides a microenvironment for much of the maturation process of B lymphocytes and for the initial maturation of T lymphocytes.

The marrow of the newborn is **red marrow** because of the great number of erythrocytes being produced there. However, by age 20, the diaphyses of long bones house only **yellow marrow** because of the accumulation of large quantities of fat and the absence of hemopoiesis in the shafts of these bones.

The vascular supply of bone marrow is derived from the nutrient arteries that pierce the diaphysis via the nutrient foramina, tunnels leading from the outside surface of bone into the medullary cavity. These arteries enter the marrow cavity and give rise to a number of small, peripherally located vessels that provide numerous branches both centrally, to the marrow, and peripherally, to the cortical bone. Those entering the cortical bone distribute through the haversian and Volkmann's canals to serve the compact bone. The centrally directed branches deliver their blood to the extensive network of large **sinusoids** (45 to 80 μm in diameter). The sinusoids drain into a **central longitudinal vein,** which is

A

B

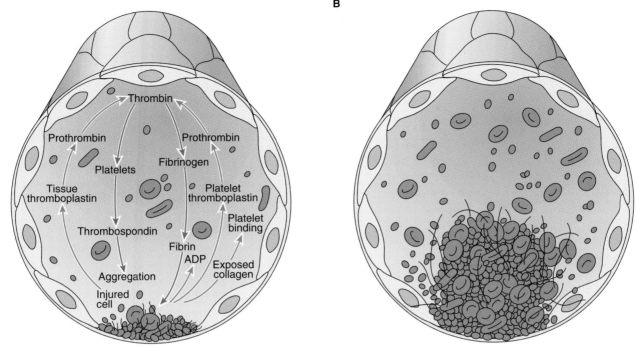

Figure 10–12. Schematic diagram of clot formation. (Modified from Fawcett, D.W.: Bloom and Fawcett's A Textbook of Histology. 12th ed. New York, Chapman and Hall, 1994.)

drained by veins leaving the bone via the nutrient canal. It is interesting to note that the veins are *smaller* than the arteries, thus establishing high hydrostatic pressure within the sinusoids, preventing their collapse. The veins, arteries, and sinusoids form the **vascular compartment,** and the intervening spaces are filled with pleomorphic **islands of hemopoietic cells** that merge with each other, forming the **hemopoietic compartment** (Fig. 10–13).

The sinusoids are lined by endothelial cells and are surrounded by slender threads of **reticular fibers** and a large number of **adventitial reticular cells.** Processes of adventitial reticular cells touch the sparse basement membrane of the endothelial cells, covering a large portion of the sinusoidal surface. Additional processes of these cells are directed away from the sinusoids and are in contact with similar processes of other adventitial reticular cells, forming a three-dimensional network surrounding discrete hemopoietic cords (islands).

The islands of hemopoietic cells are composed of blood cells in various stages of maturation as well as **macrophages,** which destroy the extruded nuclei of erythrocyte precursors, malformed cells, and excess cytoplasm. Frequently, processes of macrophages penetrate the spaces between endothelial cells to enter the sinusoidal lumina.

As adventitial reticular cells accumulate fat in their cytoplasm, they resemble adipose cells. Their large size reduces the hemopoietic compartment in size, transforming the red marrow to yellow marrow.

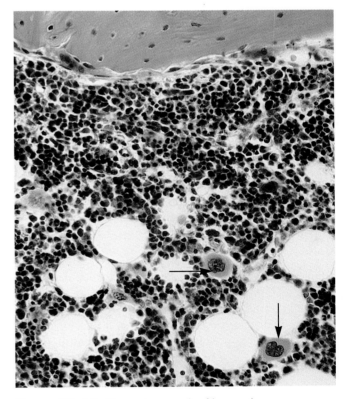

Figure 10–13. Photomicrograph of human bone marrow, displaying two megakaryocytes (*arrows*) (× 270).

CLINICAL CORRELATIONS

In certain leukemias or in severe bleeding, adventitial reticular cells may lose their lipids and decrease in size, transforming yellow marrow to red marrow, thus making more space available for hemopoiesis.

Prenatal Hemopoiesis

Blood cell formation begins 2 weeks after conception (**mesoblastic phase**) in the mesoderm of the yolk sac, where mesenchymal cells aggregate into clusters known as **blood islands.** The peripheral cells of these islands form the vessel wall, and the remaining cells become **erythroblasts,** which differentiate into nucleated **erythrocytes.**

The mesoblastic phase begins to be replaced by the **hepatic phase** by the sixth week of gestation. The erythrocytes still possess nuclei, and leukocytes appear by the eighth week of gestation. The **splenic phase** begins during the second trimester, and both hepatic and splenic phases continue until the end of gestation.

Hemopoiesis begins in the bone marrow (**myeloid phase**) by the end of the second trimester. As the skeletal system continues to develop, the bone marrow assumes an increasing role in blood cell formation. Although the liver and the spleen are not active in hemopoiesis postnatally, they both can revert back to forming new blood cells if the need arises.

Postnatal Hemopoiesis

Because all blood cells have a finite lifespan, they must be replaced continuously. This replacement is accomplished by hemopoiesis, starting from a common population of stem cells within the bone marrow (Fig. 10–14). During hemopoiesis, stem cells undergo multiple cell divisions and differentiate through several intermediate stages, eventually giving rise to the mature blood cells discussed earlier. Table 10–5 outlines the numerous intermediate cells in the formation of each type of mature blood cell. The whole process is regulated by various growth factors that act at different steps to control the type of cells formed and their rate of formation.

Stem Cells, Progenitor Cells, and Precursor Cells

All blood cells arise from **pluripotential hemopoietic stem cells (PHSCs),** which account for about 0.1% of the nucleated cell population of bone marrow. They are usually amitotic but may undergo bursts of cell division, giving rise to more PHSCs as well as to two types of **multipotential hemopoietic stem cells (MHSCs).** The two populations of MHSCs, **colony-forming unit—spleen (CFU-S)** and **colony-forming unit—lymphocyte (CFU-Ly),** are responsible for the formation of various progenitor cells. CFU-S cells are predecessors of the **myeloid cells** (erythrocytes,

granulocytes, monocytes, and platelets), whereas CFU-Ly are predecessors of the **lymphoid cells** (T cells and B cells). Both PHSCs and MHSCs resemble lymphocytes and constitute a small fraction of the null-cell population of circulating blood.

Progenitor cells also resemble small lymphocytes, but they are **unipotential** (i.e., committed to forming a single cell line, such as eosinophils). Their mitotic activity and differentiation is controlled by specific hemopoietic factors. These cells have only limited capacity for self-renewal.

Precursor cells arise from progenitor cells and are incapable of self-renewal. They have specific morphological characteristics that permit them to be recognized as the first cell of a particular cell line. Precursor cells undergo cell division and differentiation, eventually giving rise to a clone of mature cells. As cell maturation and differentiation proceed, succeeding cells become smaller, their nucleoli disappear, their chromatin network becomes denser, and the morphological characteristics of their cytoplasm approximate those of the mature cells (Fig. 10–15).

Researchers studying hemopoiesis have isolated individual lymphocyte-like cells that, under proper conditions, occasionally give rise to groups *(colonies)* of cells composed of granulocytes, erythrocytes, monocytes, lymphocytes, and platelets. Thus, it has been shown that all blood cells are derived from a single **pluripotential stem cell.** More frequently, however, isolated individual cells give rise to only

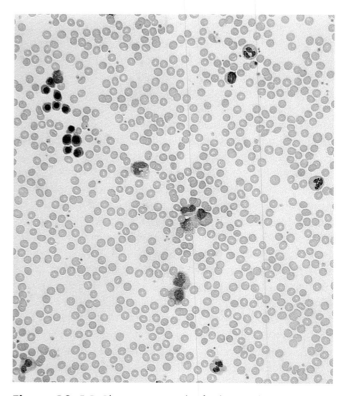

Figure 10–14. Photomicrograph of a human bone-marrow smear (× 270).

Table 10–5. Cells of Hemopoiesis

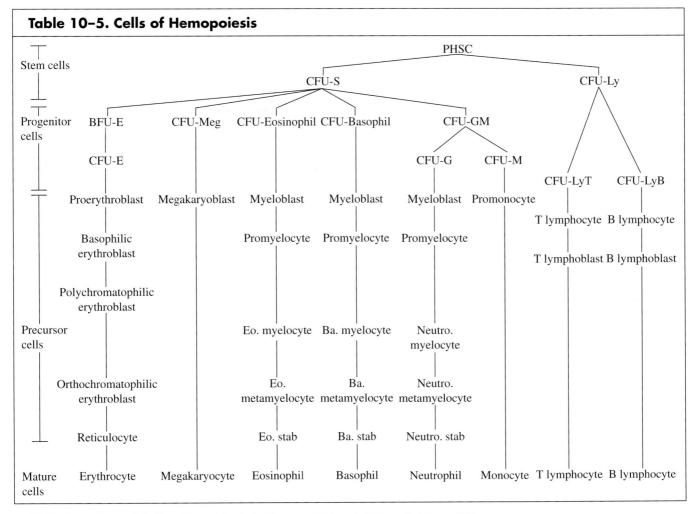

Modified from Gartner, L.P., Hiatt, J.L., and Strum, J.: Histology. Williams & Williams, Baltimore, 1988.

erythrocytes or eosinophils or another type of blood cell. Because these experiments used the spleen as the site of hemopoiesis, the individual lymphocyte-like cells were called **colony-forming units—spleen** (CFU-S). Careful observations have shown that there are two types of multipotential cells, CFU-S and CFU-Ly, which give rise to the myeloid series of cells and lymphocytes, respectively. Additional research has demonstrated that each precursor cell had a unipotential colony-forming unit as its predecessor, as listed in Table 10–5. Precursor cells undergo a series of cell divisions and differentiations to yield the mature cell.

CLINICAL CORRELATIONS

Patients who require bone marrow transplants subsequent to therapeutic procedures (such as irradiation or chemotherapy) must be matched for the major histocompatibility complex of the donor. Unless an identical twin is available for the transplant, grafting failure is common. This can be circumvented by freezing the patient's own bone marrow in liquid nitrogen and reintroducing it to the patient (**autologous transplant**) subsequent to the irradiation or chemotherapy. Because the number of stem cells per unit volume of bone marrow is relatively small, large volumes of marrow have to be harvested from the patient. Recent procedures that permit the isolation of pluripotential hemopoietic stem cells by the use of monoclonal antibodies against the CD34 molecule, which is expressed only by these cells, permit the use of small volumes of bone marrow enriched in pluripotential hemopoietic stem cells. These procedures are currently being investigated clinically, using patients suffering from various types of malignancies.

In the relatively near future, persons with hereditary blood cell disorders (e.g., sickle cell anemia) may be treated by the use of genetically engineered stem cells. Pluripotential hemopoietic stem cells isolated from the patient may be transfected with the normal gene (e.g., for hemoglobin) and reintroduced as an autologous transplant. These genetically engineered cells bearing the "normal

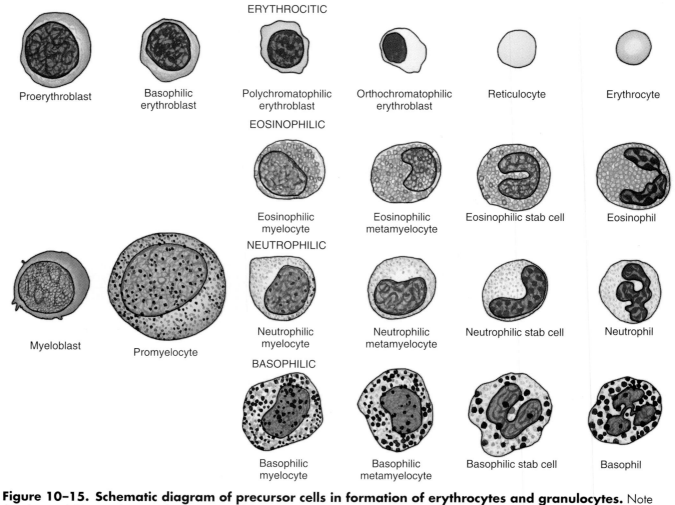

Figure 10–15. Schematic diagram of precursor cells in formation of erythrocytes and granulocytes. Note that the myeloblast and promyelocyte intermediaries in the formation of eosinophils, neutrophils, and basophils are indistinguishable for the three cell types.

gene" would proliferate, and their progeny would produce normal blood cells. Although the patient would still be producing some defective cells, it is hoped that enough normal cells would be produced to minimize the hereditary defect.

Hemopoietic Growth Factors (Colony-Stimulating Factors)

Hemopoiesis is regulated by numerous growth factors produced by various cell types. Each factor acts on specific stem cells, progenitor cells, and precursor cells, generally inducing rapid mitosis, differentiation, or both (Table 10–6). Some of these growth factors also promote the functioning of mature blood cells. Most hemopoietic growth factors are glycoproteins. Three routes are used to deliver them to their target cells: transport via the bloodstream (as endocrine hormones), secretion by stromal cells of the bone marrow near the hemopoietic cells (as paracrine hormones), and direct cell–cell contact (as surface signaling molecules).

Some growth factors, mostly three **interleukins (IL-1, IL-3, IL-6),** stimulate proliferation of pluripotential and multipotential stem cells, thus maintaining their populations. Additional factors, not as yet identified, are responsible for the differentiation of these cells into unipotential progenitor cells. **Colony-stimulating factors** are responsible for the stimulation of cell division and for the differentiation of unipotential cells of the granulocytic and monocytic series. **Erythropoietin** activates cells of the erythrocytic series, whereas **thrombopoietin** stimulates platelet production.

An additional factor, **stem cell factor (steel factor),** which acts on pluripotential, multipotential, and unipotential stem cells, has also been described. It is produced by stromal cells of the bone marrow and is inserted into their cell membranes. Stem cells must contact these stromal cells before they can become mitotically active. It is believed that hemopoiesis cannot occur without the presence of cells that express stem cell factors, which is why postnatal blood cell formation is restricted to the bone marrow (and liver and spleen, if the need arises).

Table 10–6. Hemopoietic Growth Factors

Factors	Principal Action	Site of Origin
Stem cell factor	Promotes hemopoiesis	Stromal cells of bone marrow
GM-CSF	Promotes CFU-GM mitosis and differentiation; facilitates granulocyte activity	T cells; endothelial cells
G-CSF	Promotes CFU-G mitosis and differentiation; facilitates neutrophil activity	Macrophages; endothelial cells
M-CSF	Promotes CFU-M mitosis and differentiation	Macrophages; endothelial cells
IL-1	In conjunction with IL-3 and IL-6, it promotes proliferation of PHSC, CFU-S, and CFU-Ly; suppresses erythroid precursors	Monocytes; macrophages, endothelial cells
IL-2	Stimulates activated T- and B-cell mitosis; induces differentiation of NK cells	Activated T cells
IL-3	In conjunction with IL-1 and IL-6, it promotes proliferation of PHSC, CFU-S, and CFU-Ly as well as all unipotential precursors (except for LyB and LyT)	Activated T and B cells
IL-4	Stimulates T- and B-cell activation and development of mast cells and basophils	Activated T cells
IL-5	Promotes CFU-Eo mitosis and activates eosinophils	T cells
IL-6	In conjunction with IL-1 and IL-3, it promotes proliferation of PHSC, CFU-S, and CFU-Ly; also facilitates CTL and B-cell differentiation	Monocytes and fibroblasts
IL-7	Promotes differentiation of CFU-LyB; enhances differentiation of NK cells	Adventitial reticular cells?
IL-8	Induces neutrophil migration and degranulation	Leukocytes, endothelial cells, and smooth muscle cells
IL-9	Induces mast cell activation and proliferation; modulates IgE production; promotes T helper cell proliferation	T helper cells
IL-10	Inhibits cytokine production by macrophages, T cells, and NK cells; facilitates CTL differentiation and proliferation of B cells and mast cells	Macrophages and T cells
IL-12	Stimulates NK cells; enhances TCL and NK cell function	Macrophages
γ-Interferons	Activates B cells and monocytes; enhances TCL differentiation; augments the expression of class II HLA	T cells and NK cells
Erythropoietin	CFU-E differentiation; BFU-E mitosis	Endothelial cells of the peritubular capillary network of kidney; hepatocytes
Thrombopoietin	Proliferation and differentiation of CFU-meg and megakaryoblasts	Not known

CTL, cytotoxic T cells; CFU, colony-forming unit (Eo, eosinophil; G, granulocyte; GM, granulocyte-monocyte; Ly, lymphocyte; S, spleen); CSF, colony-stimulating factor (G–, granulocyte; GM–, granulocyte-monocyte; M–, monocyte); IL, interleukin; NK, natural killer; PHSC, pluripotential hemopoietic stem cells.

Hemopoietic cells are programmed to die by undergoing **apoptosis,** unless they come into contact with growth factors. Such dying cells display clumping of the chromatin in their shrunken nuclei and a dense, granular-appearing cytoplasm. On their cell surface they express specific macromolecules that are recognized by receptors of the macrophage plasma membrane. These phagocytic cells engulf and destroy the apoptotic cells.

It has been suggested that there are factors responsible for the release of mature (and almost mature) blood cells from the marrow. These proposed factors have not as yet been characterized.

CLINICAL CORRELATIONS

Pathologically increased secretion of erythropoietin can cause **secondary polycythemia,** an increase in the total number of red blood cells in the blood, increasing its viscosity, reducing its flow rate, and thus impeding circulation. The increased secretion is usually due to tumors of erythropoietin-secreting cells. Persons suffering from this disease may have an erythrocyte count of 10 million red blood cells per mm³.

Erythropoiesis

The process of **erythropoiesis,** red blood cell formation, generates 2.5×10^{11} erythrocytes every day. In order to produce such a tremendous number of cells, two types of unipotential progenitor cells arise from the CFU-S. These are the **burst-forming units—erythrocyte (BFU-E)** and **colony-forming units—erythrocyte (CFU-E).**

If the circulating red blood cell level is low, the kidney produces a high concentration of **erythropoietin,** which, in the presence of IL-3 and granulocyte–monocyte colony-stimulating factor (GM-CSF), induces CFU-S to differentiate into BFU-E. These cells undergo a "burst" of mitotic activity, forming a large number of CFU-E.

CFU-E require low concentrations of erythropoietin not only to survive but to form the first recognizable erythrocyte precursor, the **proerythroblast** (see Figs. 10–15, 10–16). The proerythroblasts and their progeny (Figs. 10–17, 10–18) form spherical clusters around macrophages (**nurse cells**), which phagocytose extruded nuclei and excess or deformed erythrocytes. Nurse cells may also provide growth factors to assist erythropoiesis. The properties of the cells in the erythropoietic series are presented in Table 10–7.

CLINICAL CORRELATIONS

Iron deficiency anemia, the most common form of anemia due to nutritional deficiency, affects about 10% of the United States population. Although the cause may be low dietary intake of iron, that is usually not the case in the United States; instead, it is caused by either malabsorption

or chronic blood loss. The erythrocytes of iron-deficient anemic persons are smaller than usual, the patient presents a whitish pallor, and the nails appear spoon-shaped with accentuated longitudinal ridges. The patient complains of generalized weakness, constant tiredness, and lack of energy.

Granulocytopoiesis

Although the granulocytic series is usually discussed under a single heading, as it is here, it must be kept in mind that each of the three types of granulocytes are derived from their own unipotential (or bipotential, as in the case of neutrophils) stem cells (see Table 10–5). Each of these stem cells is a descendant of the pluripotential stem cell CFU-S. Thus, CFU-Eo, of the eosinophil lineage, and CFU-Ba, of the basophil lineage, each undergo cell division, giving rise to the precursor cell, or **myeloblast.** Neutrophils originate

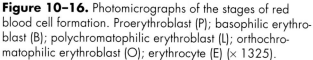

Figure 10–16. Photomicrographs of the stages of red blood cell formation. Proerythroblast (P); basophilic erythroblast (B); polychromatophilic erythroblast (L); orthochromatophilic erythroblast (O); erythrocyte (E) (× 1325).

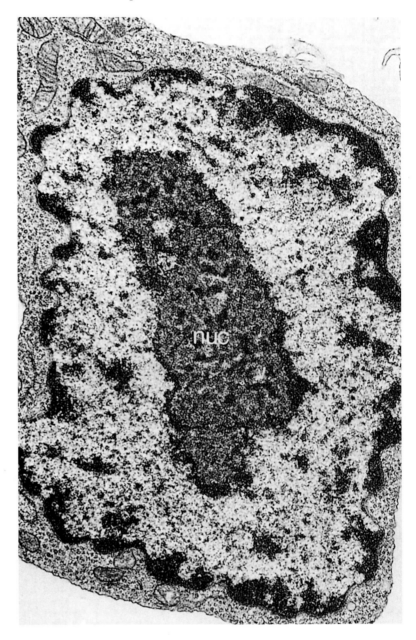

Figure 10–17. Electron micrograph of the nucleus of a proerythroblast (× **14,000**). nuc, nucleolus. (From Hopkins, C.R.: Structure and Function of Cells. Philadelphia, W.B. Saunders Company, 1978.)

from the bipotential stem cell, **CFU-GM,** whose mitosis produces two unipotential stem cells, **CFU-G** (of the neutrophil line) and **CFU-M,** responsible for the monocyte lineage. Similar to CFU-Ba and CFU-Eo, CFU-G divides to give rise to myeloblasts.

Myeloblasts (see Figs. 10–15, 10–19) are precursors of all three types of granulocytes, and they cannot be differentiated from one another. It is not known if a single myeloblast can produce all three types of granulocytes or if there is a specific myeloblast for each type of granulocyte. Myeloblasts undergo mitosis, giving rise to promyelocytes, which in turn divide to form myelocytes. It is at the myelocyte step that specific granules are present and the three granulocyte lines may be recognized. Each day the average

adult produces approximately 800,000 neutrophils, 170,000 eosinophils, and 60,000 basophils.

Table 10–8 details the neutrophil lineage. The eosinophil and basophil lineages appear to be identical to the neutrophil lineage, except for the differences in their specific granules.

Newly formed neutrophils leave the hemopoietic cords by *piercing* the endothelial cells lining the sinusoids, rather than by migrating between them. Once neutrophils enter the circulatory system they **marginate**—that is, they adhere to the endothelial cells of the blood vessels and remain there until they are needed. Thus, there are always many more neutrophils within the circulatory system than in the circulating blood.

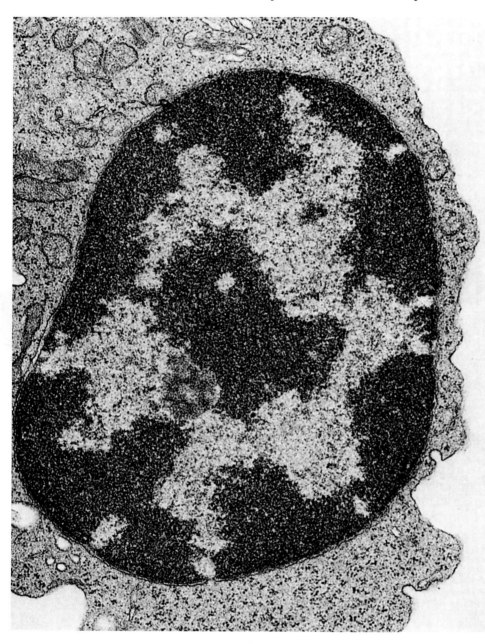

Figure 10–18. Electron micrograph of an orthochromatophilic erythroblast (× 26,500). (From Hopkins, C.R.: Structure and Function of Cells. Philadelphia, W.B. Saunders Company, 1978.)

CLINICAL CORRELATIONS

Acute myeloblastic leukemia results from uncontrolled mitosis of a transformed stem cell whose progeny do not differentiate into the mature cell. The cells involved may be the CFU-GM, CFU-Eo, or CFU-Ba, whose differentiation stops at the myeloblast stage. The disease affects young adults between 15 and 40 and is treated with intensive chemotherapy and recently by bone marrow transplantation.

Monocytopoiesis

Monocytes share their bipotential cells with neutrophils. CFU-GM undergoes mitosis and gives rise to CFU-G and CFU-M (monoblasts). The progeny of CFU-M are **promonocytes,** large cells (16 to 18 μm in diameter) that have a kidney-shaped, acentrically located nucleus. The cytoplasm of promonocytes is bluish and houses numerous azurophilic granules.

Electron micrographs of promonocytes disclose a well-developed Golgi apparatus, abundant RER, and numerous mitochondria. The azurophilic granules are resolved to be lysosomes, about 0.5 μm in diameter. The average adult forms more than 10^{10} monocytes every day, most of which enter the circulation. Within a day or two the newly formed monocytes enter the connective tissue spaces of the body and differentiate into **macrophages.**

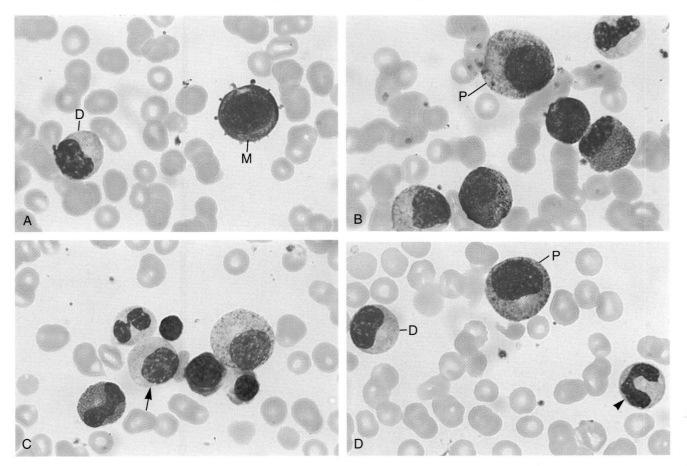

Figure 10–19. Photomicrographs of granulocytopoiesis. A, Myeloblast (M), neutrophilic metamyelocyte (D). **B,** Promyelocyte (P). **C,** Neutrophilic myelocyte (*arrow*). **D,** neutrophilic metamyelocyte (D); neutrophilic stab cell (*arrowhead*) (× 1,325).

Platelet Formation

The unipotential platelet progenitor, **CFU-Meg,** gives rise to a very large cell, the **megakaryoblast** (25 to 40 μm in diameter), whose single nucleus has several lobes. These cells undergo **endomitosis,** whereby the cell does not divide; instead, it becomes larger and the nucleus becomes polyploid, as much as 64 N. The bluish cytoplasm accumulates azurophilic granules.

Megakaryoblasts differentiate into **megakaryocytes** (see Fig. 10–13), which are large cells (40 to 100 μm in diameter), each with a single lobulated nucleus. Electron micrographs of megakaryocytes display a well-developed Golgi apparatus, numerous mitochondria, abundant RER, and many lysosomes (Fig. 10–20).

Megakaryocytes are located next to sinusoids, into which they protrude their cytoplasmic processes. These cytoplasmic processes fragment along complex, narrow invaginations of the plasmalemma, known as **demarcation channels,** into clusters of **proplatelets.** Shortly after the proplatelets are released they disperse into individual platelets. Each mega-karyocyte can form several thousand platelets. The remaining cytoplasm and nucleus of the megakaryocyte degenerate and are phagocytosed by macrophages.

Lymphopoiesis

The multipotential stem cell, **CFU-Ly,** divides in the bone marrow to form the two unipotential progenitor cells, CFU-LyB and CFU-LyT, neither of which is immunocompetent.

In birds, the **CFU-LyB** migrates to a diverticulum attached to the gut, known as the **bursa of Fabricius** (thus, B cell). Here CFU-LyB divides several times, giving rise to **immunocompetent** B lymphocytes expressing specific surface markers, including antibodies. A similar event occurs in mammals, but in the absence of a bursa, this development of immunocompetence occurs in a bursa-equivalent location, probably in the bone marrow.

CFU-LyT cells undergo mitosis, forming immunoincompetent T cells, which travel to the cortex of the thymus where they proliferate, mature, and begin to express cell sur-

Table 10–7. Cells of the Erythropoietic Series

Cell	Size (μm)	Nucleus* and Mitosis	Nucleoli	Cytoplasm*	Electron Micrographs
Proerythroblast	14–19	Round, burgundy-red; chromatin network: fine; mitosis	3–5	Gray-blue, peripheral clumping	Scant RER; lot of polysomes, few mitochondria; ferritin
Basophilic erythroblast	12–17	Same as above but chromatin network is coarser; mitosis	1–2?	Similar to above but slight pinkish background	Similar to above but some hemoglobin is present
Polychromatophilic erythroblast	12–15	Round and densely staining; very coarse chromatin network; mitosis	None	Yellowish-pink in bluish background	Similar to above but more hemoglobin is present
Orthochromatophilic erythroblast	8–12	Small, round, dense; excentric or is being extruded; no mitosis	None	Pink in a slight bluish background	Few mitochondria and polysomes; lots of hemoglobin
Reticulocyte	7–8	None	None	Like mature RBC but when stained with cresyl blue; display bluish reticulum in pink cytoplasm	Clusters of ribosomes; cell is filled with hemoglobin
Erythrocyte	7.5	None	None	Pink cytoplasm	Only hemoglobin

RBC, red blood cell; RER, rough endoplasmic reticulum.
*Colors as appear using Romanovsky-type stains (or their modifications).

Table 10–8. Cells of the Neutrophilic Series

Cell	Size (μm)	Nucleus* and Mitosis	Nucleoli	Cytoplasm*	Granules	Electron Micrographs
Myeloblast	12–14	Round, reddish-blue; chromatin network: fine; mitosis	2–3	Blue clumps in a pale-blue background; cytoplasmic blebs at cell periphery	None	RER, small Golgi, many mitochondria and polysomes
Promyelocyte	16–24	Round to oval, reddish-blue; chromatin network: coarse; mitosis	1–2	Bluish cytoplasm; no cytoplasmic blebs at cell periphery	Azurophilic granules	RER, large Golgi, many mitochondria, numerous lysosomes (0.5 μm in diameter)
Neutrophilic myelocyte	10–12	Flattened, acentric; chromatin network: coarse; mitosis	0–1	Pale-blue cytoplasm	Azurophilic and specific granules	RER, large Golgi, numerous mitochondria, lysosomes (0.5 μm) and specific granules (0.1 μm)
Neutrophilic metamyelocyte	10–12	Kidney-shaped, dense; chromatin network: coarse; no mitosis	None	Pale-blue cytoplasm	Azurophilic and specific granules	Organelle population is reduced, but granules are as above
Neutrophilic band (stab; juvenile)	9–12	Horseshoe-shaped; chromatin network: very coarse; no mitosis	None	Pale-blue cytoplasm	Azurophilic and specific granules	Same as above
Neutrophil	9–12	Multilobed; chromatin network: very coarse; no mitosis	None	Pale bluish-pink	Azurophilic and specific granules	Same as above

RER, rough endoplasmic reticulum.
*Colors as appear using Romanovsky-type stains (or their modifications).

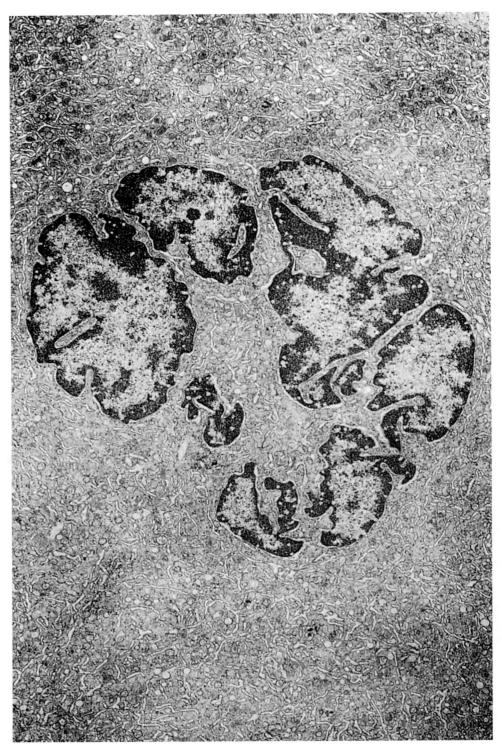

Figure 10–20. Electron micrograph of a mega-karyocyte displaying segmentation in the formation of platelets. Note that although this cell possesses a single nucleus, it is lobulated, which gives the appearance of the cell possessing several nuclei (× 4,000). (From Hopkins, C.R.: Structure and Function of Cells. Philadelphia, W.B. Saunders Company, 1978.)

face markers. As these surface markers appear on the T-cell plasmalemma (such as T-cell receptors and clusters of differentiation markers), the cells become immunocompetent T lymphocytes. Most of these newly formed T cells are destroyed in the thymus and phagocytosed by resident macrophages.

Both B lymphocytes and T lymphocytes proceed to lymphoid organs (such as the spleen and lymph nodes), where they form clones of immunocompetent T and B cells in well-defined regions of the organs.

Circulatory System

11

The circulatory system is composed of two separate but related components: the cardiovascular system and the lymphatic vascular system. The function of the **cardiovascular system** is to carry blood in both directions between the heart and the tissues. The function of the **lymphatic vascular system** is to collect **lymph,** the excess extracellular tissue fluid, and deliver it back to the cardiovascular system. Thus the lymphatic system provides one-way transport, whereas the cardiovascular system provides two-way circulation.

Cardiovascular System

The **cardiovascular system** is composed of the **heart,** a muscular organ that pumps the blood into two separated circuits: the **pulmonary circuit,** which carries blood to and from the lungs, and the **systemic circuit,** which distributes blood to and from all of the organs and tissues of the body. These circuits consist of **arteries,** a series of vessels that transport blood away from the heart by branching into vessels of smaller and smaller diameter, eventually to supply all regions of the body with blood; **capillaries,** which form capillary beds, a network of thin-walled vessels in which gases, nutrients, metabolic wastes, hormones, and signaling substances are interchanged or passed between the blood and the tissues of the body to sustain normal metabolic activities; and **veins,** vessels that drain capillary beds and form larger and larger vessels returning blood to the heart.

General Structure of Blood Vessels

Most blood vessels have several features that are structurally similar, although dissimilarities exist and are the bases for classifying the vessels into different identifiable groups. For example, the walls of high-pressure vessels (e.g., subclavian arteries) are thicker than vessels conducting blood at low pressure (e.g., subclavian veins). It should be remembered, however, that arterial diameters continue to decrease at each branching, whereas vein diameters increase at each convergence, thus altering the respective layers of the walls of the vessels. Therefore, the descriptions used as distinguishing characteristics for a particular type of artery or vein are not always absolute. Indeed, the walls of the capillaries and venules are completely modified and less complex compared with larger vessels. Generally, arteries have thicker walls and are smaller in diameter than the corresponding veins. Moreover, in histological sections, arteries are round and have no blood in their lumina.

Vessel Tunics

Three separate concentric layers of tissue, **tunics,** make up the wall of the typical blood vessel (Fig. 11–1). The innermost layer, the **tunica intima,** is composed of a single layer of flattened, squamous endothelial cells, which form a tube

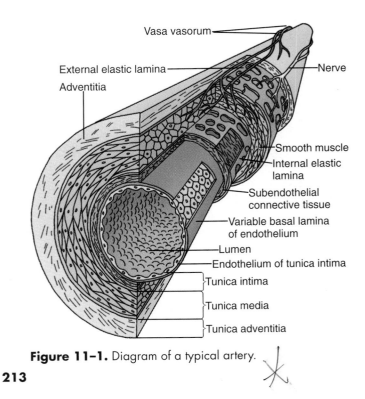

Figure 11–1. Diagram of a typical artery.

lining the lumen of the vessel, and the underlying subendothelial connective tissue. The intermediate layer, the **tunica media,** is composed mostly of smooth muscle cells oriented concentrically around the lumen. The outermost layer, the **tunica adventitia,** is composed mainly of fibroelastic connective tissue arranged longitudinally. The tunica intima houses in its outermost layer the **internal elastic lamina,** a thin band of elastic fibers that is well developed in medium-sized arteries. The outermost layer of the tunica media houses another band of elastic fibers, the **external elastic lamina,** although it is not distinguishable in all arteries.

TUNICA INTIMA. The endothelial cells (simple squamous epithelium) lining the lumen of the blood vessel rest on a basal lamina. These flattened cells are elongated into a sheet such that their long axis is more or less parallel to the long axis of the vessel, which nearly permits each endothelial cell to surround the lumen of a small-caliber vessel. In larger-bore vessels, several to many individual endothelial cells are required to line the circumference of the lumen.

A **subendothelial layer** lies immediately beneath the endothelial cells. It is composed of loose connective tissue and a few scattered smooth muscle cells, both arranged longitudinally. Beneath the subendothelial layer is an **internal elastic lamina** that is especially well developed in muscular arteries. Separating the tunica intima from the tunica media, it is composed of **elastin,** which is a fenestrated sheet that permits the diffusion of substances into the deeper regions of the arterial wall to nourish the cells there.

TUNICA MEDIA. The concentric cell layers forming the **tunica media** comprise mostly helically arranged smooth muscle cells. Interspersed within the layers of smooth muscle are some elastic fibers, type III collagen, and proteoglycans. The fibrous elements form lamellae within the ground substance secreted by smooth muscle cells. Larger muscular arteries have an **external elastic lamina,** which is more delicate than the internal elastic lamina and separates the tunica media from the overlying tunica adventitia. Capillaries and postcapillary venules do not have a tunica media; in these small vessels, **pericytes** replace the tunica media.

TUNICA ADVENTITIA. Covering the vessels on their outside surface is the **tunica adventitia,** composed mostly of fibroblasts, type I collagen fibers, and longitudinally oriented elastic fibers. This layer becomes continuous with the connective tissue elements surrounding the vessel.

Vasa Vasorum

The thickness and muscularity of larger vessels prevent the cells composing the tunics from being nourished by diffusion from the lumen of the vessel. The deeper cells of the tunica media and tunica adventitia are nourished by the **vasa vasorum,** small arteries that enter the vessel walls and branch profusely to serve the cells located primarily in the tunica media and tunica adventitia. Compared with arteries, veins have more cells that cannot be supplied with oxygen and nutrients by diffusion because venous blood contains less oxygen and nutrients than arterial blood. For this reason, vasa vasorum are more prevalent in the walls of veins than arteries.

Nerve Supply to Vessels

A network of **vasomotor** nerves of the sympathetic component of the autonomic nervous system supplies smooth muscle cells of blood vessels. These unmyelinated, postganglionic sympathetic nerves are responsible for **vasoconstriction** of the vessel walls. Because the nerves seldom enter the tunica media of the vessel, they do not synapse directly on the smooth muscle cells. Instead, they release the neurotransmitter **norepinephrine,** which diffuses into the media and acts on smooth muscle cells nearby. These impulses are propagated throughout all of the smooth muscle cells via their gap junctions, thereby orchestrating contractions of the entire smooth muscle cell layer and thus reducing the diameter of the vessel lumen. Arteries are more heavily endowed with vasomotor nerves than the veins are, but veins also receive vasomotor nerve endings in the tunica adventitia. It is important to remember that arteries supplying skeletal muscles also receive cholinergic (parasympathetic) nerves to effect vasodilation.

Arteries

Arteries are efferent vessels that transport blood away from the heart to the capillary beds. The two major arteries that arise from the right and left ventricles of the heart are the pulmonary trunk and the aorta, respectively. The **pulmonary trunk** branches, shortly after exiting the heart, into right and left pulmonary arteries that enter the lungs for distribution. (See Chapter 15 for a description of the branching and blood supply to the lungs.) The right and left coronary arteries, which supply the heart muscle, arise from the aorta as it exits the left ventricle. The **aorta,** upon leaving the heart, courses in an obliquely posterior arch to descend in the thoracic cavity, where it sends branches to the body wall and the viscera; it then enters the abdominal cavity, where it sends branches to the body wall and viscera. The abdominal aorta terminates by bifurcating into the right and left common iliac arteries in the pelvis. Three major arterial trunks—right brachiocephalic, left common carotid, and left subclavian—arise from the arch of the aorta to supply the superior extremities and the head and neck. Continued branching of all of these arteries into large numbers of smaller and smaller arteries continues until the vessel walls contain a single layer of endothelial cells. The resulting vessels, called capillaries, are the smallest functional vascular elements of the cardiovascular system.

Classification of Arteries

Arteries are grouped or classified into three major types based on relative size, morphological characteristics, or both (Table 11–1). From largest to smallest, they are: **elastic arteries,** also known as **conducting arteries; muscular arteries,** known also as **distributing arteries;** and **arterioles.** It should be remembered that artery size is a continuum; thus there is a gradual change in morphological characteristics in going from one type to another.

ELASTIC ARTERIES. The aorta and the branches originating from the aortic arch (common carotid and the subclavian arteries), the common iliac arteries, and the pulmonary trunk are **elastic arteries (conducting arteries)** (Fig. 11–2). The walls of these vessels may be yellow in the fresh state because of the abundance of elastin in their walls. The **tunica intima** of elastic arteries contains an endothelium that is supported by a narrow layer of underlying connective tissue containing a few fibroblasts, occasional smooth muscle cells, and collagen fibers. Thin laminae of elastic fibers, the **internal elastic lamina,** are also present.

The endothelial cells of the elastic arteries are 10 to 15 μm wide and 25 to 50 μm long; their long axes are oriented in the longitudinal plane. These cells are connected to each other mostly by occluding junctions. Their plasma membranes contain small vesicles thought to be related to transport of water, macromolecules, and electrolytes. Occasional blunt processes may extend from the plasma membrane through the internal elastic lamina to form junctions with smooth muscle cells located in the tunica media. The endothelial cells contain **Weibel-Palade bodies,** membrane-bound inclusions, 0.1 μm in diameter and 3 μm long, that have a dense matrix housing tubular elements containing the glycoprotein **von Willebrand factor.** This factor, which facilitates the coagulation of platelets during clot formation, is manufactured by most endothelial cells, but it is stored only in arteries.

CLINICAL CORRELATIONS

Persons with **von Willebrand disease,** an inherited disorder, have prolonged coagulation times and excessive bleeding at an injury site.

(handwritten note: listed by size biggest → smallest)

Table 11–1. Characteristics of Various Types of Arteries

Artery	Tunica Intima	Tunica Media	Tunica Adventitia
Elastic artery **(conducting)** (e.g., aorta)	Endothelium with Weibel-Palade bodies, basal lamina, subendothelial layer, incomplete internal elastic lamina	40–70 fenestrated elastic membranes, smooth muscle cells interspersed between elastic membranes, thin external elastic lamina, vasa vasorum in outer half	Thin layer of fibro-elastic connective tissue, vasa vasorum, lymphatic vessels, nerve fibers
Muscular artery **(distributing)** (e.g., femoral)	Endothelium with Weibel-Palade bodies, basal lamina, subendothelial layer, thick internal elastic lamina	Up to 40 layers of smooth muscle cells, thick external elastic lamina	Thin layer of fibro-elastic connective tissue, vasa vasorum not prominent, lymphatic vessels, nerve fibers
Arteriole	Endothelium with Weibel-Palade bodies, basal lamina, subendothelial layer not prominent, some elastic fibers instead of a defined internal elastic lamina	1 or 2 layers of smooth muscle cells	Loose connective tissue, nerve fibers
Metarteriole	Endothelium, basal lamina	Smooth muscle cells form precapillary sphincter	Sparse loose connective tissue

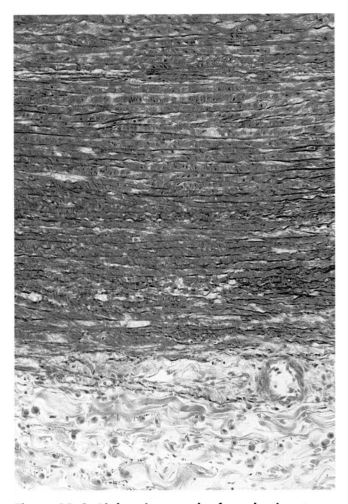

Figure 11-2. Light micrograph of an elastic artery (× 132). Observe the fenestrated membranes and the adventitia.

The **tunica media** of elastic arteries consists of many fenestrated lamellae of elastin, known as the **fenestrated membranes,** alternating with circularly oriented layers of smooth muscle cells. The number of lamellae of elastin increases with age, there being about 40 in newborns and 70 in adults, each being thicker because of the continued deposition of elastin. Elastin constitutes much of the tunica media; smooth muscles cells are less abundant than in some of the muscular arteries. The extracellular matrix, secreted by the smooth muscle cells, is composed mostly of chondroitin sulfate, collagen, and reticular and elastin fibers. The **external elastic laminae** is also present in the tunica media.

The **tunica adventitia** of elastic arteries is relatively thin and composed of loose fibroelastic connective tissue housing some fibroblasts. Vasa vasorum are abundant throughout the adventitia. Capillary beds arise from the vasa vasorum and extend to the tissues of the tunica media, where they supply the cells with oxygen and nutrients. Fenestrations in the elastic laminae permit some diffusion of oxygen and nu-

trients to the cells in the tunica media from the blood flowing through the lumen, although most of the nourishment is derived from the vasa vasorum.

MUSCULAR ARTERIES. The **muscular arteries (distributing arteries)** include most of those arising from the aorta, except the major trunks originating from the arch of the aorta and the terminal bifurcation of the abdominal aorta, which are identified as elastic arteries. Indeed, most of the named arteries, even those with a diameter of only 0.1 mm, are classified as muscular arteries (e.g., brachial, ulnar, renal). The identifying characteristic of muscular arteries is a relatively thick tunica media composed mostly of smooth muscle cells (Fig. 11–3).

The **tunica intima** in muscular arteries is thinner than in the elastic arteries, but the subendothelial layer contains a few smooth muscle cells. In contrast with that of elastic arteries, the **internal elastic lamina** of muscular arteries is prominent and displays an undulating surface to which the endothelium conforms. Occasionally the internal elastic lamina is duplicated and is then known as bifid internal elastic lamina. As in elastic arteries, the endothelium has processes that pass through fenestrations within the internal elastic lamina and make gap junctions with smooth muscle cells of the tunica media that are near the interface with the tunica intima. It is thought that these gap junctions serve to couple metabolically the endothelium and the smooth muscle cells.

The **tunica media** of muscular arteries is composed predominantly of smooth muscle cells, but these cells are con-

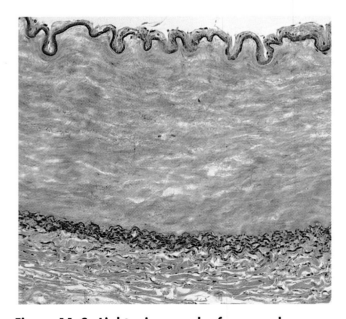

Figure 11-3. Light micrograph of a muscular artery (× 132). Note the internal and external elastic laminae and the thick tunica media.

siderably smaller than those located in the walls of the viscera. The orientation of most of the smooth muscle cells is circular; where the tunica media interfaces the tunica intima and the tunica adventitia, however, a few bundles of smooth muscle fibers are arranged longitudinally. Small muscular arteries have three or four layers of smooth muscle cells, whereas larger muscular arteries have as many as 40 layers of circularly arranged smooth muscle cells. The number of cell layers decreases as artery diameter diminishes.

Each smooth muscle cell is enveloped by an **external lamina (basal lamina),** although muscle cell processes extend through intervals in the basal lamina to make gap junctions with other muscle cells, ensuring coordinated contractions within the tunica media. Interspersed within the layers of smooth muscle cells are elastic fibers, type III collagen fibers, and chondroitin sulfate, all secreted by the smooth muscle cells. Type III collagen fibers (30 nm) are located in bundles within the intercellular spaces.

An **external elastic lamina** is identifiable in histological sections of larger muscular arteries as several layers of thin elastic sheets; in electron micrographs these sheets display fenestrations.

The **tunica adventitia** of muscular arteries consists of elastic fibers, collagen fibers (60 to 100 nm), and a ground substance composed mostly of dermatan sulfate and heparan sulfate. This extracellular matrix is produced by fibroblasts in the adventitia. The collagen and elastic fibers are oriented longitudinally and blend into the surrounding connective tissues. Located at the outer regions of the adventitia are vasa vasorum and unmyelinated nerve endings. Neurotransmitter released at the nerve endings diffuses through fenestrations in the external elastic lamina into the tunica media to depolarize some of the superficial smooth muscle cells. Depolarization is propagated to all of the muscle cells of the tunica media via gap junctions.

ARTERIOLES. Arteries with a diameter of less than 0.1 mm are considered to be **arterioles** (Fig. 11–4). In histological sections the width of the wall of an arteriole is approximately equal to the diameter of its lumen. The endothelium of the **tunica intima** is supported by a thin subendothelial layer consisting of type III collagen and a few elastic fibers embedded in ground substance. A thin fenestrated **internal elastic lamina** is absent in small and terminal arterioles but present in larger arterioles (Fig. 11–5). In small arterioles, the **tunica media** is composed of a single smooth muscle cell layer that completely encircles the endothelial cells (Fig. 11–6). In larger arterioles the tunica media consists of two to three layers of smooth muscle cells. Arterioles do not have an external elastic lamina. The **tunica adventitia** of arterioles is scant and is represented by fibroelastic connective tissue housing a few fibroblasts.

Arteries that supply blood to capillary beds are called **metarterioles.** These differ structurally from arterioles in that the smooth muscle layer is not continuous; rather, the

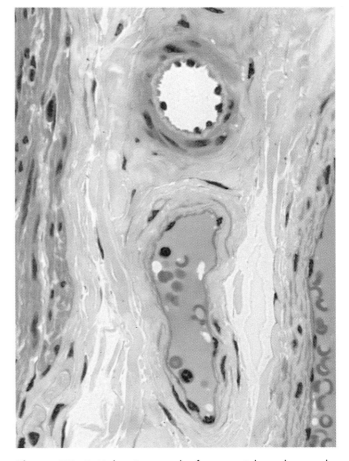

Figure 11–4. Light micrograph of an arteriole and a venule containing blood cells (× 540).

individual muscle cells are spaced apart, and each encircles the endothelium of a capillary arising from the metarteriole. It is thought that this arrangement permits these smooth muscle cells to function as a sphincter upon contraction, thus controlling blood flow into the capillary bed.

CLINICAL CORRELATIONS

Vessel walls that are weakened from embryological defects or damaged from diseases such as atherosclerosis, syphilis, and connective tissue disorders (e.g., **Marfan's syndrome** and **Ehler-Danlos syndrome**) may balloon out at the affected site, forming an **aneurysm.** Further weakening may cause the aneurysm to rupture, a grave condition that may lead to death.

Specialized Sensory Structures in Arteries

The major arteries of the body have three types of specialized sensory structures: carotid sinuses, carotid bodies, and aortic bodies. The nerve endings in these structures monitor

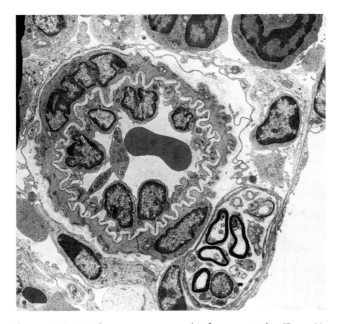

Figure 11-5. Electron micrograph of an arteriole. (From Yamazaki, K., and Allen, T.D.: Ultrastructural morphometric study of efferent nerve terminals on murine bone marrow stromal cells, and the recognition of a novel anatomical unit: The "neuro-reticular complex." Am. J. Anat. **187:**261–276, 1990. Copyright © 1990. Reprinted by permission of John Wiley & Sons, Inc.)

blood pressure and blood composition, providing essential inputs to the brain for controlling heart beat, respiration, and blood pressure.

CAROTID SINUSES. The **carotid sinuses** are baroreceptors; that is, they perceive changes in blood pressure. These structures are specializations within the walls of the internal carotid arteries just above the bifurcation of the common carotid arteries. At this site, the adventitia of these vessels is relatively thicker and heavily endowed with sensory nerve endings from the glossopharyngeal nerve (cranial nerve IX). The tunica media at this site is relatively thinner, thus permitting it to be distended during increases in blood pressure; this distention stimulates the nerve endings. The afferent impulses, received at the vasomotor center in the brain, trigger adjustments in vasoconstriction, resulting in maintenance of proper blood pressure. Additional small baroreceptors are located in the aorta and in some of the larger vessels.

CAROTID BODIES. Located at the bifurcation of the common carotid arteries are the **carotid bodies,** which have specialized chemoreceptor nerve endings responsible for monitoring changes in oxygen, carbon dioxide, and the concentrations of H^+ ions in the blood. These oval structures, about 3 × 5 mm, are composed of multiple clusters of pale-staining cells embedded in connective tissue. Two types of parenchymal cells are clearly distinguishable in electron mi-

crographs: **glomus cells (type I cells)** and **sheath cells (type II cells).**

Glomus cells have a large nucleus and the usual array of organelles. They are distinguished by the presence of dense-cored vesicles, 60 to 200 nm in diameter, that resemble vesicles located in the chromaffin cells of the adrenal medulla. Cell processes contain longitudinally oriented microtubules, dense-cored vesicles, and a few small electron-lucent vesicles. These processes contact other glomus cells and capillaries.

Sheath cells are more complex and have long processes that almost completely ensheath the processes of the glomus cells. Their nuclei are irregular and contain more heterochromatin than glomus cells; moreover, these cells contain no dense-cored vesicles. As nerve terminals enter clusters of glomus cells, they lose their Schwann cells and become covered by the sheath cells in much the same way as glial cells would ensheath neurons in the central nervous system.

It is now accepted that carotid bodies contain catecholamines (as in the adrenal medulla and paraganglia), but whether they produce hormones is unclear. The glossopharyngeal and vagus nerves supply the carotid bodies with numerous afferent fibers. In some of the synapses, the glomus cells appear to function as the presynaptic portion of the synapse. The facts surrounding this complexity are yet to be sorted out.

AORTIC BODIES. Aortic bodies are located on the arch of the aorta between the right subclavian and the left com-

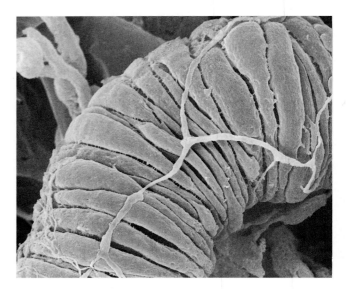

Figure 11-6. Scanning electron micrograph of an arteriole illustrating its compact layer of smooth muscle and its attendant nerve fibers (x 4200). (From Fujiwara, T., and Uehara, Y.: The cytoarchitecture of the wall and innervation pattern of the microvessels in the rat mammary gland: A scanning electron microscopic observation. Am. J. Anat. **170:**39–54, 1984. Copyright © 1984. Reprinted by permission of John Wiley & Sons, Inc.)

mon carotid artery and between the left common carotid artery and the left subclavian artery. Their structure and function are the same as those of carotid bodies.

Regulation of Arterial Blood Pressure

The heart, which serves as the cardiovascular pump, rests between each stroke, thus developing a pressurized burst of blood that first enters into the elastic arteries, then moves into the muscular arteries and arterioles, and finally into capillaries, which serve the tissues. The **vasomotor center** in the brain responds to the continual monitoring of blood pressure by controlling **vasomotor tone.** Vasomotor tone is the constant state of contraction of the vessel walls, which is modulated via vasoconstriction and vasodilation. **Vasoconstriction** is accomplished via **vasomotor nerves** of the sympathetic nervous system. **Vasodilation** is a function of the parasympathetic system. During vasodilation, acetylcholine from the nerve terminals in the vessel walls initiates release of **nitric oxide** from the endothelium to diffuse into the smooth muscle cells, which activates the cGMP system, resulting in relaxing the muscle cells, thus dilating the vessel lumen.

Smooth muscle cells of the arteries have receptors for substances besides the neurotransmitter norepinephrine. When the blood pressure is low, the kidneys secrete **renin,** which cleaves **angiotensinogen** circulating in the blood, forming **angiotensin I.** This mild vasoconstrictor is converted to angiotensin II by an enzyme located on the luminal plasmalemma of capillary endothelia (especially in the lungs). Angiotensin II is a potent vasoconstrictor that initiates smooth muscle contraction, thereby reducing vessel lumen diameter, resulting in increased blood pressure. Severe hemorrhage induces pituitary secretion of **ADH (vasopressin),** which is another powerful vasoconstrictor.

The structure of elastic arteries permits distension of their walls during systole (heart contraction), followed by recoil of their walls during diastole (heart relaxation), which assists in delivering a more constant blood pressure and flow of blood. Muscular arteries branching from the elastic arteries distribute blood to the body and are subject to constant changes in diameter resulting from vasoconstriction and vasodilation. To assist in accommodating for these events, the tunica adventitia blends loosely into the surrounding connective tissue, thus preventing restraint on the vessel during contractions and expansions for changes in blood pressure.

Artery location also dictates the thickness of the various tunics. For example, the thickness of the tunica media in the arteries of the legs is greater than that found in the arteries of the upper extremity. This is in response to the continued pressure resulting from gravitational forces. Also, the coronary arteries, serving the heart, are high-pressure arteries and, as such, have a thick tunica media. On the other hand, the arteries in the pulmonary circulation are under low pressure; thus the tunica media in these vessels is thinner.

CLINICAL CORRELATIONS

Normal and Pathological Changes in Vessels

The largest arteries continue to grow until about age 25, although there is progressive thickening of their walls and an increase in the number of elastic laminae. In muscular arteries, from middle age on, deposits of collagen and proteoglycans increase in the walls, thus reducing their flexibility. The coronary vessels are the first to display the effects of aging, with the intima displaying the greatest age-related changes. These natural changes are not unlike the regressive changes observed in **arteriosclerosis** (hardening of the arteries).

The largest of the arteries are prone to **atherosclerosis,** a disease that is the forerunner to heart attack and stroke. Atherosclerosis is distinguished by infiltrations of soft noncellular lipid material into the intima walls; these infiltrations can reduce the luminal diameter appreciably even by age 25. It is not clear whether these conditions are physiological or a manifestation of a disease process. The fibrous plaques that form in the intima of older persons, however, are pathological.

The smooth muscle cell layer of a healthy person's tunica media undergoes renewal, but when the endothelium is injured, platelets that accumulate at the site release **platelet-derived growth factor,** stimulating proliferation of smooth muscle cells. As a consequence, these cells begin to get packed with cholesterol-rich lipids, which stimulate the muscle cells to manufacture additional collagen and proteoglycans, resulting in a cycle whereby the tunica intima becomes thickened. This further damage to the endothelium leads to necrosis, which attracts more platelets, and finally clotting, forming a thrombus that may occlude the vessel at that site or get into the general circulation and occlude a more dangerous vessel (e.g., a coronary vessel or a cerebral vessel).

The pathogenesis of this disease process is still unclear, although current research theories point to the role of cholesterol, lipoproteins, and certain mitogens.

Capillaries

Arising from the terminal ends of the arterioles are **capillaries,** which form, by branching and anastomosing, a capillary bed (network) between the arterioles and the venules. Electron micrographs have revealed three types of capillaries: continuous, fenestrated, and sinusoidal. The differences among them will be discussed later.

General Capillary Structure

Capillaries are usually short, ranging from 0.25 μm up to 1 mm in muscle cells. Capillaries are formed by a single layer of squamous endothelial cells with dimensions of about 10 × 30 μm; the long axis of these cells lies in the same direction as the blood flow. These endothelial cells are flattened with the attenuated ends tapering to a thickness to 0.2 μm or less, although an elliptical nucleus bulges out into the lumen of the capillary. The cytoplasm contains a Golgi complex, a few mitochondria, some rough endoplasmic reticulum, and free ribosomes (Figs. 11–7, 11–8). Intermediate filaments (9 to 11 nm), located about the perinuclear zone, vary in filament composition. For example, some cells contain filaments composed of **desmin,** whereas others contain filaments composed of **vimentin,** yet some endothelial cells contain both kinds of filaments. These filaments provide structural support to endothelial cells, but the significance of their variation is unclear.

The large number of pinocytotic vesicles associated with the entire plasmalemma is an identifying characteristic of capillaries. These vesicles may be in singular array, two single vesicles may be fused together, or several vesicles may be fused, forming a transient channel. Where the endothelial cells are the thinnest, a single vesicle may span from the adluminal plasmalemma across the cytoplasm to the abluminal plasmalemma of the endothelial cell.

The endothelial cells of capillaries are rolled into a tube, giving the lumen a diameter that ranges from 8 to 10 μm but remains constant throughout the entire length of a capillary. This diameter is sufficient to permit individual cells of the blood to pass without being hindered. Although all of the capillary beds are not open at any one time, increased demand initiates the opening of more beds, thus increasing blood flow to meet physiological needs. The external sur-

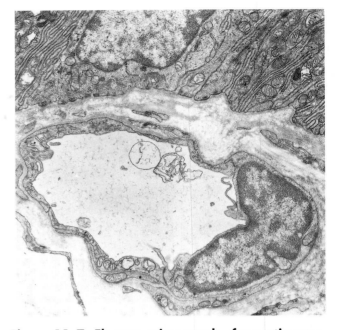

Figure 11–7. Electron micrograph of a continuous capillary in the rat submandibular gland (× 13,000). Observe that the pericyte shares the endothelial cell's basal lamina. (From Sato, A., and Miyoshi, S.: Morphometric study of the microvasculature of the main excretory duct subepithelia of the rat parotid, submandibular and sublingual salivary glands. Anat. Rec. **226:**288–294, 1990. Copyright © 1990. Reprinted with permission of John Wiley & Sons, Inc.)

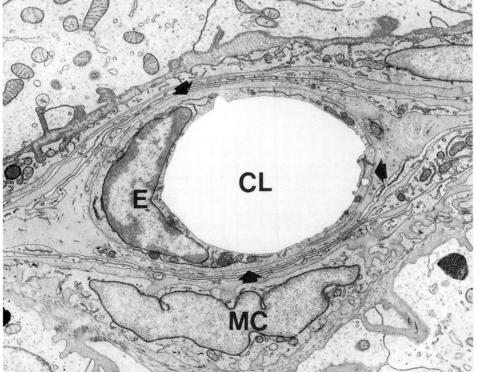

Figure 11–8. Electron micrograph of a testicular capillary. CL, capillary lumen; MC, myoid cell; E, nucleus of endothelial cell; arrows, basal lamina. (From Meyerhofer, A., Hikim, A.P.S., Bartke, A., and Russell, L.D.: Changes in the testicular microvascular during photoperiodrelated seasonal transition from reproductive quiescence to reproductive activity in the adult golden hampster. Anat. Rec. **224:**495–507, 1989. Copyright © 1989. Reprinted with permission of John Wiley & Sons, Inc.)

face of the endothelial cells are surrounded by a basal lamina secreted by the endothelial cells (see Fig. 11–8). When viewed in cross-section, the endothelial walls making up small capillaries are formed by one endothelial cell, whereas portions of two or three endothelial cells contribute to forming the endothelial wall of larger capillaries. At these cellular junctions, the endothelial cells tend to overlap, forming a **marginal fold** that projects into the lumen. Endothelial cells are joined together by **fasciae occludentes.**

Pericytes are located along the outside of the capillaries and small venules, where pericytes seem to be surrounding them (Figs. 11–9, 11–10). They have long primary processes, which are located along the long axis of the capillary and from which secondary processes arise to wrap around the capillary, forming a few **gap junctions** with the endothelial cells. The pericytes share the basal lamina of the endothelial cells. Pericytes possess a small Golgi complex, mitochondria, rough endoplasmic reticulum, microtubules, and filaments extending into the processes. Pericytes also contain tropomyosin, isomyosin, and protein kinase, which are all related to contraction that regulates blood flow through the capillaries. Further, as discussed in Chapter 6, there is evidence that after injury pericytes may undergo differentiation to become smooth muscle cells and endothelial cells in the walls of arterioles and venules.

Classification of Capillaries

Figure 11–11 illustrates the three types of capillaries, which differ in their location and structure.

CONTINUOUS CAPILLARIES. As the name suggests, **continuous capillaries** have no interruptions (pores or fenestrae) in their walls. This type of capillary is present in muscle, nervous, and connective tissues. The capillaries in the brain tissue are classified as modified continuous capillaries. The intercellular junctions between their endothelial cells are a type of **fasciae occludentes (tight junctions),** which prevent passage of many molecules. Substances such as amino acids, glucose, nucleosides, and purines move across the capillary wall via carrier-mediated transport. Also, it has been demonstrated that the cells exhibit a polarity with the transport systems such that Na+-K+ ATPase is located in the adluminal cell membrane only. There is evidence that barrier regulation resides within the endothelial cells but is influenced by products produced by the astrocytes associated with the capillaries.

FENESTRATED CAPILLARIES. Fenestrated capillaries have pores, or fenestrae, in their walls that are 60 to 80 nm in diameter and covered by a pore diaphragm. These capillaries are found in the pancreas, intestines, and endocrine glands.

The **pores** in fenestrated capillaries are bridged by an ultrathin diaphragm. When viewed after processing with platinum-carbon shadowing, the diaphragm displays eight fibrils radiating out from a central area and forming wedge-like channels, each with an opening of about 5.5 nm. These pore/diaphragm complexes are regularly spaced about 50 nm apart, but they are located in clusters; thus most of the endothelial wall of the fenestrated capillary is without fenestrae (see Fig. 11–11B). An exception is the endothelial pores of the renal glomerulus, which lack diaphragms.

SINUSOIDAL CAPILLARIES. The vascular channels in certain organs of the body, including the bone marrow, liver, spleen, lymphoid organs, and certain of the endocrine glands are called **sinusoids.** These are irregular blood pools or channels that conform to the shape of the structure in which they are located. The peculiar conformation of a sinusoid is determined by its being shaped between the parenchymal components of the organ during organogenesis.

Because of their location, sinusoid capillaries have an enlarged diameter of 30 to 40 μm (see Fig. 11–11C). They also contain many large fenestrae that lack diaphragms; the endothelial wall may be discontinuous, as is the basal lamina,

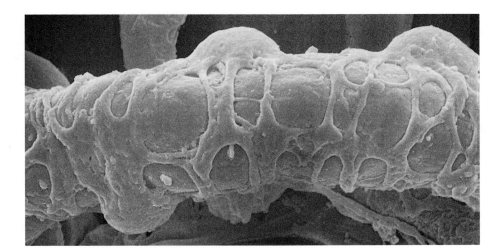

Figure 11–9. Scanning electron micrograph of a capillary displaying pericytes on its surface (× 5,000). (From Fujiwara, T., and Uehara, Y.: The cytoarchitecture of the wall and innervation pattern of the microvessels in the rat mammary gland: A scanning electron microscopic observation. Am. J. Anat. **170:**39–54, 1984. Copyright © 1984. Reprinted with permission of John Wiley & Sons, Inc.)

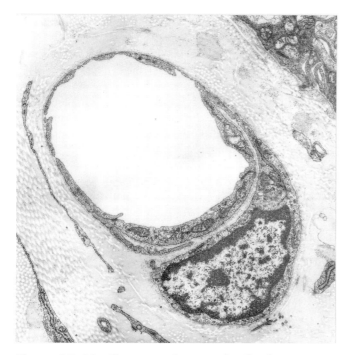

Figure 11–10. Electron micrograph of a fenestrated capillary and its pericyte in cross-section. Note that the capillary endothelial cells and the pericyte share the same basal lamina. (From Sato, A., and Miyoshi, S.: Morphometric study of the microvasculature of the main excretory duct subepithelia of the rat parotid, submandibular and sublingual salivary glands. Anat. Rec. **226:**288–294, 1990. Copyright © 1990. Reprinted with permission of John Wiley & Sons, Inc.)

permitting enhanced exchange between the blood and the tissues. Sinusoids are lined by endothelium, but in certain organs the endothelium is thin and continuous (some lymphoid organs), whereas in others it may have continuous areas mixed with fenestrated areas (endocrine glands). Although the endothelial cells lack pinocytic vesicles, macrophages may be located either in or along the outside of the endothelial wall.

Regulation of Blood Flow into a Capillary Bed

ARTERIOVENOUS ANASTOMOSES. Terminals of most arteries end in capillary beds, which deliver their blood to venules for the return back to the venous side of the cardiovascular system. In many parts of the body, however, the artery simply joins with a venous channel, forming an **arteriovenous anastomosis (AVA).** The structures of the arterial and venous ends of the AVA are similar to those of an artery and vein, respectively, whereas the intermediate segment has thickened tunica media, and its subendothelial layer is composed of plump polygonal cells that are modified longitudinally arranged smooth muscle cells.

When the arteriovenous anastomoses are closed, the blood passes through the capillary bed, but when these

shunts are open a large amount of blood bypasses the capillary bed and flows through the AVA. It is important to note that these shunts are useful in thermoregulation and are abundant in skin. The intermediate segments of the AVAs are richly innervated with adrenergic and cholinergic nerves. Whereas most peripheral nerves are controlled somewhat by local environmental stimuli, those nerves of AVAs are controlled by the thermoregulatory system in the brain.

GLOMERA. Nail beds and the tips of the fingers and toes are vascularized by **glomera.** The glomus is a small organ that receives an arteriole devoid of an elastic lamina and ac-

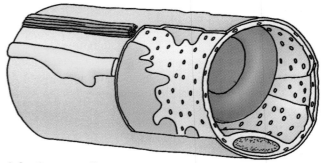

A Continuous capillary

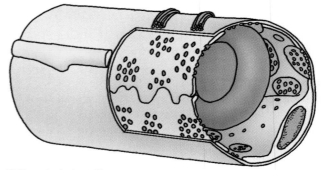

B Fenestrated capillary

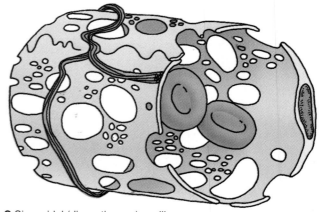

C Sinusoidal (discontinuous) capillary

Figure 11–11. Diagram of the three types of capillaries: **A,** continuous; **B,** fenestrated; and **C,** sinusoidal.

quires a richly innervated smooth muscle cell layer, which surrounds the vessel lumen, thus directly controlling blood flow to the region before emptying into a venous plexus. The entire glomera complex is not fully understood.

CENTRAL CHANNEL. Blood flow from the arterial system is controlled either by metarterioles (with precapillary sphincters) or by terminal arterioles. Thus, metarterioles form the proximal portion of a **central channel**, whereas its distal portion is formed by the **thoroughfare channel**, a structure so named because it is without precapillary sphincters. The thoroughfare channels drain the capillary bed and empty the blood into **small venules** of the venous system (Fig. 11–12). When the precapillary sphincters are contracted, blood flows through the central channels, bypassing the capillary bed and entering into the venules.

Capillary Histophysiology

The endothelial cells of capillaries may contain two distinct pore systems: small pores about 9 to 11 nm in diameter and large pores about 50 to 70 nm in diameter. The smaller pores are thought to be discontinuities between endothelial cell junctions, whereas the large pores are represented by fenestrae and transport vesicles. Oxygen, carbon dioxide, and glucose may diffuse or be transported across the plasmalemma, then diffuse through the cytoplasm and finally through the abluminal plasmalemma into the extravascular space. Water and hydrophilic molecules of about 1.5 nm simply diffuse through these intercellular junctions.

It has been shown that water-soluble molecules greater than 11 nm in diameter are transported from the adluminal plasmalemma to the abluminal plasmalemma by the numerous pinocytic vesicles adjacent to the plasmalemma. This process is called **transcytosis** (Fig. 11–13) because the material traverses the entire cell rather than remaining within the cell. In continuous capillaries, substances are taken up by open vesicles located on the adluminal plasmalemma. The vesicles are then transported across the cytoplasm to the abluminal plasmalemma, where the vesicles fuse with it to deliver their contents into the extravascular space. This is an efficient process because the number of vesicles in these endothelial cells may exceed $1000/\mu m^2$. Recent evidence indicates that these vesicles are members of a stable population arising from the Golgi complex via a fusion/fission mechanism of renewal.

Leukocytes leave the bloodstream to enter the extravascular space by passing through the junctions via a process called **diapedesis.** It should be pointed out that **histamine** and **bradykinin,** whose levels are increased during the inflammatory process, increase capillary permeability, thus causing excessive fluid passage into the extravascular spaces. This excess extravascular fluid causes the tissues to swell and is known as edema.

The endothelial cells of capillaries also secrete a number of substances including **types II, IV, and V collagen, fibronectin,** and **laminin,** all of which are released into and become part of the extracellular matrix. Additionally, endothelial cells produce several other important substances related to **clotting, vascular smooth muscle tone, lymphocyte circulation,** and **neutrophil movement.**

A vasoconstrictor substance, **endothelin I,** secreted by the capillary endothelial cells, attaches to vascular smooth muscle cells. It acts as a hypertensive agent, keeping the smooth muscle cells contracted for long periods and thus elevating blood pressure. Although endothelin I is much more effective than angiotensin II, it is unclear how widespread its effects are.

Adhesion molecules (L-selectin and B$_2$-integrins) expressed on the plasma membranes of migrating leukocytes bind to receptors on the plasma membranes of capillary endothelial cells at sites of inflammation. The bound leukocytes then enter the connective tissue spaces, where they perform their duties in the inflammatory process. **Prostacyclin,** a potent vasodilator and inhibitor of platelet aggregation, is released by capillaries.

In addition to these functions, capillaries also serve a maintenance role in converting such substances as serotonin, norepinephrine, bradykinin, prostaglandins, and thrombin into inactive compounds.

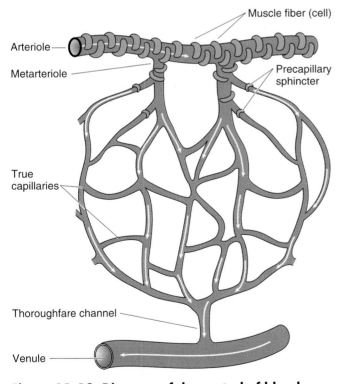

Figure 11–12. Diagram of the control of blood flow through a capillary bed. The central channel, composed of the metarteriole on the atrial side and the thoroughfare channel on the venous side, can bypass the capillary bed by closure of the precapillary sphincters.

A

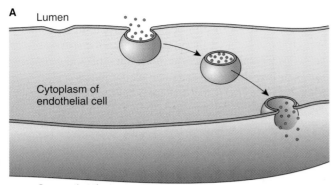

B

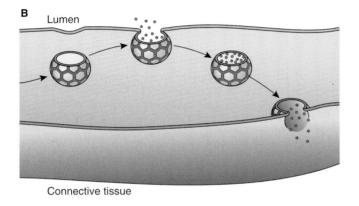

C

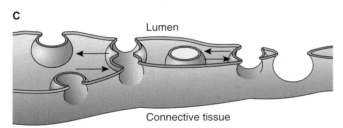

Figure 11–13. Diagram of the various methods of transport across capillary endothelia. A, Pinocytotic vesicles, which form on the luminal surface, traverse the endothelial cell, and their contents are released on the opposite surface into the connective tissue spaces. **B,** Trans Golgi network–derived vesicles possessing clathrin coats and receptor molecules fuse with the luminal surface of the endothelial cells and pick up specific ligands from the capillary lumen. Then they detach and traverse the endothelial cell, fuse with the membrane of the opposite surface, and release their contents into the connective tissue spaces. **C,** In regions where the endothelial cells are highly attenuated, the pinocytotic (or trans Golgi–derived) vesicles may fuse with each other to form transient fenestrations through the entire thickness of the endothelial cell, permitting material to travel between the lumen and the connective tissue spaces. (Based on Simionescu, N., and Simionescu, M.: *In* Ussing, H., Bindslev, N., and Sten-Knudsen, O. [eds.]: Water Transport Across Epithelia. Copenhagen, Munksgaard, 1981. Copyright © 1981 Munksgaard International Publishers Ltd., Copenhagen, Denmark.)

Enzymes on the luminal surface of endothelial cells of the capillaries in adipose tissue break down lipoproteins into triglycerides and fatty acids for storage within adipocytes.

Veins

At the discharging ends of capillaries are small venules, the beginning of the venous return, which conducts blood away from the organs and tissues to the heart. These venules empty their contents into larger veins, and the process continues as the vessels become larger and larger back to the heart. Because veins not only outnumber arteries but usually have larger luminal diameters, almost 70% of the total blood volume is in these vessels. In histological sections, veins parallel arteries, but their walls are usually collapsed because they are thinner and less elastic than arterial walls owing to the fact that the venous return is a low-pressure system.

Classification of Veins

Veins are grouped into three categories based on size: small, medium, and large veins (Table 11–2). However, their structure is not necessarily uniform for veins of the same size or for the same vein along its entire length. Veins are described as having the same three tunics (i.e., intima, media, and adventitia) as arteries. Although the muscular and elastic layers are not as well developed, the connective tissue component is more pronounced than in arteries. In certain areas of the body where the structures housing the veins protect them from pressure (e.g., retina, meninges, placenta, penis), the veins have little or no smooth muscle in their walls. Also, the boundaries between the tunica intima and the tunica media of most veins are not clearly distinguishable.

VENULES AND SMALL VEINS. As the blood pools from the capillary bed, it is discharged into **postcapillary venules,** which are 15 to 20 μm in diameter. Their walls are similar to those of capillaries, with a thin endothelium surrounded by reticular fibers and pericytes (see Fig. 11–4). The pericytes of postcapillary venules form an intricate, loose network surrounding the endothelium. Pericytes are replaced by smooth muscle cells in larger venules (whose diameter is > 1 mm)—first as scattered smooth muscle cells, then, as venule diameter increases, the smooth muscle cells become more closely spaced, forming a continuous layer in the largest venules and small veins. Materials are exchanged between the connective tissue spaces and vessel lumina not only in the capillaries but also in the postcapillary venules, whose walls are even more permeable. Indeed, this is the preferred location for emigration of the leukocytes from the bloodstream into the tissue spaces. Also, these vessels respond to pharmacological agents such as histamine and serotonin.

Table 11-2. Vein Characteristics

Veins	Tunica Intima	Tunica Media	Tunica Adventitia
Large veins	Endothelium, basal lamina, valves in some, subendothelial connective tissue	Connective tissue, smooth muscle cells	Smooth muscle cells oriented in longitudinal bundles, cardiac muscle cells near their entry into the heart, collagen layers with fibroblasts
Medium and small veins	Endothelium, basal lamina, valves in some, subendothelial connective tissue	Reticular and elastic fibers, some smooth muscle cells	Collagen layers with fibroblasts
Venules	Endothelium, basal lamina (pericytes, postcapillary venules)	Sparse connective tissue and a few smooth muscle cells	Some collagen and a few fibroblasts

The endothelial cells of venules located in certain lymphoid organs are cuboidal rather than squamous and are named **high-endothelial venules.** These function in lymphocyte recognition and segregation by type-specific receptors on their luminal surface, ensuring that specific lymphocytes migrate into the proper regions of the lymphoid parenchyma.

MEDIUM VEINS. Medium veins are less than 1 cm in diameter and include those draining most of the body, including most of the regions of the extremities. Their tunica intima includes the endothelium and its basal lamina and reticular fibers. Sometimes an elastic network surrounds the endothelium, but these elastic fibers do not form laminae characteristic of an internal elastic lamina. The smooth muscle cells of the tunica media are in a loosely organized layer interwoven with collagen fibers and fibroblasts. The tunica adventitia, the thickest of the tunics, is composed of longitudinally arranged collagen bundles and elastic fibers along with a few scattered smooth muscle cells.

LARGE VEINS. The large veins are those major veins returning blood to the heart from the extremities, head, gut, and the body wall. These include the venae cava and the pulmonary, portal, renal, internal jugular, iliac, and azygos veins. The tunica intima of the large veins is similar to that of the medium veins, except that large veins have a thick subendothelial connective tissue layer, containing fibroblasts and a network of elastic fibers. Whereas only a few major vessels such as the pulmonary veins have a well-developed smooth muscle layer, most large veins are without a tunica media; in its place is a well-developed tunica adventitia. An exception to this are the superficial veins of the legs, which have a well-defined muscular wall, perhaps to resist the distension caused by gravity.

The tunica adventitia of large veins contains many elastic fibers, abundant collagen fibers, and vasa vasorum, whereas the inferior vena cava has longitudinally arranged smooth muscle cells in its adventitia. As the pulmonary veins and the venae cava approach the heart, their adventitia contains some cardiac muscle cells.

Valves of Veins

Many medium veins have valves that function to prevent the back-flow of blood. These **valves** are especially abundant in the veins of the legs, where they act against the force of gravity. A venous valve is composed of two leaflets, each composed of a thin fold of the intima jutting out from the wall into the lumen. The thin leaflets are structurally reinforced by collagen and elastic fibers that are continuous with those of the wall. As blood flows to the heart, the valve cusps are deflected in the direction of the blood flow toward the heart. Backward flow of blood forces the cusps to approximate each other, thus blocking back-flow.

CLINICAL CORRELATIONS

Varicose veins are abnormally enlarged, tortuous veins usually affecting the superficial veins in the legs of older persons. This condition results from loss of muscle tone, degeneration of vessel walls, and valvular incompetence. Varicose veins may also occur in the lower end of the esophagus (**esophageal varices**) or at the terminus of the anal canal (**hemorrhoids**).

Heart

The **heart** is the pump for the cardiovascular system. Its muscular wall (**myocardium**) is composed of cardiac muscle, which is described in Chapter 8. The heart consists of four chambers, two **atria,** which receive blood, and two **ventricles,** which discharge blood from the heart (Fig. 11–14). The **superior** and **inferior venae cavae** return systemic blood to the **right atrium** of the heart. From here, the blood passes through the **right atrioventricular valve (tricuspid valve)** into the **right ventricle.** As the ventricles contract, blood from the right ventricle is pumped out the **pulmonary trunk,** which bifurcates into the right and left pulmonary arteries, from which the blood is delivered to the lungs for gaseous exchange. Oxygenated blood from the lungs returns to the heart via the **pulmonary veins** that empty into the **left atrium.** From here, the blood passes through the **left atrioventricular valve (bicuspid or mitral valve)** to enter the **left ventricle.** Again, ventricular contraction expels the blood from the left ventricle into the aorta, from which many branches emanate to deliver blood to the tissues of the body.

The atrioventricular valves prevent the regurgitation of the ventricular blood back into the atria. **Semilunar valves** located in the pulmonary trunk and the aorta near their origins prevent back–flow from these vessels into the heart.

Layers of the Heart Wall

The three layers making up the heart wall are the **endocardium, myocardium,** and **epicardium,** homologous to the tunica intima, tunica media, and the tunica adventitia, respectively, of the blood vessels.

ENDOCARDIUM. The lining of the heart lumen is the **endocardium,** which is continuous with the tunica intima of the blood vessels entering and leaving the heart. The endocardium is made up of an **endothelium** composed of simple

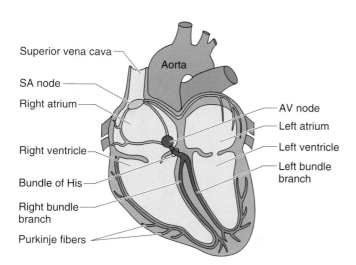

Superior vena cava
Aorta
SA node
Right atrium
AV node
Left atrium
Left ventricle
Right ventricle
Left bundle branch
Bundle of His
Right bundle branch
Purkinje fibers

Figure 11–14. Diagram of the locations of the sinoatrial and atrioventricular nodes, Purkinje fibers, and bundle of His of the heart.

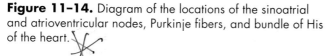

squamous epithelium, beneath which is a layer of collagenous and elastic fibers and scattered fibroblasts. Lying deeper is a layer of dense connective tissue heavily endowed with elastic fibers interspersed with smooth muscle cells. A **subendocardial layer** of loose connective tissue contains small blood vessels, nerves, and Purkinje fibers from the conduction system. It forms the boundary of the endocardium as it attaches to the endomysium of the cardiac muscle.

CLINICAL CORRELATIONS

Children who have had **rheumatic fever** may later develop **rheumatic heart-valve disease** due to scarring of the valves during the episode with rheumatic fever. This condition develops because the valves cannot close (incompetence) or open properly (stenosis) because of reduced elasticity as a result of rheumatic fever. The bicuspid (mitral) valve is the most commonly affected valve, followed by the aortic valves.

MYOCARDIUM. The **myocardium,** the middle and thickest of the three layers of the heart, contains cardiac muscle cells, arranged in complex spirals around the orifices of the chambers. Certain of the cardiac muscle cells attach the myocardium to the fibrous cardiac skeleton; others are specialized for endocrine secretions; still others are specialized for impulse generation or impulse conduction.

The heart rate (normally about 70 beats a minute) is controlled by the **sinoatrial node (pacemaker)** located at the junction of the superior vena cava and the right atrium (see Fig. 11–14). These specialized nodal cardiac muscle cells can spontaneously depolarize 70 times per minute, creating an impulse that spreads over the atrial chamber walls by internodal pathways to the **atrioventricular node,** located in the septal wall just above the tricuspid valve. Modified cardiac muscle cells of the atrioventricular node, regulated by impulses arriving from the sinoatrial node, transmit signals to the myocardium of the atria via the **atrioventricular bundle (bundle of His).** Fibers from the atrioventricular bundle pass down the interventricular septum to conduct the impulse to the cardiac muscle, thus producing a rhythmic contraction. The atrioventricular bundle travels in the subendocardial connective tissue as large, modified cardiac muscle cells, forming **Purkinje fibers** (Fig. 11–15), which transmit impulses to the cardiac muscle cells located at the apex of the heart. It should be noted that although the autonomic nervous system does not initiate the heart beat, it does modulate the rate and stroke volume of the heart beat. Stimulation of sympathetic nerves accelerates the heart rate, whereas stimulation of the parasympathetic nerves serving the heart slows the heart rate.

Specialized cardiac muscle cells located primarily in the atrial wall and in the interventricular septum produce an array of small secreted peptides (Fig. 11–16). These include

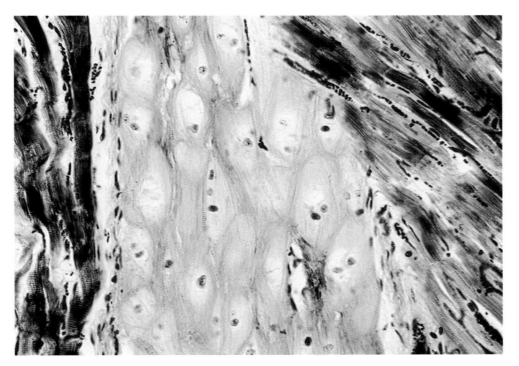

Figure 11-15. Light micrograph of Purkinje fibers (× 270).

atriopeptin, atrial natriuretic polypeptide, cardiodilatin, and **cardionatrin,** which are released into the surrounding capillaries. These hormones aid fluid maintenance and electrolyte balance and decrease blood pressure.

EPICARDIUM. The **epicardium,** the homologue of the tunica adventitia in blood vessels, is also called the **visceral layer of the pericardium** (composed of a simple squamous epithelium known as a **mesothelium**). The subepicardial layer of loose connective tissue contains the coronary vessels, nerves, and ganglia. It also is the region where fat is stored on the surface of the heart. At the roots of the vessels entering and leaving the heart, the visceral pericardium becomes continuous with the serous layer of the parietal pericardium. These two layers of the pericardium enclose the pericardial cavity, a space containing a small amount of

Figure 11-16. Electron micrograph of a cardiac muscle cell containing clusters of vesicles with atrial natriuretic peptide (ANP). (From Mifune, H., Suzuki, S., Honda, J., Kobayashi, Y., Noda, Y., Hayashi, Y., and Mochizuki, K.: Atrial natriuretic peptide (ANP): A study of ANP and its mRNA in cardiocytes, and of plasma ANP levels in non-obese diabetic mice. Cell Tiss. Res. **267:**267–272, 1992. Copyright Springer-Verlag.)

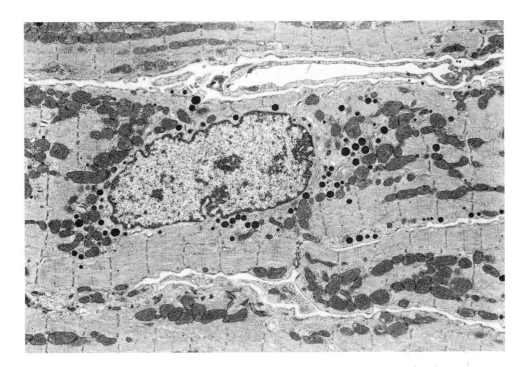

serous fluid for lubricating the serous layer of the pericardium and the visceral pericardium.

CLINICAL CORRELATIONS

Infection in the pericardial cavity, called **pericarditis,** severely restricts the heart from beating properly because the space is obliterated by adhesions between the serous layer of the pericardium and the epicardium.

Cardiac Skeleton

The cardiac skeleton, composed of dense connective tissue, includes three main components: the **annuli fibrosi,** formed around the base of the aorta, pulmonary artery, and the atrioventricular orifices; the **trigonum fibrosum,** formed primarily about some of the cuspal area of the aortic valve; and the **septum membranaceum,** constituting the upper portion of the interventricular septum. In addition to providing a structural framework for the heart and attachment sites for the cardiac muscle, the cardiac skeleton provides a discontinuity between the myocardia of the atria and ventricles, thus ensuring a rhythmic and cyclic beating of the heart controlled by the conduction mechanism of the atrioventricular bundles.

CLINICAL CORRELATIONS

Ischemic (coronary) heart disease, especially prevalent in older persons, is related to **atherosclerosis of the coronary vessels** serving the myocardium. As atherosclerotic plaques reduce the lumina of the coronary vessels, the patient may experience referred pain and pressure, known as **angina,** from lack of oxygen. Continued narrowing will result in ischemia of the heart wall, which may be fatal.

Lymphatic Vascular System

The **lymphatic vascular system** is a series of vessels that remove excess tissue fluid **(lymph)** from the interstitial tissue spaces and return it to the cardiovascular system. Lymphatic vessels are found throughout the body except in the central nervous system and a few other areas, including the orbit, internal ear, epidermis, cartilage, and bone. Unlike the cardiovascular system, which contains a pump (the heart) and circulates blood in a closed system, the lymphatic vascular system is an open system in that there is no pump and no circulation of fluid. The lymphatic vascular system begins in the tissues of the body as blind-ended **lymphatic capillaries,** which simply act as drain fields for excess interstitial fluid. The lymphatic capillaries empty their contents into **lymphatic vessels,** which empty into successively larger vessels until one of the two **lymphatic ducts** is reached. From either of these ducts the lymph is emptied into the venous portion of the cardiovascular system at the junctions of the internal jugular and the subclavian veins.

Lymph nodes are interposed along the paths of lymphatic vessels, and lymph must pass through them to be filtered. **Afferent lymphatic vessels** deliver lymph into the lymph nodes, where lymph is distributed into labyrinthine channels lined by an endothelium and abundant macrophages. Here the lymph is filtered and cleared of particulate matter; lymphocytes are added to the lymph as it leaves by **efferent lymphatic vessels,** eventually reaching a lymphatic duct. Lymph nodes are discussed in Chapter 12.

Lymphatic Capillaries and Vessels

The blind-ended, thin-walled **lymphatic capillaries** are composed of a single layer of attenuated endothelial cells with an incomplete basal lamina (Fig. 11–17). The endothelial cells overlap each other in places but have intercellular clefts that permit easy access to the lumen of the vessel. These cells do not have fenestrae, nor do they make tight junctions with each other. Bundles of **lymphatic anchoring filaments** (5 to 10 nm in diameter) terminate on the abluminal plasma membrane. It is thought that these filaments play a role in maintaining the luminal patency of these flimsy vessels.

Small and medium lymphatic vessels are characterized by closely spaced valves. Large lymphatic vessels resemble

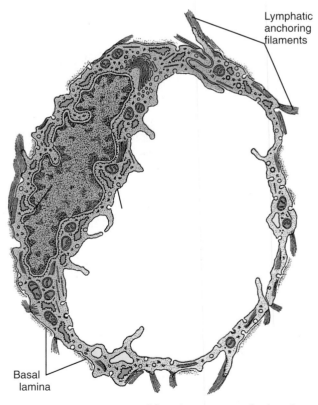

Figure 11–17. Diagram of the ultrastructure of a lymphatic capillary. (From Lentz, T.L.: Cell Fine Structure. An Atlas of Drawings of Whole-Cell Structure. W.B. Saunders Company, Philadelphia, 1971.)

small veins structurally, except that their lumina are larger and their walls thinner. Large lymphatic vessels have a thin layer of elastic fibers beneath their endothelium and a thin layer of smooth muscle cells. This smooth muscle layer is then overlaid with elastic and collagen fibers that blend with the surrounding connective tissue, much like a tunica adventitia. Although some histologists describe tunics similar to those in blood vessels, most do not concur because there are no clear boundaries between the layers and because the walls are so varied.

Lymphatic Ducts

The **lymphatic ducts,** which are similar in structure to large veins, are the final two collecting vessels of the lymphatic vascular system. The short **right lymphatic duct** empties its contents into the venous system at the junction of the right internal jugular and subclavian veins. The larger, the **thoracic duct,** begins in the abdomen as the **cisterna chyli** and ascends through the thorax and neck to empty its contents at the junction of the left internal jugular and subclavian veins. The right lymphatic duct collects lymph from the upper right quadrant of the body, whereas the thoracic duct collects lymph from the remainder of the body.

The tunica intima of lymphatic ducts is composed of an endothelium and several layers of elastic and collagen fibers. At the interface with the tunica media, a layer of condensed elastic fibers resembles an internal elastic lamina. Both longitudinal and circular layers of smooth muscle are present in the media. The tunica adventitia contains longitudinally oriented smooth muscle cells and collagen fibers that blend into the surrounding connective tissue. Piercing the walls of the thoracic duct are small vessels homologous to the vasa vasorum of the arteries.

CLINICAL CORRELATIONS

Malignant tumor cells (especially carcinomas) are spread throughout the body by lymphatic vessels. When the malignant cells reach a lymph node, they will be slowed and multiply there, eventually leaving to **metastasize** at a secondary site. Therefore, in surgical removal of a cancerous growth, examination of the lymph nodes and the removal of both enlarged lymph nodes in the pathway and associated lymphatic vessels is essential in preventing secondary growth of the tumor.

Lymphoid (Immune) System

12

The lymphoid system is responsible for the immunological defense of the body. Some of its component organs, **lymph nodes, thymus,** and **spleen,** are bounded by connective tissue capsules, whereas its other components, members of the **diffuse lymphoid system,** are not encapsulated. The cells of the lymphoid system protect the body against foreign macromolecules, viruses, bacteria and other invasive microorganisms, and transformed cells.

Overview of the Immune System

The immune response exhibits four distinctive properties: **specificity, diversity, memory,** and **self/nonself recognition** (the ability to distinguish between structures that belong to the organism, **self,** and those that are foreign, **nonself).** The **B** and **T lymphocytes** are responsible for these four features. The lymphocytes, along with **antigen-presenting cells,** initiate and participate in the immune response. These cells communicate with each other by signaling molecules, known as **cytokines,** which are released in response to encounters with foreign substances, called **antigens.**

The recognition of a substance as foreign stimulates a complex sequence of reactions that results either in the production of immunoglobulins, or **antibodies,** that bind to the antigen, or in the induction of a group of cells that specialize in killing the foreign cell or altered self-cell (e.g., tumor cell). The immune response that depends on the formation of antibodies is called the **humoral immune response,** whereas the cytotoxic response is known as the **cell-mediated immune response.**

The three types of cells that constitute the functional components of the immune system (T cells, B cells, antigen-presenting cells) are all formed in the bone marrow. B cells become immunocompetent in the bone marrow, whereas T cells migrate to the thymus to become immunocompetent; thus these two organs are called the **primary (central) lymphoid organs.** After lymphocytes become immunocompetent in the bone marrow or in the thymus, they migrate to the

secondary (peripheral) lymphoid organs, namely diffuse lymphoid tissue, lymph nodes, and spleen, where they come into contact with antigens.

Immunogens and Antigens

A foreign structure that can elicit an immune response in a particular host is known as an **immunogen;** an **antigen** is a molecule that can react with an antibody, irrespective of its ability to elicit an immune response. Although not all antigens are immunogens, in this textbook the two terms will be assumed to be synonymous, and only the term *antigen* will be used.

The region of the antigen that reacts with the antibody (or T-cell receptor) is known as its **epitope,** or antigenic determinant. Each epitope is a small portion of the antigen molecule, consisting of only four to six hydrophilic amino acid or sugar residues that are accessible to the immune apparatus. Large foreign invaders, such as bacteria, have several epitopes, each capable of binding a different antibody.

CLINICAL CORRELATIONS

The complexity of a foreign substance is also important in determining its antigenicity. Hence, large polymeric molecules that have relatively simple chemical compositions, such as certain man-made plastics, have minimal immunogenicity, and are therefore used in the manufacture of artificial implants (as in hip replacement).

Clonal Selection and Expansion

The immune system can recognize and combat an astonishing number of different antigens. The explanation for this capability is that during embryonic development, an enormous number of lymphocyte **clones** are formed by rearrangement of the genes encoding immunoglobulins or

T-cell receptors. All the cells in a particular clone have identical surface markers and can react with a specific antigen, even though they have not yet been exposed to that antigen. The cell-surface proteins that enable lymphocytes to interact with antigens are **membrane-bound antibodies** in the case of B cells and **T-cell receptors** in the case of T cells. Although the molecular structure of antibodies and T-cell receptors differ, they are functionally equivalent in their ability to recognize and interact with specific epitopes.

The first time the organism encounters an antigen, the immune response is slow to begin and not very robust and is called the **primary immune response.** Subsequent exposures to the same antigen elicit the **secondary immune response,** which begins rapidly and is much more intense than the primary response. The increased potency of the secondary reaction is due to the process of **immunological memory** inherent to the immune system. Both B and T cells are said to be **virgin cells** (naive cells) before exposure to antigens. Once a virgin cell comes in contact with an antigen, it proliferates to form activated cells and memory cells.

Activated cells, also known as **effector cells,** are responsible for carrying out an immune response. Effector cells called **plasma cells,** which are derived from B cells, produce and release antibodies. Effector cells derived from T cells either secrete cytokines or destroy foreign cells or altered self-cells.

Like virgin lymphocytes, **memory cells** express either membrane-bound antibodies or T-cell receptors, which can interact with specific antigens. Memory cells are not directly involved in the immune response during which they are generated. However, these cells live for months or years and have a higher affinity for antigens than do virgin lymphocytes. Moreover, formation of memory cells following first exposure to an antigen increases the size of the original clone, a process called **clonal expansion.** Because of the presence of an expanded population of memory cells with high affinity for the antigen, subsequent exposure to the same antigen induces a secondary response that is much faster, more potent, and longer in duration than the primary response.

Immunological Tolerance

The immune system can recognize macromolecules that belong to the self and does not attempt to mount an immune response against them. This lack of action is due to **immunological tolerance.** The mechanism of immunological tolerance depends on killing or disabling cells that would react against the self. If during development a lymphocyte encounters the substance to which it is designed to react, the cell is either killed (**clonal deletion**), so that that particular clone does not form, or the lymphocyte is disabled (**clonal anergy**) and cannot mount an immune response, even though it is present.

CLINICAL CORRELATIONS

Autoimmune diseases involve a malfunction of the immune system that results in the loss of immunological tolerance. One example is **Graves disease,** in which the receptors for thyroid-stimulating hormone receptors on the follicular cells of the thyroid gland are perceived to be antigens. Antibodies formed against thyroid-stimulating hormone receptors bind to these receptors and stimulate the cells to release an excess amount of thyroxin. Persons suffering from Graves disease present with enlarged thyroid glands and exophthalmos (protruding eyeballs).

Immunoglobulins

Immunoglobulins (antibodies) are glycoproteins that inactivate antigens (including viruses) and elicit an extracellular response against invading microorganisms. The response may involve phagocytosis in the connective tissue spaces by macrophages (or neutrophils) or the activation of the blood-borne **complement system.**

CLINICAL CORRELATIONS

The complement system is composed of 20 plasma proteins that assemble in a specific sequence and fashion on the surface of invading microorganisms to form a **membrane attack complex** that lyses the foreign cell. The key component of the complement system is the **protein C3.** Deficiency of protein C3 predisposes a person to recurring bacterial infections.

Immunoglobulins are manufactured in large number by plasma cells, which release them into lymph or blood circulation. As noted earlier, small amounts of immunoglobulins are made by B cells and inserted into their plasmalemma; these are known as **surface immunoglobulins (SIGs)** and function as antigen-receptor molecules.

Each antibody is a Y-shaped molecule, composed of two long, identical 55- to 70-kDa polypeptides, known as **heavy chains,** and two shorter, identical 25-kDa polypeptides, the **light chains.** The four chains are bound to each other by several disulfide bonds and noncovalent bonds such that the stem of the Y is composed only of heavy chains, and the diverging arms consist of both light and heavy chains (Fig. 12–1).

The region in the vicinity of the sulfide bonds between the two heavy chains—known as the **hinge region**—is flexible, permitting the arms to move away from or toward each other. The distal regions on the tips of the arms (the four amino-terminal segments) are responsible for binding to the epitope; hence each antibody molecule can bind two epitopes.

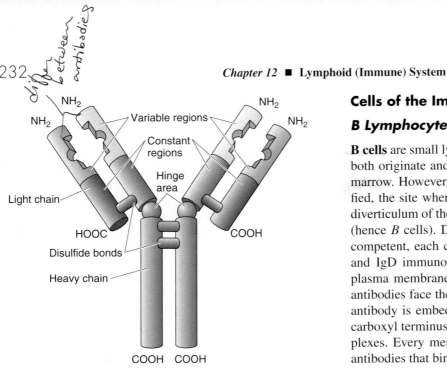

Figure 12–1. Schematic diagram of an antibody, indicating its regions.

The enzyme papain cleaves the antibody molecule at its hinge regions (see Fig. 12–1), forming three fragments: one **Fc fragment** composed of the stem of the Y and containing equal parts of the two heavy chains, and two **Fab fragments,** each composed of the remaining part of one heavy chain and one entire light chain. Fc fragments are easily crystallized (hence the "c" designation), whereas the Fab fragment is the *a*ntigen-*b*inding region of the antibody (hence the "ab" designation).

The amino acid sequence of the Fc fragment is mostly constant in its class; thus the stem of an antibody will bind to Fc receptors of many different cells. The amino acid sequence of the Fab region is variable, and it is the alterations of that sequence that determine the **specificity** of the antibody molecule for a specific antigen.

Each antibody is specific against a particular epitope; thus the Fab regions of all antibodies against that epitope are identical. It is believed that there are 10^6 to 10^9 different types of antibodies in a person, each specific against a different antigen. Each type of antibody is manufactured by members of the same **clone.** Thus there are 10^6 to 10^9 clones, whose members discern and react to a particular epitope (or a small number of similar epitopes).

Classes of Immunoglobulins

Humans have five **isotypes** (classes) of immunoglobulins: immunoglobulin G (IgG), immunoglobulin M (IgM), immunoglobulin A (IgA), immunoglobulin D (IgD), and immunoglobulin E (IgE), determined by the amino acid sequences of their heavy chains. The various heavy chains are designated by the Greek letters α, δ, γ, ε, and μ. The characteristics of the five isotypes of immunoglobulins are detailed in Table 12–1.

Cells of the Immune System

B Lymphocytes

B cells are small lymphocytes (described in Chapter 10) that both originate and become **immunocompetent** in the bone marrow. However, in birds, where B cells were first identified, the site where B cells become immunocompetent is a diverticulum of the cloaca, known as the **bursa of Fabricius** (hence *B* cells). During the process of becoming immunocompetent, each cell manufactures 50,000 to 100,000 IgM and IgD immunoglobulins (SIGs) and inserts these in its plasma membrane, so that the epitope-binding sites of the antibodies face the extracellular space. The Fc region of the antibody is embedded in the phospholipid bilayer, with its carboxyl terminus in contact with intracellular protein complexes. Every member of a particular clone of B cells has antibodies that bind to the same epitope.

When the surface immunoglobulin reacts with its epitope, the intracellular portion of the Fc region of the antibody transduces the information to the intracellular protein complex with which it is in contact, initiating a chain of events that results in **activation** of the B cell. The activated B cell undergoes mitosis, forming antibody-producing **plasma cells** and **B memory cells,** as discussed earlier. Because the antibodies produced by plasma cells are released either into the blood or into the lymph circulation, B cells are said to be responsible for the **humorally mediated immune response.**

The antibody produced during the primary response is IgM. After subsequent antigen stimulation, plasma cells preferentially release IgG, IgA, and IgE antibodies, a process called **class switching.** IgG appears to be more effective than IgM in combating antigens.

Most antigens require participation of a T-cell intermediary before they can induce a humoral immune response, a process described later in this chapter. Certain antigens (e.g., polysaccharides of microbial capsules), however, can elicit a humoral immune response without a T-cell intermediary. These are known as **thymic-independent antigens.** They cannot induce formation of B memory cells and can elicit only IgM-antibody formation.

T Lymphocytes

T cells are also formed in the bone marrow, but they migrate to the thymic cortex where they become immunocompetent by expressing on their cell membranes specific molecules that permit them to perform their functions. The process whereby T cells become immunocompetent is discussed later in the section detailing the thymus.

Although histologically T cells appear to be identical to B cells, there are important differences between them:

- T cells possess T-cell receptors, rather than antibodies, on their cell surface

Table 12–1. Properties of Human Immunoglobulins

Class	Heavy Chain	Number of Units*	% of Ig in Blood	Crosses Placenta	Binds to Cells	Biological Characteristics
IgA	α	1 or 2	10–15%	No	Temporarily to epithelial cells during secretion	Also known as **secretory antibody** because it is secreted into tears, saliva, the lumen of the gut, and the nasal cavity as **dimers;** individual units of the dimer are held together by **J protein** manufactured by plasma cells and protected from enzymatic degradation by a **secretory component** manufactured by the epithelial cell; combats antigens and micro-organisms in the lumen of gut, nasal cavity, vagina, and conjunctival sac; secreted into milk, thus protects neonate with passive immunity; **monomeric** form in bloodstream; assists eosinophils in recognizing and killing parasites
IgD	δ	1	< 1%	No	B-cell plasma membrane	Surface immunoglobulin (SIG); assists B cells in recognizing antigens for which they are specific; functions in the activation of B cells subsequent to antigenic challenge to differentiate into plasma cells
IgE	ε	1	< 1%	No	Mast cells and basophils	Reaginic antibody; when several membrane bound antibodies are cross-linked by antigens, IgE facilitates degranulation of basophils and mast cells, with subsequent release of pharmacological agents, such as heparin, histamine, eosinophil and neutrophil chemotactic factors, and leukotrienes; elicits immediate hypersensitivity reactions; assists eosinophils in recognizing and killing parasites
IgG	γ	1	80%	Yes	Macro-phages and neutrophils	Crosses placenta, thus protects fetus with passive immunity; secreted in milk, thus protects neonate with passive immunity; activates complement cascade; functions as **opsonins,** that is, by coating microorganisms, facilitates their phagocytosis by macrophages and neutrophils, cells that possess Fc receptors for the Fc region of these antibodies; also participates in **antibody-dependent cell-mediated cytotoxicity** by activating NK cells; produced in large quantities during secondary immune responses
IgM	μ	1 or 5	5–10%	No	B cells (in monomeric form)	Pentameric form is maintained by J-protein links, which bind Fc regions of each unit; activates complement system; is the first isotype to be formed in the primary immune response

*A unit is a single immunoglobulin composed of two heavy and two light chains; thus, IgA exists both as a monomer and as a dimer.

- T cells recognize only epitopes presented to them by other cells
- T cells perform their functions only at short distances

Like the surface immunoglobulins on B cells, **T-cell receptors (TCRs)** on the plasmalemma of T cells function as antigen receptors. The constant regions of the TCR are membrane-bound, whereas the variable amino-terminal regions containing the antigen-binding sites extend from the cell surface. The membrane-bound portion of the TCR associates with another membrane protein, CD3, forming the **TCR–CD3 complex.** Several other membrane proteins also play roles in strengthening the interaction between the TCR and an epitope and in signal transduction, thus facilitating antigen-stimulated T-cell activation.

TCRs can recognize epitopes only if the epitopes are bound to **major histocompatibility complex (MHC) molecules** present in the plasmalemma of other cells. There are two classes of these glycoproteins: class-I MHC and class-II MHC molecules. Most nucleated cells express MHC I molecules on their surface, whereas antigen-presenting cells (discussed later) can express both MHC I and MHC II on their plasmalemma. The MHC molecules are unique to each individual (except for identical twins), and T cells must recognize not only the foreign epitope but also the MHC molecule as self to become activated. If a T cell recognizes the epitope but not the MHC molecule, it does not become stimulated; hence the T cell's capability of acting against an epitope is **MHC-restricted.**

There are several subtypes of T cells: T helper cells 1 and 2 (T_H1 and T_H2), cytotoxic T cells, suppressor T cells, and T memory cells. Activated T helper cells secrete a variety of cytokines, which modulate the activity of other lymphoid cells. In general, the cytokines secreted by **T_H1 cells** regulate the cellularly mediated immune response, whereas those secreted by **T_H2 cells** regulate the humorally mediated immune response. **Cytotoxic T lymphocytes (CTLs)** kill cells they recognize as foreign, such as cells transformed by viruses. **T suppressor cells** repress the immune response by inhibiting the capabilities of other T and B cells. **T memory cells** are members of clones with immunological memory for a particular epitope.

In addition to TCR molecules, T cells express on their plasmalemma **clusters of differentiation proteins (CD proteins).** These accessory proteins bind to specific ligands on target cells. Although many CD molecules are known, Table 12–2 lists only those that are immediately pertinent to the subsequent discussion of cellular interactions in the immune process.

*[handwritten margin note: * T suppressor cells don't exit]*

Antigen-Presenting Cells (APC)

Antigen-presenting cells phagocytose, catabolize, and process antigens, attach their epitopes to MHC II molecules, and present this complex to T cells. Most antigen-presenting cells are monocyte-derived and thus belong to the mononuclear phagocyte system. Antigen-presenting cells include macrophages, dendritic cells, Langerhans cells of the epidermis and oral mucosa, and two types of non–monocyte-derived cells (epithelial reticular cells of the thymus and B cells).

Like T helper cells, antigen-presenting cells manufacture and release **cytokines.** These signaling molecules are required to activate target cells to perform their specific functions not only in the immune response but also in other processes. Table 12–3 lists some of these cytokines but includes only those properties that relate specifically to the immune response.

Natural Killer Cells

Natural killer (NK) cells account for a portion of the null-cell population of lymphocytes. These cells are similar to CTLs in that they kill some tumor and virally altered cells. However, NK cells are not MHC-restricted, do not enter the thymus to become immunologically competent, and they act nonspecifically.

NK cells can recognize the Fc region of antibodies and preferentially kill cells coated with antibodies, a process called **antibody-dependent cell-mediated cytotoxicity (ADCC).** The mode of killing depends on the release of **perforins** and **fragmentins** by NK cells. The released per-

Table 12–2. Selected Surface Markers Involved in the Immune Process

Protein	Cell Surface	Ligand and Target Cell	Function
CD3	All T cells	None	Transduces epitope–MHC complex binding into intracellular signal, activating T cell
CD4	T helper cells	MHC II on antigen-presenting cells	Coreceptor for TCR binding to epitope–MHC II complex, activation of T helper cell
CD8	Cytotoxic T cells and suppressor T cells	MHC I on most nucleated cells	Coreceptor for TCR binding to epitope–MHC I complex; activation of cytotoxic T cell
CD28	T helper cells	B7 on antigen-presenting cells	Assists in the activation of T helper cells
CD40	B cells	CD40 receptor molecule expressed on activated helper T cells	Binding of CD40 to CD40 receptor permits T helper cell to activate B cell to proliferate into B memory cells and plasma cells

[handwritten margin note: don't bind to epitope, just receptor]

MHC, major histocompatibility complex; TCR, T-cell receptors.

Table 12–3. Origin and Selected Functions of Some Cytokines

Cytokine	Cell Origin	Target Cell	Function
IL-1α and IL-1β	Macrophages and epithelial cells	T cells and macrophages	Activates T cells and macrophages
IL-2	T$_H$1 cells	Activated T cells and activated B cells	Promotes proliferation of activated T cells and B cells
IL-4	T$_H$2 cells	B cells	Promotes proliferation of B cells and their maturation to plasma cells; also facilitates switch from production of IgM to IgG and IgE
IL-5	T$_H$2 cells	B cells	Promotes B-cell proliferation and maturation
IL-6	Antigen-presenting cells and T$_H$2 cells	T cells and activated B cells	Activates T cells and promotes B-cell maturation to IgG-producing plasma cells
IL-12	B cells and macrophages	NK cells and T cells	Activates NK cells and induces the formation of T$_H$1-like cells
γ-IFN	T$_H$1 cells	Macrophages and T cells	Promotes cell killing by cytotoxic T cells and phagocytosis by macrophages

IL, interleukin; γ-INF, gamma interferon; NK, natural killer.

forins assemble in the plasma membrane of the target cell, forming pores through which fragmentins can enter the cytoplasm. Fragmentins induce apoptosis, a form of programmed cell death.

Natural killer cells possess receptors for IL-12, for interferon-α, and for interferon-β. These cytokines greatly enhance the cytotoxic capabilities of NK cells, which in turn release large quantities of interferon-γ, a cytokine that activates macrophages to kill bacteria. NK cells also can kill cells that do not present Fc regions of antibodies. The antibody-independent mode of killing is regulated by the presence of receptors on tumor or virally transformed cells recognized by NK cells.

Interaction Among the Lymphoid Cells

Cells of the lymphoid system interact with each other to effect an immune response. The process of interaction is regulated by recognition of surface molecules; if the molecules are not recognized, the cell is eliminated to prevent an incorrect response. If the surface molecules are recognized, the lymphocytes proliferate and differentiate. The initiation of these two responses is called **activation.** Activation requires at least two signals:

1. Recognition of the antigen (or epitope)
2. Recognition of a second, co-stimulatory signal, which may be mediated by a cytokine or by a membrane-bound signaling molecule

T Helper Cell–Mediated (T$_H$2) Humoral Immune Response

Except for thymic-independent antigens, B cells can respond to an antigen only if instructed to do so by the T$_H$2 subtype of T helper cells (Fig. 12–2). When the B cell binds antigens on its surface immunoglobulins (SIGs), it internalizes the antigen–antibody complex, removes the epitope, attaches it to MHC II molecules, places the epitope-MHC II complex on its surface, and presents it to a T$_H$2 cell.

Signal 1: The T$_H$2 cell not only has to recognize the epitope with its T-cell receptor (TCR) but must recognize the MHC II molecule with its CD4 molecule

Signal 2: The T$_H$2 cell's CD40 receptor must bind to the B cell's CD40 molecule

If both signaling events are properly executed, the B cell becomes activated and rapidly proliferates. During proliferation, the T$_H$2 cell releases interleukins 4, 5, and 6. These cytokines facilitate the differentiation of the newly formed B cells into **B memory cells** and antibody-secreting **plasma cells.**

T Helper Cell–Mediated (T$_H$1) Killing of Virally Transformed Cells

In most cases, cytotoxic T lymphocytes (CTLs) need to receive a signal from a T$_H$1 cell to be capable of killing virally transformed cells. However, before that signal can be given, the T$_H$1 cell must be activated by an antigen-presenting cell offering the proper epitope (Fig. 12–3).

Thymus-Dependent Antigen-Induced B-Memory and Plasma Cell Formation

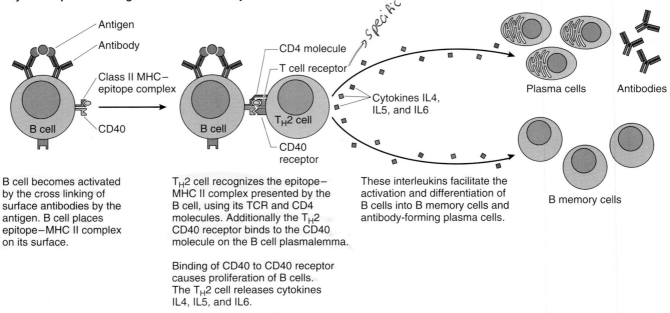

B cell becomes activated by the cross linking of surface antibodies by the antigen. B cell places epitope–MHC II complex on its surface.

T$_H$2 cell recognizes the epitope–MHC II complex presented by the B cell, using its TCR and CD4 molecules. Additionally the T$_H$2 CD40 receptor binds to the CD40 molecule on the B cell plasmalemma.

Binding of CD40 to CD40 receptor causes proliferation of B cells. The T$_H$2 cell releases cytokines IL4, IL5, and IL6.

These interleukins facilitate the activation and differentiation of B cells into B memory cells and antibody-forming plasma cells.

Figure 12–2. Schematic diagram of the interaction between B cells and T$_H$2 cell in a thymic-dependent, antigen-induced B-memory and plasma-cell formation.

Signal 1: The TCR and the CD4 molecule of a T$_H$1 cell must recognize the epitope–MHC II complex on the surface of an antigen-presenting cell. If these events occur, the antigen-presenting cell expresses on its surface a molecule called **B7.**

Signal 2: The CD28 molecule of the T$_H$1 cell binds to the B7 molecule of the antigen-presenting cell.

The T$_H$1 cell is now activated and releases **interleukin-2 (IL-2),** which will cause activation and proliferation of the cytotoxic T cell (CTL), *if* that CTL is bound to the same

T$_H$1 Cell Activation of Cytotoxic T Cells to Kill Virus-Transformed Cells

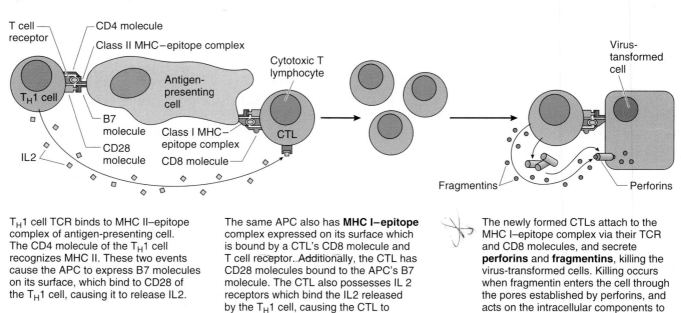

T$_H$1 cell TCR binds to MHC II–epitope complex of antigen-presenting cell. The CD4 molecule of the T$_H$1 cell recognizes MHC II. These two events cause the APC to express B7 molecules on its surface, which bind to CD28 of the T$_H$1 cell, causing it to release IL2.

The same APC also has **MHC I–epitope** complex expressed on its surface which is bound by a CTL's CD8 molecule and T cell receptor. Additionally, the CTL has CD28 molecules bound to the APC's B7 molecule. The CTL also possesses IL 2 receptors which bind the IL2 released by the T$_H$1 cell, causing the CTL to undergo proliferation.

The newly formed CTLs attach to the MHC I–epitope complex via their TCR and CD8 molecules, and secrete **perforins** and **fragmentins,** killing the virus-transformed cells. Killing occurs when fragmentin enters the cell through the pores established by perforins, and acts on the intracellular components to drive the cell into apoptosis.

Figure 12–3. Schematic diagram of the activation of cytotoxic T cells in killing virus-transformed cells.

antigen-presenting cell and if the following conditions are met:

Signal 1: The TCR and the **CD8 molecule** of the CTL must recognize the epitope–**MHC I complex** of the antigen-presenting cell; also, the CD28 molecule of the CTL must bind with the B7 molecule of the antigen-presenting cell.

Signal 2: IL-2 released by the T_H1 cell binds to the IL-2 receptors of the CTL.

The CTL is now activated and rapidly proliferates. The newly formed CTLs seek out virally transformed cells by binding with their TCR and CD8 to the transformed cell's epitope–MHC I complex. Binding causes release of perforins and fragmentins by the killer cells. **Perforins** are a group of glycoproteins that enter the cell membranes of the transformed cells, forming hydrophilic pores. **Fragmentins** are enzymes that enter the transformed cells via these pores and drive the cells into apoptosis, a form of programmed cell death, killing the cells within a few minutes.

Certain highly vigorous antigen-presenting cells can act as the first signal. In this case the CTL does not require a T helper cell intermediary but can release IL-2 and activate itself.

T_H1 Cells Assist Macrophages in Killing Bacteria

Bacteria phagocytosed by macrophages can readily proliferate within the phagosome (becoming infected), because macrophages cannot destroy these microorganisms unless they are activated by T_H1 cells (Fig. 12–4).

Signal 1: The TCR and CD4 molecules of the T_H1 cell must recognize the epitope–MHC II complex of the macrophage that phagocytosed the bacteria.

Signal 2: The T_H1 cell expresses IL-2 receptors on its surface and releases IL-2, which binds to the receptors, thus activating itself.

The activated T_H1 cell rapidly proliferates, and the newly formed T_H1 cells contact macrophages infected with bacteria.

Signal 1: The TCR and CD4 molecules of the T_H1 cell must recognize the epitope–MHC II complex of the infected macrophage, and the T cell releases γ-interferon (IFN-γ).

Signal 2: The γ-IFN activates the macrophage, which then expresses tumor necrosis factor α (TNF-α) receptors on its surface and releases the cytokine TNF-α.

When these two factors, γ-IFN and TNF-α, bind to their receptors on macrophages, they facilitate the production of oxygen radicals by the macrophage, resulting in bacterial killing.

CLINICAL CORRELATIONS

Human immunodeficiency virus (HIV), the cause of **acquired immunodeficiency syndrome (AIDS),** binds to CD4 molecules of T helper cells and injects its core into the cell. The virus incapacitates the cell, and as the virus spreads, it infects other T helper cells, reducing their number. As a result, infected persons eventually become incapable of mounting an immune response against bacterial or viral infections. Victims succumb to secondary infections due to opportunistic microorganisms or to malignancies.

Lymphoid Organs

Thymus

The **thymus,** situated in the superior mediastinum and extending over the great vessels of the heart, is a small encap-

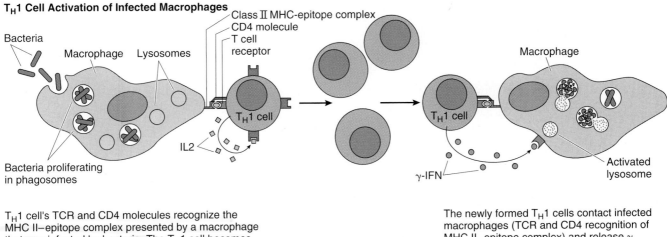

T_H1 Cell Activation of Infected Macrophages

T_H1 cell's TCR and CD4 molecules recognize the MHC II–epitope complex presented by a macrophage that was infected by bacteria. The T_H1 cell becomes activated, expresses IL2 receptors on its surface, and releases IL2. Binding of IL2 results in proliferation of the T_H1 cells.

The newly formed T_H1 cells contact infected macrophages (TCR and CD4 recognition of MHC II–epitope complex) and release γ interferon. The γ IFN activates the macrophage so that it can kill the bacteria in its phagosomes.

Figure 12–4. Schematic diagram of macrophage activation by T cells.

sulated organ composed of two **lobes.** Each lobe arises separately from the third (and possibly fourth) pharyngeal pouches of the embryo. The T lymphocytes that enter the thymus to become instructed to achieve immunological competence arise from mesoderm.

The thymus originates early in the embryo, and continues to grow until puberty, when it may weigh as much as 35 to 40 g. After the first few years of life, the thymus begins to **involute** (atrophy), and becomes infiltrated by adipose cells. However, it possibly continues to function even in older adults.

The capsule of the thymus, composed of dense, irregular collagenous connective tissue, sends septa into the lobes, subdividing them into incomplete **lobules** (Fig. 12–5). Each lobule is composed of a cortex and a medulla, although the medullae of adjacent lobules are confluent with each other.

Cortex

The **cortex** of the thymus appears much darker histologically than the medulla because of the presence of large number of **T lymphocytes (thymocytes)** (see Fig. 12–5; Fig. 12–6). Immunologically incompetent T cells leave the bone marrow and migrate to the periphery of the thymic cortex, where they undergo extensive proliferation and instruction to become immunocompetent T cells. In addition to the lymphocytes, the cortex houses macrophages and endodermally derived **epithelial reticular cells.** Three types of epithelial reticular cells are present in the thymic cortex:

- **Type I epithelial reticular cells** separate the cortex from the connective tissue capsule and trabeculae as well as surround vascular elements in the cortex. These cells form occluding junctions with each other, completely isolating

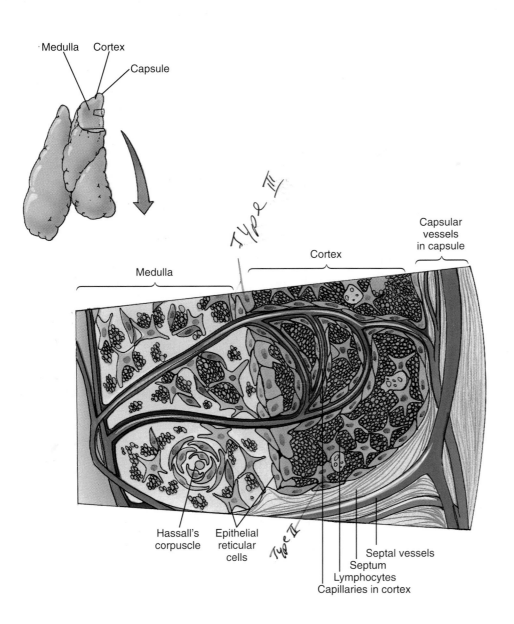

Figure 12–5. Diagram of the thymus, demonstrating its blood supply and histological arrangement.

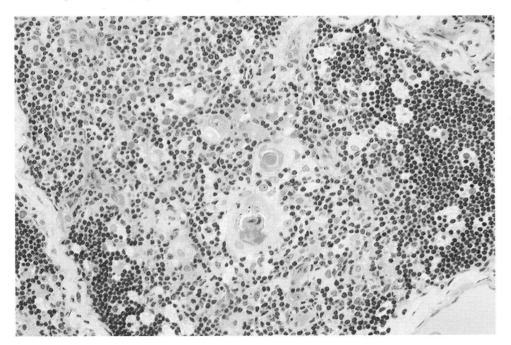

Figure 12–6. Photomicrograph of a lobule of the thymus (× 132).

the thymic cortex from the remainder of the body. The nuclei of type I cells are polymorphous and have a well-defined nucleolus.

- **Type II epithelial reticular cells** are located in the midcortex. These cells possess long, wide, sheath-like processes that form desmosomal junctions with each other. Their processes form a cytoreticulum that subdivides the thymic cortex into small lymphocyte-filled compartments. The nuclei of type II cells are large, pale structures with little heterochromatin. The cytoplasm is also pale and richly endowed with tonofilaments.
- **Type III epithelial reticular cells** are located in the deep cortex and at the corticomedullary junction. The cytoplasm and the nuclei of these cells are denser than those of type I and type II epithelial reticular cells. The rough endoplasmic reticulum of type III cells displays dilated cisternae, indicative of protein synthesis. Type III epithelial reticular cells also possess wide, sheath-like processes that form lymphocyte-filled compartments. These cells participate in the formation of occluding junctions with each other and with epithelial reticular cells of the medulla, isolating the cortex from the medulla.

The three types of epithelial reticular cells completely isolate the thymic cortex and in this fashion prevent developing T cells from contacting foreign antigens. Type II and III cells also present **self-antigens, MHC I,** and **MHC II** molecules to the developing T cells. T lymphocytes whose TCRs recognize self-proteins, or whose CD4 or CD8 molecules cannot recognize the MHC I or MHC II molecules, are killed before they can leave the cortex. It is interesting to note that 98% of T cells die in the cortex and are phagocytosed by resident macrophages. The surviving T cells enter

the medulla of the thymus as naive T lymphocytes and are distributed to secondary lymphoid organs via the vascular system.

Medulla

The thymic **medulla** stains much lighter than the cortex, because its lymphocyte population is not nearly as profuse and houses a large number of endothelially derived epithelial reticular cells (see Figs. 12–5, 12–6). There are three types of epithelial reticular cells in the medulla:

- **Type IV epithelial reticular cells** are found in close association with type III cells of the cortex and assist in the formation of the corticomedullary junction. The nuclei of these cells have a coarse chromatin network, and their cytoplasm is dark-staining and richly endowed with tonofilaments.
- **Type V epithelial reticular cells** form the cytoreticulum of the medulla. The nuclei of these cells are polymorphous, with a well-defined perinuclear chromatin network and conspicuous nucleolus.
- **Type VI epithelial reticular cells** compose the most characteristic feature of the thymic medulla. These large, pale-staining cells coalesce around each other, forming whorl-shaped **thymic corpuscles (Hassall's corpuscles),** whose numbers increase with a person's age (see Figs. 12–5, 12–6). Type VI cells may become highly cornified and even calcified. It has been suggested that unlike types IV and V, type VI epithelial reticular cells may be ectodermal in origin. The function of thymic corpuscles is not known, although they have been suggested to be the site of T lymphocyte cell death in the medulla.

Vascular Supply

The thymus receives numerous small arteries, which enter the capsule and are distributed throughout the organ via the trabeculae between adjacent lobules. Branches of these vessels do not gain access to the cortex directly; instead, from the trabeculae, they enter the corticomedullary junction, where they form capillary beds that penetrate the cortex.

The capillaries of the cortex are of the **continuous** type, possess a thick basal lamina, and are invested by a sheath of type I epithelial reticular cells, forming a **blood–thymus barrier.** Thus the developing T cells of the cortex are protected from contacting bloodborne macromolecules. However, self-macromolecules are permitted to cross the blood–thymus barrier (probably controlled by the epithelial reticular cells), possibly to eliminate those T cells that are programmed against self-antigens. The cortical capillary network drains into small venules in the medulla.

Newly formed, immunologically incompetent T cells arriving from the bone marrow leave the vascular supply at the corticomedullary junction and migrate to the periphery of the cortex. As these cells mature they move deeper and deeper into the cortex and enter the medulla as naive but immunocompetent cells. They leave the medulla via veins draining the thymus.

Histophysiology of the Thymus

The primary function of the thymus is to instruct immunoincompetent T cells to achieve immunocompetence. The developing T cells proliferate extensively in the cortex, begin to express their surface markers, and are tested for their ability to recognize **self-MHC molecules** and **self-epitopes.** T cells incapable of recognizing self–MHC I and self–MHC II molecules are destroyed. Additionally, those T lymphocytes whose TCRs are programmed against self-macromolecules are also destroyed.

The process of testing for MHC molecules and self-epitopes is believed to be a function of type II and type III epithelial reticular cells, because they express both classes of epitope–MHC molecule complex on their surface.

The epithelial reticular cells of the thymus produce at least four hormones that are required for the maturation of T cells. These are probably paracrine hormones, acting at short range, although some are believed to be released into the bloodstream. These hormones include thymosin, thymopoietin, thymulin, and thymic humoral factor, and they facilitate T cell proliferation and the expression of their surface markers. Additionally, hormones from extrathymic sources, especially the pituitary, thyroid, and suprarenal glands and the gonads influence T cell maturation. The most potent effects are due to **adrenocorticosteroids,** which decrease T cell numbers in the thymic cortex; **thyroxin,** which stimulates the cortical epithelial reticular cells to increase thymulin production; and **somatotropin,** which promotes T cell development in the thymic cortex.

CLINICAL CORRELATIONS

Congenital failure of the thymus to develop is called **DiGeorge's syndrome.** Persons afflicted with this disease cannot produce T cells. Hence, their cellularly mediated immune response is nonfunctional, and they die at an early age from infection. Because these persons also lack parathyroid glands, death also may be caused by **tetany.**

Lymph Nodes

Lymph nodes are small, encapsulated, oval structures interposed in the path of lymph vessels to serve as filters for the removal of bacteria and other foreign substances. They are located in various regions of the body but are most prevalent in the neck, in the axilla, in the groin, along major vessels, and in the body cavities. Their parenchyma is composed of collections of T and B lymphocytes, antigen-presenting cells, and macrophages. These lymphoid cells react to the presence of antigens by mounting an immunological response in which macrophages phagocytose bacteria and other microorganisms that enter the node by way of the lymph.

Each lymph node is a relatively small, soft structure, less than 3 cm in diameter, possessing a fibrous connective tissue capsule, usually surrounded by adipose tissue (Fig. 12–7). It has a convex surface, perforated by **afferent lymph vessels** that have **valves,** ensuring that lymph from those vessels enters the substance of the node. The concave surface of the node, the **hilum,** is the site of arteries and veins entering and exiting the node. Additionally, lymph leaves the node via the **efferent lymph vessels** also located at the hilum. The efferent lymph vessels have valves, preventing regurgitation of lymph back into the node.

CLINICAL CORRELATIONS

In the presence of antigens or bacteria, lymphocytes of the lymph node rapidly proliferate, and the node may increase to several times its normal size, becoming hard and palpable to the touch.

Histologically, the lymph node is subdivided into three regions: cortex, paracortex, and medulla; all three regions possess a rich supply of sinusoids, enlarged endothelially lined spaces through which lymph percolates.

Cortex

The dense irregular collagenous connective tissue **capsule** of the lymph node sends **trabeculae** into the substance of the node, subdividing the outer region of the **cortex** into incomplete compartments that extend to the vicinity of the hilum (see Fig. 12–7; Fig. 12–8). The capsule is thickened at the hilum, and as vessels enter the substance of the node, they are surrounded by a connective tissue sheath derived

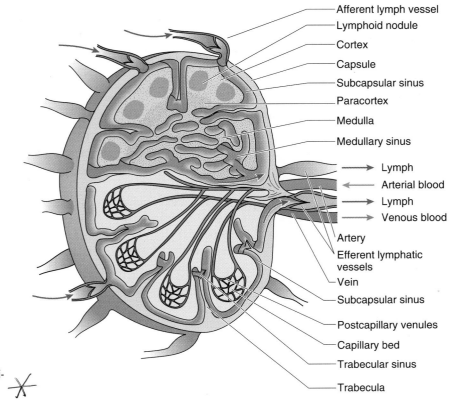

Afferent lymph vessel
Lymphoid nodule
Cortex
Capsule
Subcapsular sinus
Paracortex
Medulla
Medullary sinus

→ Lymph
← Arterial blood
→ Lymph
→ Venous blood

Artery
Efferent lymphatic vessels
Vein
Subcapsular sinus
Postcapillary venules
Capillary bed
Trabecular sinus
Trabecula

Figure 12–7. Schematic diagram of a typical lymph node.

from the capsule. Suspended from the capsule and trabeculae is a three-dimensional network of reticular connective tissue that forms the architectural framework of the entire lymph node.

The afferent lymph vessels pierce the capsule on the convex surface of the node and empty their lymph into the **subcapsular sinus,** located just deep to the capsule. This sinus is continuous with the **cortical sinuses (paratrabecular sinuses)** that parallel the trabeculae and deliver the lymph into the **medullary sinuses,** eventually to enter the **efferent lymphatic vessels.** These sinuses have a network of **stellate reticular cells** whose processes contact those of other cells and the endothelial-like simple squamous epithelium. **Macrophages,** attached to the stellate reticular cells, avidly phagocytose foreign particulate matter. Additionally, lymphoid cells can enter or leave the sinusoids by passing between their squamous cell lining.

LYMPHOID NODULES. The incomplete compartments within the cortex house **primary lymphoid nodules,** spherical aggregates of **B lymphocytes** (both virgin B cells and B memory cells) that are in the process of entering or leaving the lymph node (see Figs. 12–7, 12–8). Frequently the centers of these primary nodules are stained paler and are called **secondary nodules (housing germinal centers).** Secondary nodules form only in response to an antigenic challenge, and it is believed that they are the site of B memory cell and plasma cell generation.

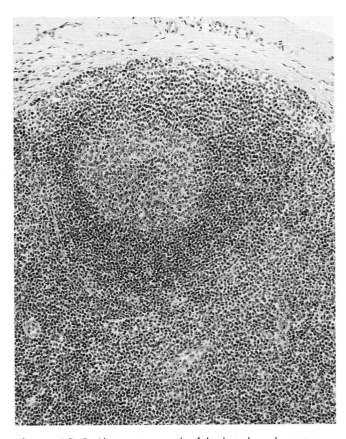

Figure 12–8. Photomicrograph of the lymph node cortex (× 132).

The region of the lymphoid nodule peripheral to the germinal center is composed of a dense accumulation of small lymphocytes that are migrating away from their site of origin within the secondary nodules. This peripheral region is called the **cortex (mantle).**

Germinal centers display three zones: a dark zone, a basal light zone, and an apical light zone. The **dark zone** is the site of most intense proliferation of closely packed B cells, called **centroblasts.** It also houses processes of antigen-presenting **follicular dendritic cells.** The newly formed B memory cells and plasma cells migrate from the dark zone into the **basal light zone** and then into the **apical light zone,** regions that also house follicular dendritic cells and occasional T helper cells. Cells in the two paler regions are less tightly packed, but B cells (centrocytes) still have some mitotic activity. Cell death also occurs in the pale regions, as evidenced by B cells undergoing **apoptosis.**

Paracortex

The region of the lymph node between the cortex and the medulla is the **paracortex,** housing mostly **T cells,** and is the thymus-dependent zone of the lymph node (see Fig. 12–7). Antigen-presenting cells migrate to this region of the lymph node to present their epitope–MHC II complex to T helper cells. If T helper cells become activated, they proliferate, increasing the width of the paracortex to such an extent that it may intrude deep into the medulla. Newly formed T cells then migrate to the medullary sinuses, leave the lymph node, and proceed to the area of antigenic activity.

High endothelial venules (HEVs) are located in the paracortex. Lymphocytes leave the vascular supply by migrating between the cuboidal cells of this unusual endothelium and enter the substance of the lymph node. B cells migrate to the outer cortex, whereas most T cells will remain in the paracortex.

The lymphocyte plasma membrane expresses surface molecules known as **selectins** that aid the cell in recognizing the endothelial cells of HEVs and permit it to roll along the surface of these cells. When the lymphocyte contacts additional signaling molecules located on the endothelial cell plasmalemma, the selectins become activated and bind firmly to the endothelial cell, stopping the rolling action of the lymphocyte. Then, via **diapedesis,** the lymphocyte migrates between the cuboidal endothelial cells to leave the lumen of the postcapillary venule and enter the lymph node parenchyma.

Medulla

The **medulla** is composed of large, tortuous lymph sinuses surrounded by lymphoid cells organized in clusters, known as **medullary cords** (see Fig. 12–7; Fig. 12–9). The cells of the medullary cords (lymphocytes, plasma cells, and macrophages) are enmeshed in a network of reticular fibers and

reticular cells. The lymphocytes are in the process of migrating from the cortex to enter the medullary sinuses. Histological sections of the medulla also display the presence of trabeculae, arising from the thickened capsule of the hilum, conveying blood vessels into and out of the lymph node.

Vascularization of the Lymph Node

The arterial supply enters the substance of lymph nodes at the hilum. The vessels course through the medulla within trabeculae and become smaller as they repeatedly branch. Eventually they will lose their connective tissue sheath, travel within the substance of medullary cords, and contribute to the formation of the medullary capillary beds. The small branches of the arteries continue in the medullary cords until they reach the cortex. Here they form a cortical capillary bed, which is drained by **postcapillary venules.** Blood from postcapillary venules drains into larger veins, which exit the lymph node at the hilum.

Histophysiology of Lymph Nodes

As lymph enters the lymph node, the flow rate is reduced, giving the macrophages that reside in (or have their pro-

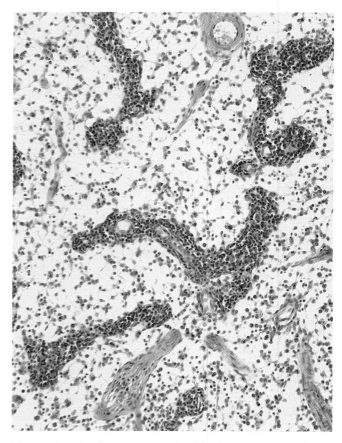

Figure 12–9. Photomicrograph of the lymph node medulla (× 132).

cesses intrude into) the sinuses more time to phagocytose foreign particulate matter. In this fashion, 99% of the impurities found in lymph are removed.

Lymph nodes also function as sites of antigen recognition, because antigen-presenting cells that contact antigens migrate to the nearest lymph node and present their epitope–MHC complex to lymphocytes. Additionally, antigens percolating through the lymph node are trapped by follicular dendritic cells, and lymphocytes that are either present in or migrate into the lymph node recognize the antigen.

If an antigen is recognized and a B cell becomes activated, that B cell migrates to a primary lymphoid nodule and proliferates, forming a secondary lymphoid nodule. The newly formed cells differentiate into B memory and plasma cells, leave the cortex, and form the medullary cords. About 10% of the newly formed plasma cells stay in the medulla and release antibodies into the medullary sinuses. The remainder of the plasma cells enter the sinuses and go to the bone marrow, where they will continue to manufacture antibodies until they die. Some B memory cells stay in the primary lymphoid nodules of the cortex, but most leave the lymph node to take up residence in other secondary lymphatic organs of the body. In this fashion, in case of a second exposure to the same antigen, a large number of memory cells are available so that the body can mount a prompt and potent secondary response.

CLINICAL CORRELATIONS

Because lymph nodes are located along the paths of lymph vessels, they form a chain of lymph nodes, so lymph flows from one node to the next. For this reason infection can spread, and malignant cells may metastasize through a chain of nodes to remote regions of the body.

Spleen

The **spleen,** the largest lymphoid organ in the body, is located intraperitoneally, in the upper left quadrant of the abdominal cavity. Its dense, irregular fibroelastic connective tissue capsule, housing occasional **smooth muscle cells,** is surrounded by visceral peritoneum, whose simple squamous epithelium provides a smooth surface for this organ. The spleen functions not only in the immunological capacity of T-cell and B-cell proliferation and antibody formation but also as a filter of the blood in destroying old erythrocytes. During fetal development, the spleen is a hemopoietic organ; if necessary, it can resume that function in the adult. Additionally, in some animals (but not in humans), the spleen also acts as a reservoir of red blood cells, which may be released into circulation as the need arises.

The spleen possesses a convex surface as well as a concave aspect, the **hilum.** The capsule of the spleen is thickened at the hilum where arteries and their accompanying nerve fibers enter, whereas veins and lymph vessels leave the spleen at this region.

The trabeculae, arising from the capsule, carry blood vessels into and out of the parenchyma of the spleen (Fig. 12–10). Histologically, the spleen has a three-dimensional network of **reticular fibers** and associated reticular cells. The reticular fiber network is attached to the capsule as well as to the trabeculae and forms the architectural framework of this organ (Fig. 12–11).

The interstices of the reticular tissue network are occupied by **venous sinuses,** trabeculae conveying blood vessels, and the splenic parenchyma. The cut surface of a fresh spleen shows gray areas surrounded by red areas. The former are called the white pulp, whereas the latter are known as red pulp. Central to the appreciation of the organization and function of the spleen is understanding of its blood supply.

Vascular Supply of the Spleen

The splenic artery branches repeatedly as it pierces the connective tissue capsule at the hilum of the spleen. Branches of these vessels, **trabecular arteries,** are conveyed into the substance of the spleen by trabeculae of decreasing sizes (see Fig. 12–10). When the trabecular arteries are reduced to about 0.2 mm in diameter, they leave the trabeculae. The tunica adventitia of these vessels become loosely organized, and they become infiltrated by a sheath of lymphocytes, the **periarterial lymphatic sheath (PALS).** Because the vessel occupies the center of the PALS, it is called the **central artery.**

At its termination, the central artery loses its lymphatic sheath and subdivides into several short, parallel branches, known as **penicillar arteries,** which enter the red pulp. The penicillar arteries have three regions, **pulp arteriole, sheathed arteriole** (a thickened region of the vessel surrounded by a sheath of macrophages, the Schweigger-Seidel sheath), and **terminal arterial capillaries.**

Although it is known that the terminal arterial capillaries deliver their blood into the splenic sinuses, the method of delivery is incompletely understood and has prompted the formulation of three theories of circulation in the spleen: closed circulation, open circulation, and a combination of the two theories.

Proponents of the **closed circulation** theory believe that the endothelial lining of the terminal arterial capillaries is continuous with the sinus endothelium (Fig. 12–12). Investigators who subscribe to the **open circulation** theory believe that the terminal arterial capillaries terminate prior to reaching the sinusoids, and blood from these vessels percolates through the red pulp into the sinuses. Still other investigators believe that some vessels connect to the sinusoids, whereas other vessels terminate as open-ended channels in the red pulp, suggesting that the spleen has both an open and a closed system of circulation.

Splenic sinuses are drained by small **veins of the pulp,** which are tributaries of larger and larger veins that merge to form the **splenic vein,** a tributary of the **portal vein.**

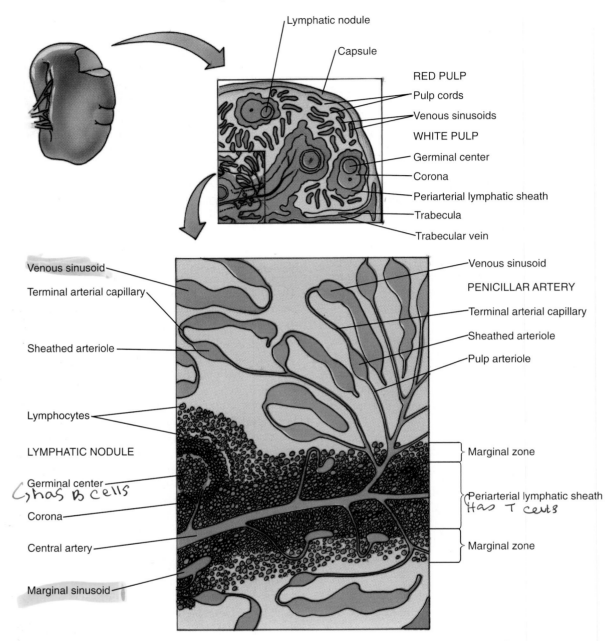

Figure 12–10. Schematic diagram of the spleen. Top, Low-magnification view of white pulp and red pulp. **Bottom,** Higher-magnification view of the central arteriole and its branches.

White Pulp and Marginal Zone

The structure of the **white pulp** is closely associated with the central arteriole. The PALS that surrounds the central arteriole is composed of T lymphocytes. Frequently, enclosed within the PALS are **lymphoid nodules** composed of B cells, displacing the central arteriole to a peripheral position. Lymphoid nodules may display **germinal centers,** indicative of antigenic challenge (see Fig. 12–10; Fig. 12–13). The PALS and lymphoid nodules constitute the white pulp, and as in the lymph node, the T and B cells are stationed in specific locations.

The white pulp is surrounded by a 100-μm-wide **marginal zone** that separates the white pulp from the red pulp (see Figs. 12–10, 12–13; Fig. 12–14). This zone is composed of plasma cells, T and B lymphocytes, macrophages, and **interdigitating dendritic cells** (antigen-presenting cells). Additionally, numerous small vascular channels, **marginal sinuses,** are present in the marginal zone, especially surrounding lymphoid nodules. Slender blood vessels, radiating from the central arteriole, pass into the red pulp, recur, and deliver their blood into the marginal sinuses.

Because the intercellular spaces between the endothelial

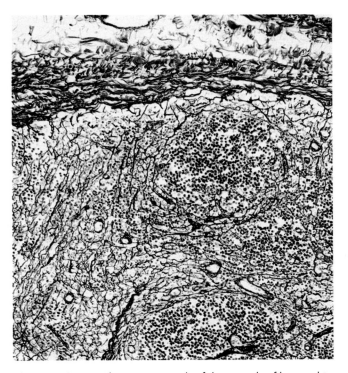

Figure 12–11. Photomicrograph of the reticular fiber architecture of the spleen. Silver stain (× 132).

cells of these sinuses may be as wide as 2 to 3 μm, it is here that bloodborne cells, antigens, and particulate matter have their first free access to the parenchyma of the spleen. Thus the following events occur at the marginal zone:

- Antigen-presenting cells sample the material traveling in blood, searching for antigens
- Macrophages attack microorganisms present in blood
- The circulating pool of T and B lymphocytes leave the

bloodstream to enter their preferred locations within the white pulp

- Lymphocytes come into contact with the interdigitating dendritic cells; in the event that they recognize their epitope–MHC complex, the lymphocytes initiate an immune response within the white pulp

Red Pulp

The **red pulp** of the spleen is composed of splenic sinuses and **splenic cords (of Billroth)** (see Fig. 12–10). The red pulp resembles a sponge in that the spaces within the sponge represent the sinuses and the sponge material among the spaces denotes the splenic cords.

The endothelial lining of **splenic sinuses** is unusual in that its cells are fusiform, resembling staves of a barrel (Fig. 12–15). Moreover, 2- to 3-μm-wide spaces between adjoining cells are common. The sinuses are surrounded by reticular fibers (continuous with those of the splenic cords) that wrap around the sinuses as individual, thin strands of thread. The reticular fibers are arranged perpendicular to the longitudinal axis of the sinuses and are coated by **basal lamina.** Thus splenic sinuses have a discontinuous basal lamina.

The **splenic cords** are composed of a loose network of reticular fibers, whose interstices are permeated by extravasated blood. The reticular fibers are enveloped by **stellate reticular cells,** which isolate the type III collagen fibers from blood, preventing a platelet reaction to the collagen (coagulation). **Macrophages** are particularly numerous in the vicinity of the sinusoids.

Histophysiology of the Spleen

The functions of the spleen, as alluded to during the discussion of its structure, are the filtration of the blood, formation

Figure 12–12. Diagram of open and closed circulation in the spleen.

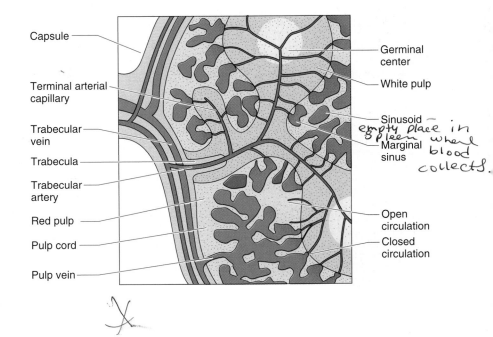

Capsule

Terminal arterial capillary

Trabecular vein

Trabecula

Trabecular artery

Red pulp

Pulp cord

Pulp vein

Germinal center

White pulp

Sinusoid

Marginal sinus

Open circulation

Closed circulation

empty place in spleen where blood collects.

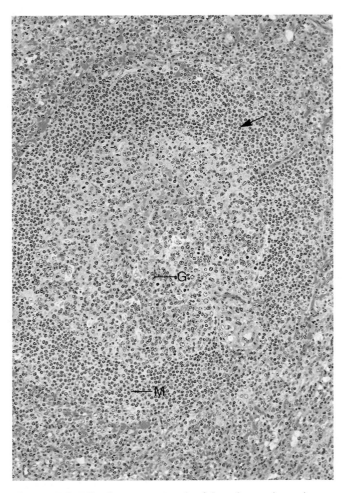

Figure 12-13. Photomicrograph of the white pulp and marginal zone of the spleen (× 132). Germinal center (G); marginal zone (M); central artery (*arrow*).

of lymphoid cells, elimination or inactivation of bloodborne antigens, destruction of erythrocytes, and hemopoiesis.

As blood enters the marginal sinuses of the marginal zone, it flows by a macrophage-rich zone. These cells phagocytose bloodborne antigens, bacteria, and other foreign particulate matter. Material that is not eliminated in the marginal zone is cleared in the red pulp at the periphery of the splenic sinuses.

Lymphoid cells are formed in the white pulp in response to an antigenic challenge. B memory cells and plasma cells are formed in lymphoid nodules, whereas T cells of various subcategories are formed in the PALS. The newly formed B and T cells enter the marginal sinuses and migrate to the site of antigenic challenge or become part of the circulating pool of lymphocytes. Some plasma cells may stay in the marginal zone, manufacture antibodies, and release the immunoglobulins into the marginal sinuses. However, most plasma cells migrate to the bone marrow to manufacture and release their antibodies into the bone marrow sinuses.

Soluble bloodborne antigens are inactivated by the antibodies formed against them, whereas bacteria become **opsonized** and are eliminated by macrophages or neutrophils. Virus-transformed cells are killed by CTLs formed in the PALS of the white pulp.

Macrophages monitor erythrocytes as they migrate from the splenic cords between the endothelial cells into the sinuses (Fig. 12–16). Because older erythrocytes lose their flexibility (as do erythrocytes infected by the malarial parasite), they cannot penetrate the spaces between the endothelial cells and are phagocytosed by macrophages. The phagocytes also monitor the surface coats of red blood cells. Old erythrocytes tend to lose sialic acid residues from their

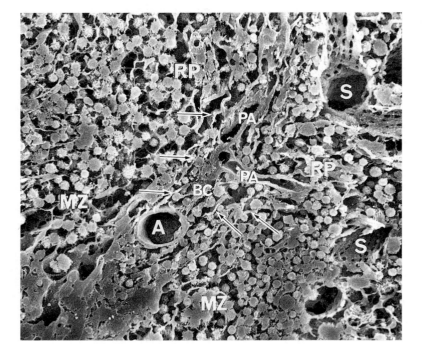

Figure 12-14. Scanning electron micrograph of the marginal zone and adjoining red pulp of the spleen (× 680). A, central artery; MZ, marginal zone; BC, marginal zone bridging channel; RP, red pulp; PA, penicillar artery; S, venous sinus; arrows point to periarterial flat reticular cells. (From Sasou, S., and Sugai, T.: Periarterial lymphoid sheath in the rat spleen: A light, transmission, and scanning electron microscopic study. Anat. Rec. **232:**15–24, 1992. Copyright © 1992. Reprinted by permission of John Wiley & Sons, Inc.)

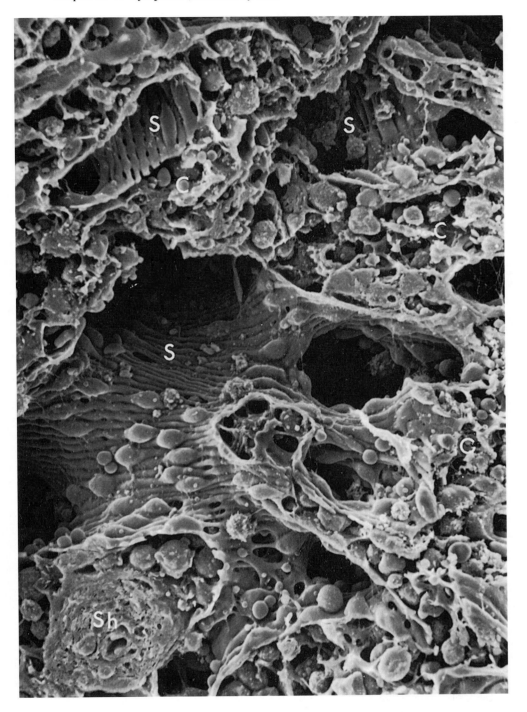

Figure 12–15. Scanning electron micrograph of the sinusoidal lining cells bounded by splenic cords (× 700). S, venous sinuses; C, splenic cords; Sh, sheathed arteriole. (From Leeson, T.S., Leeson, C.R., and Paparo, A.A.: Text/Atlas of Histology. Philadelphia, W.B. Saunders Company, 1988.)

surface macromolecules, exposing galactose moieties, which induce their phagocytosis. Engulfed erythrocytes are destroyed within phagosomes. Hemoglobin is catabolized into its heme and globin portions. The globin moiety is disassembled into its constituent amino acids, which become part of the circulating amino acid pool of the blood. The iron molecules are conveyed to the bone marrow by **transferrin** and are used in the formation of new red blood cells,

whereas the heme is converted to **bilirubin** and excreted by the liver in **bile.** Macrophages are also noted to phagocytose damaged or defunct platelets and neutrophils.

During the second trimester of gestation, the spleen actively participates in hemopoiesis; however, after birth, blood cell formation occurs only in the bone marrow. If the necessity arises, the spleen can resume its hemopoietic function.

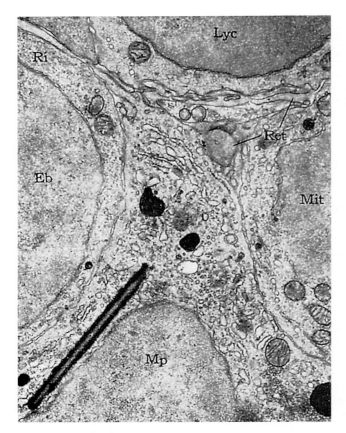

Figure 12–16. Electron micrograph of a macrophage containing phagocytosed materials, including a crystalloid body. Mp, macrophage; Mit, cell undergoing mitosis; Lyc, lymphocyte; Eb, erythroblast; Ri, ribosomes; Ret, reticular fibers in the interstitial spaces. (From Rhodin, J.A.G.: An Atlas of Ultrastructure. Philadelphia, W.B. Saunders Company, 1963.)

CLINICAL CORRELATIONS

Because the spleen is a friable (fragile) organ, major trauma to the upper-left abdominal quadrant may cause rupture of the spleen. In severe cases, the spleen may be removed surgically, without compromising a person's life. Aged red blood cells are then phagocytosed by macrophages of the liver and bone marrow.

Diffuse Lymphoid System

The diffuse lymphoid system is composed of localized lymphocyte infiltration and lymphoid nodules in the mucosa of the gastrointestinal, respiratory, and urinary tracts. These nonencapsulated lymphoid tissues are collectively called **mucosa-associated lymphoid tissue (MALT).** The best depicted of these accumulations are those associated with the mucosa of the gut, gut-associated lymphoid tissue (GALT) and the bronchus-associated lymphatic tissue (BALT).

Gut-Associated Lymphoid Tissue (GALT)

GALT is composed of lymphoid follicles along the length of the gastrointestinal tract. Most of the lymphoid follicles are isolated from each other; however, in the ileum, they form lymphoid aggregates, known as **Peyer's patches.** The lymphoid follicles of Peyer's patches are composed of B cells surrounded by a looser region of T cells and numerous antigen-presenting cells.

Although the ileum is lined by a simple columnar epithelium, the regions immediately adjacent the lymphoid follicles are lined by squamous-like cells, known as **M cells (microfold cells).** It is believed that M cells capture antigens and present their epitopes to lymphocytes of Peyer patches (see Chapter 17 for a more complete discussion).

Peyer's patches have no afferent lymphatic vessels, but they do have efferent lymph drainage. They receive small arterioles that form a capillary bed, drained by high endothelial lined venules (HEVs). Lymphocytes destined to enter Peyer's patches have homing receptors that are specific for the HEVs of gut-associated lymphoid tissue.

Bronchus-Associated Lymphoid Tissue (BALT)

BALT is similar to Peyer's patches, except it is located in the walls of bronchi, especially in regions where bronchi and bronchioles bifurcate. As in GALT, the epithelial cover over these lymphoid nodules changes from a pseudostratified ciliated columnar with goblet cells to **M cells.**

Afferent lymph vessels are absent, although lymph drainage has been demonstrated. The rich vascular supply of BALT indicates its possible systemic as well as localized role in the immune process. Most of the cells are B cells, although antigen-presenting cells and T cells are known to be present. Lymphocytes destined to enter BALT have homing receptors specific for the HEVs of this lymphoid tissue.

Tonsils

The **tonsils** (palatine, pharyngeal, and lingual) are incompletely encapsulated aggregates of lymphoid nodules that guard the entrance to the oral pharynx. Because of their locations, the tonsils are interposed into the path of airborne and ingested antigens. They react to these antigens by forming lymphocytes and mounting an immune response.

Palatine Tonsils

The bilateral **palatine tonsils** are located at the boundary of the oral cavity and the oral pharynx, between the palatoglossal and the palatopharyngeal folds. The deep aspect of each palatine tonsil is isolated from the surrounding connective tissue by a dense, fibrous **capsule.** The superficial aspect of the tonsils is covered by a stratified squamous nonkera-

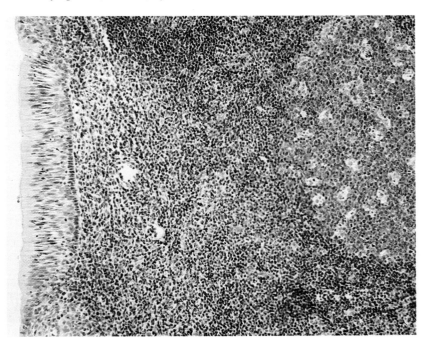

Figure 12–17. Photomicrograph of a lymphoid nodule of the pharyngeal tonsil (× 132).

tinized epithelium that dips into the 10 to 12 deep **crypts** that invaginate the tonsilar parenchyma. The crypts frequently contain desquamated epithelial cells, dead leukocytes, bacteria and other antigenic substances, and food debris.

The parenchyma of the tonsil is composed of numerous lymphoid nodules, many of which display germinal centers, indicative of B cell formation.

Pharyngeal Tonsil

The single **pharyngeal tonsil** is in the roof of the nasal pharynx. It is similar to the palatine tonsils, but its incomplete capsule is thinner. Instead of crypts, the pharyngeal tonsil has shallow, longitudinal infoldings, called **pleats.** Ducts of seromucous glands open into the base of the pleats. Its superficial surface is covered by a pseudostratified ciliated columnar epithelium, interspersed with patches of stratified squamous epithelium (Fig. 12–17).

The parenchyma of the pharyngeal tonsil is composed of lymphoid nodules, with occasional germinal centers. When this tonsil is inflamed, it is called the **adenoid.**

Lingual Tonsils

The **lingual tonsils** are on the dorsal surface of the posterior one third of the tongue. They are several and are covered on their superficial aspect by a stratified squamous nonkeratinized epithelium. The deep aspects of the lingual tonsils have flimsy capsules that separate them from the underlying connective tissue. Each tonsil has a single crypt, whose base receives the ducts of seromucous minor salivary glands.

The parenchyma of the lingual tonsils is composed of lymphoid nodules, which frequently have germinal centers.

Endocrine System

13

The **endocrine system** regulates metabolic activities in certain organs and tissues of the body, thereby helping to bring about homeostasis. The autonomic nervous system regulates certain organs and tissues via impulses that cause release of neurotransmitter substances, which produce rapid responses in the tissues affected. The endocrine system, on the other hand, produces a slow and diffused effect via chemical substances called **hormones,** which are released into the bloodstream to influence target cells at remote sites. Although the nervous and endocrine systems function in different ways, the two interact to modulate and coordinate the metabolic activities of the body.

The **endocrine system** consists of **ductless glands,** distinct clusters of cells within certain organs of the body, and **endocrine cells** isolated in the epithelial lining of the digestive tract and in the respiratory system. The latter are discussed in Chapter 17 and 15, respectively. The **endocrine glands,** the subject of this chapter, are abundantly and richly vascularized so that their secretory product may be released into slender connective tissue spaces between cells and the capillary beds from which they enter the bloodstream. The endocrine glands include the **pituitary, thyroid, parathyroid,** and **suprarenal glands** and the **pineal body.** Unlike the endocrine glands, which are ductless, the various exocrine glands (discussed in other chapters) empty their secretions in a duct system and exert only local effects.

Hormones

Hormones are chemical messengers secreted by endocrine glands and delivered via the bloodstream to their target cells or organs. The chemical nature of a hormone dictates its mechanism of action. Most hormones elicit multiple effects on their target cells (e.g., short-term and long-term effects). Hormones are classified into three types based on their composition:

- **Proteins and polypeptides**—mostly water-soluble (e.g., **insulin, glucagon,** and **follicle-stimulating hormone (FSH)**

- **Amino acid derivatives**—mostly water soluble (e.g., **thyroxine** and **epinephrine)**
- **Steroid and fatty acid derivatives**—mostly lipid soluble (e.g., **progesterone, estradiol,** and **testosterone)**

Once a hormone has been released into the bloodstream and arrived in the vicinity of its target cells, it first binds to specific receptors on (or in) the target cell. Receptors for certain hormones (mostly protein and peptide hormones) are located on the plasmalemma **(cell-surface receptors)** of the target cell, whereas other receptors are located in the cytoplasm and bind only to hormones that have diffused through the plasmalemma. The binding of a hormone to its receptor communicates a message to the target cell, initiating **signal transduction**—that is, translation of the signal into a biochemical reaction.

Thyroid and steroid hormones bind to cytoplasmic receptors. The resulting hormone–receptor complex translocates to the nucleus, where it binds directly to DNA close to a promoter site, thereby stimulating gene transcription. Neither the hormone nor the receptor alone can initiate the target-cell response.

Hormones that bind to cell-surface receptors located in the plasmalemma use several different mechanisms to elicit a response in their target cells. In each instance, the hormone–receptor complex is believed to induce a protein kinase to phosphorylate certain regulatory proteins, thereby generating a biological response to the hormone. For example, some hormone–receptor complexes stimulate adenylate cyclase to synthesize cyclic adenosine monophosphate (cAMP), which stimulates protein kinase A in the cytosol. In this case cAMP acts as a **second messenger.** Several second messengers have been identified, including **guanosine 3', 5'-monophosphate (cGMP), metabolites of phosphatidylinositol, calcium ions,** and **sodium ions** (in neurons).

Some hormone receptors are associated with guanosine triphosphate binding proteins **(G proteins),** which couple the receptor to the hormone-induced responses of the target cells. The receptors for epinephrine, thyroid-stimulating hormone (TSH), and serotonin, for example, utilize G proteins to activate a second messenger, which elicits a metabolic response. Other hormones, such as insulin and growth hormone, employ **catalytic receptors** that activate protein kinases to phosphorylate target proteins.

Once a hormone has activated its target cell, an inhibitory signal is generated and returned to the endocrine gland **(feedback mechanism),** either directly or indirectly, to halt hormone secretion. The feedback mechanism also operates in another way: when the hormone level is inadequate to elicit a sufficient metabolic response in the target, a positive feedback signal is released, which travels to the endocrine gland and initiates an increase in hormone secretion. Thus, through the feedback mechanism, regulation of the endocrine glands maintains homeostasis.

Many of the hormones that circulate in the bloodstream are in oversupply. They are usually bound to plasma proteins, which makes them biologically inactive, but they can be released from their bound state quickly, thus becoming active. Hormones become permanently inactivated in their target tissue; additionally they may be degraded and destroyed in the liver and kidneys.

Pituitary Gland (Hypophysis)

The **pituitary gland,** or **hypophysis,** is an endocrine gland that produces several hormones responsible for regulating growth, reproduction, and metabolism. It has two subdivisions, which develop from different embryologic sources: the **adenohypophysis** develops from an evagination **(Rathke's pouch)** of the oral ectoderm lining the primitive oral cavity (stomodeum); the **neurohypophysis** develops from neural ectoderm as a downgrowth of the diencephalon. Subsequently, both the adenohypophysis and the neurohypophysis are joined and encapsulated into a single organ. But, because each subdivision has a distinctly different embryonic origin, the cellular constituents and the functions of each differ.

The pituitary gland lies below the hypothalamus, to which it is connected extending inferiorly from the diencephalon. It sits in the hypophyseal fossa, a bony depression in the sella turcica of the sphenoid bone that is lined by dura mater and covered over by a portion of the dura called the diaphragma sellae. The gland measures about 1 cm × 1 to 1.5 cm; it is 0.5 cm thick and weighs about 0.5 g in men and slightly more in women.

The pituitary is connected by neural pathways to the brain; it also has a rich vascular supply from vessels supplying the brain, attesting to the intercoordination of the two systems in maintaining a physiological balance. Indeed, secretion of nearly all of the hormones produced by the pituitary gland is controlled by either hormonal or nerve signals from the hypothalamus. It is interesting to note that in addition to controlling the pituitary, the hypothalamus also receives input from various areas of the central nervous system: information regarding plasma circulating levels of electrolytes and hormones, and controls the autonomic nervous system; therefore, it is the brain center for the maintenance of homeostasis.

Within each subdivision of the hypophysis are various regions, with different names, that have specialized cells that release different hormones. The subdivisions of the hypophysis and the named regions of each are as follows (Figs. 13–1, 13–2):

- Adenohypophysis (anterior pituitary)
    Pars distalis (pars anterior)
    Pars intermedia
    Pars tuberalis
- Neurohypophysis (posterior pituitary)
    Median eminence
    Infundibulum
    Pars nervosa

Interposed between the anterior and posterior lobes are remnants of Rathke's pouch (epithelial cells) surrounding an amorphous colloid. The pars tuberalis forms a sleeve around the stem of the infundibulum.

Blood Supply and Control of Secretion

The arterial supply for the pituitary gland is provided from two pairs of vessels arising from the internal carotid artery (see Fig. 13–2). The **superior hypophyseal arteries** supply the pars tuberalis and infundibulum. They also form an extensive capillary network, the **primary capillary plexus,** in the median eminence. **Inferior hypophyseal arteries** supply mostly the posterior lobe, although they send a few branches to the anterior lobe.

Hypophyseal portal veins drain the **primary capillary plexus** of the median eminence, delivering its blood into the **secondary capillary plexus** located in the pars distalis (see Fig. 13–2). The capillaries of both plexuses are fenestrated. **Hypothalamic neurosecretory hormones** manufactured in the hypothalamus and stored in the median eminence enter the primary capillary plexus and are drained by the hypophyseal portal veins, which course through the infundibulum and connect to the secondary capillary plexus in the anterior lobe. Here the neurosecretory hormones leave the blood to stimulate or inhibit the parenchymal cells. Thus, the hypophyseal portal system is the vascular system used for hormonal regulation of the pars distalis by the hypothalamus.

Axons of neurons originating in various portions of the hypothalamus terminate around these capillary plexuses. The endings of these axons are different, because instead of delivering a signal, they release either **releasing** or **inhibiting hormones (factors)** directly into the primary capillary bed. These hormones are immediately taken into the hy-

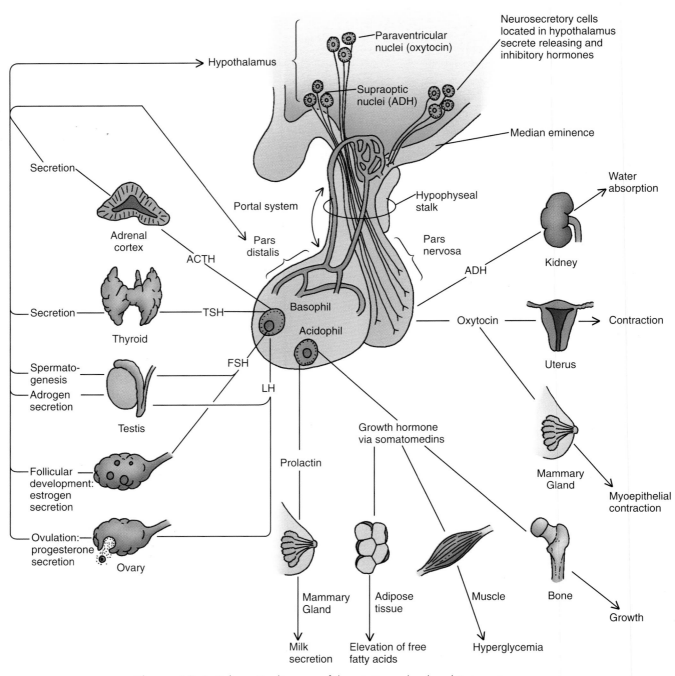

Figure 13–1. Schematic diagram of the pituitary gland and its target organs.

pophyseal portal system and delivered to the pars distalis, where they regulate secretion of various anterior pituitary hormones. The following are the main releasing and inhibitory hormones (factors):

- **Thyroid–stimulating hormone–releasing hormone (TRH)** stimulates release of thyroid-stimulating hormone
- **Corticotropin-releasing hormone (CRH)** stimulates release of adrenocorticotropin
- **Somatotropin (growth hormone–releasing hormone—**

(SRH) stimulates release of somatotropin (growth hormone)
- **Gonadotropin-releasing hormone (GnRH)** stimulates release of luteinizing hormone (**LH**) and follicle-stimulating hormone (**FSH**)
- **Prolactin-releasing hormone (PRH)** stimulates release of prolactin
- **Prolactin inhibitory factor (PIF)** inhibits prolactin secretion

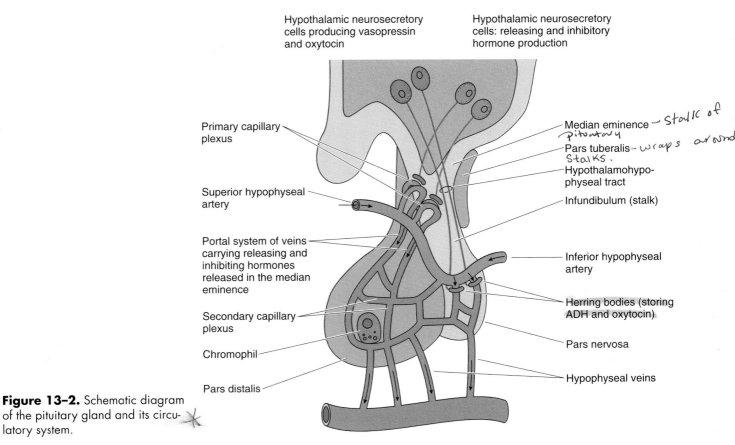

Figure 13–2. Schematic diagram of the pituitary gland and its circulatory system.

The physiological effects of pituitary hormones are summarized in Table 13–1.

Adenohypophysis

As noted already, the anterior pituitary gland, the **adenohypophysis,** develops from Rathke's pouch, a diverticulum of the oral ectoderm.

Pars Distalis

The **pars distalis,** or anterior lobe, is covered by a fibrous capsule and composed of cords of parenchymal cells surrounded by reticular fibers, which also surround the large sinusoidal capillaries. Scant connective tissue is located mostly around the hypophyseal arteries and the portal veins. The endothelial lining of the sinusoids is fenestrated, facilitating the diffusion of releasing factors to the parenchymal cells and providing entry sites for their released secretions. The parenchymal cells of the pars distalis that have an affinity for dyes are called **chromophils**. Those that have no affinity for dyes are called **chromophobes**. Chromophils are further subdivided into **acidophils** (staining with acid dyes) or **basophils** (staining with basic dyes), which constitute the main secretory cells of the pars distalis (Fig. 13–3). It should be remembered, however, that these latter designa-

tions refer to the affinity of the secretory granules within the cells to the dyes, not to the parenchymal cell cytoplasm.

CHROMOPHILS. Acidophils. The most abundant cells in the pars distalis are **acidophils,** whose granules, large enough to be seen by the light microscope, stain orange to red with eosin dye. These small, rounded acidophils are of two kinds: somatotrophs and mammotrophs (Fig. 13–4).

Somatotrophs have a centrally placed nucleus, a moderate Golgi complex, small rod-shaped mitochondria, abundant rough endoplasmic reticulum (RER), and numerous secretory granules 300 to 400 nm in diameter. These cells secrete **somatotropin (growth hormone);** thus they are stimulated by the releasing factor for this hormone **(SRH)** and inhibited by **somatostatin.** Somatotropin has a generalized effect of increasing cellular metabolic rates. This hormone also induces liver cells to produce **stomatomedins,** which stimulate the mitotic rates of epiphyseal plate chondrocytes, thus promoting elongation of long bones and, hence, a person's growth.

Mammotrophs are arranged as individual cells rather than as clumps or clusters. These small, polygonal acidophils have the usual unremarkable organelle population, but during lactation the organelles enlarge and the Golgi complex may become as large as the nucleus. These cells can be distinguished by their large secretory granules,

Table 13-1. Physiological Effects of Pituitary Hormones

Hormones	Releasing/Inhibiting Hormones	Hormone Function
Pars Distalis		
Somatotropin (growth hormone)	*Releasing,* SRH *Inhibiting,* somatostatin	Generalized effect on most cells is to increase metabolic rates, stimulate liver cells to release **somatomedins,** which increases proliferation of cartilage, and assists in growth in long bones
Prolactin	*Releasing,* PRH *Inhibiting,* PIF	Promotes development of mammary glands during pregnancy; stimulates milk production after parturition (prolactin secretion is stimulated by suckling)
Adrenocorticotropic hormone (ACTH) (corticotropin)	*Releasing,* CRH	Stimulates synthesis and release of hormones (cortisol and corticosterone) from suprarenal cortex
Follicle stimulating hormone (FSH)	*Releasing,* GnRH *Inhibiting,* inhibin (in males)	Stimulates secondary ovarian follicle growth and estrogen secretion; stimulates Sertoli cells in seminiferous tubules to produce androgen binding protein
Luteinizing hormone (LH) **Interstitial cell-stimulating hormone (ISCH) in men**	*Releasing,* GnRH	Assists FSH in promoting ovulation, formation of the corpus luteum, and secretion of progesterone and estrogen, forming a negative feedback to the hypothalamus to inhibit GnRH in women; stimulates Leydig cells to secrete and release testosterone, which forms a negative feedback to the hypothalamus to inhibit GnRH in men
Thyroid stimulating hormone (TSH) (thyrotropin)	*Releasing,* TRH *Inhibiting,* negative feedback suppresses via CNS	Stimulates synthesis and release of thyroid hormone, which increases metabolic rate
Pars Nervosa		
Oxytocin		Stimulates smooth muscle contractions of the uterus during orgasm; causes contractions of pregnant uterus at parturition (stimulation of cervix sends signal to hypothalamus to secrete more oxytocin); suckling sends signals to hypothalamus, resulting in more oxytocin, causing contractions of myoepithelial cells of the mammary glands, assisting in milk ejection
Vasopressin (antidiuretic hormone—ADH)		Conserves body water by increasing resorption of water by kidneys; thought to be regulated by osmotic pressure; causes contraction of smooth muscles in arteries, thus raising the blood pressure; may restore normal blood pressure after severe hemorrhage

CNS, central nervous system; CRH, corticotropin-releasing hormone; FSH, follicle stimulating hormone; GnRH, gonadotropin-releasing hormone; PIF, prolactin inhibitory factor; PRH, prolactin-releasing hormone; SRH, somatotropin-releasing hormone; TRH, thyroid-stimulating hormone–releasing hormone.

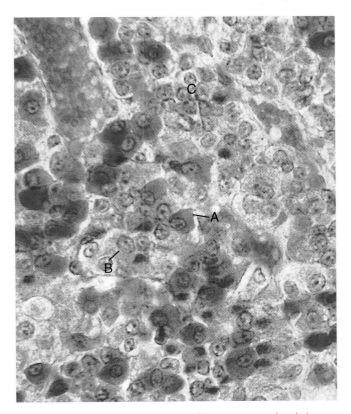

Figure 13–3. Light micrograph of the pituitary gland displaying chromophobes (C), acidophils (A), and basophils (B) (× 540).

formed by the fusion of smaller granules released by the trans-Golgi network. These fused granules, which may be 600 nm in diameter, contain the hormone **prolactin,** which promotes mammary gland development during pregnancy as well as lactation after birth. During pregnancy, circulating estrogen and progesterone inhibit secretion of prolactin. At birth the levels of estrogen and progesterone drop; thus their inhibitory effect is lost. The number of mammotrophs also increases following birth. At the conclusion of nursing, the granules are degraded and the excess mammotrophs regress. Release of prolactin from mammotrophs is stimulated by the releasing factor **(PRH)** and oxytocin, especially when nursing is taking place, and is inhibited by **PIF.**

Basophils. Basophils stain blue with basic dyes (especially with periodic acid–Schiff reagent) and are mostly located at the periphery of the pars distalis (see Fig. 13–3). There are three subtypes of basophils: **corticotrophs, thyrotrophs,** and **gonadotrophs.**

Corticotrophs, which are scattered throughout the pars distalis, are round to ovoid cells with an eccentric nucleus and relatively few organelles. Their secretory granules are 250 to 400 nm in diameter. Corticotrophs secrete **adrenocorticotropic hormone (ACTH)** and **lipotropic hormone (LPH).** Secretion is stimulated by **corticotropin-releasing**

hormone (CRH). The hormone ACTH stimulates cells of the suprarenal cortex to release their secretory products.

Thyrotrophs are deeply embedded within cords of the parenchymal cells at a distance from sinusoids. These cells can be distinguished by their small secretory granules (about 150 nm in diameter), which contain **thyroid-stimulating hormone (TSH),** also known as **thyrotropin.** Secretion is stimulated by **TRH** and inhibited by the presence of thyroxin (T_4) and triiodothyronine (T_3) (thyroid hormones) in the blood.

Gonadotrophs are round cells that have abundant RER and mitochondria and a well-developed Golgi complex. Their secretory granules vary in diameter from 200 to 400 nm. Gonadotrophs, situated near sinuses, secrete **FSH** and **LH;** sometimes the latter is called **interstitial cell–stimulating hormone (ICSH),** because it stimulates steroid hormone production in interstitial cells of the testes. It remains unclear whether there are two subpopulations of gonadotrophs, one secreting FSH and the other LH, or whether both hormones are produced by one cell in different phases of the secretory cycle. Secretion is stimulated by gonadotropin-releasing hormone **(GnRH)** and inhibited by various hormones produced by the ovaries and testes.

CHROMOPHOBES. Groups of small, weakly staining cells in the pars distalis are called **chromophobes** (see Fig. 13–3). These cells generally have less cytoplasm than chromophils and they may represent either nonspecific stem cells or partially degranulated chromophils, although some do retain secretory granules.

FOLLICULOSTELLATE CELLS. Nonsecretory **folliculostellate cells** constitute a large population of cells in the pars distalis. Although their function is not clear, they have been noted to have long processes that form gap junctions with those of other folliculostellate cells. Whether they physically support parenchymal cells of the anterior pituitary or provide a network of intercommunication with each other is not known.

Pars Intermedia

Lying between the pars distalis and the pars nervosa is the **pars intermedia,** characterized by many cuboidal, cell-lined, colloid-containing cysts (Rathke's cysts), which are remnants of the ectoderm of the evaginating Rathke's pouch from the developing oral ectoderm. The pars intermedia sometimes contains basophils in cords along the networks of capillaries. These basophils synthesize the prohormone **proopiomelanocortin,** which undergoes posttranslational cleavage to form α- and β-**melanocyte stimulating hormone (MSH).** Although this hormone stimulates melanin production in lower animals, its function in humans is not understood.

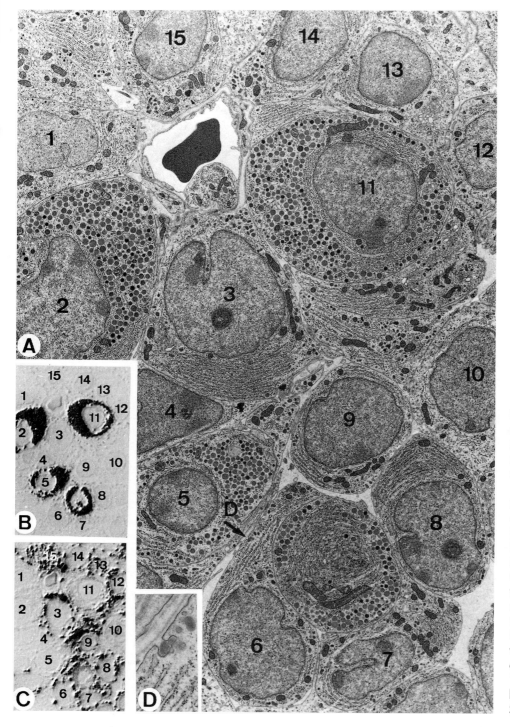

Figure 13–4. Light and electron micrograph of mouse adenohypophysis (× 5000). Observe the mammotropes (cells 3, 6–9, 12–15) and somatotropes (cells 2, 5, 11). Note the secretory granules of these cells. (From Yamaji, A., Sasaki, F., Iwama, Y. and Yamauchi, S.: Mammotropes and somatotropes in the adenophyophysis of androgenized female mice: Morphological and immunohistochemical studies by light microscopy correlated with routine electron microscopy. Anat. Rec. **233:** 103–110, 1992. Reprinted by permission of John Wiley & Sons, Inc.)

Pars Tuberalis

The **pars tuberalis** surrounds the hypophyseal stalk but frequently is absent on its posterior aspect. Thin layers of pia arachnoid–like connective tissue separate the pars tuberalis from the infundibular stalk. The pars tuberalis is highly vascularized by arteries and the hypophyseal portal system, along which lie longitudinal cords of cuboidal to low columnar epithelial cells. The cytoplasm of these basophilic cells contains small dense granules, lipid droplets, occasional colloid droplets, and glycogen. Although no specific hormones are known to be secreted by the pars tuberalis, some cells contain secretory granules that possibly contain **FSH** and **LH**.

Neurohypophysis

The posterior pituitary gland, the **neurohypophysis,** develops from a downgrowth of the hypothalamus. The neurohypophysis is divided into the median eminence, infundibulum (continuation of the hypothalamus), and pars nervosa (see Fig. 13–1).

Hypothalamohypophyseal Tract

Unmyelinated axons of neurosecretory cells whose cell bodies lie in the **supraoptic** and **paraventricular nuclei** of the hypothalamus enter the posterior pituitary to end in the vicinity of the capillaries. These axons form the **hypothalamohypophyseal tract** and constitute the bulk of the posterior pituitary. The neurosecretory cells of the supraoptic and paraventricular nuclei synthesize two hormones: **vasopressin (antidiuretic hormone, ADH)** and **oxytocin.** A carrier protein, **neurophysin,** also produced by the cells of these nuclei, binds to each of these hormones as they travel down the axons to the posterior pituitary, where they are released into the bloodstream from the axon terminals.

Pars Nervosa

The **pars nervosa** of the posterior pituitary gland receives the distal terminals of the axons of the **hypothalamohypophyseal tract** (Fig. 13–5). These axons are supported by glial-like cells known as **pituicytes.** Although only the nuclei of the pituicytes stain well enough for light microscopy, electron micrographs reveal that one population of the nerve terminals contains membrane-bound granules of **vasopressin** and that another population contains **oxytocin.** Special staining for light microscopy (chrome-alumhematoxylin), reveals blue-black–colored distensions of the axons; these are called **Herring bodies,** which represent accumulations of neurosecretory granules (see Fig. 13–5). Herring bodies are observed along the length of the axons, not only at their termini. The contents of these granules are released into the perivascular space near the fenestrated capillaries of the capillary plexus in response to nerve stimulation.

Pituicytes occupy about 25% of the volume of the pars nervosa. They are similar to neuroglial cells and function in supporting the axons of the pars nervosa by ensheathing them as well as their dilations. Pituicytes contain lipid droplets as well as some pigment and intermediate filaments; they have numerous cytoplasmic processes that contact and form gap junctions with each other. Beyond supporting the neural elements in the pars nervosa, additional functions of pituicytes have not been elucidated.

CLINICAL CORRELATIONS

Pituitary adenomas are common tumors of the anterior pituitary gland. Their growth and enlargement may sup-

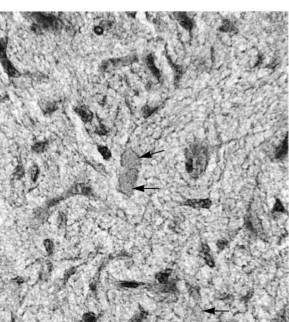

Figure 13–5. Light micrograph of the pars nervosa of the pituitary gland displaying pituicytes and Herring bodies (*arrow*) (× 132).

press hormonal production in other secretory cells of the pars distalis. When left unattended, these adenomas may erode surrounding bone and other neural tissues.

Thyroid Gland

The **thyroid gland,** located in the anterior portion of the neck, secretes the hormones **thyroxine (T_4)** and **triiodothyronine (T_3),** which stimulate metabolic rate. It also secretes **calcitonin,** a hormone that probably aids in controlling blood calcium levels and storage of calcium in bones. Secretion of T_4 and T_3 is under the control of **TSH** secreted by the anterior pituitary gland.

The thyroid gland lies just inferior to the larynx, anterior to the junction of the thyroid and cricoid cartilages (Fig. 13–6). It is composed of **right** and **left lobes** connected across the midline by an **isthmus.** In some persons the gland has an additional **pyramidal lobe** ascending from the left side of the isthmus toward the head. The pyramidal lobe is an embryological remnant of the descent of the thyroid primordia from its origin at the base of the tongue by way of the thyroglossal duct to its final adult resting place.

The gland is surrounded by a slender, dense, irregular collagenous connective tissue capsule, a derivative of the deep cervical fascia. Septa derived from the capsule subdivide the

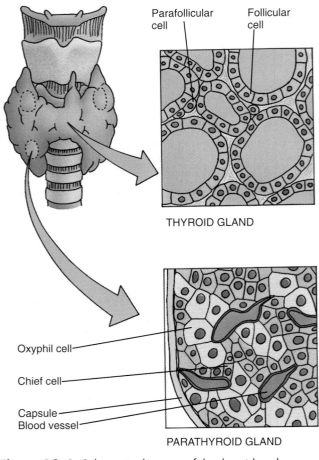

THYROID GLAND

Parafollicular cell

Follicular cell

Oxyphil cell

Chief cell

Capsule
Blood vessel

PARATHYROID GLAND

Figure 13–6. Schematic diagram of the thyroid and parathyroid glands.

gland into lobules. Embedded within the capsule, on the posterior aspect of the gland, are the parathyroid glands.

Cellular Organization

Unlike most of the endocrine glands, which store their secretory substances within the parenchymal cells, the thyroid gland stores its secretory substances in the lumina of **follicles** (Fig. 13–7). These cyst-like structures, ranging from 0.2 to 0.9 mm in diameter, are composed of a simple cuboidal epithelium surrounding a central colloid-filled lumen. Each follicle can hold several weeks' supply of hormone within the **colloid.** The hormones T_4 and T_3 are stored in the colloid bound to a large (660,000 MW) secretory glycoprotein called **thyroglobulin.** When the hormones are to be released, the hormone-bound thyroglobulin is endocytosed and the hormones are cleaved from it by lysosomal proteases.

Connective tissue septa derived from the capsule invade the parenchyma and continue thinning to surround and separate each follicle with a thin connective tissue composed mostly of reticular fibers. The septa also provide a conduit for blood vessels, lymphatic vessels, and nerves. Each follicle is ensheathed in a thin **basal lamina,** some **reticular fibers,** and a **capillary plexus.** Occasionally, follicular cells of neighboring follicles may come into contact with each other without an intervening basal lamina. Most cells constituting the follicle are **follicular cells.** A few **parafollicular cells** also are located at the periphery of the follicles as individual cells or in small clumps.

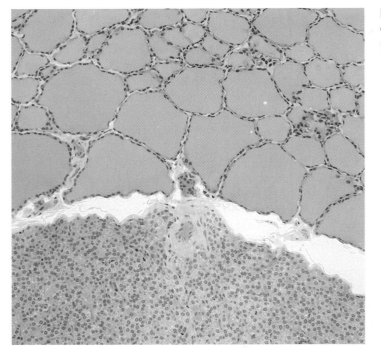

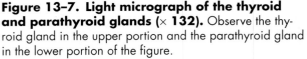

Figure 13–7. Light micrograph of the thyroid and parathyroid glands (× 132). Observe the thyroid gland in the upper portion and the parathyroid gland in the lower portion of the figure.

Follicular Cells (Principal Cells)

Follicular cells range from squamous to low columnar in shape, being tallest when stimulated. These cells have a round to ovoid nucleus with two nucleoli, basophilic cytoplasm, distended RER with zones that are ribosome-free, numerous apically located lysosomes, rod-shaped mitochondria, a supranuclear Golgi complex, and numerous short villi extending into the colloid (Fig. 13–8). Numerous small vesicles, dispersed throughout the cytoplasm, are thought to contain thyroglobulin packaged in the Golgi and destined for exocytosis into the follicle lumen. **Iodide** is essential for the synthesis of the thyroid hormones (T_3 and T_4); iodination of tyrosine residues occurs in the follicles.

During great demand for thyroid hormone, follicular cells extend pseudopods into the follicles to envelop the colloid, which is absorbed. When demand declines, colloid accumulates.

Parafollicular Cells (Clear Cells, C Cells)

The pale-staining **parafollicular cells** lie in clusters or singly within the epithelium, but they do not reach the lumen of the follicle. Although these cells are two to three times larger than follicular cells, they account for only about 0.1% of the epithelium. They have a round nucleus, moderate RER, elongated mitochondria, a well-developed Golgi complex, and small dense secretory granules (0.1 to 0.4 μm in diameter), which accumulate in the basal cytoplasm and are clearly displayed only in electron micrographs. These granules contain **calcitonin (thyrocalcitonin),** a peptide hormone that inhibits bone resorption by osteoclasts, thereby lowering calcium concentrations in blood. When the circulating level of calcium is high, release of calcitonin is stimulated.

Synthesis and Release of Thyroid Hormones (T_3 and T_4)

Figure 13–9 outlines the pathway for synthesis and release of thyroid hormones. Thyroglobulin is synthesized on the RER and subsequently glycosylated in both the RER and the Golgi apparatus. The modified protein is packaged in the trans-Golgi network. The vesicles containing thyroglobulin are transported to the apical plasmalemma, where their contents are released into the colloid and stored in the lumen of the follicle.

Iodide is actively transported via iodide pumps located in the basal plasmalemma of the follicular cells into the cytosol, where it is oxidized by the enzyme **thyroid peroxidase.** The activated iodide enters the colloid and iodinates tyrosine residues of thyroglobulin at the interface of the colloid and the apical plasmalemma of the thyroid follicular cell.

TSH, released from the basophils of the anterior pituitary, binds to TSH receptors on the basal plasmalemma of the follicular cells. Binding of TSH facilitates formation of filopodia at the apical cell membrane, resulting in endocytosis of aliquots of the colloid. Cytoplasmic vesicles containing colloid fuse with early (or late) endosomes. Within the endosomes, iodinated residues are cleaved from thyroglobulin by

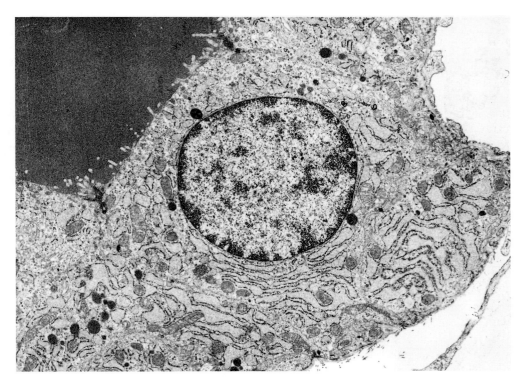

Figure 13–8. Electron micrograph of a thyroid follicular cell bordering the colloid (the black area in the upper left hand corner) (× 11,600). (From Mestdagh, C., Many, M.C., Haalpern, S., Briancon, C., Fragu, P., and Denef, J.F.: Correlated autoradiographic and ion-microscopic study of the role of iodine in the formation of "cold" follicles in young and old mice. Cell Tiss. Res. **260:**449–457, 1990. © Springer-Verlag.)

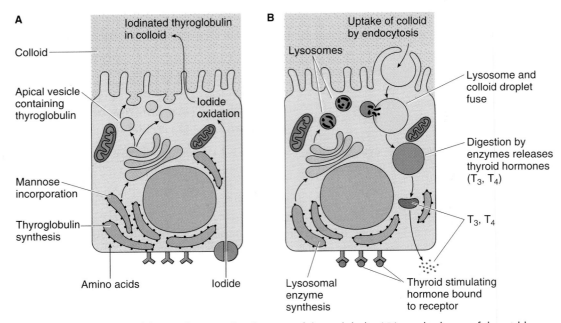

Figure 13–9. Schematic diagram of the synthesis and iodination of thyroglobulin **(A),** and release of thyroid hormone **(B).**

proteases and are transferred into the cytosol as free mono-iodotyrosine, diiodotyrosine, T_3 and T_4.

Monoiodotyrosine and diiodotyrosine are stripped of their iodine by the enzyme **iodotyrosine dehaloginase,** and both the iodine and the amino acid tyrosine become part of their respective pools within the cytosol for later use.

T_3 and T_4 are released at the basal plasmalemma of the follicular cells, entering the connective tissue spaces of the thyroid for distribution by the bloodstream. T_4 constitutes about 90% of the released hormone, although it is not as effective as T_3.

Physiological Effects of T_3 and T_4

Once released into the blood, T_4 and T_3 bind to plasma-binding proteins and are released to the tissues slowly, especially T_4. Only half of what is released into the blood is taken up by the tissues in 6 days. Once in the tissues, the hormone is once again bound to intracellular proteins and slowly used over several days to weeks.

These hormones stimulate transcription of many genes encoding various kinds of proteins. As a result, these hormones induce a generalized increase in cellular metabolism up to 100%. They also increase the growth rate in the young, facilitate mental processes, and stimulate endocrine gland activity.

Generally, the thyroid hormones stimulate carbohydrate metabolism. They decrease synthesis of cholesterol, phospholipids, and triglycerides, but they increase synthesis of fatty acids. Because thyroid hormones increase synthesis of various enzymes, more vitamins are required when thyroid hormone levels are increased. Increased thyroid hormone

production also decreases body weight and increases heart rate, metabolism, respiration, muscle function, and appetite. Excessive amounts of thyroid hormone cause muscle tremor, tiredness, and impotence in men and frequent and excessive menstrual bleeding in women.

CLINICAL CORRELATIONS

Graves' disease is characterized by hyperplasia of the follicular cells, increasing the size of the thyroid gland two to three times above normal. Thyroid hormone production is also greatly increased from 5 to 15 times normal (**hyperthyroidism**). Other symptoms include **exophthalmos,** or protrusion of the eyeballs. Although Graves' disease may develop from several causes, the most common agent is the binding of autoimmune IgG antibodies to TSH receptors, stimulating thyroid follicular cells.

Insufficient dietary intake of iodine will cause the thyroid gland to enlarge, a condition called **simple goiter.** It usually is not associated with hyperthyroidism or hypothyroidism. This condition can be treated with iodine in the diet.

Hypothyroidism is characterized by such conditions as fatigue, sleeping for up to 14 to 16 hours a day, muscular sluggishness, slowed heart rate, decreased cardiac output and blood volume, mental sluggishness, failure of body functions, constipation, and loss of hair growth. Those with severe hypothyroidism may develop **myxedema,** characterized by bagginess under the eyes and a swollen face due to nonpitting edema of the skin caused by infiltration of excess glycosaminoglycans and proteoglycans into the tissue spaces. **Cretinism** is an extreme form of hypothyroidism in fetal life through childhood characterized by failure of growth and mental retardation due to a congenitally missing thyroid gland.

The nerves supplying the laryngeal musculature (i.e., external laryngeal and recurrent laryngeal nerves) are closely applied to the thyroid gland and must be isolated and protected during **thyroidectomy.** Damage to either of these two nerves results in hoarseness and possibly loss of speech.

Parathyroid Glands

The **parathyroid glands,** usually four in number, are located on the posterior surface of the thyroid gland, each enveloped in its own thin, collagenous connective tissue capsule (see Fig. 13–6). The glands function in producing **parathyroid hormone (PTH),** which acts on bone, kidneys, and the intestines in maintaining the optimal concentrations of calcium within the interstitial tissue fluid.

Normally, one parathyroid gland is located on each pole (superior and inferior) of the right and left lobes of the thyroid gland. Because of their embryological origin and descent in the neck with the primordium of the thymus and thyroid tissues, however, parathyroid glands may be located anywhere along the pathway of descent, even into the thorax, and there may be supernumerary glands.

The parathyroid glands develop from the third and fourth pharyngeal pouches of the pharyngeal arch (branchial arch) formation during embryogenesis. The parathyroid glands that develop in the third pharyngeal pouches descend with the thymus, which also develops in the third pouches, to become the inferior parathyroid glands. The parathyroid glands that develop in the fourth pharyngeal pouches descend only a short distance to become the superior parathyroid glands. The glands grow slowly, reaching the adult size at about 20 years of age.

Parathyroid Cellular Organization

Each parathyroid gland is a small ovoid structure that is about 5 mm in length, 4 mm wide, and 2 mm in thickness and weighs about 25 to 50 mg. Extensions of the connective tissue capsule enter the gland as septa, accompanied by blood vessels, lymphatics, and nerves. The septa serve mostly to support the parenchyma, consisting of cords or clusters of epithelial cells surrounded by reticular fibers, which also support the parenchyma and a rich capillary network. The connective tissue stroma in older adults often contains several to many adipose cells, which may occupy up to 60% of the gland in elderly persons. The parenchyma of the parathyroid glands is composed of two cell types: **chief cells** and **oxyphil cells** (see Fig. 13–7).

Chief Cells

The major functional parenchymal cells of the parathyroid glands are the slightly eosinophilic-staining **chief cells** (5 to

8 μm in diameter), which contain granules of lipofuscin pigment scattered throughout the cytoplasm. Smaller dense granules, 200 to 400 nm in diameter, arising from the Golgi and moving to the cell periphery, represent the secretory granules containing **parathyroid hormone.** Electron micrographs also reveal a juxtanuclear Golgi complex, elongated mitochondria, and abundant RER. Occasionally, desmosomes join adjacent chief cells. A single cilium may extend into the intercellular space. Some chief cells have a smaller Golgi complex, scant secretory granules, and large amounts of glycogen; these cells are thought to be in an inactive phase.

The precursor of **preproparathyroid hormone** is synthesized on ribosomes of the RER and rapidly cleaved as it is transported to the lumen of the RER to form **proparathyroid hormone** and a polypeptide. On reaching the Golgi, the proparathyroid hormone is cleaved again into PTH and a small polypeptide. The hormone is packaged into secretory granules and released from the cell surface by exocytosis.

Oxyphil Cells

The second cell type located in the parathyroid glands are the **oxyphil cells.** Their function is unknown, although it is believed that oxyphil cells and a third cell, described as an **intermediate cell,** probably represent inactive phases of a single cell type, with chief cells being the actively secreting phase.

Oxyphil cells are less numerous, larger (6 to 10 μm in diameter) and more deeply stained with eosin than chief cells. Oxyphils appear in groups and as single cells. They possess more abundant mitochondria than chief cells, but their Golgi apparatus is small and there is little RER. Glycogen is also located in the cytosol surrounded by mitochondria.

Physiological Effect of Parathyroid Hormone

PTH, produced by chief cells of the parathyroid glands, helps to maintain the proper extracellular fluid concentration of calcium ions (8.5 to 10.5 mg/100 ml). This hormone acts on cells of the bones, kidneys, and indirectly on the intestines, leading to an increase in the calcium ion concentration in body fluids. When calcium ion concentration in body fluids falls below normal, the chief cells increase their production and release of PTH, quickly increasing their normal secretion rate tenfold. This rapid response is especially important because of the many functions that calcium has in homeostasis, including its role in stabilizing ion gradients across the plasmalemmae of muscle and nerve cells and its role in the release of neurotransmitter at axon terminals.

Note that the interplay of PTH and calcitonin represents a dual mechanism for regulating calcium levels in the blood. PTH acts to increase calcium levels in the serum, whereas calcitonin has the opposite effect.

In bone, PTH binds to receptors on osteoblasts, signaling

the cells to increase their secretion of **osteoclast-stimulating factor.** This factor induces activation of these cells, thereby increasing bone resorption and the ultimate release of calcium ions into the blood (see Chapter 7). In the kidneys, PTH prevents loss of calcium in the urine. Finally, PTH controls the rate of calcium uptake in the gastrointestinal tract. It does this by indirectly regulating the production of vitamin D in the kidneys; vitamin D is necessary for intestinal uptake of calcium.

CLINICAL CORRELATIONS

A condition called **primary hyperparathyroidism,** which may be caused by a tumor in one of the parathyroid glands, is marked by high blood calcium, low blood phosphate, loss of bone mineral, and sometimes kidney stones. **Secondary hyperparathyroidism** may develop in patients with **rickets,** because calcium cannot be absorbed from the intestines due to vitamin D deficiency; therefore, these patients have a low calcium ion concentration in the blood.

Hypoparathyroidism results from deficiency in secretion of PTH, commonly due to injury of the parathyroid glands or their removal during thyroid gland surgery. This condition is marked by low blood calcium levels, retention of bone calcium, and increased phosphate resorption in the kidney. The main symptoms are numbness, tingling, **carpopedal spasms** (muscle cramps) in the hands and feet, **muscle tetany** (tremors) in the facial and laryngeal muscles, mental confusion, and memory loss. The only treatment for survival is large intravenous doses of calcium gluconate, much vitamin D, and oral calcium.

Suprarenal (Adrenal) Glands

The **suprarenal glands** are located at the superior poles of the kidneys embedded in adipose tissue. The right and left suprarenal glands are not mirror images of each other. Rather, the right suprarenal gland is pyramid-shaped and sits directly on top of the right kidney, whereas the left suprarenal gland is more crescent-shaped and lies along the medial border of the left kidney from the hilus to its superior pole.

Both glands are about 1 cm in thickness, 2 cm in width at the apex, and up to 5 cm at the base; each weighs 7 to 10 g. The parenchyma of the gland is divided into two histologically and functionally different regions: an outer yellowish portion, accounting for about 80% to 90% of the organ, called the **suprarenal cortex,** and a small, dark, inner portion called the **suprarenal medulla** (Fig. 13–10). Although both entities are endocrine in function, each develops from a different embryological origin and performs a different function. The **suprarenal cortex** produces a group of hormones called **corticosteroids,** which are synthesized from **cholesterol.** Secretion of these hormones, namely **cortisol** and **corticosterone,** is regulated by **ACTH,** a hormone secreted by the anterior pituitary gland. The **suprarenal**

medulla is functionally related to and regulated by the sympathetic nervous system; it produces the hormones **epinephrine** and **norepinephrine.**

The suprarenal glands are retroperitoneal, located behind the peritoneum and surrounded by a connective tissue capsule containing large amounts of adipose tissue. Each gland has a thick capsule of connective tissue that sends septa into the parenchyma of the gland accompanied by blood vessels and nerves.

Blood Supply to the Suprarenal Gland

The suprarenal glands have one of the richest blood supplies in the body (Fig. 13–11). Each suprarenal gland is supplied by three separate arteries arising from three separate sources: the **inferior phrenic arteries,** from which the **superior suprarenal arteries** originate; the **aorta,** from which the **middle suprarenal arteries** originate; and the **renal arteries,** from which the **inferior suprarenal arteries** originate. These branches pass over the capsule, penetrate it, and form a **subcapsular plexus.** Arising from the plexus are **short cortical arteries,** which form a network of sinusoidal fenestrated capillaries (with diaphragms in the cortical parenchyma). The pore diameters of the fenestrated endothelial walls of the capillaries increase from 100 nm at the outer cortex to 250 nm in the deep cortex, where the sinusoidal capillaries become confluent with a venous plexus. Small venules arising from this area pass through the suprarenal medulla and drain into a suprarenal vein, emerging from the hilus. The right joins the inferior vena cava, whereas the left drains into the left renal vein. Additional **long cortical arteries** pass unbranched through the cortex and into the medulla, where they form networks of capillaries. Thus the medulla receives a dual blood supply, an arterial supply from the long cortical arteries and numerous vessels from the cortical capillary beds.

Suprarenal Cortex

The **suprarenal cortex** contains parenchymal cells that synthesize and secrete several steroid hormones without storing them. The cortex, developed from mesoderm, is subdivided histologically into three concentric zones; named from the capsule inward, they are the **zona glomerulosa, zone fasciculata,** and **zona reticularis** (see Fig. 13–10; Fig. 13–12).

The three classes of adrenocortical hormones—**mineralocorticoids, glucocorticoids,** and **androgens**—are all synthesized from **cholesterol.** The major component of **low-density lipoprotein,** cholesterol is taken up from the blood and stored esterified in lipid droplets within the cytoplasm of the cortical cells. When these cells are stimulated, cholesterol is freed and utilized in hormone synthesis in the smooth endoplasmic reticulum (SER) by enzymes located there as well as in the mitochondria. The intermediate products of the hormone being synthesized are transferred between the SER and mitochondria until the final hormone is produced.

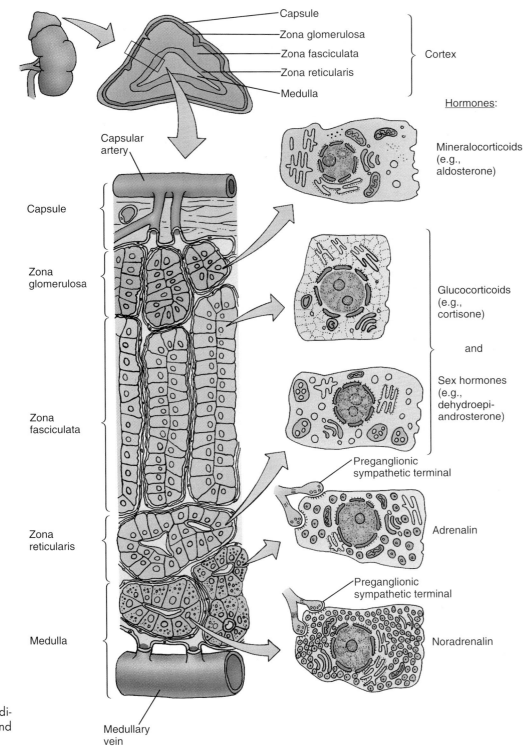

Figure 13–10. Schematic diagram of the suprarenal gland and its cell types.

Zona Glomerulosa

The outer concentric ring of capsular parenchymal cells just beneath the suprarenal capsule is the **zona glomerulosa,** constituting about 13% of the total adrenal volume (see Fig. 13–10). The small columnar cells composing this zone are arranged in cords and clusters. Their small, dark-staining nuclei contain one or two nucleoli, and their acidophilic cytoplasm contains an abundant and extensive SER, short mitochondria with shelf-like cristae, a well-developed Golgi complex, abundant RER, and free ribosomes. Some lipid droplets also are dispersed in the cytoplasm. Occasional desmosomes and small gap junctions join cells to each other, and some cells have short microvilli.

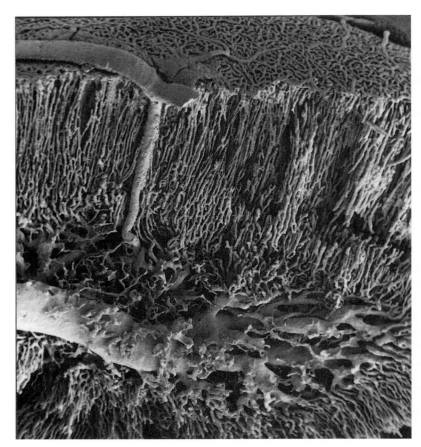

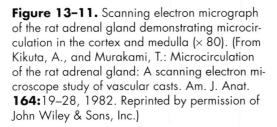

Figure 13–11. Scanning electron micrograph of the rat adrenal gland demonstrating microcirculation in the cortex and medulla (× 80). (From Kikuta, A., and Murakami, T.: Microcirculation of the rat adrenal gland: A scanning electron microscope study of vascular casts. Am. J. Anat. **164:**19–28, 1982. Reprinted by permission of John Wiley & Sons, Inc.)

The parenchymal cells of the zona glomerulosa synthesize and secrete the **mineralocorticoid hormones,** mostly **aldosterone** and some **deoxycorticosterone.** Synthesis of these hormones is stimulated by **angiotensin II** and **ACTH,** both of which are required for normal existence of glomerulosa cells. The mineralocorticoid hormones function in controlling fluid and electrolyte balance in the body by affecting the function of the renal tubules (see Chapter 19).

Zona Fasciculata

The intermediate concentric layer of cells in the suprarenal cortex is the **zona fasciculata,** the largest layer of the cortex, accounting for up to 80% of the total volume of the gland. This zone contains sinusoidal capillaries arranged longitudinally between the columns of parenchymal cells. The polyhedral cells in this layer are larger than the cells of the zona glomerulosa and are arranged in radial columns, one to two layers thick, and stain lightly acidophilic. Because they have many lipid droplets in their cytoplasm, which are extracted during histological processing, these cells appear vacuolated and are called **spongiocytes.** These cells have spherical mitochondria with tubular and vesicular cristae, extensive networks of SER, some RER, lysosomes, and granules of lipofuscin pigment.

Cells of the zona fasciculata synthesize and secrete the **glucocorticoid hormones—cortisol** and **corticosterone.** The synthesis of these hormones is stimulated by ACTH. Glucocorticoids function in the control of carbohydrate, fat, and protein metabolism.

Zona Reticularis

The innermost layer of the suprarenal cortex is the **zona reticularis,** constituting about 7% of gland volume. The darkly staining acidophilic cells in this layer are arranged in anastomosing cords. They are similar to the spongiocytes of the zona fasciculata, but smaller and with fewer lipid droplets. They frequently contain large amounts of lipofuscin pigment granules. Several cells near the suprarenal medulla are dark with electron-dense cytoplasm and pyknotic nuclei, suggesting that this zone contains degenerating parenchymal cells.

Cells of the zona reticularis synthesize and secrete **androgens,** mostly **dehydroepiandrosterone** and some **androstenedione.** Additionally, these cells of the zona reticularis may synthesize and secrete small amounts of glucocorticoids. The secretion of these hormones is stimulated by ACTH. Both dehydroepiandrosterone and androstenedione are weak masculinizing hormones with negligible effects under normal conditions.

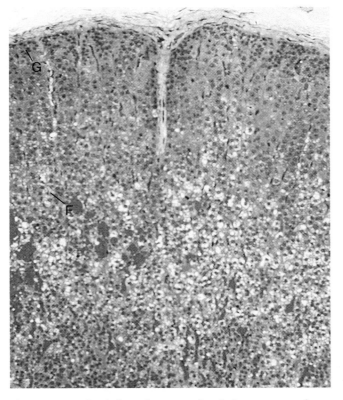

Figure 13–12. Light micrograph of the cortex of the suprarenal gland (× 132). Observe the zona glomerulosa (G) and the zona fasciculata (F).

CLINICAL CORRELATIONS

Addison's disease is characterized by decreased secretion of the adrenocortical hormones due to destruction of the suprarenal cortex. This disease is most often caused by an autoimmune disease; it also can develop as a sequela of tuberculosis or from some other infectious diseases. Death will occur if steroid treatment is not provided.

Cushing's disease (hyperadrenocorticism) is caused by small tumors in the basophils of the anterior pituitary gland that lead to an increase in the output of **ACTH.** The excess ACTH causes enlargement of the suprarenal glands and hypertrophy of the suprarenal cortex, resulting in overproduction of cortisol. Individuals with this disease are obese, mostly in the face, neck, and trunk. Males become impotent and females have amenorrhea.

Suprarenal Medulla

The central portion of the suprarenal gland is the **suprarenal medulla,** which is completely invested by the suprarenal cortex. The suprarenal medulla, which develops from ectodermal neural crest cells, comprises two populations of parenchymal cells: **chromaffin cells** (Fig. 13–13), which produce the **catecholamines (epinephrine and norepinephrine),** and **sympathetic ganglion cells,** which are scattered throughout the connective tissue.

Chromaffin Cells

Chromaffin cells of the suprarenal medulla are large epithelioid cells, arranged in clusters or short cords, that contain granules that stain intensely with chromaffin salts. The reac-

Figure 13–13. Light micrograph of the medulla of the suprarenal gland (× 270). Note the chromaffin cells.

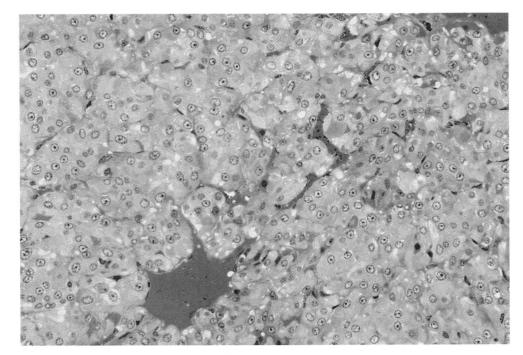

tion of the granules, which turn deep brown when exposed to chromaffin salts, indicates that the cells contain **catecholamines,** transmitters produced by postganglionic cells of the sympathetic nervous system. Thus, the suprarenal medulla functions as a modified sympathetic ganglion, housing postganglionic sympathetic cells that lack dendrites and axons. The catecholamines synthesized by the chromaffin cells are the sympathetic transmitters, **epinephrine** and **norepinephrine.** These transmitters are secreted by the chromaffin cells in response to stimulation by **preganglionic sympathetic (cholinergic) splanchnic nerves.**

Two types of chromaffin cells have been identified via histochemical staining: those producing and storing **norepinephrine** and those producing and storing **epinephrine.**

The granules of the norepinephrine-storing cells have an eccentric electron-dense core within the limiting membrane of the granule, whereas the granules of those chromaffin cells storing epinephrine are more homogeneous and less dense (Fig. 13–14). Both types of chromaffin cells have a well-developed juxtanuclear Golgi complex, some RER, and numerous mitochondria. The identifying characteristic of the chromaffin cells are the 30,000 or so small, membrane-bound, dense granules in the cytoplasm; about 20% of these granules contain either epinephrine or norepinephrine, but not both. The remaining granules are composed of soluble proteins called **chromagranins,** along with **adenosine triphosphate** and **enkephalins.** Chromagranins are proteins that are believed to bind epinephrine and norepinephrine.

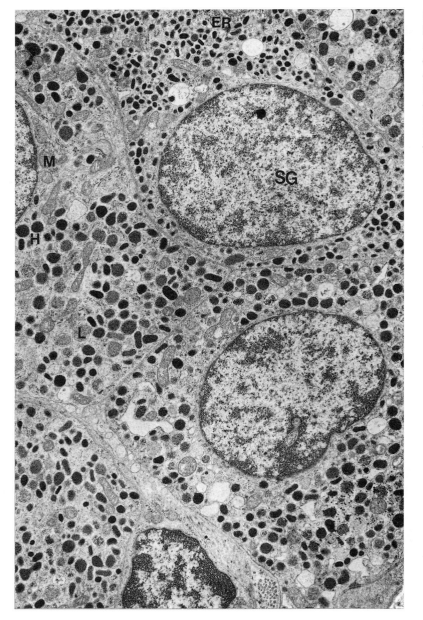

Figure 13–14. Electron micrograph of baboon adrenal medulla (× 14,000). SG, small granule cell; H, high–electron-density vesicle; L, low–electron-density vesicle; M, mitochondrion; ER, endoplasmic reticulum. (From Al-Lami, F., and Carmichael, S.W.: Microscopic anatomy of the baboon *(Papio hamadryas)* adrenal medulla. J. Anat. **178:**213–221, 1991. Reprinted with the permission of Cambridge University Press.)

Histophysiology of the Suprarenal Medulla

The secretory activity of the suprarenal medulla is controlled by the hypothalamus via the splanchnic nerves. Release of the aggregated catecholamines from chromaffin cells is induced by stimulation of the sympathetic ganglion cells in the suprarenal medulla. Release of acetylcholine from these preganglionic sympathetic nerve endings depolarizes the chromaffin cell membranes, leading to an influx of calcium ions. The rise in intracellular calcium then induces release of secretory granules containing epinephrine or norepinephrine via exocytosis. Because the relative amounts of the two catecholamines released at any one time is not constant, it is believed that the epinephrine-producing cells and norepinephrine-producing cells are separately innervated. Indeed, when the stimulus is derived from an emotional source, secretion of norepinephrine predominates, whereas epinephrine secretion predominates when the stimulus is, for example, pain.

In severe fear or stress, increased epinephrine is released to prepare the body for "fight or flight." The resulting plasma levels of epinephrine, up to 300 times the normal level, increase alertness, cardiac output and heart rate, and release of glucose from the liver for energy.

Epinephrine is most effective in controlling cardiac output, heart rate, and increasing blood flow through organs, whereas norepinephrine has little effect on these but effects an elevation in blood pressure by vasoconstriction.

Norepinephrine is produced also in the brain and in peripheral nerves, functioning as a neurotransmitter; however, norepinephrine produced in the suprarenal medulla has a short half-life because it is destroyed in the liver shortly after its release.

Pineal Gland

The **pineal gland** (also known as the **pineal body**) is an endocrine gland whose secretions are influenced by the light and dark periods of the day. It is a conically shaped midline projection from the roof of the diencephalon with a recess of the third ventricle extending into the stalk attaching to it. It is 5 to 8 mm in length and 3 to 5 mm in width; it weighs about 120 mg. The gland is covered by pia mater forming a capsule from which septa extend, dividing the pineal gland into incomplete lobules. Blood vessels enter the gland via the connective tissue septa. The parenchymal cells of the gland are composed primarily of **pinealocytes** and **interstitial cells.**

Pinealocytes

Pinealocytes are slightly basophilic cells with one or two long processes whose terminal dilations approximate capillaries and occasionally other parenchymal cells. Their spherical nuclei have a single prominent nucleolus. The cytoplasm contains SER and RER, a small Golgi apparatus, numerous mitochondria, and small secretory vesicles, some with electron-dense cores. Pinealocytes also contain a well-developed cytoskeleton composed of microtubules, microfilaments, and dense tubular structures invested by spherical vesicular elements. These unusual structures, known as **synaptic ribbons,** increase in number during the dark period of the diurnal cycle, but their function is not understood.

The pineal gland produces **melatonin** and several other substances (e.g., serotonin), which may influence reproduction. It is interesting to note that melatonin is secreted at night, whereas serotonin is produced during the day.

CLINICAL CORRELATIONS

Recent evidence has shown that melatonin, which freely enters the brain tissue, may act to protect the central nervous system by its ability to scavenge and eliminate free radicals produced during oxidative stress.

Interstitial Cells

Interstitial cells, believed to be astrocyte-like neuroglia cells, are scattered about the pinealocytes and are particularly abundant in the pineal stalk leading to the diencephalon. These cells have deeply staining, elongated nuclei and well-developed rough endoplasmic reticulum; some have deposits of glycogen. Their long cellular processes are rich in intermediate filaments, microtubules, and microfilaments.

The pineal gland also contains concretions of calcium phosphates and carbonates deposited in concentric rings around an organic matrix. These structures, called **corpora arenacea (brain sand),** appear in early childhood and increase in size throughout life. Although it is unclear how they are formed or function, it is known that they do increase during short photoperiods, and they are reduced as the pineal gland is actively secreting.

Histophysiology of the Pineal Gland

The pineal gland is innervated by **postganglionic sympathetic nerves** from the superior cervical ganglion in the neck. As the axons enter the gland, their myelin is lost and they synapse on the pinealocytes. **Norepinephrine** released at the pinealocytes controls production of **melatonin.** It is interesting to note that melatonin is released into the connective tissue spaces to be distributed by blood vessels, whereas serotonin is taken up by presynaptic axon terminals.

Recent research on the pineal gland has focused on the pineal hormones and their functions. Synthesis of pineal hormones exhibits a diurnal rhythm in that it is increased during dark periods and inhibited during light periods.

Table 13–2 identifies the hormones and secretory cells of the thyroid, parathyroid, adrenal, and pineal glands and summarizes their functions.

Table 13–2. Summary of Hormones, Cells of Origin, Regulating Hormones, and Functions of the Thyroid, Parathyroid, Adrenal, and Pineal Glands

Hormone	Cell Source	Regulating Hormone	Function
Thyroid Gland			
Thyroxine (T_4) Triiodothyronine (T_3)	Follicular cells	Thyroid stimulating hormone (TSH)	Nuclear transcription of genes responsible for protein synthesis; increased cellular metabolism, growth rates; facilitate mental processes; increase in endocrine gland activity; stimulates carbohydrate and fat metabolism; decreases cholesterol, phospholipids, and triglycerides; increases fatty acids; decreases body weight; increases heart rate, respiration, muscle action
Calcitonin (thyrocalcitonin)	Parafollicular cells	Feedback mechanism with parathyroid hormone	Lowers plasma calcium concentration by suppressing bone resorption
Parathyroid Gland			
Parathyroid hormone (PTH)	Chief cells	Feedback mechanism with calcitonin	Increases calcium concentration in body fluids
Suprarenal (Adrenal) Glands			
Suprarenal Cortex Mineralocorticoids: aldosterone and deoxycorticosterone	Cells of the zona glomerulosa	Angiotensin II and adrenocorticotropic hormone (ACTH)	Controls body fluid volume and electrolyte concentrations by acting on distal tubules of the kidney, causing excretion of potassium and resorption of sodium
Glucocorticoids: cortisol and corticosterone	Cells of the zona fasciculata (spongiocytes)	Adrenocorticotropic hormone (ACTH)	Regulates metabolism of carbohydrates, fats, and proteins; decreases protein synthesis—increasing amino acids in blood; stimulates gluconeogenesis by activating liver to convert amino acids to glucose; releases fatty acid and glycerol; acts as an anti-inflammatory; reduces capillary permeability; suppresses immune response
Androgens: dehydroepiandrosterone and androstenedione	Cells of the zona reticularis	Adrenocorticotropic hormone (ACTH)	Weak masculinizing characteristics
Suprarenal Medulla			
Catecholamines: epinephrine and norepinephrine	Chromaffin cells	Preganglionic Sympathetic Splanchnic Nerves	Epinephrine: operates "fight or flight" mechanism preparing the body for severe fear or stress; increases cardiac heart rate and output, augmenting blood flow to the organs, and release of glucose from the liver for energy. Norepinephrine: effects an elevation in blood pressure by vasoconstriction
Pineal Gland			
Melatonin	Pinealocytes	Norepinephrine	May influence cyclic gonadal activity

Integument

14

The **integument,** composed of **skin** and its appendages, **sweat glands, sebaceous glands, hair,** and **nails,** is the largest organ, constituting 16% of the body weight. It invests the entire body, becoming continuous with the mucous membranes of the digestive system at the lips and the anus, the respiratory system in the nose, and the urogenital systems where they surface. Additionally, the skin of the eyelids becomes continuous with the conjunctiva lining the anterior portion of the orb. Skin also lines the external auditory meatus and covers the external surface of the tympanic membrane.

Skin

Besides providing a cover for the underlying soft tissues, skin performs many additional functions, including **protection** against injury, bacterial invasion, and desiccation; **regulation of body temperature; reception** of continual sensations from the environment (e.g., touch, temperature, and pain); **excretion** from sweat glands; and **absorption** of ultraviolet radiation from the sun for vitamin D synthesis.

Skin consists of two layers, an outer epidermis and a deeper connective tissue layer, the dermis (Fig. 14–1). The **epidermis** is composed of stratified squamous keratinized epithelium derived from **ectoderm.** Lying directly below and interdigitating with the epidermis is the **dermis,** derived from **mesoderm** and composed of dense, irregular collagenous connective tissue. The interface between the epidermis and dermis is formed by raised ridges of the dermis, the **dermal ridges (papillae),** which interdigitate with invaginations of the epidermis, called **epidermal ridges.** Additional downgrowths of the epidermal derivatives (i.e., hair follicles, sweat and sebaceous glands) that come to lie in the dermis cause the interface to have an irregular contour. The **hypodermis,** a loose connective tissue containing varying amounts of fat, underlies the skin. The hypodermis is not part of the skin but is the **superficial fascia** that covers the entire body, immediately deep to the skin. In persons who are overnourished or live in cold climates, a large amount of fat is deposited in the superficial fascia (hypodermis), named **panniculus adiposus.**

In certain regions of the body the skin displays different textures and thicknesses. For example, skin of the eyelid is soft, fine, and thin and has fine hairs, whereas only a short distance away, on the eyebrow, the skin is thicker and produces coarse hair. Skin of the forehead produces oily secretions; the skin on the chin lacks oily secretions but develops much hair.

The palms of the hands and soles of the feet are thick and do not produce hair but contain many sweat glands. In addition, finger and toe pad surfaces have well-defined, alternating ridges and grooves that form patterns of loops, curves, arches, and whorls called **dermatoglyphs** (fingerprints), which develop in the fetus and remain unchanged throughout life. They are so individualized that they are used for identification purposes in forensic medicine and in criminal investigation. Although fingerprints are determined genetically, perhaps by multiple genes, other grooves and flexure lines about the knees, elbows, and hands are, for the most part, related to habitual use and physical stresses in one's environment.

Epidermis

The **epidermis** is 0.07 to 0.12 mm in thickness over most of the body, with localized thickening on the palms of the hands (0.8 mm) and the soles of the feet (1.4 mm). Although thicker skin on the palms and soles is evident in the fetus, use, applied pressure, and friction over time result in continued increases in skin thickness in these areas.

The stratified squamous keratinized epithelium of skin is composed of four populations of cells: **keratinocytes, melanocytes, Langerhans cells,** and **Merkel cells.** Keratinocytes form the largest population and are arranged in five recognizable layers; the other three cell types are interspersed among keratinocytes in specific locations. Because

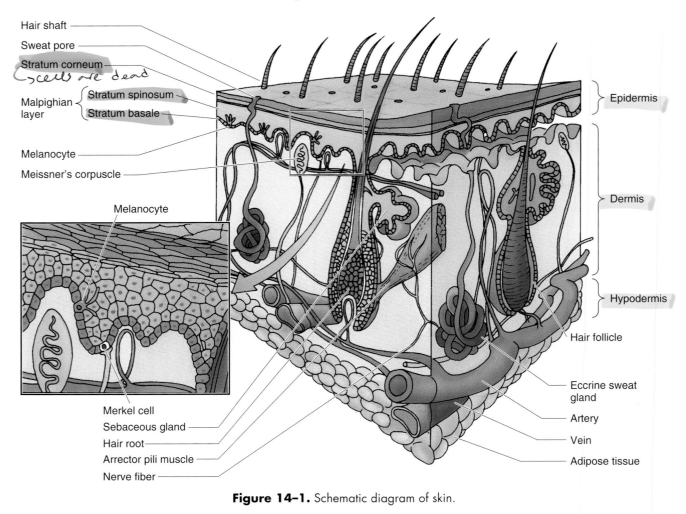

Hair shaft
Sweat pore
Stratum corneum
↳ cells are dead
Malpighian layer
  Stratum spinosum
  Stratum basale
Melanocyte
Meissner's corpuscle

Melanocyte

Merkel cell
Sebaceous gland
Hair root
Arrector pili muscle
Nerve fiber

Epidermis
Dermis
Hypodermis
Hair follicle
Eccrine sweat gland
Artery
Vein
Adipose tissue

Figure 14-1. Schematic diagram of skin.

keratinocytes are being continually sloughed from the surface of the epidermis, this cell population must continually be renewed. This is accomplished through mitotic activity of the keratinocytes in the basal layer of the epidermis. Keratinocytes undergo mitosis at night, and while the new cells are forming, the cells above get pushed toward the surface, passing from one layer to another until the surface is reached, a process that takes 20 to 30 days. On their way, the cells become enlarged and more differentiated, and they begin to accumulate **keratin filaments** in their cytoplasm. Eventually, as the surface is neared, the cells die and are sloughed off.

Because of the **cytomorphosis** of keratinocytes during their migration from the basal layer of the epidermis to its surface, five morphologically distinct zones of the epidermis can be identified. From the inner to the outer layer, these are called the stratum basale (germinativum), stratum spinosum, stratum granulosum, stratum lucidum, and stratum corneum. Skin is classified as **thick** or **thin** based on the thickness of the epidermis. However, these two types also are distinguished by the presence or absence of certain epidermal layers.

Thick skin covers the palms and soles. The epidermis of thick skin, which is 400 to 600 μm thick, is characterized by the presence of all five layers. Thick skin lacks hair follicles, arrector pili muscles, and sebaceous glands but does have sweat glands (Fig. 14-2).

Thin skin covers most of the remainder of the body. The epidermis of thin skin, which ranges from 75 to 150 μm in thickness, has a thin stratum corneum and lacks a definite stratum lucidum and stratum granulosum, although individual cells of these layers are present in the proper location. Thin skin contains **hair follicles, arrector pili muscles, sebaceous glands,** and **sweat glands.**

Stratum Basale (Stratum Germinativum)

The deepest layer of the epidermis, the **stratum basale,** is supported by a **basal lamina** and sits on the dermis, forming an irregular interface. The stratum basale consists of a single layer of mitotically active, cuboidal to low columnar-shaped cells containing basophilic cytoplasm and a large nucleus (Fig. 14-3). Many desmosomes are located in the lateral compart-

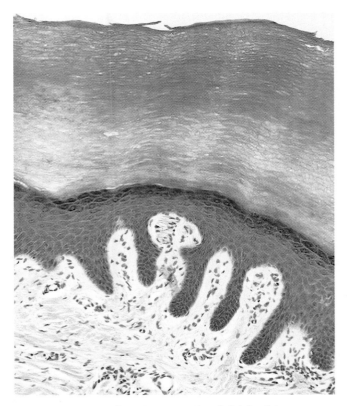

Figure 14–2. Light micrograph of thick skin
(× **132).** Observe the epidermis and dermis as well as the
dermal ridges interdigitating with epidermal ridges.

ments attaching stratum basale cells to each other and to cells
of the stratum spinosum. Basally located hemidesmosomes
attach the cells to the basal lamina. Electron micrographs reveal a few mitochondria, a small Golgi complex, a few rough
endoplasmic reticulum (RER) profiles, and abundant free ribosomes. Numerous bundles and single (10-nm) **intermediate filaments** course through the plaques of the laterally
placed desmosomes and end in plaques of hemidesmosomes.

Mitotic figures should be common in the stratum basale
because this layer is partially responsible for cell renewal in
the epithelium. However, mitosis occurs mostly during the
night, and histological specimens are procured during the
day, thus mitotic figures are rarely seen in histological slides
of skin. When new cells are formed from mitosis, the previous layer of cells is pushed surfaceward to become a new
layer, the stratum spinosum, where the cells begin to flatten
and the intermediate filaments continue to accumulate.

Stratum Spinosum

The thickest layer of the epidermis is the **stratum spinosum,** composed of polyhedral to flattened cells. The
basally located keratinocytes in the stratum spinosum also
are mitotically active like those of the stratum basale, and
the two strata together are responsible for the turnover of
epidermal keratinocytes. Keratinocytes of the stratum spi-

nosum have the same organelles as those described in the
stratum basale. However, they contain more bundles of intermediate filaments **(tonofilaments),** representing **cytokeratin,** than do stratum basale cells. In the stratum spinosum
cells, these bundles radiate outward from the perinuclear region toward highly interdigitated cellular processes, which
attach adjacent cells to each other by desmosomes. These
processes, called intercellular bridges by early histologists,
give cells of the stratum spinosum a "prickle-cell" appearance (see Fig. 14–3). As keratinocytes move upward
through the stratum spinosum, they continue to produce
tonofilaments, which become grouped in bundles called
tonofibrils, causing the cytoplasm to become eosinophilic
(Fig. 14–4). Cells of the stratum spinosum also contain cytoplasmic secretory granules (0.1 to 0.4 μm in diameter)
called **membrane-coating granules (lamellar granules).**
These flattened vesicles house lipid substance arranged in a
closely packed, lamellar configuration. Some histologists
refer to the two layers, the stratum basale and the stratum
spinosum, as the **Malpighian layer.**

Stratum Granulosum

The **stratum granulosum,** consisting of three to five layers
of flattened keratinocytes, is the most superficial layer of the
epidermis in which cells possess nuclei. The cytoplasm of
the keratinocytes in this layer contains large, irregularly
shaped, coarse, basophilic **keratohyalin granules,** which
are not membrane-bound. Keratin filaments are associated
with these granules, with some filaments passing through

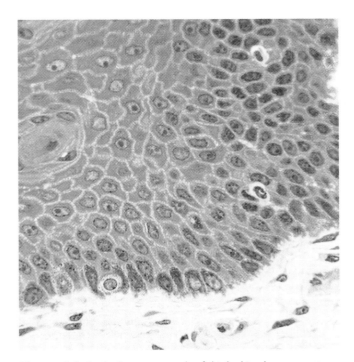

Figure 14–3. Light micrograph of thick skin demonstrating
the stratum basale and stratum spinosum (× 540).

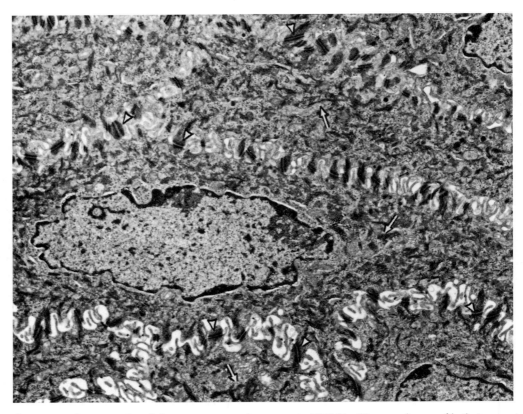

Figure 14-4. Electron micrograph of the stratum spinosum (×7500). Observe the tonofibrils (*arrows*) and the cytoplasmic processes bridging the intercellular spaces. (From Leeson, T.S., Leeson, C.R., and Paparo, A.A.: Text/Atlas of Histology. Philadelphia, W.B. Saunders Company, 1988.)

them. These filaments are believed to be precursors of the keratin located in cells of the stratum corneum.

Cells of the stratum granulosum contain more membrane-coating granules than do those in the stratum spinosum. The contents of these granules are released by exocytosis, forming a layer of lipid-rich substance over the plasma membranes. This coating acts as a waterproof barrier, one of the functions of skin. Additionally, it prevents cells lying superficial to this region from receiving nutrients, thus hastening their death.

Stratum Lucidum

The clear, homogeneous, lightly staining thin layer of cells immediately superficial to the stratum granulosum is the **stratum lucidum.** This layer is present only in thick skin (i.e., palms of the hands and soles of the feet). Although the flattened cells of the stratum lucidum lack organelles and nuclei, they contain densely packed keratin filaments orientated parallel to the skin surface and **eleidin,** a transformation product of keratohyalin.

Stratum Corneum

The most superficial layer of skin, the **stratum corneum,** is composed of numerous layers of flattened, keratinized cells

with a thickened plasmalemma. These cells lack nuclei and organelles but have numerous keratin filaments embedded in an amorphous matrix. Those cells farther away from the skin surface display desmosomes, whereas cells near the surface of the skin, called **squames** or **horny cells,** are without desmosomes and are to be **desquamated** (sloughed).

Nonkeratinocytes in the Epidermis

In addition to keratinocytes, specific layers of the epidermis contain three other cell types.

Langerhans Cells

Scattered throughout the epidermis but located primarily in the stratum spinosum are **Langerhans cells,** sometimes called **dendritic cells** because of their numerous long processes. These cells also may be found in the dermis as well as in the stratified squamous epithelia of the oral cavity, esophagus, and vagina. However, they are most prevalent in the epidermis, where their numbers may reach as many as 800 per mm².

Viewed with light microscopy, Langerhans cells display a dense nucleus, pale cytoplasm, and long slender processes that radiate out from the cell body into the intercellular spaces between keratinocytes. Electron micrographs reveal the nucleus to be polymorphous; the electron-lucent cytoplasm houses few mitochondria, sparse RER, and no intermediate filaments, but contains lysosomes, multivesicular bodies, and small vesicles. Although the irregularly contoured nucleus and the absence of tonofilaments distinguish Langerhans cells from surrounding keratinocytes, the most unique feature of Langerhans cells are the membrane-bound **Birbeck granules (vermiform granules),** which in section resemble a ping-pong paddle (15 to 50 nm in length, 4 nm thick). The function of these granules is not known.

Langerhans cells, once thought to be derived from neural crest cells, are now known to originate from precursors in the bone marrow. Although they are capable of mitosis, this activity is restricted; thus they are continually replaced by precursor cells leaving the bloodstream to migrate into the epidermis and differentiate into Langerhans cells.

Langerhans cells function in the immune response. These cells have cell-surface Fc (antibody) and C3 (complement) receptors and phagocytose and process foreign antigens. Langerhans cells migrate to lymph nodes in the vicinity, where they present epitopes of processed foreign antigens to T lymphocytes; thus they are **antigen-presenting cells.**

Merkel Cells

Merkel cells, which are interspersed among the keratinocytes of the stratum basale of the epidermis, are especially abundant in the fingertips. Their origin has not been elucidated. Although Merkel cells are usually found as single cells orientated parallel to the basal lamina, they may extend their processes between keratinocytes, to which they are attached by desmosomes (Fig. 14–5). Merkel cell nuclei are deeply indented, and three types of cytokeratins within the cytoplasm make up the cytoskeletal filaments. Dense-cored granules located in the perinuclear zone and in the processes, whose function is unclear, are the distinguishing feature of Merkel cells.

Unmyelinated sensory nerves traverse the basal lamina to approximate the Merkel cells, thus forming **Merkel cell–neurite complexes.** These complexes may function as **mechanoreceptors.**

Melanocytes

Also present in the stratum basale are **melanocytes,** which originate from neural crest cells. These cells may also reside

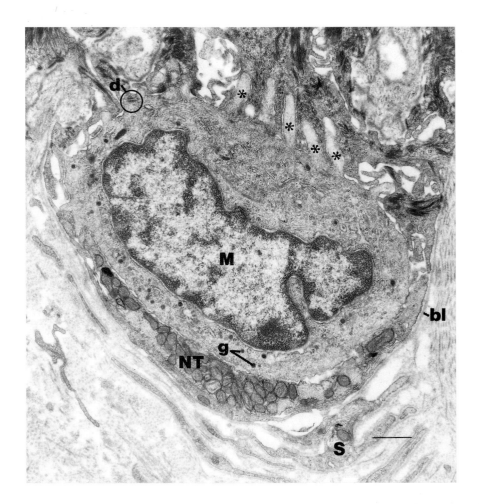

Figure 14–5. Electron micrograph of a Merkel cell (M) and its nerve terminal (NT) from an adult rat. × **Scale bar = 0.5 μm.** Note the spine-like processes (*) that project into the intercellular spaces of the stratum spinosum. Merkel cells form desmosomes (d) with cells of the stratum spinosum and share the basal lamina (bl) of cells of the stratum basale. (From English, K.B., Wang, Z.Z., Stayner, N., Stensaas, L.J., Martin, H., and Tuckett, R.P.: Serotonin-like immunoreactivity in Merkel's cells and their afferent neurons in touch domes from hairy skin of rats. Anat. Rec. **232**:112–120, 1991. Copyright © 1991. Reprinted by permission of John Wiley & Sons, Inc.)

in the superficial portions of the dermis and extend their processes into the epidermis between keratinocytes (Fig. 14–6). Melanocytes produce **melanin,** the brown pigment imparting various shades of brown to skin color. **Tyrosinase,** an enzyme possessed by melanocytes, is essential for melanin synthesis. It is located in specialized organelles, known as **melanosomes,** within the cytoplasm of melanocytes. **Tyrosine** transported into melanosomes is converted by tyrosinase into **melanin** via a series of reactions progressing through 3,4-dihydroxyphenylalanine and dopaquinone. Melanosomes containing melanin are transferred via melanocyte dendritic processes to the cytoplasm of keratinocytes via a special secretory process called **cytocrine secretion.** This process is not completely understood. However, it appears that melanosomes move to the tip of the melanocyte processes, which are pinched off by the keratinocytes and become incorporated into their cytoplasm. Thus, a melanocyte serves a number of keratinocytes with which it is associated, constituting an **epidermal melanin unit.**

The number of melanocytes in the skin varies in different areas of the body, ranging from 800 to 2300/mm². For ex-

ample, there are far fewer melanocytes on the insides of the arms and thighs than on the face. The difference in skin pigmentation is related more to location of the melanin than to the total number of melanocytes in the skin, which is nearly the same for all races. In whites melanosomes are smaller and fewer, and they congregate in the vicinity of the nucleus, whereas in blacks melanosomes are large, more numerous, and dispersed throughout the keratinocytes' cytoplasm.

Dermis (Corium)

The region of the skin lying directly beneath the epidermis, called the **dermis,** is derived from the mesoderm and is divided into two layers: the superficial, loosely woven **papillary layer** and the deeper, much denser **reticular layer.** The dermis is composed of dense, irregular collagenous connective tissue, containing mostly type I collagen fibers and networks of elastic fibers, which support the epidermis and bind the skin to the underlying **hypodermis.** The dermis ranges in thickness from 0.6 mm in the eyelids to 3 mm or so on the palms and soles. However, there is not a sharp line of demarcation at its interface with the underlying connective tissue of the superficial fascia. Normally the dermis is thicker in men than in women; it also is thicker on the dorsal than on the ventral surfaces of the body.

Papillary Layer of the Dermis

bumps are referred to as epidermal ridges & dermatoglyphs

This superficial layer of the dermis is uneven where it interdigitates with the epidermis, forming the dermal ridges (papillae) (see Fig. 14–2). It is composed of a loose connective tissue whose thin **type III collagen fibers** (reticular fibers) and **elastic fibers** are arranged in loose networks. **Anchoring fibrils,** composed of type VII collagen, extend from the basal lamina into the papillary layer, binding the epidermis to the dermis (see Figs. 4–13, 4–14). The papillary layer contains fibroblasts, macrophages, mast cells, and other cells common to connective tissue.

The papillary layer also possesses many capillary loops, which extend to the epidermis–dermis interface. These capillaries regulate body temperature and nourish the cells of the avascular epidermis. Located in some dermal papillae are pear-shaped encapsulated **Meissner corpuscles,** mechanoreceptors specialized to respond to slight deformations of the epidermis. These receptors are most common in areas of the skin especially sensitive to tactile stimulation (e.g., lips, external genitalia, nipples). Another encapsulated mechanoreceptor present in the papillary layer is **Krause end bulb.** Although it was once thought to respond to cold, presently its function is unclear.

Reticular Layer of the Dermis

The interface between the papillary layer and **reticular layer** of the dermis is indistinguishable because the two lay-

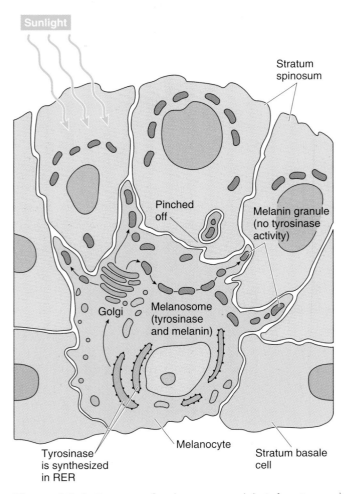

Figure 14–6. Diagram of melanocytes and their function.

Labels in figure: Sunlight · Stratum spinosum · Pinched off · Melanin granule (no tyrosinase activity) · Golgi · Melanosome (tyrosinase and melanin) · Tyrosinase is synthesized in RER · Melanocyte · Stratum basale cell

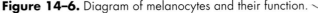

ers are continuous with each other. Characteristically, the reticular layer is composed of dense, irregular collagenous connective tissue, displaying thick **type I collagen fibers,** which are closely packed into large bundles lying mostly parallel to the skin surface. Networks of **thick elastic fibers** are intermingled with the collagen fibers, appearing especially abundant near sebaceous and sweat glands. Proteoglycans, rich in **dermatan sulfate,** fill the interstices of the reticular layer. Cells are more sparse in this layer than in the papillary layer. They include fibroblasts, mast cells, lymphocytes, macrophages, and frequently fat cells in the deeper aspects of the reticular layer.

Sweat glands, sebaceous glands, and **hair follicles,** all derived from the epidermis, invade the dermis and hypodermis during embryogenesis, where they remain permanently (see Fig. 14–1). Groups of **smooth muscle cells** are located in the deeper regions of the reticular layer at particular sites, such as the skin of the penis and scrotum and the areola around the nipples; contractions of these muscle groups wrinkle the skin in these regions. Other smooth muscles, called **arrector pili muscles,** are inserted into the hair follicles; contractions of these muscles erect the hairs when the body is cold or suddenly exposed to a cold environment, giving the skin "goose bumps." Additionally, a particular group of striated muscles located about the face, parts of the anterior neck, and scalp (**muscles of facial expression**) originate in the superficial fascia and insert into the dermis.

At least two types of encapsulated mechanoreceptors are located in the deeper portions of the dermis: **pacinian corpuscles,** which respond to pressure and vibrations, and **Ruffini corpuscles,** which respond to tensional forces. The latter are most abundant in the dermis of the soles of the feet.

Epidermis–Dermis Interface

At the epidermis–dermis interface, as described previously, the line of demarcation is irregular because interdigitations of the epidermal and dermal layers are translated through the epidermis to become visible on the surface of the skin, especially in the palms and soles where they are represented by the whorls, arches, and loops called **dermatoglyphs.** Because these interdigitations are not easily visualized from two-dimensional histological sections, a technique employing ethylenediaminetetraacetic acid (EDTA) is used. EDTA chelates the Ca²⁺ located at the hemidesmosomes, which frees the epidermis from the dermis. Once the epidermis and dermis are dissociated, the three-dimensional surface of the papillary layer of the dermis may be examined more completely by scanning electron microscopy.

The papillary layer presents parallel **primary dermal ridges** on its surface separated by **primary grooves,** which house projections of the epidermis (see Fig. 14–2). Also in the center of each primary dermal ridge is a **secondary groove** that receives a downgrowth of the epidermis known as an **interpapillary peg.** Along this and other adjacent ridges are rows of round-topped **dermal papillae** that project into concavities in the epidermis, thus firmly interlocking the epidermis and dermis at the interface. The epidermis–dermis interface in thin skin is much less complex, lacking such deep and widespread interlocking.

Histophysiology of Skin

The structural protein produced by the keratinocytes is **keratin,** which forms 10-nm filaments within the cytoplasm. Ten or so different species of keratin have been identified in the body; four of these are found within the skin.

Stratum basale cells synthesize two of the four keratins, whereas the cells of the stratum spinosum synthesize the other two different keratins, which form coarser bundles of filaments. Cells of this stratum also produce **involucrin** and additional proteins that are deposited on the cytoplasmic aspect of their plasmalemma. The cells of the stratum spinosum also form the **membrane-coating granules,** which later release their lipid-rich contents into the intercellular spaces, forming a permeability barrier.

The keratin-synthesizing machinery shuts down after keratinocytes enter the stratum granulosum. The cells in this layer produce **filaggrin,** a protein thought to function in assembling keratin filaments into coarser bundles. Once keratinocytes reach this stratum they also become permeable to calcium ions, which assist in cross-linking involucrin with other proteins, thereby forming a tough layer beneath the plasmalemma. As keratinocytes move through the stratum granulosum, enzymes, released by lysosomes, digest the organelles and the nucleus, and the cells then progress through the stratum lucidum. When the cells finally enter the stratum corneum, they are nonliving, tough shells filled with bundles of keratin filaments and lacking nuclei and organelles.

Epidermal growth factor (EGF) and **interleukin-1 alpha (IL-1α)** influence the growth and development of keratinocytes, at least in tissue culture. In contrast, **transforming growth factor (TGF)** suppresses keratinocyte proliferation and differentiation.

CLINICAL CORRELATIONS

Freckles are hyperpigmented spots located on sun-exposed areas of the skin, especially in persons who sunburn easily. They are usually exhibited by the age of 3 and are the result of increased melanin production and accumulation in the basal area of the epidermis without an increase in melanocytes. They tend to fade in the winter and darken with exposure to ultraviolet light.

Psoriasis is a disease characterized by patchy lesions caused by increased keratinocyte proliferation and an accelerated cell cycle (turnover is increased as much as seven times), resulting in accumulations of keratinocytes and stratum corneum. The lesions are common on the scalp, elbows, and knees, but they may occur most anywhere on the body. In some cases, the nails may also be involved. Psoriasis is an incurable but manageable chronic condition whose symptoms periodically escalate and then diminish with no apparent cause.

Warts are benign epidermal growths caused by infection of the keratinocytes with **papillomaviruses.** The resulting epidermal hyperplasia thickens the epidermis with scaling. Deeper ingrowth of the dermis brings capillaries closer to the surface. Warts are common in children, young adults, and immunosuppressed patients.

Basal cell carcinoma, the most common human malignancy, arises in the **stratum basale cells** of the epidermis and usually is caused by exposure to ultraviolet radiation. Although basal cell carcinomas do not usually metastasize, they are destructive to local tissue. Of the several types of lesions that occur, the most common is the nodular variety, characterized by a papule or nodule with a central depressed "crater," which eventually ulcerates and crusts. These lesions are most frequent on the face, especially the nose. Surgery is the usual treatment, and up to 90% of patients recover with no additional sequelae.

Squamous cell carcinoma, the second most common skin cancer, arises in the keratinocytes of the epidermis. It is locally invasive and may metastasize. It is characterized by a hyperkeratotic scaly plaque or nodule that often bleeds or ulcerates. It invades deeply, resulting in fixation to the underlying tissues. Several factors may cause this disease, including ultraviolet radiation, x-irradiation, soot, chemical carcinogens, and arsenic. The lesions are most common on the head and neck. Surgery is the usual treatment of choice.

Glands of the Skin

The glands of the skin include eccrine and apocrine sweat glands, sebaceous glands, and the mammary gland (a modified and highly specialized type of sweat gland). The mammary gland is described in Chapter 20 on the female reproductive system.

Eccrine Sweat Glands

Eccrine sweat glands are about 0.4 mm in diameter and located in the skin throughout most of the body, numbering as many as 3 to 4 million. Eccrine sweat glands develop as invaginations of the epithelium of the dermal ridge that grows down into the dermis with its deep aspect becoming the glandular portion of the sweat gland. These glands, which begin to function soon after birth, excrete sweat, as much as 10 liters a day under extreme conditions in highly active persons engaged in vigorous exercise.

Eccrine sweat glands are **simple coiled tubular glands** located deep in the dermis or in the underlying hypodermis

(Figs. 14–7, 14–8). Passing from the secretory portion of the gland is a slender, coiled **duct** that traverses the dermis and epidermis to open on the surface of the skin at a **sweat pore.** Eccrine sweat glands are merocrine in their method of releasing their secretory product (sweat). The eccrine glands are innervated by cholinergic fibers.

Secretory Unit

The secretory portion of the gland is said to be a simple cuboidal to low columnar epithelium composed of **dark cells** and **clear cells;** however, some investigators consider it to be pseudostratified.

DARK CELLS (MUCOID CELLS). *Dark cells* line the lumen of the gland and secrete a **mucus-rich substance.** Their shape resembles an inverted cone with the broad ends lining the lumen. The narrowed ends, which seldom reach the basal lamina, conform to fit between adjacent clear cells. Electron micrographs reveal some RER, numerous free ribosomes, elongated mitochondria, and a well-developed Golgi complex. Moderately dense glycoprotein-containing secretory granules are located in the apical cytoplasm of the dark cells.

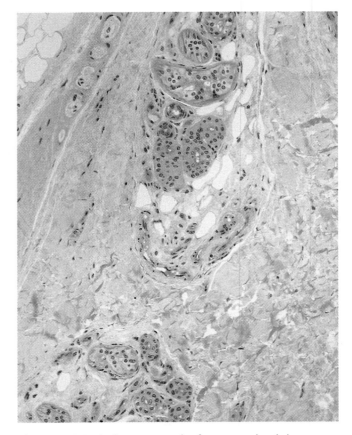

Figure 14–7. Light micrograph of a sweat gland demonstrating secretory units and ducts (× 132).

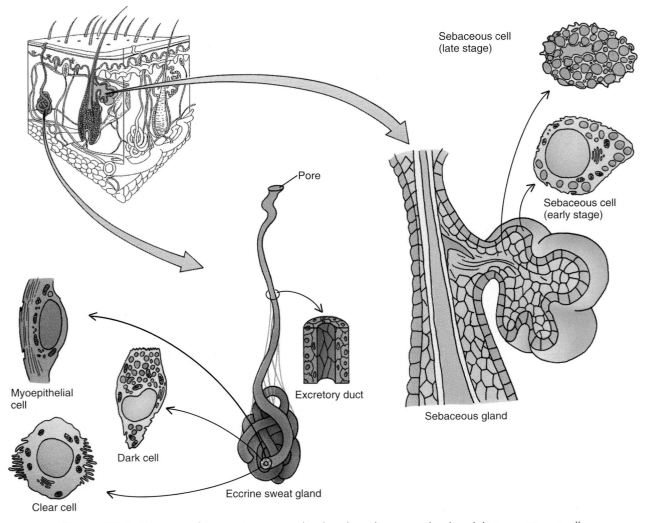

Figure 14-8. Diagram of an eccrine sweat gland and a sebaceous gland and their constituent cells.

CLEAR CELLS. Clear cells have a narrow apical area and a broader base that extends to the basal lamina. Unlike dark cells, **clear cells** do not contain secretory granules, but they do contain accumulations of **glycogen,** and their organelles are similar to those of dark cells, except that they have little ER. The bases of the clear cells are tortuously infolded, similar to other cell types involved in transepithelial transport. Clear cells have limited access to the lumen of the gland because of the dark cells; therefore, their **watery secretion** enters **intercellular canaliculi** interposed between adjacent clear cells, where it mixes with the mucous secretion of the dark cells.

MYOEPITHELIAL CELLS. The **myoepithelial cells** surrounding the secretory portion of the eccrine sweat glands are enveloped by the basal lamina of the secretory cells. The cytoplasm of myoepithelial cells has many deeply acidophilic-staining **actin** filaments, which give the cell contractile capability. Contractions of the myoepithelial cells assist in expressing the fluid from the gland.

SECRETORY DUCT. The **secretory duct** is continuous with the secretory unit at its base but narrows as it passes through the dermis on its way to the epidermal surface. The duct is composed of a stratified cuboidal epithelium made up of two layers (see Figs. 14–7, 14–8). The **cells of the basal layer** have a large, heterochromatic nucleus and abundant mitochondria. The **cells of the luminal layer** have an irregularly-shaped nucleus, little cytoplasm, only a few organelles, and a terminal web immediately deep to the apical plasma membrane.

The ducts follow a helical path through the dermis. As a duct reaches the epidermis, keratinocytes envelop the duct on its way to the sweat pore. The fluid secreted by the secretory portion of the gland is similar to blood plasma in regard to electrolyte balance. However, most of the potassium, sodium, and chloride ions are resorbed by cells of the duct as the secretion travels through its lumen. The cells of the duct excrete ions, urea, lactic acid, and some drugs into the lumen.

Apocrine Sweat Glands

Apocrine sweat glands are found only in certain locations: the axilla (arm pit), the areola of the nipple, and the anal region. Modified apocrine sweat glands constitute the **ceruminous (wax) glands** of the external auditory canal and the **glands of Moll** in the eyelids. Apocrine sweat glands are much larger than eccrine sweat glands, up to 3 mm in diameter. These glands are embedded in the deeper portions of the dermis and hypodermis. Unlike eccrine sweat glands, whose ducts open onto the skin surface, the ducts of apocrine sweat glands open into canals of the hair follicles just superficial to the entry of the sebaceous gland ducts.

The secretory cells of apocrine glands are simple cuboidal to low columnar in profile. When the lumen of the gland is filled with secretory product, these cells may become squamous. The lumina of these glands are much larger than those of eccrine glands, and the secretory cells contain granules that are isolated from the apical membrane by the presence of a prominent terminal web. The viscous secretory product of apocrine glands is odorless upon secretion, but when metabolized by bacteria, it presents a distinctive odor. Myoepithelial cells surround the secretory portion of the apocrine sweat glands and assist in expressing the secretory product into the duct of the gland.

Apocrine sweat glands arise from the epithelium of the hair follicles as an epithelial bud that develops into a gland. Secretion by apocrine glands is under the influence of hormones and does not begin until puberty. Their innervation is provided by adrenergic nerves. Because of the similarity of their location and histology, it is speculated that apocrine sweat glands evolved from glands that secrete sex attractants in lower animals. As an interesting note, apocrine sweat glands in women undergo cyclic changes, which seem to be related to the menstrual cycle, such that the secretory cells and lumina grow before the premenstrual period and shrink during menstruation.

The name given to these special sweat glands, apocrine sweat glands, implies that the secretion contains a portion of the cytoplasm of the secreting cells, which was originally thought to be true. Electron microscopic evidence, however, has shown that no part of the secretory cell is secreted; thus the mode of secretion is merocrine instead. However, the gland still retains the original name.

Sebaceous Glands

Except for the palms of the hands, soles of the feet, and sides of the feet inferior to the hair line, **sebaceous glands** are found all over the body embedded in the dermis and hypodermis. These glands are most abundant on the face, scalp, and the forehead. The secretory product of the sebaceous glands, **sebum,** is a wax-like mixture of cholesterol and triglycerides. Sebum is thought to assist in maintaining skin texture and hair flexibility.

Like apocrine sweat glands, sebaceous glands are appendages of hair follicles. The ducts of the sebaceous glands open into the upper one third of the follicular canal, where they discharge their secretory product (see Fig. 14–8). The ducts of sebaceous glands in certain regions of the body lacking hair follicles (i.e., the lips, glans penis, areola of the nipples, labia minora, and mucous surface of the prepuce) open onto the surface of the skin to empty their secretions. Sebaceous glands are under the influence of sex hormones and become active after puberty.

Sebaceous glands are lobular with clusters of acini opening into single short ducts. Each acinus is composed of peripherally located small basal cells (resting on the basal lamina), which surround larger round cells that fill the remainder of the acinus (Fig. 14–9). The basal cells have a spherical nucleus, both smooth and rough ER, glycogen, and lipid droplets. These cells undergo cell division to form more basal cells and larger round cells. The larger cells have abundant smooth ER and cytoplasm filled with lipid droplets. The central region of the acinus is filled with cells in different stages of degeneration. These pale-staining cells display only strands of cytoplasm, deeply staining pyknotic nuclei, ruptured plasmalemmae, and coalescing lipid droplets. Lipid synthesis continues for a short time, followed by necrosis of the cells and the ultimate release of lipid and cellular debris, which form the secretory product (i.e., holocrine secretion). The secretory product is released into a duct lined with a stratified squamous epithelium that is continuous with the follicular canal at the hair follicle.

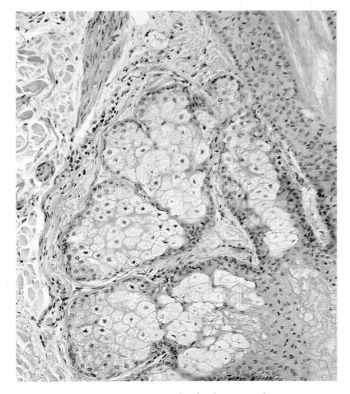

Figure 14–9. Light micrograph of a human sebaceous gland and the arrector pili muscle (× 132).

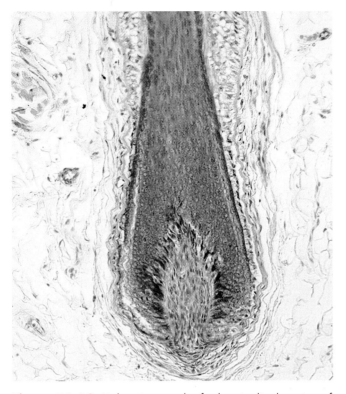

Figure 14-10. Light micrograph of a longitudinal section of a hair follicle with its hair root and papilla (× 132).

CLINICAL CORRELATIONS

Acne, the most common disease seen by dermatologists, is a chronic inflammatory disease involving the sebaceous glands and hair follicles. Obstructions resulting from impaction of sebum and keratinous debris within hair follicles is one cause of acne lesions. Anaerobic bacteria near these obstructions may contribute to development of acne, although the role of bacteria is not clear. However, the efficacy of antibiotic treatment for acne supports the idea of bacterial involvement in its pathogenesis. The disease is most severe in boys, with onset commonly from age 9 to 11 when increasing levels of sex hormones begin to stimulate the sebaceous glands. Acne usually subsides through the later teen years, but it may not resolve until the fourth decade of life. In some persons acne does not begin until adulthood.

Hair

Hairs are filamentous, keratinized structures that project from the epidermal surface of the skin (see Fig. 14–1). Hair grows over most of the body except on the vermilion zone of the lips, palms and sides of the palms, soles and sides of the feet, dorsum of the distal phalanges of the fingers and toes, glans penis, glans clitoris, labia minora, and vestibular aspect of the labia majora.

Two types of hairs are present on the human body. Hairs that are soft, fine, short, and pale (e.g., those covering the eyelids) are called **vellus hairs;** the hard, large, coarse, long, and dark hairs (e.g., those of the scalp and eyebrows) are called **terminal hairs.** Additionally, very fine hair, called **lanugo,** is present on the fetus.

The number of hairs on humans is essentially the same as on other primates, but most of human hair is of the vellus type, whereas terminal hairs predominate on other primates. Also, human hair does not provide the thermal insulation that animals with fur have. Instead, human hairs serve in tactile sensation, such that any stimulus that deforms the hair is translated down the shaft to sensory nerves about the hair follicle.

Hair growth is optimal from about 16 to 46 years of age; after the age of 50, hair growth begins to diminish. During pregnancy hair growth is normal; after delivery, the cycle of hair growth subsides and hair loss is temporarily increased.

Hair Follicles

Hair follicles, the organs from which hairs develop, arise from invaginations of the epidermis invading the dermis, hypodermis, or both. Hair follicles are surrounded by dense accumulations of fibrous connective tissue belonging to the dermis (Fig. 14–10). A thickened basal lamina, the **glassy membrane,** separates the dermis from the epithelium of the hair follicle (Fig. 14–11). The expanded terminus of the hair

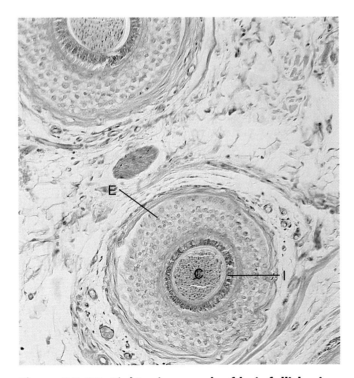

Figure 14-11. Light micrograph of hair follicles in cross-section (× 132). Observe the external root sheath (E), the internal root sheath (I), and the cortex (C).

follicle, the **hair root,** is indented to conform to the shape of the **dermal papilla** pushing into it. These two structures together are known as the **hair bulb.** The dermal papilla contains a rich supply of capillaries that nourish the cells of the hair follicle. Also, the dermal papilla acts as an inductive force controlling the physiological activities of the hair follicle.

The bulk of the cells composing the hair root is called the **matrix.** Proliferation of these cells accounts for the growth of hair: thus they are homologous to the stratum basale of the epidermis. The outer layers of follicular epithelium form the **external root sheath,** which is composed of a single layer at the hair bulb and several layers near the surface of the skin (Fig. 14–12).

Internal to the external root sheath are a number of layers of cells forming the **internal root sheath,** consisting of three components: (1) an outer single row of cuboidal cells, **Henle's layer,** which contacts the innermost layer of cells of the external root sheath, (2) one or two layers of flattened cells forming **Huxley's layer,** and (3) the **cuticle of the internal root sheath,** formed by overlapping scale-like cells whose free ends project toward the base of the hair follicle. The internal root sheath ends where the duct of the sebaceous gland attaches to the hair follicle (see Fig. 14–12).

The hair shaft is the long slender filament that extends to and through the surface of the epidermis (Fig. 14–13). It consists of three regions: **medulla, cortex,** and the **cuticle** of the hair. As the cells of the matrix within the hair root proliferate and differentiate, they move upward, eventually developing into the hair shaft. The cells in the center of the matrix are closest to the underlying dermal papilla and thus are most influenced by it; cells lying more and more peripheral to the matrix center are progressively less influenced by the dermal papilla. The distinctive layers of the follicle develop from different matrix cells as follows:

- The *most central* matrix cells give rise to large vacuolated cells that form the core of the hair shaft, known as the **medulla.** This layer is present only in thick hair.
- Matrix cells *slightly peripheral* to the center become the **cortex** of the hair shaft.
- *More peripheral* matrix cells become the **cuticle** of the hair shaft.
- *Most peripheral* matrix cells develop into the cells of the **internal root sheath.**

As the cells of the cortex are displaced upward, they synthesize abundant **keratin filaments** and **trichohyalin granules** (resembling keratohyalin granules of the epidermis). These granules coalesce, forming an amorphous substance in which the keratin filaments are embedded. Scattered among the cells of the matrix nearest to the dermal papilla

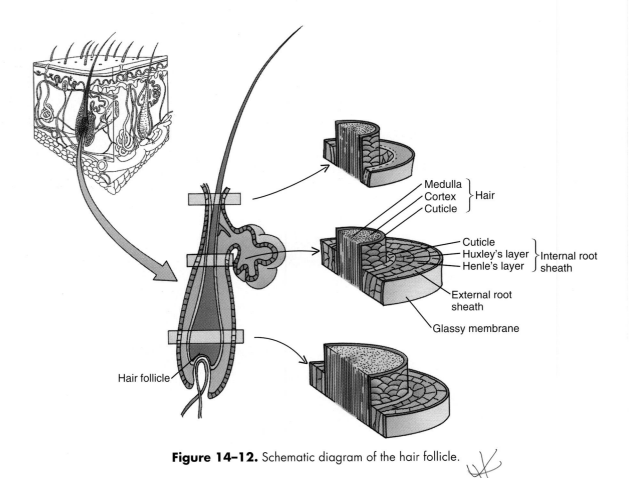

Figure 14–12. Schematic diagram of the hair follicle.

Medulla ⎫
Cortex ⎬ Hair
Cuticle ⎭

Cuticle ⎫
Huxley's layer ⎬ Internal root
Henle's layer ⎭ sheath

External root sheath

Glassy membrane

Hair follicle

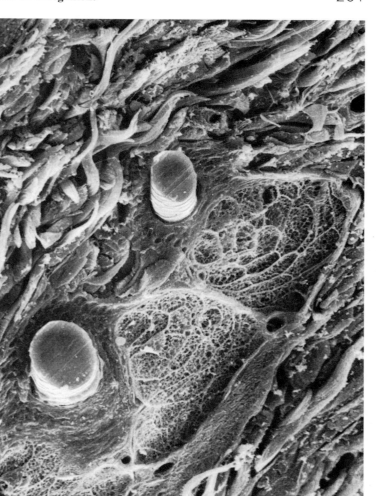

Figure 14–13. Scanning electron micrograph of monkey scalp showing three hair shafts and their sebaceous glands surrounded by the dense, irregular collagenous connective tissue of the dermis (× 300). (From Leeson, T.S., Leeson, C.R., and Paparo, A.A.: Text/Atlas of Histology. Philadelphia, W.B. Saunders Company, 1988.)

are large **melanocytes,** with long dendritic processes that transfer **melanosomes** to the cells of the cortex. The melanosomes remain in these cells, imparting to the hair a color based on the amount of melanin present. With age, the melanocytes gradually lose their ability to produce **tyrosinase,** which is essential for the production of melanin, so that the hair becomes gray.

Arrector Pili Muscles

Attached to the connective tissue sheath surrounding the hair follicles and to the papillary layer of the dermis are the **arrector pili muscles** (see Fig. 14–1). These smooth muscles attach to the hair follicle slightly above its middle, in-

clined at an angle to the epidermal surface. Contractions of these muscles depress the skin over their attachment and elevate the skin around the hair shaft, forming tiny "goose bumps" on the surface of the skin. These are easily observed when one is chilled or suddenly frightened.

Histophysiology of Hair

Hair grows at an average rate of about 1 cm per month, but hair growth is not continuous. The hair growth cycle includes three successive phases: the growth period, the **anagen phase,** which is followed by a brief period of involution, the **catagen phase;** during the final phase of rest, the **telogen phase,** the mature, aged hair is shed (falls out or is pulled out). Hairs shed in this fashion are called **club hairs** because they retain their club-shaped root. Soon afterward, a new hair is formed by the hair follicle and the cycle begins again.

The duration of the hair growth cycle varies in different areas of the body. For example, the life span of an axillary hair is roughly 4 months, whereas scalp hair may remain in the anagen phase for as long as 6 years and in the telogen phase for 4 months.

Hair follicles in certain regions of the body respond to male sex hormones. For this reason, men begin to develop more dark-pigmented terminal hairs about the chin, cheeks, and upper lip at puberty. Although women possess the same number of hair follicles in these regions, the hairs remain of the fine, pale, vellus type. In both sexes at puberty, however, heavily pigmented, coarse terminal hairs begin to grow in the axillary and pubic regions.

The keratinization processes in hair and in skin, although generally similar, differ in some respects. The superficial cell layers of the epidermis of the skin form a **soft keratin,** consisting of keratin filaments embedded in filaggrin; the keratinized cells are sloughed continuously. In contrast, keratinization of hair forms a **hard keratin,** consisting of keratin filaments embedded in trichohyalin; moreover, the keratinizing cells are not shed but accumulate, compressing and becoming hard.

The arrangement of cells composing the cuticle of the hair and cuticle of the internal root sheath interlock the opposing free edges of these cells, making it difficult to pull the hair shaft out of its follicle (Fig 14–14).

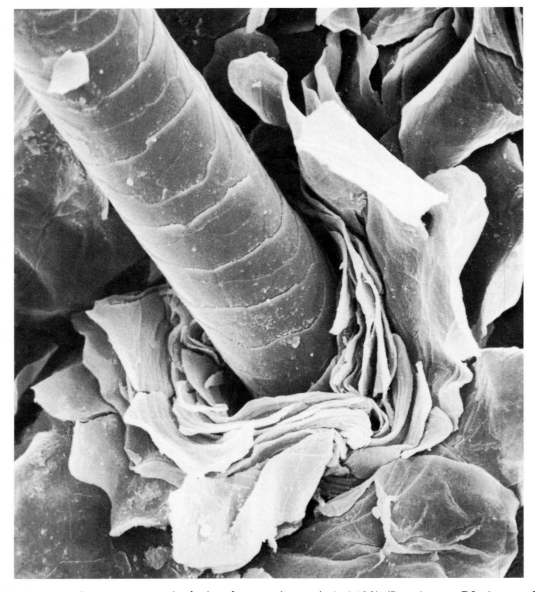

Figure 14–14. Scanning electron micrograph of a hair from monkey scalp (× 1400). (From Leeson, T.S., Leeson, C.R., and Paparo, A.A.: Text/Atlas of Histology. Philadelphia, W.B. Saunders Company, 1988.)

Nails

The **nails,** located on the distal phalanx of each finger and toe, are composed of plates of heavily compacted, highly keratinized epithelial cells, called the **nail plate,** lying on the epidermis, known as the **nail bed** (Fig. 14–15). The nails develop from cells of the **nail matrix** that proliferate and become keratinized. The nail matrix, a region of the **nail root,** is located beneath the **proximal nail fold.** The stratum corneum of the proximal nail fold forms the **eponychium (cuticle),** which extends from the proximal end up on the nail for about 0.5 to 1 mm. Laterally, the skin turns under as **lateral nail folds,** forming the **lateral nail grooves;** the epidermis continues beneath the nail plate as the **nail bed,** with the nail plate occupying the position (and function) of the stratum corneum. The **lunula,** the white crescent, is observed at the proximal end of the nail. The distal end of the nail plate is not attached to the nail bed, which becomes continuous with the skin of the finger (or toe) tip. Near this junction is an accumulation of stratum corneum, called the **hyponychium.** The fingernails grow continuously at the rate of about 0.5 mm per week, whereas the toenails grow somewhat more slowly. The translucency of the fingernails provides a quick indication of the health of an individual; pinkness indicates a good oxygenated blood supply.

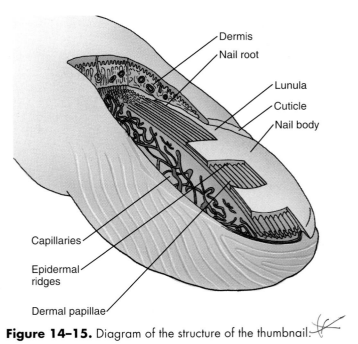

Figure 14–15. Diagram of the structure of the thumbnail.

Respiratory System

15

The respiratory system, composed of the lungs and a sequence of airways leading to the external environment, functions in providing oxygen to and eliminating carbon dioxide from the cells of the body. The realization of this goal requires the fulfillment of the following four discrete events, collectively known as **respiration:**

- Movement of air in and out of the lungs **(breathing or ventilation)**
- Exchange of oxygen in the inspired air for carbon dioxide in the blood **(external respiration)**
- Conveyance of oxygen and carbon dioxide to and from the cells **(transport of gases)**
- Exchange of carbon dioxide for oxygen in the vicinity of the cells **(internal respiration)**

The first two of these events—ventilation and external respiration—occur within the confines of the respiratory system. The circulatory system carries out the transport of gases. Internal respiration occurs in the tissues throughout the body.

The respiratory system is subdivided into two major segments, the conducting portion and the respiratory portion. The **conducting portion,** situated both outside and within the lungs, conveys air from the external milieu to the lungs. The **respiratory portion,** located strictly within the lungs, functions in the actual exchange of oxygen for carbon dioxide (external respiration).

Conducting Portion of the Respiratory System

The **conducting portion** of the respiratory system, listed in order from the exterior to the inside of the lung, is composed of the nasal cavity, mouth, nasopharynx, pharynx, larynx, trachea, primary bronchi, secondary bronchi (lobar bronchi), tertiary bronchi (segmental bronchi), bronchioles, and terminal bronchioles. These structures not only transport but also filter, moisten, and warm the inspired air before it reaches the respiratory portion.

The patency of the conducting airways is maintained by a combination of bone, cartilage, and fibrous elements. As the air progresses along the airway during inspiration, it encounters a branching system of tubules. Although the luminal diameter of each succeeding tubule continues to decrease, the *total* cross-sectional diameter of the various branches increases at each level of branching. As a result the velocity of air flow for a given volume of inhaled air decreases as the air proceeds toward the respiratory portion.

Nasal Cavity

The **nasal cavity** is divided into right and left halves by the cartilaginous and bony nasal septum. Each half of the nasal cavity is bounded laterally by a bony wall and a cartilaginous ala (wing) of the nose; it communicates with the outside, anteriorly, via the **nares** (nostrils) and with the nasopharynx by way of the **choana.** Projecting from the bony lateral wall are three thin, scroll-like bony shelves, situated one above the other: the superior, middle, and inferior **nasal conchae.**

Anterior Portion of the Nasal Cavity (Vestibule)

The anterior portion of the nasal cavity, in the vicinity of the nares, is dilated and is known as the **vestibule.** This region is lined with skin and has **vibrissae,** short stiff hairs that prevent larger dust particles from entering the nasal cavity. The dermis of the vestibule houses numerous sebaceous and sweat glands; it is anchored by numerous collagen bundles to the perichondria of the hyaline cartilage segments constituting the substance of the ala.

Posterior Aspect of the Nasal Cavity

Except for the vestibule and the olfactory region, the nasal cavity is lined by pseudostratified ciliated columnar epithelium, frequently called the **respiratory epithelium** (discussed later in the section describing the trachea). The goblet cell population of this epithelium increases in the deeper regions of the nasal cavity.

The subepithelial connective tissue (**lamina propria**) is richly vascularized, especially in the region of the conchae and anterior aspect of the nasal septum, housing large arterial plexuses and venous sinuses. The lamina propria has many seromucous glands and abundant lymphoid elements, including occasional lymphoid nodules, mast cells, and plasma cells. Antibodies produced by plasma cells (IgA, IgE, and IgG) protect the nasal mucosa against inhaled antigens and microbial invasion.

CLINICAL CORRELATIONS

Nasal bleeding usually occurs from Kiesselbach's area, the anteroinferior region of the nasal septum, the site of anastomosis of the arterial supply of the nasal mucosa. The bleeding may be arrested by applying pressure on the region or by packing the nasal cavity with cotton.

Olfactory Region of the Nasal Cavity

The roof of the nasal cavity, the superior aspect of the nasal septum, and the superior concha are covered by the 60-μm-thick olfactory epithelium. The underlying lamina propria houses collections of axons from the olfactory epithelium, a rich vascular plexus, and Bowman's glands. The **olfactory epithelium,** which is yellow in the living person, is composed of three types of cells: olfactory cells, sustentacular cells, and basal cells (Fig. 15–1).

OLFACTORY CELLS. Olfactory cells are bipolar neurons whose apical aspect, the distal terminus of its slender dendrite, is modified to form a bulb, the **olfactory vesicle,** which projects above the surface of the sustentacular cells (Figs. 15–2, 15–3). The nucleus of the cell is spherical and is closer to the basal lamina than to the olfactory vesicle. Most of the organelles of the cell are in the vicinity of the nucleus.

Scanning electron micrographs demonstrate that six to eight long, nonmotile olfactory cilia extend from the olfactory vesicle and lie on the epithelial surface. Transmission electron micrographs of these cilia display an unusual axoneme pattern that begins as a typical peripheral ring of nine **doublet** microtubules surrounding two central **singlets** (9 + 2 configuration) but distally changes so that it is composed of nine **singlets** surrounding the two central singlets.

The basal region of the olfactory cell is its **axon,** which penetrates the basal lamina and joins similar axons to form bundles of nerve fibers. Each axon, although unmyelinated, has a sheath composed of Schwann cells. The nerve fibers pass through the cribriform plate in the roof of the nasal cavity to synapse with secondary neurons in the olfactory bulb.

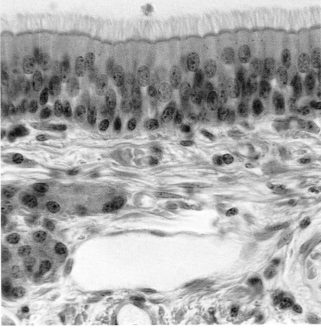

Figure 15–1. Photomicrograph of the human olfactory mucosa (× 540).

SUSTENTACULAR AND BASAL CELLS. Sustentacular cells are 50- to 60-μm-tall columnar cells whose apical aspects have a striated border composed of microvilli. Their oval nuclei are in the apical one third of the cell, somewhat superficial to the location of the olfactory cell nuclei. The apical cytoplasm of these cells has secretory granules housing a yellow pigment characteristic of the color of the olfactory mucosa. Electron micrographs of sustentacular cells demonstrate that they form junctional complexes with the olfactory vesicle regions of olfactory cells as well as with contiguous sustentacular cells. The morphology of sustentacular cells is not remarkable, although they do display a prominent terminal web of actin microfilaments. These cells are believed to provide physical support, nourishment, and electrical insulation for the olfactory cells.

Basal cells are short, basophilic, pyramid-shaped cells whose apical aspects do not reach the epithelial surface. Their nuclei are centrally located, but because these are short cells, these nuclei occupy the basal one third of the epithelium. Basal cells have considerable proliferative capacity and have been shown to replace both sustentacular and olfactory cells. In a healthy person, the olfactory and sustentacular cells have a lifespan of less than a year.

LAMINA PROPRIA. The lamina propria of the olfactory mucosa is composed of a richly vascularized, loose-to-dense irregular collagenous connective tissue that is firmly attached to the underlying periosteum. It houses numerous lymphoid elements as well as the collection of axons of the

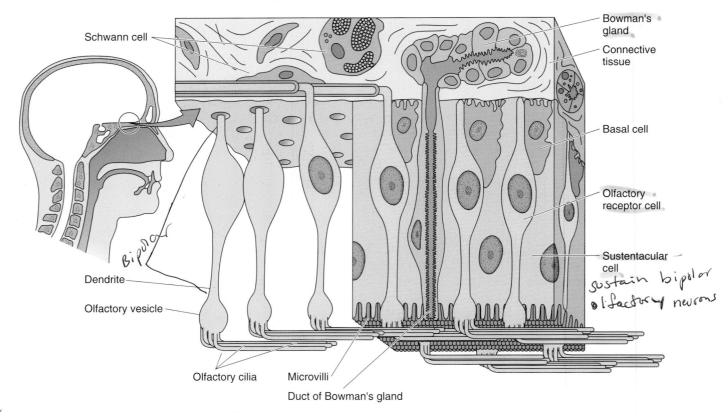

Figure 15–2. Schematic diagram of the olfactory epithelium displaying basal, olfactory, and sustentacular cells.

olfactory cells, which form fascicles of unmyelinated nerve fibers. **Bowman's glands,** which produce a serous secretory product, are also indicative of the olfactory mucosa.

Histophysiology of the Nasal Cavity

The moist nasal mucosa filters inhaled air. Particulate matter, such as dust, is trapped by the mucus produced by the goblet cells of the epithelium and the seromucous glands of the lamina propria. The serous fluid, produced by the seromucous glands, is situated between the mucus and the apical plasmalemmae of the respiratory epithelial cells. The cilia of the ciliated columnar cells do not reach the mucous layer, so their movement is restricted to the serous fluid layer. As the cilia move within that watery fluid, the mucus is swept along ("hydroplaned") between the interface of the two fluids. The particulate matter trapped in mucus is thus delivered, by ciliary action, to the pharynx to be swallowed or expectorated.

In addition to being filtered, the air is also warmed and humidified by passing over the mucosa, which is kept warm and moist by its rich blood supply. Warming of the inspired air is facilitated by the presence of an extensive network of rows of arched vessels grouped in an anteroposterior arrangement. Capillary beds arising from these vessels lie just beneath the epithelium. Blood flows into this vascular network from posterior to anterior, antiparallel to the flow of air; thus heat is continuously being transferred to the inspired air by a countercurrent mechanism.

Antigens and allergens carried by the air are combatted by lymphoid elements of the lamina propria. Secretory immunoglobulin (IgA), produced by plasma cells, is transported across the epithelium into the nasal cavity by ciliated columnar cells and by the acinar cells of the seromucous glands. IgE, also produced by plasma cells, binds to IgE receptors of mast cell and basophil plasmalemmae. Subsequent binding of a specific antigen or allergen to the bound IgE causes the mast cell (and basophil) to release various mediators of inflammation. These, in turn, act on the nasal mucosa, inducing the symptoms associated with colds and hay fever.

CLINICAL CORRELATIONS

The nasal mucosa is protected from dehydration by alternating blood flow to the venous sinuses of the lamina propria overlying the conchae of the right and left nasal cavities. The erectile tissue–like region (**swell bodies**) of one side expands when its venous sinuses become engorged with blood, reducing the flow of air through that side. Seepage of plasma from the sinuses and seromucous secretions from the glands thus rehydrate the mucosa approximately every half hour.

Chemical irritants and particulate matter are removed

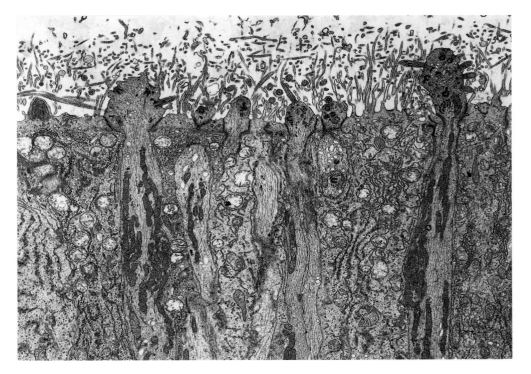

Figure 15–3. Transmission electron micrograph of the apical region of the rat olfactory epithelium. Note the olfactory vesicles and the cilia projecting from them (× 8,260). (From Mendoza, A.S., and Kühnel, W.: Postnatal changes in the ultrastructure of the rat olfactory epithelium: The supranuclear region of supporting cells. Cell Tissue Res. **265:**193–196, 1991. Copyright Springer-Verlag.)

from the nasal cavity by the **sneeze reflex.** The sudden explosive expulsion of air clears the nasal passage of the irritant.

The olfactory epithelium is responsible for the perception of odors, which also makes a major contribution to taste discrimination. The mechanism of odor discernment is poorly understood, although it is known that the plasmalemma of the olfactory cilia of a particular olfactory cell has numerous copies of one particular **odor receptor molecule.** Molecules of an odoriferous substance dissolved in the serous fluid bind to its specific receptor. When a threshold number of odor receptors are occupied, the olfactory cell becomes stimulated, an action potential is generated, and the information is transmitted via its axon to the olfactory bulb, a projection of the central nervous system, for processing. Axons of olfactory cells synapse with dendrites of 1 of 30 mitral cells within small spherical regions of the olfactory bulb, known as **glomeruli.** If a threshold level of impulses reaches a mitral cell, it becomes depolarized and relays the signal to the olfactory cortex for further processing.

Each glomerulus receives input (information) from approximately 2000 olfactory neurons, each specific for the same odoriferous substance. Like antigens, which may have several epitopes, each of which binds a specific antibody, odoriferous substances possess several small regions, each of which binds to a specific odor receptor molecule. Thus one particular odoriferous substance may bind to several odor receptor molecules, activating a number of olfactory neurons and providing input to several glomeruli. Although

there are only about 1000 glomeruli, each receiving information concerning a single odor receptor molecule, the olfactory cortex can differentiate about 10,000 different scents. It does so by recognizing information arising from a particular combination of glomeruli as a single scent. Thus a particular glomerulus may be active in the recognition of several scents.

To ensure that a single stimulus does not produce repeated responses, the continuous flow of serous fluid from Bowman's glands ensures a constant refreshing of the olfactory cilia.

Paranasal Sinuses

The ethmoid, sphenoid, frontal, and maxilla bones of the skull house large, mucoperiosteal-lined spaces, the **paranasal sinuses** (named after their location), which communicate with the nasal cavity. The mucosa of each sinus is composed of a vascular connective tissue lamina propria fused with the periosteum. The thin lamina propria resembles that of the nasal cavity in that it houses seromucous glands as well as lymphoid elements. The respiratory epithelial lining of the paranasal sinuses, like that of the nasal cavity, has numerous ciliated columnar cells, whose cilia sweep the mucous layer toward the nasal cavity.

Nasopharynx

The pharynx begins at the choana and extends to the opening of the larynx. This continuous cavity is subdivided into three regions: the superior **nasopharynx,** the middle oral pharynx, and the inferior laryngeal pharynx. The nasopharynx is lined by a respiratory epithelium, whereas the oral and laryngeal regions are lined by a stratified squamous epithelium. The lamina propria is composed of a loose-to-dense irregular type of vascularized connective tissue housing seromucous glands and lymphoid elements. It is fused with the epimysium of the skeletal muscle components of the pharynx. The lamina propria of the posterior aspect of the nasopharynx houses the **pharyngeal tonsil,** an unencapsulated collection of lymphoid tissue described in Chapter 12.

Larynx

The **larynx,** situated between the pharynx and the trachea, is a rigid, short, cylindrical tube, 4 cm in length and 4 cm in diameter. It is responsible for phonation and prevents the entry of solids or liquids into the respiratory system during swallowing. The wall of the larynx is reinforced by several hyaline cartilages (the unpaired thyroid and cricoid cartilages, and the inferior aspect of the paired arytenoids) and elastic cartilages (the unpaired epiglottis, the paired corniculate and cuneiform cartilages, and the superior aspect of the arytenoids). These cartilages are connected to each other by ligaments, and their movements with respect to one another are controlled by **intrinsic** and **extrinsic** skeletal muscles.

The thyroid and cricoid cartilages form the cylindrical support for the larynx, whereas the epiglottis provides a cover over the laryngeal aditus (opening). During respiration the epiglottis is in the vertical position permitting the flow of air, but during swallowing of food, fluids, or saliva it is positioned horizontally, closing the laryngeal aditus. The arytenoid and corniculate cartilages are occasionally fused to each other, and most of the intrinsic muscles of the larynx move the two arytenoids with respect to each other and to the cricoid cartilage.

The lumen of the larynx is characterized by two pairs of shelf-like folds, the superiorly positioned vestibular folds and the inferiorly placed vocal folds. The **vestibular folds** are immovable. Their lamina propria, composed of loose connective tissue, houses seromucous glands, adipose cells, and lymphoid elements. The free edge of each **vocal fold** is reinforced by dense, regular elastic connective tissue, the **vocal ligament.** The vocalis muscle, attached to the vocal ligament, assists the other intrinsic muscles of the larynx in altering the tension on the vocal folds. These muscles also regulate the width of the space between the vocal folds (the **rima glottidis),** thus permitting precisely regulated vibrations of their free edges by the exhaled air.

During silent respiration the vocal folds are partially abducted (pulled apart), and during forced inspiration they are fully abducted, but during phonation they are strongly adducted, forming a narrow interval between them. The movement of air against the edges of the strongly adducted vocal folds produces and modulates sound (but not speech, which

is formed by movements of the pharynx, soft palate, tongue, and lips). The longer and more relaxed the vocal fold, the deeper the **pitch** of the sound. Because the larynx of a postpubescent male is larger than that of a female, men tend to have deeper voices than women.

The larynx is lined by pseudostratified ciliated columnar epithelium, except on the superior surfaces of the epiglottis and vocal folds, which are covered by stratified squamous nonkeratinized epithelium. The cilia of the larynx beat toward the pharynx, transporting mucus and trapped particulate matter toward the mouth to be expectorated or swallowed.

CLINICAL CORRELATIONS

Laryngitis, inflammation of the laryngeal tissues, including the vocal folds, prevents the vocal folds from vibrating freely. Persons suffering from laryngitis sound hoarse or can only whisper.

The presence of chemical irritants or particulate matter in the upper air passages, including the trachea or bronchi, elicits the **cough reflex,** producing an explosive rush of air that removes the irritant. The cough reflex begins with the inhalation of a large volume of air and the closure of the epiglottis and glottis (abduction of the vocal folds), followed by powerful contraction of the muscles responsible for forced expiration (intercostal and abdominal muscles). Sudden opening of the glottis and epiglottis generates a rush of air whose velocity can exceed 100 miles per hour, removing the irritant with an enormous force.

Trachea

The **trachea** is a tube, 12 cm long and 2 cm in diameter, that begins at the cricoid cartilage of the larynx and ends when it bifurcates to form the primary bronchi. The wall of the trachea is reinforced by 10 to 12 horseshoe-shaped hyaline cartilage rings **(C-rings).** The open ends of these rings face posteriorly and are connected to each other by smooth muscle, the trachealis muscle. Because of this arrangement of the C-rings, the trachea is rounded anteriorly, whereas it is flattened posteriorly. The perichondria of the C-rings are connected to one another by fibroelastic connective tissue that provides flexibility to the trachea and permits its elongation during inspiration. Contraction of the trachealis muscle decreases the diameter of the tracheal lumen, resulting in faster air flow, which assists in the dislodging of foreign material (or mucus or other irritants) from the larynx by coughing.

The trachea has three layers: the mucosa, the submucosa, and an adventitia (Fig. 15–4).

Mucosa

The **mucosal lining** of the trachea is composed of pseudostratified ciliated columnar (respiratory) epithelium, the

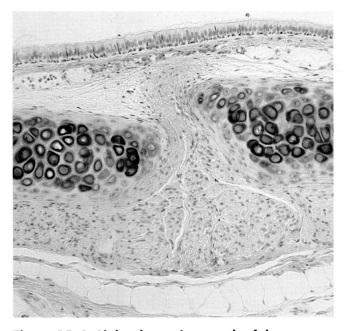

Figure 15–4. Light photomicrograph of the monkey trachea. Note the presence of the hyaline cartilage C-ring in the adventitia (× 135).

subepithelial connective tissue (lamina propria), and a relatively thick bundle of elastic fibers separating the mucosa from the submucosa.

RESPIRATORY EPITHELIUM. The **respiratory epithelium,** a pseudostratified ciliated columnar epithelium, is separated from the lamina propria by a thick basement membrane. The epithelium is composed of six cell types: goblet cells, ciliated columnar cells, basal cells, brush cells, serous cells, and cells of the diffuse neuroendocrine system (DNES). All of these cells come into contact with the basement membrane, but they do not all reach the lumen (Fig. 15–5).

Goblet cells constitute about 30% of the total cell population of the respiratory epithelium. These cells produce mucinogen, which becomes hydrated and is known as **mucin** when released into an aqueous environment. Like goblet cells elsewhere, those in the respiratory epithelium have a narrow, basally positioned **stem** and an expanded **theca** containing secretory granules. Electron micrography demonstrates that the nucleus and most organelles are located in the stem. This region displays a rich network of rough endoplasmic reticulum (RER), a well-developed Golgi complex, numerous mitochondria, and an abundance of ribosomes. The theca is filled with numerous mucinogen-containing secretory granules of varied diameters. The apical plasmalemma has a few short blunt microvilli (see Fig. 15–5).

Ciliated columnar cells constitute approximately 30% of the total cell population. These tall, slender cells have a basally located nucleus and possess cilia and microvilli on the apical cell membrane (Fig. 15–6). The cytoplasm just below these structures is rich in mitochondria and has a Golgi complex. The remainder of the cytoplasm presents some RER and a few ribosomes. These cells move the mucus and its trapped particulate matter, via ciliary action, toward the nasopharynx for elimination.

The short **basal cells** compose about 30% of the total cell population. They are located on the basement membrane, but their apical surfaces do not reach the lumen (see Fig. 15–5). These relatively undifferentiated cells are considered to be stem cells that proliferate to replace defunct goblet, ciliated columnar, and brush cells.

Brush cells (small-granule mucous cells) constitute about 3% of the total cell population. They are narrow, columnar cells with tall microvilli. Their function is unknown, but they have been associated with nerve endings; thus some investigators suggest that they may have a sensory role. Other investigators believe that they are merely goblet cells that have released their mucinogen.

Serous cells, which make up about 3% of the total cell population of the respiratory epithelium, are columnar cells. They have apical microvilli and apical granules containing an electron-dense secretory product, a serous fluid of unknown composition.

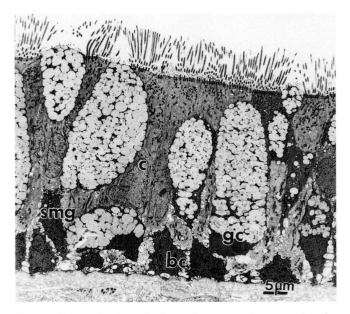

Figure 15–5. Transmission electron micrograph of the monkey respiratory epithelium from the anterior nasal septum. Note the presence of goblet cell (GC), ciliated cell (C), basal cell (BC), and small granule mucous cell (SMG). (From Harkema, J.R., Plopper, C.G., Hyde, D.M., Wilson, D.W., St. George, J.A., and Wong, V.J.: Nonolfactory surface epithelium of the nasal cavity of the bonnet monkey: A morphologic and morphometric study of the transitional and respiratory epithelium. Am. J. Anat. **180:**266–279, 1987. Copyright © 1987. Reprinted by permission of John Wiley & Sons, Inc.)

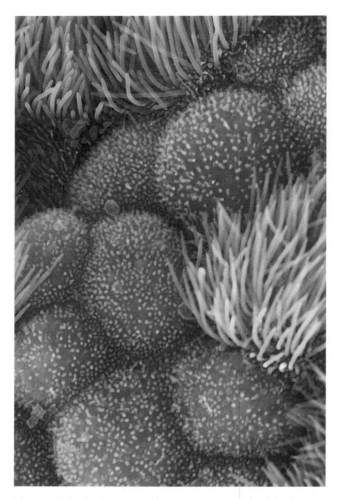

Figure 15–6. Scanning electron micrograph of the human fetal trachea displaying ciliated and nonciliated cells (× 7000). (From Montgomery, P.Q., Stafford, N.D., and Stolinski, C.: Ultrastructure of the human fetal trachea. A morphologic study of the luminal and glandular epithelia at the mid-trimester. J. Anat. **173:**43–59, 1990.)

DNES cells, also known as small-granule cells, make up about 3% to 4% of the total cell population. They are probably derived from neural crest cells and contain numerous granules in their basal cytoplasm. The contents of these granules probably are released into the connective tissue spaces of the lamina propria. These cells are of various types and release pharmacological agents thought to control the functioning of other cells of the respiratory epithelium. These cells are discussed in greater detail in Chapter 17.

LAMINA PROPRIA AND ELASTIC FIBERS. The **lamina propria** of the trachea is composed of a loose, fibroelastic connective tissue. It contains lymphoid elements (e.g., lymphoid nodules, lymphocytes, and neutrophils) as well as mucous and seromucous glands, whose ducts open onto the epithelial surface. A dense layer of elastic fibers, the **elastic**

lamina, separates the lamina propria from the underlying submucosa.

Submucosa

The tracheal **submucosa** is composed of a dense, irregular fibroelastic connective tissue housing numerous mucous and seromucous glands. The short ducts of these glands pierce the elastic lamina and the lamina propria to open onto the epithelial surface. Lymphoid elements are also present in the submucosa. Moreover, this region has a rich blood and lymph supply, whose smaller branches reach the lamina propria.

Adventitia

The **adventitia** of the trachea is composed of a fibroelastic connective tissue (see Fig. 15–4). The most prominent features of the adventitia are the hyaline cartilage C-rings and the intervening fibrous connective tissue. The adventitia also is responsible for anchoring the trachea to the adjacent structures (i.e., esophagus and connective tissues of the neck).

CLINICAL CORRELATIONS

The respiratory epithelium of persons chronically exposed to irritants such as cigarette smoke and coal dust undergoes reversible alterations known as **metaplasia,** associated with an increase in the number of goblet cells relative to ciliated cells. The increased number of goblet cells produces a thicker layer of mucus to remove the irritants, but the reduction in the number of cilia retards the rate of mucus elimination, resulting in congestion. Moreover, the seromucous glands of the lamina propria and submucosa increase in size, forming a more copious secretion. A few months after elimination of the pollutants, the cell ratio returns to normal (1:1) and the seromucous glands revert to their previous size.

Bronchial Tree

The **bronchial tree** begins at the bifurcation of the trachea, as the right and left primary bronchi, which arborize, forming branches that gradually decrease in size. The bronchial tree is composed of airways located outside the lungs (the primary bronchi, extrapulmonary bronchi) and airways located inside the lungs: the intrapulmonary bronchi (secondary and tertiary bronchi), bronchioles, terminal bronchioles, and respiratory bronchioles (Fig. 15–7). As the airways progressively decrease in size, several trends are observed, including a *decrease* in the amount of cartilage, glands, goblet cells, and height of epithelial cells and an *increase* in smooth muscle and elastic tissue (with respect to the thickness of the wall).

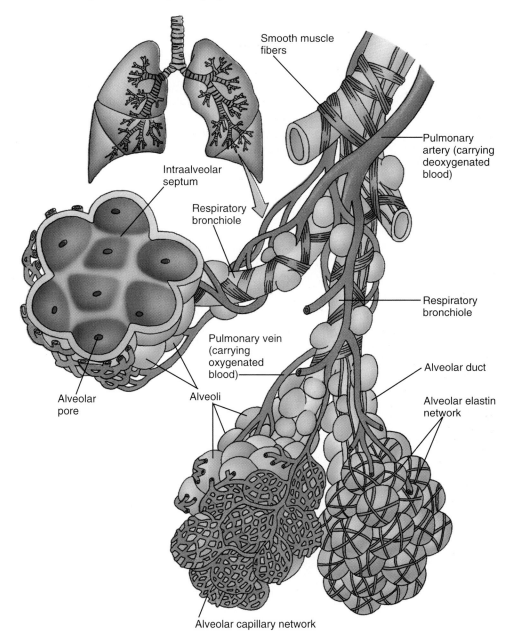

Smooth muscle fibers

Pulmonary artery (carrying deoxygenated blood)

Intraalveolar septum

Respiratory bronchiole

Respiratory bronchiole

Pulmonary vein (carrying oxygenated blood)

Alveolar duct

Alveolar elastin network

Alveolar pore

Alveoli

Alveolar capillary network

Figure 15–7. Schematic diagram of the respiratory system, displaying bronchioles, terminal bronchioles, respiratory bronchioles, alveolar ducts, sacs, and alveoli.

Primary (Extrapulmonary) Bronchi

The structure of the **primary bronchi** is identical to that of the trachea, except that they are smaller in diameter and their walls are thinner. Each primary bronchus, accompanied by the pulmonary arteries, veins, and lymph vessels, pierces the root of the lung. The right bronchus is straighter than the left bronchus. The right bronchus trifurcates to lead to the three lobes of the right lung, and the left bronchus bifurcates, sending a branch to the two lobes of the left lung. These branches then enter the substance of the lungs as intrapulmonary bronchi.

Intrapulmonary (Secondary and Tertiary) Bronchi

Each **intrapulmonary bronchus** is the airway to a lobe of the lung. These airways are similar to primary bronchi with the following exceptions. The cartilage C-rings are replaced by irregular plates of hyaline cartilage that completely surround the lumina of the intrapulmonary bronchi; thus these airways do not have a flattened region but are completely round. The smooth muscle is located at the interface of the fibroelastic lamina propria and submucosa as two distinct smooth muscle layers spiraling in opposite directions. Elastic fibers, which radiate from the adventitia, connect to elastic fibers arising from the adventitia of other parts of the bronchial tree.

As in the primary bronchi and in the trachea, seromucous glands and lymphoid elements are present in the lamina propria and the submucosa of the intrapulmonary bronchi. Ducts of these glands deliver their secretory products onto the surface of the pseudostratified ciliated epithelial lining of the lumen. Lymphoid nodules are particularly evident where these airways branch to form increasingly smaller intrapulmonary bronchi. The smaller intrapulmonary bronchi have thinner walls, decreasing amounts of hyaline cartilage plates, and shorter epithelial-lining cells.

Secondary bronchi, direct branches of the primary bronchi, leading to the lobes of the lung, are also known as **lobar bronchi.** The left lung has two lobes—thus it has two secondary bronchi, whereas the right lung has three lobes and therefore has three secondary bronchi.

As secondary bronchi enter the lobes of the lung they subdivide into smaller branches, **tertiary (segmental) bronchi.** Each tertiary bronchus will arborize but will lead to a discrete section of lung tissue, known as a **bronchopulmonary segment.** Each lung has 10 bronchopulmonary segments that are completely separated from each other by connective tissue elements and are clinically important in surgical procedures involving the lungs.

As the arborized branches of intrapulmonary bronchi decrease in diameter, they eventually lead to bronchioles.

Bronchioles

Each **bronchiole** (also known as a **primary bronchiole**) supplies air to a pulmonary lobule. Bronchioles are considered to be the 10th to 15th generation of dichotomous branching of the bronchial tree. Their diameter commonly is described as less than 1 mm, although this number varies among authors from 5 mm to 0.3 mm. This disagreement concerning the diameter of bronchioles may lead to confusion in the descriptions of their structure (but should not be considered a cause to complicate the life of the student).

The epithelial lining of bronchioles ranges from ciliated simple columnar with occasional goblet cells in larger bronchioles to simple cuboidal (many with cilia) with occasional Clara cells and no goblet cells in smaller bronchioles.

Clara cells are columnar with dome-shaped apices that have short, blunt microvilli (Fig. 15–8). Their apical cytoplasm houses numerous secretory granules containing glycoproteins manufactured on their abundant RER. Clara cells are believed to protect the bronchiolar epithelium by lining it with their secretory product. Additionally, these cells degrade toxins in the inhaled air via cytochrome P-450 enzymes in their smooth endoplasmic reticulum. Some investigators also suggest that Clara cells produce a surfactant-like material that reduces the surface tension of bronchioles and facilitates the maintenance of their patency. Finally, Clara cells divide to regenerate the bronchiolar epithelium.

The lamina propria of bronchioles has no glands; it is surrounded by a loose meshwork of helically oriented smooth muscle layers (Fig. 15–9). The walls of bronchioles and their branches have no cartilage. Elastic fibers radiate from the fibroelastic connective tissue that surrounds the smooth muscle coats of bronchioles. These elastic fibers connect to elastic fibers ramifying from other branches of the bronchial tree. During inhalation, as the lung expands in volume, the elastic fibers exert tension on the bronchiolar walls, and by pulling uniformly in all directions, they help maintain the patency of the bronchioles.

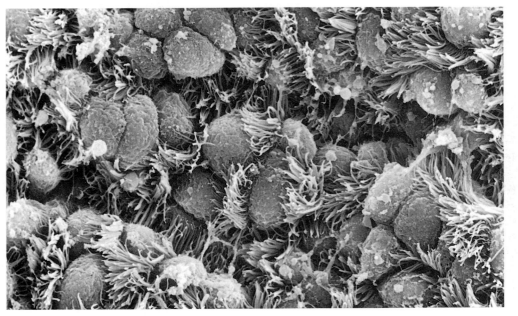

Figure 15–8. Scanning electron micrograph of Clara cells and ciliated cuboidal cells of rat terminal bronchioles (× 2000). (From Peao, M.N.D., Aguas, A.P., De Sa, C.M., and Grande, N.R.: Anatomy of Clara cell secretion: Surface changes observed by scanning electron microscopy. J. Anat. **183:**377–388, 1993. Reprinted with the permission of Cambridge University Press.)

Respiratory Portion of the Respiratory System

The respiratory portion of the respiratory system is composed of respiratory bronchioles, alveolar ducts, alveolar sacs, and alveoli.

Respiratory Bronchioles

Respiratory bronchioles are similar in structure to terminal bronchioles, except that their wall is interrupted by the presence of thin-walled, pouch-like structures known as **alveoli,** where gas can be exchanged. As respiratory bronchioles branch they become narrower in diameter and their population of alveoli increases. Subsequent to several branchings, each respiratory bronchiole terminates in an alveolar duct (Fig. 15–10).

Alveolar Ducts, Atria, and Alveolar Sacs

Alveolar ducts do not have walls of their own; they are merely linear arrangements of alveoli (Figs. 15–11A, 15–12). The alveolar duct that arises from the respiratory bronchiole branches, and each of the resultant alveolar ducts usually ends as a blind outpouching composed of two or

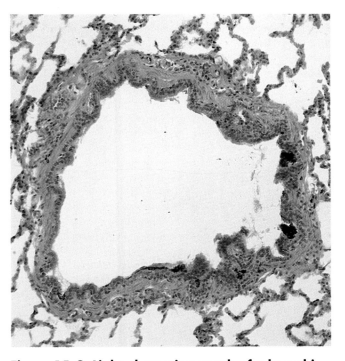

Figure 15–9. Light photomicrograph of a bronchiole (× 132). Note the presence of smooth muscle and the absence of cartilage in its wall.

CLINICAL CORRELATIONS

The smooth muscle layers of bronchioles are controlled by the parasympathetic nervous system. Normally, the smooth muscle coats contract at the end of expiration and relax during inspiration. In persons suffering from **asthma** the smooth muscle coat undergoes prolonged contraction during expiration; thus they have difficulties in expelling air from their lungs. Steroids and beta-2-agonists relax bronchiolar smooth muscle and are frequently used to relieve asthmatic attacks.

Terminal Bronchioles

Each bronchiole subdivides to form several smaller **terminal bronchioles,** which are less than 0.5 mm in diameter and constitute the terminus of the conducting portion of the respiratory system. These structures supply air to lung acini, subdivisions of the lung lobule. The epithelium of terminal bronchioles is composed of Clara cells and cuboidal cells, some with cilia. The narrow lamina propria consists of fibroelastic connective tissue and is surrounded by one or two layers of smooth muscle cells. Elastic fibers radiate from the adventitia and, as with the bronchioles, bind to elastic fibers radiating from other members of the bronchial tree. Terminal bronchioles branch to give rise to respiratory bronchioles.

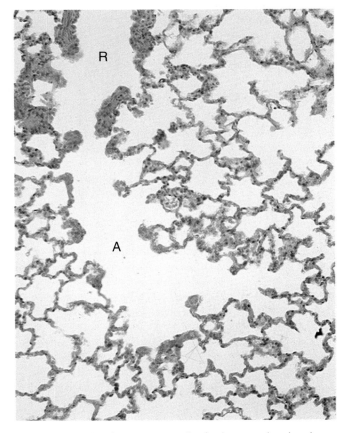

Figure 15–10. Photomicrograph of a human alveolar duct. Respiratory bronchiole (R); alveolar duct (A) (× 132).

Diffusion of CO_2 into blood and conversion to HCO_3^-

Diffusion of CO_2 out of blood into alveolus

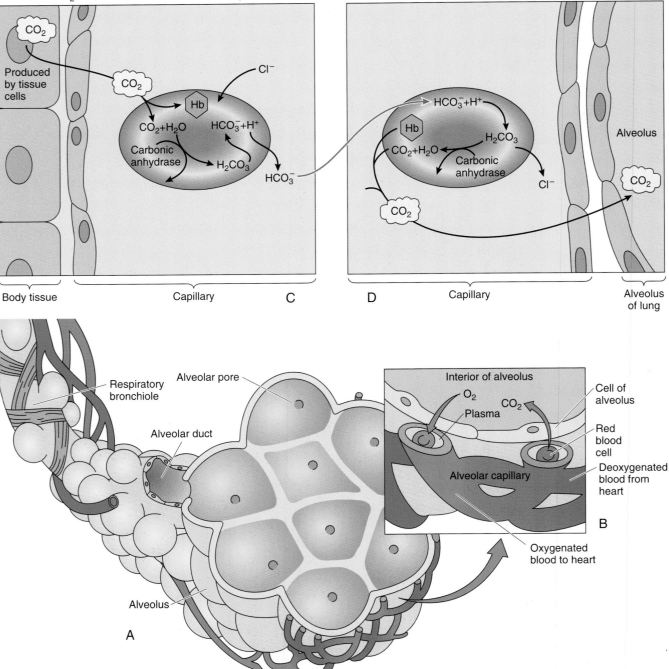

Figure 15–11. Schematic diagram of **A,** a respiratory bronchiole, alveolar sac, alveolar pore, and alveoli, **B,** interalveolar septum, **C,** carbon dioxide uptake from body tissues by erythrocytes and plasma, and **D,** carbon dioxide release by erythrocytes and plasma in the lung.

more small clusters of alveoli, where each cluster is known as an **alveolar sac.** These alveolar sacs thus open into a common space, which some investigators call the **atrium.**

Slender connective tissue elements between alveoli, the **interalveolar septa,** reinforce the alveolar duct, stabilizing

it somewhat. Additionally, the opening of each alveolus is controlled by a single smooth muscle cell (smooth muscle "knob"), embedded in type III collagen, that forms a delicate sphincter regulating the diameter of that opening.

Fine elastic fibers ramify from the periphery of alveolar

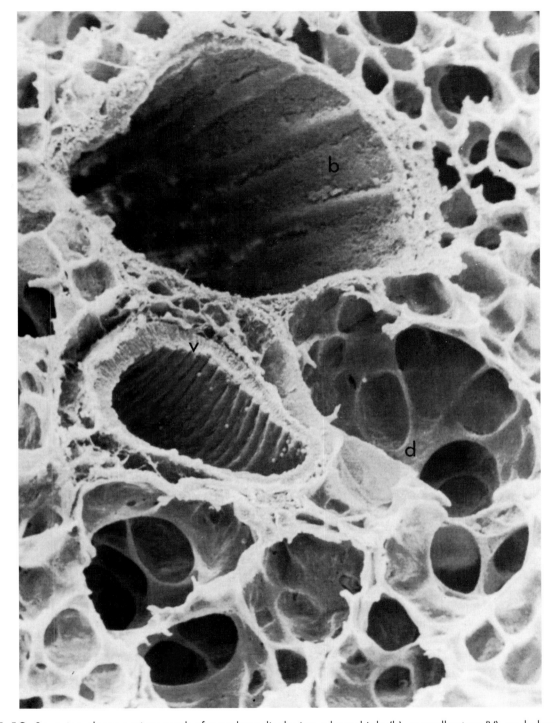

Figure 15-12. Scanning electron micrograph of a rat lung displaying a bronchiole (b), a small artery (V), and alveoli (d), some of which present alveolar pores. (From Leeson, T.S., Leeson, C.R., and Paparo, A.A.: Text/Atlas of Histology. Philadelphia, W.B. Saunders Company, 1988.)

ducts and sacs to intermingle with elastic fibers radiating from other intrapulmonary elements. This network of elastic fibers not only maintains the patency of these delicate structures during inhalation but also protects them against damage during distention and is responsible for nonforced exhalation.

Alveoli

Alveoli are small outpocketings, about 200 µm in diameter, of respiratory bronchioles, alveolar ducts, and alveolar sacs (see Figs. 15–11A and B; 15–12; 15–13). They form the primary structural and functional unit of the respiratory sys-

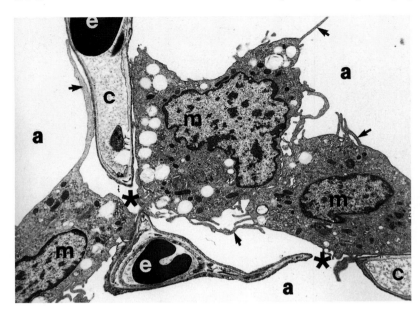

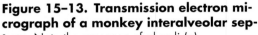

Figure 15–13. Transmission electron micrograph of a monkey interalveolar septum. Note the presence of alveoli (a), erythrocytes (e) within capillaries (c), and alveolar macrophages (m), whose filopodia (*arrows*) are evident. Asterisks indicate the presence of alveolar pores. (From Maina, J.N.: Morphology and morphometry of the normal lung of the adult vervet monkey (Cercopithecus aethiops). Am. J. Anat. **183**:258–267, 1988. Copyright © 1988. Reprinted with permission of John Wiley & Sons, Inc.)

tem, because their thin walls permit exchange of CO_2 for O_2 between the air in their lumina and blood in adjacent capillaries. Although each alveolus is a small structure, about 0.002 mm³, their total number approximates 300 million, conferring on the lung its sponge-like consistency. It has been estimated that the total surface area of all the alveoli available for gas exchange exceeds 140 m².

Because of their large number, alveoli are frequently pressed against each other, eliminating the connective tissue interstitium between them. In such areas of contact, the airspaces of the two alveoli communicate with each other through an **alveolar pore (of Kohn),** whose diameter varies from 8 to 60 μm (see Fig. 15–12). These pores presumably function to equilibrate air pressure within pulmonary segments. The region between adjacent alveoli is known as the **interalveolar septum.** It is occupied by an extensive capillary bed composed of **continuous capillaries,** supplied by the pulmonary artery and drained by the pulmonary vein. The connective tissue of the interalveolar septum is rich in elastic fibers and type III collagen (reticular) fibers.

Because alveoli and capillaries are composed of epithelial cells, they are invested by a prominent basal lamina. The openings of alveoli associated with alveolar sacs, unlike those of respiratory bronchioles and alveolar ducts, are devoid of smooth muscle cells. Instead, their orifice is circumscribed by elastic and especially reticular fibers. Walls of alveoli are composed of two types of cells: type I pneumocytes and type II pneumocytes.

Type I Pneumocytes

Approximately 95% of the alveolar surface is composed of simple squamous epithelium, whose cells are known as **type I pneumocytes** (also called type I alveolar cells or squamous

alveolar cells). The cells of this epithelium are highly attenuated, so that their cytoplasm may be as thin as 80 nm in width (see Fig. 15–12; Fig. 15–14). The region of the nucleus is much wider and it houses much of the cell's organelle population, composed of a small number of mitochondria, a few profiles of RER, and a modest Golgi apparatus.

These cells form occluding junctions with each other, thus preventing the seepage of extracellular fluid (tissue fluid) into the alveolar lumen. The adluminal aspect of these cells is covered by a well-developed basal lamina, which is absent in areas of alveolar pores. The rim of each alveolar pore is formed by the fusion of the cell membranes of two closely apposed type I pneumocytes that belong to two discrete alveoli.

Type II Pneumocytes

Although **type II pneumocytes** (also known as great alveolar cells, septal cells, and type II alveolar cells) are more numerous than type I pneumocytes, they occupy only about 5% of the alveolar surface. These cuboidal cells are interspersed among and form occluding junctions with type I pneumocytes. Their dome-shaped apical surface juts into the lumen of the alveolus (Figs. 15–15, 15–16). They are usually located in regions where adjacent alveoli are separated from each other by a septum (hence the name septal cells), and their adluminal surface is covered by basal lamina.

Electron micrographs of type II pneumocytes display short apical microvilli. They have a centrally placed nucleus, an abundance of RER profiles, a well-developed Golgi apparatus, and mitochondria. The most distinguishing feature of these cells is the presence of membrane-bounded **lamellar bodies** that contain **pulmonary surfactant,** the secretory product of these cells.

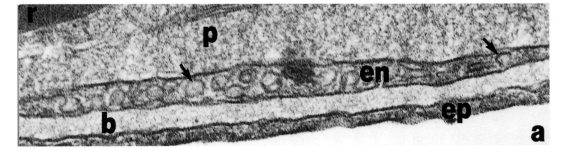

Figure 15–14. Transmission electron micrograph of the blood–gas barrier (× 71,250). Note the presence of the alveolus (a), the attenuated type I pneumocytes (ep), the fused basal laminae (b), the attenuated endothelial cell of the capillary (en) with pinocytotic vesicles (*arrows*), the plasma (p), and the erythrocyte (r) within the capillary lumen. (From Maina, J.N.: Morphology and morphometry of the normal lung of the adult vervet monkey (*Cercopithecus aethiops*). Am. J. Anat. **183:**258–267, 1988. Copyright © 1988. Reprinted with permission of John Wiley & Sons, Inc.)

Pulmonary surfactant, synthesized on the RER of type II pneumocytes, is composed primarily of the phospholipids, **dipalmitoyl phosphatidylcholine** and **phosphatidylglycerol,** and four unique proteins, **surfactant protein A, B, C, and D.** It is modified in the Golgi apparatus and is then released from the *trans*-Golgi network into secretory vesicles, known as **composite bodies,** the immediate precursors of lamellar bodies.

The surfactant is released by exocytosis into the lumen of the alveolus. Here, it forms a broad, lattice-like network known as **tubular myelin,** which becomes separated into lipid and protein portions. The lipid is inserted into a monomolecular phospholipid film forming an interface with air, and the protein enters an aqueous layer between the pneumocytes and the phospholipid film. The surfactant decreases surface tension, thus preventing the collapse of the alveolus. It is continuously manufactured by type II pneumocytes and, according to recent evidence, phagocytosed by type II pneumocytes and alveolar macrophages.

In addition to producing and phagocytosing surfactant, type II pneumocytes undergo mitosis to regenerate themselves as well as type I pneumocytes.

CLINICAL CORRELATIONS

At birth the infant's lungs expand upon the first intake of breath, and the presence of pulmonary surfactant permits the alveoli to remain patent. Immature infants (those born prior to 7 months of gestation) who have not as yet produced surfactant (or who have produced an inadequate supply of surfactant) suffer from the potentially fatal **respiratory distress of the newborn.** These newborns are treated with a combination of synthetic surfactant and glucocorticoid therapy. The former acts immediately to reduce surface tension, and the latter stimulates type II pneumocytes to produce surfactant.

Alveolar Macrophages

Monocytes gain access to the pulmonary interstitium, become **alveolar macrophages (dust cells),** migrate between type I pneumocytes, and enter the lumen of the alveolus.

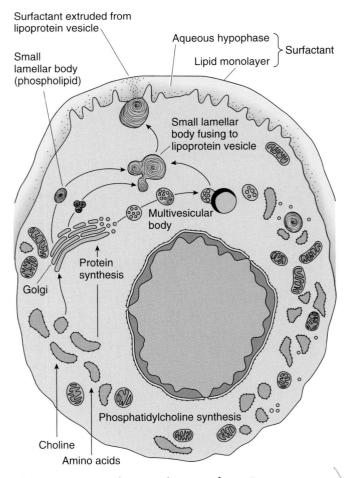

Figure 15–15. Schematic diagram of type II pneumocyte.

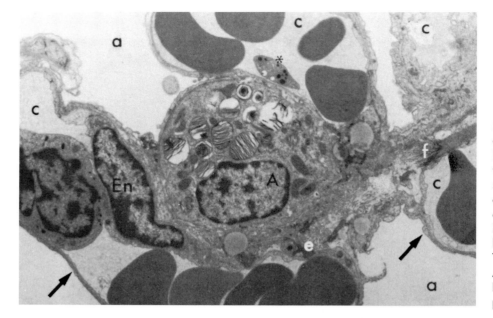

Figure 15–16. Transmission electron micrograph of a type II pneumocyte. Observe the centrally placed nucleus (A) flanked by several lamellar bodies. a, alveolus; c, capillaries; En, nucleus of endothelial cell; e, elastic fibers; f, collagen fibers; *arrows*, blood–gas barrier; *, platelet. (From Leeson, T.S., Leeson, C.R., and Paparo, A.A.: Text/Atlas of Histology. Philadelphia, W.B. Saunders Company, 1988.)

These cells phagocytose particulate matter, such as dust and bacteria, and thus maintain a sterile environment within the lungs (see Fig. 15–13). These cells also assist type II pneumocytes in the uptake of surfactant. Approximately 100 million macrophages migrate to the bronchi each day and are transported from there by ciliary action to the pharynx to be eliminated by being swallowed or expectorated. However, some alveolar macrophages reenter the pulmonary interstitium and migrate into lymph vessels to exit the lungs.

Characteristic features of the respiratory system are presented in Table 15–1.

CLINICAL CORRELATIONS

Alveolar macrophages of persons suffering from pulmonary congestion and congestive heart failure contain phagocytosed, extravasated red blood cells. These macrophages are frequently called **heart-failure cells.**

Emphysema is a disease usually associated with the sequelae of long-term exposure to cigarette smoke and other inhibitors of the protein α_1-antitrypsin. This protein safeguards the lungs against the destruction of elastic fibers by elastase synthesized by dust cells. Persons suffering from this disease have reduced elasticity of their lung tissue and display large, fluid-filled sacs that decrease the gas-exchange capability of the respiratory portion of the respiratory system.

Interalveolar Septum

The region between two adjacent alveoli, known as an **interalveolar septum,** is lined on both sides by alveolar epithelium (see Fig. 15–13). The interalveolar septum may be extremely narrow, housing only a **continuous capillary** and its basal lamina, or it may be somewhat wider, including connective tissue elements, such as type III collagen and elastic fibers, macrophages, fibroblasts (and myofibroblasts), mast cells, and lymphoid elements.

Blood–Gas Barrier

The thinnest regions of the interalveolar septum in which gases can be exchanged are called the **blood–gas barriers** (see Fig. 15–14). The narrowest blood–gas barrier, where the type I pneumocyte is in intimate contact with the endothelial lining of the capillary and the basal laminae of the two epithelia become fused, is most efficient for the exchange of oxygen (in the alveolar lumen) for carbon dioxide (in the blood). These regions are composed of the following three structures:

- Surfactant and type I pneumocytes
- Fused basal laminae of type I pneumocytes and endothelial cells of the capillary
- Endothelial cells of the continuous capillary

Exchange of Gases Between the Tissues and Lungs

During inspiration, oxygen-containing air enters the alveolar spaces of the lung. Oxygen diffuses through the blood–gas barrier to enter the lumina of the capillaries and binds to the **heme** portion of the erythrocyte hemoglobin, forming **oxyhemoglobin.** Carbon dioxide leaves the blood, diffuses through the blood–gas barrier into the lumina of the alveolus, and exits the alveolar spaces as the carbon dioxide–rich air is exhaled. The passage of oxygen and carbon dioxide across the blood–gas barrier is due to passive

Table 15-1. Characteristic Features of the Respiratory System

Division	Region	Support	Glands	Epithelium	Cell Types	Additional Features
Extra-pulmonary conducting	Nasal vestibule	Hyaline cartilage	Sebaceous and sweat glands	Stratified squamous keratinized	Epidermis	Vibrissae
Extra-pulmonary conducting	Nasal cavity: respiratory	Hyaline cartilage and bone	Seromucous glands	Respiratory	Basal, goblet, ciliated, brush, serous, and DNES	Erectile-like tissue
Extra-pulmonary conducting	Nasal cavity: olfactory	Bone	Bowman's glands (serous)	Olfactory	Olfactory, sustentacular, and basal	Olfactory vesicle
Extra-pulmonary conducting	Nasopharynx	Skeletal muscle	Seromucous glands	Respiratory	[See above]	Pharyngeal tonsils and eustachian tubes
Extra-pulmonary conducting	Larynx	Hyaline and elastic cartilages	Mucous and seromucous glands	Respiratory and stratified squamous nonkeratinized	[See above]	Epiglottis, vocal folds, and false vocal folds
Extra-pulmonary conducting	Trachea and primary bronchi	Hyaline cartilage and dense, irregular collagenous connective tissue	Mucous and seromucous glands	Respiratory	[See above]	C-rings and trachealis muscle (smooth muscle) in adventitia
Intra-pulmonary conducting	Secondary (intra-pulmonary) bronchi	Hyaline cartilage and smooth muscle	Seromucous glands	Respiratory	[See above]	Plates of hyaline cartilage and two ribbons of helically oriented smooth muscle
Intra-pulmonary conducting	(Primary) bronchioles	Smooth muscle	No glands	Simple columnar to simple cuboidal	Ciliated cells and Clara cells (and occasional goblet cells in larger bronchioles)	Less than 1 mm in diameter; supply air to lobules; two ribbons of helically oriented smooth muscle
Intra-pulmonary conducting	Terminal bronchioles	Smooth muscle	No glands	Simple cuboidal	Some ciliated cells and many Clara cells (no goblet cells)	Less than 0.5 mm in diameter; supply air to lung acini; some smooth muscle
Respiratory	Respiratory bronchioles	Some smooth muscle and collagen fibers	No glands	Simple cuboidal and highly attenuated simple squamous	Some ciliated cuboidal cells, Clara cells, and types I and II pneumocytes	Alveoli in their walls; alveoli have smooth muscle sphincters in their opening
Respiratory	Alveolar ducts	Type III collagen (reticular) fibers and smooth muscle sphincters of alveoli	No glands	Highly attenuated simple squamous	Types I and II pneumocytes of alveoli	No walls of their own, only a linear sequence of alveoli
Respiratory	Alveolar sacs	Type III collagen and elastic fibers	No glands	Highly attenuated simple squamous	Types I and II pneumocytes	Clusters of alveoli
Respiratory	Alveoli	Type III collagen and elastic fibers	No glands	Highly attenuated simple squamous	Types I and II pneumocytes	200 μm in diameter; have alveolar macrophages

DNES, diffuse neuroendocrine system.

diffusion in response to the partial pressures of these gases within the blood and alveolar lumina.

Approximately 200 ml of carbon dioxide is formed by the cells of the body per minute. It enters the bloodstream and is transported in three forms: as a dissolved gas in plasma (20 ml), bound to hemoglobin (40 ml), and as plasma bicarbonate ion (140 ml). The following sequence of events occurs (see Fig. 15–11C):

- Most of the carbon dioxide dissolved in the plasma diffuses into the cytosol of the erythrocytes.
- Some of the carbon dioxide binds to the globin moiety of hemoglobin. Although CO_2 is carried in a different region of the hemoglobin molecule, its binding capacity is greater in the absence than in the presence of O_2 in the heme portion.
- Within the cytosol of the erythrocyte, most of the carbon dioxide combines with water, a reaction catalyzed by the enzyme **carbonic anhydrase,** to form carbonic acid, which dissociates into H^+ and HCO_3^- (bicarbonate ion). The hydrogen ion binds to hemoglobin, and the bicarbonate ion leaves the erythrocyte to enter the plasma. To maintain ionic equilibrium, Cl^- enters the erythrocyte from the plasma; this exchange of bicarbonate for chloride ions is known as the **chloride shift.**

The bicarbonate-rich blood is delivered to the lungs by the pulmonary arteries. Because the level of carbon dioxide is greater in the blood than in the lumina of the alveoli, CO_2 is released (following the concentration gradient). The mechanism of release is the reverse of the previous reactions. The following sequence of events occurs (see Fig. 15–11D):

- Bicarbonate ions enter the erythrocytes (with a consequent release of Cl^- from the red blood cells into the plasma known as **chloride shift).**
- Bicarbonate ions and hydrogen ions within the erythrocyte cytosol combine to form carbonic acid.
- **Carbonic anhydrase** catalyzes the cleavage of carbonic acid to form water and carbon dioxide.
- Carbon dioxide dissolved in the plasma, bound to hemoglobin, and cleaved from carbonic acid, follows the concentration gradient to diffuse across the blood–gas barrier to enter the lumina of the alveoli.

Pleural Cavities and the Mechanism of Ventilation

The thoracic cage is separated into three regions, the left and right thoracic cavities and the centrally located mediastinum. Each thoracic cavity is lined by a serous membrane, the **pleura,** composed of simple squamous epithelium and subserous connective tissue. The pleura may be imagined as an inflated balloon; as the lung develops, it pushes against this serous membrane, as if a fist were to push against the outer surface of the balloon. In this fashion a portion of the pleura, the **visceral pleura,** covers and adheres to the lung, and the remainder of the pleura, the **parietal pleura,** lines and adheres to the walls of the thoracic cavity.

The space between the visceral and parietal pleura (inside the balloon) is known as the **pleural cavity.** This space contains a slight amount of serous fluid (produced by the serous membranes), which permits a nearly frictionless movement of the lungs during **ventilation** (breathing), which involves air moving into the lungs (inhalation) and out of the lungs (exhalation).

Inhalation is an energy-requiring process, because it involves contraction of the diaphragm, intercostal, scalenus, and other accessory respiratory muscles. As these muscles contract, the volume of the thoracic cage expands. Because the parietal pleura is firmly attached to the walls of the thoracic cage, the pleural cavities also increase in volume, and consequently the pressure within the pleural cavities decreases. The pressure differential between the atmospheric pressure outside the body and the pressure within the pleural cavities drives air into the lungs. With the influx of air the lungs expand, stretching the elastic fiber network of the pleural interstitium, and the visceral pleura is brought closer to the parietal pleura, reducing the volume of the pleural cavities and thus increasing the pressure inside the pleural cavities.

For **exhalation** to occur, the respiratory (and accessory respiratory) muscles relax, decreasing the volume of the pleural cavities, with a consequent increase in the pressure within the pleural cavities. Additionally, the stretched elastic fibers return to their resting length, driving air out of the lungs. Thus normal expiration does not require energy. In forced expiration, the internal intercostal and abdominal muscles also contract further, decreasing the volume of the pleural cavity, forcing additional air to leave the lungs.

CLINICAL CORRELATIONS

In patients afflicted with **poliomyelitis** the muscles of respiration may become so weakened that the accessory muscles hypertrophy because they become responsible for the elevation of the thoracic cage. In other diseases, such as **myasthenia gravis** and **Guillain-Barré syndrome,** the weakness of the respiratory and accessory respiratory muscles may lead to respiratory failure and consequent death even though the lungs function normally.

Gross Structure of the Lungs

The left lung is subdivided into two lobes and the right lung into three lobes. Each lung has a medial indentation, the **hilus,** where the primary bronchi, bronchiolar arteries, and pulmonary arteries enter and bronchiolar veins, pulmonary veins, and lymph vessels leave the lung. This group of vessels and the airway that enter the hilus make up the root of the lung.

Each lobe is subdivided into several **bronchopulmonary segments** supplied by a tertiary intrapulmonary (segmental) bronchus. In turn, bronchopulmonary segments are subdivided into many **lobules,** each served by a bronchiole. Lobules are separated from one another by connective tissue septa, in which lymph vessels and tributaries of pulmonary veins travel. Branches of bronchial and pulmonary arteries follow bronchioles in their passage through the center of the lobule.

Pulmonary Vascular and Lymphatic Supply

The pulmonary arteries supply deoxygenated blood to the lungs from the right side of the heart. Branches of these vessels follow the bronchial tubes into the lobules of the lung (see Fig. 15–7). When they reach the respiratory bronchioles, these vessels form an extensive pulmonary capillary network composed strictly of **continuous capillaries.** Because these capillaries are only 8 μm in diameter, erythrocytes follow each other in single file, reducing the space that gases have to traverse and maximally exposing the erythrocyte to oxygen.

The blood in the capillary bed becomes oxygenated and then drains into veins of increasing diameter. These tributaries of the pulmonary vein carry oxygenated blood and travel in the septa between lobules of the lung. Thus the veins follow a path that is different from that of the arteries, until they reach the apex of the lobule, where they accompany the bronchial tubes to the hilus of the lung to deliver oxygenated blood to the left side of the heart.

Bronchial arteries, branches of the thoracic aorta, bring nutrient-laden and oxygen-laden blood to the bronchial tree, interlobular septa, and pleura of the lungs. Many of the small branches anastomose with those of the pulmonary system. Others are drained by tributaries of the **bronchial veins,** which return the blood to the azygos system of veins.

The lung has a dual-lymph drainage, a superficial system of vessels in the visceral pleura and a deep network of vessels in the pulmonary interstitium, but these systems have numerous interconnections. The superficial system of lymph vessels forms several larger vessels, which drain into the hilar (bronchopulmonary) lymph nodes at the root of each lung. The deep network is organized into three groups following the pulmonary arteries, pulmonary veins, and bronchial tree down to the levels of the respiratory bronchioles. All of these networks drain into the hilar lymph nodes at the root of each lung. Efferent lymph vessels from these lymph nodes deliver their lymph to the thoracic duct or the right lymphatic duct, which return the lymph to the junction of the internal jugular and subclavian veins of the left and right sides, respectively.

Pulmonary Nerve Supply

The thoracic sympathetic chain ganglia provide sympathetic fibers and the vagus nerve supplies parasympathetic fibers to the smooth muscles of the bronchial tree. **Sympathetic fibers** cause *relaxation* of bronchial smooth muscles, thus bronchodilation (while causing constriction of pulmonary blood vessels: "paradoxical response"), and **parasympathetic fibers** elicit *contraction* of bronchial smooth muscles, causing bronchoconstriction.

Synapses occasionally involve type II pneumocytes, suggesting the possibility of some neural control over the production of pulmonary surfactant.

Digestive System I—
Oral Cavity

16

The digestive system, composed of the oral cavity, alimentary tract, and associated glands, functions in the ingestion, mastication, deglutition (swallowing), digestion, and absorption of food as well as the elimination of its undigestible remnants. To perform these varied tasks, regions of the digestive system are modified and have specialized structures.

This and the following two chapters detail the histology and function of the component parts of the digestive system. The present chapter discusses the contents of the oral cavity; Chapter 17 discusses the alimentary tract (esophagus, stomach, small and large intestines, rectum, and anus); and Chapter 18 considers the glands of the digestive system (major salivary glands, pancreas, and liver and gallbladder).

Oral Mucosa: Overview

The oral cavity is lined by the **oral mucosa,** composed of a wet **stratified squamous nonkeratinized epithelium** and an underlying connective tissue. Regions of the oral cavity that are exposed to considerable frictional and shearing forces (gingiva and hard palate) have a partially (parakeratinized) to completely keratinized stratified squamous epithelium.

Ducts of the three pairs of major salivary glands (parotid, submandibular, and sublingual) open into the oral cavity, delivering saliva to moisten the mouth. These glands also manufacture and release the enzyme **salivary amylase** to break down carbohydrates, **lactoferrin** and **lysozymes,** antibacterial agents, and **secretory immunoglobulin (IgA).** Additionally, minor salivary glands, located in the connective tissue elements of the oral mucosa, add to the flow of saliva into the oral cavity. It is here that food is moistened with saliva, chewed, and isolated by the tongue, ultimately forming a **bolus.** These spherical masses are about 2 cm in diameter and are forced by the tongue into the pharynx to be swallowed.

The lips form the anterior whereas the palatoglossal folds form the posterior boundaries of the oral cavity. The struc-tures of interest in and about the oral cavity are the lips, the teeth and their associated structures, the palate, and the tongue.

Lips

The upper and lower **lips** are usually in contact with one another and thus resemble a drawstring in that they guard the entrance into the oral cavity. The core of the lips is composed of skeletal muscle fibers that are responsible for the lips' mobility. Each lip may be subdivided into three regions: the external aspect, vermilion zone, and mucous (internal, wet) aspect.

The **external aspect** of the lip is covered with thin skin and is associated with sweat glands, hair follicles, and sebaceous glands. This region is continuous with the **vermilion zone,** the pink region of the lip, which is also covered by thin skin. However, the vermilion zone is devoid of sweat glands and hair follicles, although occasional, nonfunctional sebaceous glands are present here. The interdigitation between the epithelium and connective tissue components of the oral mucosa (**rete apparatus**) is highly developed, so that the capillary loops of the dermal papillae are close to the surface of the skin, imparting a pink color to the vermilion zone. The absence of functional glands in this region necessitates the occasional moistening of the vermilion zone by the tongue. The **mucous (internal) aspect** of the lip is always wet, and is lined by stratified squamous nonkeratinized epithelium. The subepithelial connective tissue is of the dense, irregular collagenous type and houses numerous, mostly mucous, minor salivary glands.

Teeth

Humans have two sets of teeth: 20 deciduous (milk) teeth, which are replaced by 32 permanent (adult) teeth, composed of 20 succedaneous teeth and 12 molars. The permanent dentition is evenly distributed between the maxillary and mandibular arches.

The various teeth have different morphologies, numbers of roots, and functions, such as seizing prey, cutting smaller pieces from large chunks, and macerating the chunks to form a bolus. However, only the general structure of teeth is discussed here.

Each tooth is suspended in its bony socket, the **alveolus,** by a dense collagenous connective tissue, the **periodontal ligament.** The gingiva also supports the tooth, and its epithelium seals the oral cavity from the subepithelial connective tissue spaces (Fig. 16–1).

The portion of the tooth that is visible in the oral cavity is called the **crown,** whereas the region housed within the alveolus is known as the **root.** The portion between the crown and the root is the **cervix.** The entire tooth is composed of three calcified substances, which enclose a soft, gelatinous connective tissue, the **pulp,** located in a continuous space subdivided into the pulp chamber and root canal. The root canal communicates with the periodontal ligament space via a small opening, the apical foramen, at the tip of each root. It is through this opening that blood and lymph vessels as well as nerves enter and leave the pulp (Fig. 16–2).

Mineralized Components

The mineralized structures of the tooth are enamel, dentin, and cementum. Dentin surrounds the pulp chamber and root canal and is covered on the crown by enamel and on the root by cementum. Thus, the bulk of the hard substance of the tooth is composed of dentin. Enamel and cementum meet each other at the cervix of the tooth.

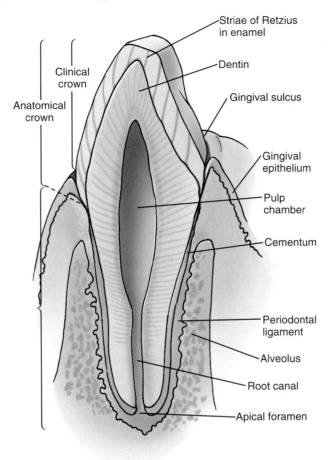

Figure 16–2. Schematic diagram of a tooth and its surrounding structures.

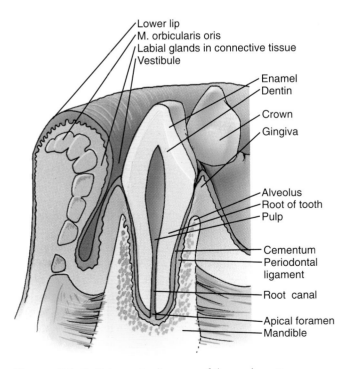

Figure 16–1. Schematic diagram of the oral cavity.

ENAMEL. Enamel is the hardest substance in the body. It is translucent, and its coloration is due to the color of the underlying dentin. Enamel consists of 96% calcium hydroxyapatite and 4% organic material and water. The calcified portion of enamel is composed of large crystals coated with a thin layer of organic matrix. The organic constituents of enamel are the keratin-like, high-molecular-weight glycoproteins tyrosine-rich **amelogens** and **enamelins.**

Enamel is produced by cells known as ameloblasts, which elaborate enamel daily in 4- to 8-μm segments. Successive **rod segments** adhere to one another, forming keyhole-shaped **enamel rods (prisms),** which extend over the complete width of the enamel, from the dentinoenamel junction to the enamel surface. The calcium hydroxyapatite crystal orientation within rods varies, permitting a subdivision of the enamel rod into a cylindrical head to which a tail (interrod enamel), in the shape of a rectangular solid, is attached. Enamel is a nonvital substance; because the ameloblasts die before the tooth enters the mouth, the body cannot repair enamel.

CLINICAL CORRELATIONS

Caries usually results from the accumulation of microorganisms in and on slight defects of the enamel surface. As these bacteria metabolize nutrients in the saliva and on the tooth surface, they produce acids that begin to decalcify the enamel. As the bacteria proliferate in the cavity that they have "excavated," they and the toxins that they release enlarge the caries.

Fluoride increases the hardness of enamel, making it more resistant to caries. The incidence of cavities has been greatly reduced by the addition of fluoride to the public water supply and to toothpastes and by its topical application in the dental office.

Because during its formation enamel is elaborated in daily segments, the quality of the enamel produced varies with the health of the mother during prenatal stages or the health of the person after birth. The enamel rod then reflects the metabolic state of the person during the time of enamel formation, resulting in successive rod segment sequences of normally calcified and hypocalcified enamel. These alternating sequences, analogous to growth rings in a tree trunk, are evident histologically and are called **striae of Retzius.**

The free surface of a newly erupted tooth is covered by a basal lamina–like substance, the **primary enamel cuticle,** manufactured by the same cells that elaborated enamel. This cuticle wears away shortly after the tooth's emergence into the oral cavity.

DENTIN. Dentin is the second hardest tissue in the body (see Figs. 16–2, 16–3). It is yellowish, and its high degree of elasticity protects the overlying brittle enamel from becoming fractured. Dentin is composed of 65% to 70% calcium hydroxyapatite, 20% to 25% organic materials, and about 10% bound water. Most of the organic substance is type I collagen associated with proteoglycans and glycoproteins.

The cells that produce dentin are known as odontoblasts. Unlike ameloblasts, they maintain their association with dentin for the life of the tooth. These cells are located at the periphery of the pulp, and their cytoplasmic extensions, **odontoblastic processes,** occupy tunnel-like spaces within dentin. These tissue fluid–filled spaces, known as **dentinal tubules,** extend from the pulp to the dentinoenamel (in the crown) or dentinocemental (in the root) junctions.

During dentinogenesis odontoblasts manufacture about 4 to 8 μm of dentin every day, and the quality of dentin, as of enamel, varies with the health of the mother prenatally or the child postnatally. Thus, along the length of the dentinal tubule, dentin displays alternating regions of normal calcification and hypocalcification. These are recognizable histologically as **lines of Owen,** analogous to the striae of Retzius in enamel.

Because odontoblasts remain functional, dentin has the capability of self-repair, and **reparative dentin** is elabo-

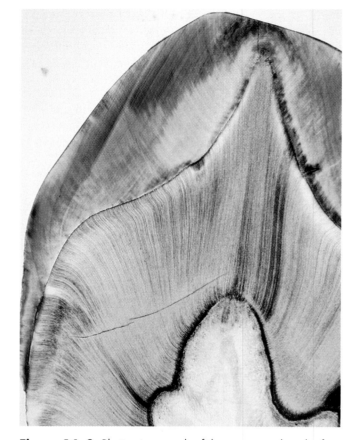

Figure 16–3. Photomicrograph of the crown and neck of a tooth (× 17).

rated on the surface of preexisting dentin within the pulp chamber, thus reducing the size of the pulp chamber with age.

CLINICAL CORRELATIONS

Dentin sensitivity is mediated by sensory nerve fibers that are closely associated with odontoblasts, their processes, and the dentinal tubules. Disturbance of the tissue fluid within dentinal tubules is thought to somehow depolarize the nerve fibers, sending a signal to the brain, where the signal is interpreted as pain.

CEMENTUM. The third mineralized tissue of the tooth is **cementum,** which is restricted to the root (see Figs. 16–2, 16–3). Cementum is composed of 45% to 50% calcium hydroxyapatite and 50% to 55% organic material and bound water. Most of the organic material is composed of type I collagen with associated proteoglycans and glycoproteins.

The apical region of cementum is similar to bone in that it houses cells, **cementocytes,** within lenticular spaces, known as lacunae. Processes of cementocytes extend from lacunae, within narrow **canaliculi,** that extend toward the vascular periodontal ligament. Because of the presence of cementocytes, this type of cementum is called **cellular cementum.** The coronal region of cementum is without cementocytes and is called **acellular cementum.** Both cellular and acellular cementum have **cementoblasts.** These cells, which are responsible for the formation of cementum, line cementum at its interface with the periodontal ligament and continue to elaborate cementum for the life of the tooth.

Collagen fibers of the periodontal ligament, known as **Sharpey's fibers,** are embedded in cementum and in the alveolus, and in this fashion the ligament suspends the tooth in its bony socket.

Cementum can be resorbed by osteoclast-like cells known as **odontoclasts.** During exfoliation, the replacement of deciduous teeth by their succedaneous counterparts, odontoclasts resorb cementum (and dentin) of the root.

CLINICAL CORRELATIONS

Cementum does not resorb as readily as does bone, a property that orthodontists use to their advantage in moving improperly positioned teeth. By placing the correct force on a tooth, the orthodontist reshapes the bony socket and consequently causes the tooth to be moved into its correct position.

Pulp

The **pulp** of the tooth is composed of a loose, gelatinous connective tissue, which is rich in proteoglycans and glycosaminoglycans, has an extensive vascular and nerve supply, and has some lymph circulatory elements (see Fig. 16–2; Fig. 16–4). The pulp communicates with the periodontal ligament through the apical foramen, a small opening at the tip of each root. Vessels and nerves enter and leave the pulp through these openings.

It is customary to subdivide the pulp into three concentric zones around a central **core.** The outermost, **odontoblastic,** zone of the pulp is composed of a single layer of **odontoblasts,** whose processes extend into the adjacent dentinal tubules of dentin. The **cell free zone** forms the layer deep to the odontoblastic zone, and as its name implies, it is devoid of cells. The **cell rich zone,** consisting of fibroblasts and mesenchymal cells, is the deepest zone of the pulp, immediately surrounding the pulp core.

The core of the pulp resembles most other loose connective tissues, except that it lacks adipose cells. An additional notable difference is that the pulp core is highly vascularized, and occasionally it houses calcified elements called **pulp stones (denticles).**

The nerve fibers of the pulp are of two types: **sympathetic** (vasomotor) fibers that control the luminal diameters of blood vessels and **sensory** fibers responsible for the transmission of pain sensation. The pain fibers are thin myelinated fibers that form **Raschkow's plexus** just deep to the cell rich zone. As nerve fibers continue through this plexus

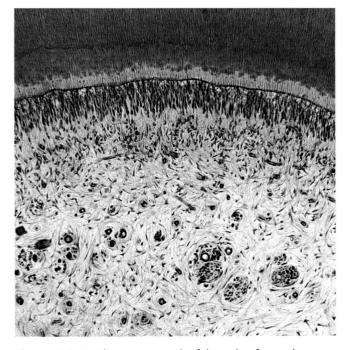

Figure 16–4. Photomicrograph of the pulp of a tooth (× 132).

they become unmyelinated, pass through the cell free zone, and penetrate the space between odontoblasts to enter the dentinal tubule. Some nerve fibers synapse on the odontoblasts or their processes instead of entering the dentinal tubules.

CLINICAL CORRELATIONS

Hemorrhage of the pulp is evident clinically as dark discoloration of the tooth. However, because the pulp may recover, hemorrhage should not be the sole determinant for performing root canal treatment.

Odontogenesis

The first sign of **odontogenesis** (tooth development) occurs between the 6th and 7th weeks of gestation, when the ectodermally derived **oral epithelium** proliferates (Fig. 16–5). The result of this mitotic activity is the formation of a horseshoe-shaped band of epithelial cells, the **dental lamina,** surrounded by **neural crest**–derived **ectomesenchyme** of the mandibular and maxillary arches. The dental lamina is separated from the ectomesenchyme by a well-defined basal lamina.

Shortly after the appearance of the dental lamina, mitotic activity increases on the inferior aspect of this epithelial band of each arch. This is responsible for the formation of 10 discrete epithelial structures, known as **buds,** initiating the **bud stage** of tooth development. These buds presage the

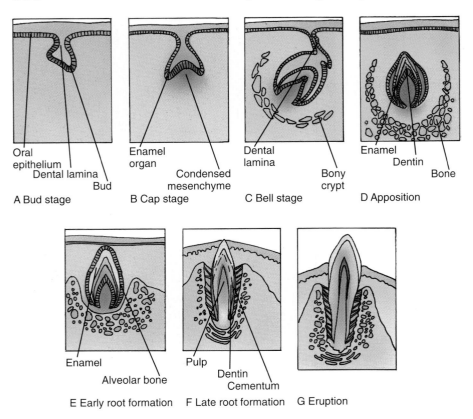

Oral
epithelium
Dental lamina
Bud
A Bud stage

Enamel
organ
Condensed
mesenchyme
B Cap stage

Dental
lamina
Bony
crypt
C Bell stage

Enamel
Dentin
Bone
D Apposition

Enamel
Alveolar bone
E Early root formation

Pulp
Dentin
Cementum
F Late root formation

G Eruption

Figure 16–5. Schematic diagram of odontogenesis.

10 deciduous teeth of both the maxillary and the mandibular arches. Further development, although similar for each bud, is asynchronous, corresponding to the order of emergence of the various teeth of the child.

As cells of the bud proliferate, this structure not only increases in size but alters its morphology to form a three-layered configuration, known as the **cap,** initiating the **cap stage** of tooth development. Two of the three layers—the convex simple squamous **outer enamel epithelium** and the concave simple squamous **inner enamel epithelium**—are continuous with each other at a rim-like region, the **cervical loop.** They enclose a third layer, the **stellate reticulum,** whose cells have numerous processes that contact one another. These epithelially derived layers, constituting the "plump" **enamel organ,** are separated from the surrounding ectomesenchyme by a basal lamina.

The concavity of the enamel organ is filled by closely grouped ectomesenchymal cells. This cluster of cells, known as the **dental papilla,** and the enamel organ are collectively called the **tooth germ.** The dental papilla, whose peripheral-most layer of cells is separated from the inner enamel epithelium by the basal lamina, is responsible for the formation of the pulp and dentin of the tooth. Ectomesenchymal cells surrounding the tooth germ form a vascularized membranous capsule, the **dental sac,** which will give rise to the cementum, periodontal ligament, and alveolus. Mature cells of the inner enamel epithelium will form enamel. Therefore,

except for enamel, the tooth and its associated structures are derived from cells of neural crest origin.

During the cap stage of tooth development, a solid cord of epithelial cells, the **succedaneous lamina,** derived from the dental lamina, grows deep into the ectomesenchyme. The cells at the tip of the succedaneous lamina proliferate to form a bud, the precursor of the **succedaneous** tooth that eventually replaces the **deciduous tooth** being developed. Because there are only 20 deciduous teeth, only the same number of succedaneous teeth can be formed. The remaining 12 permanent teeth (three molars in each quadrant) arise from the posterior extensions of the two dental laminae that begins in the fifth month of gestation.

Proliferation of the cells of the tooth germ increase its size, and the accumulation of fluid within the enamel organ increases its plump appearance. Additionally, its concavity deepens, and an additional layer of cells develops between the stellate reticulum and inner enamel epithelium of the enamel organ. This new layer of cells is the **stratum intermedium,** and its appearance characterizes the **bell stage** of tooth development. Because of changes in the morphology of the enamel organ and changes in the shape of certain cells of the tooth germ, this stage of odontogenesis is also called the **stage of morphodifferentiation and histodifferentiation.**

As most of the fluid within the enamel organ is resorbed, much of the outer enamel epithelium collapses over the stratum intermedium, bringing the vascularized dental sac close to that new layer. The proximity of blood vessels apparently causes the stratum intermedium to induce the simple squamous cells of the inner enamel epithelium to become enamel-producing columnar cells, known as **ameloblasts** (Fig. 16–6). In response to the histodifferentiation of the inner enamel epithelial cells, the peripheral-most cells of the dental papilla, in contact with the basal lamina, also differentiate to become dentin-producing columnar cells, known as **odontoblasts** (see Fig. 16–6; Fig. 16–7).

Shortly after the odontoblasts begin to elaborate the matrix of dentin into the basal lamina, the ameloblasts also begin to manufacture the matrix of enamel. The dentin and enamel adjoin each other, and the junction between them is called the **dentinoenamel junction (DEJ)** (see Fig. 16–3). The tooth germ is now said to be in the **appositional stage** of odontogenesis.

During the formation of dentin, as the odontoblasts move away from the DEJ, the distal tip of their process remains at that junction and the process continues to elongate. This cytoplasmic extension, known as the **odontoblastic process,** is surrounded by dentin. The space occupied by the odontoblastic process is the dentinal tubule.

Similarly, the ameloblasts also move away from the DEJ and form a process known as **Tomes's process.** As the ameloblasts secrete the enamel matrix, their apical region

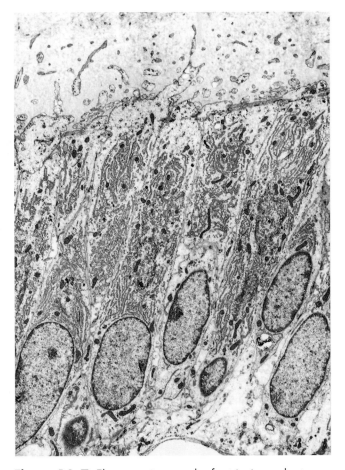

Figure 16–7. Electron micrograph of rat incisor odontoblasts (x 3600). (From Ohshima, H., and Yoshida, S.: The relationship between odontoblasts and pulp capillaries in the process of enamel- and cementum-related dentin formation in rat incisors. Cell Tissue Res. **268:**51–63, 1992. Copyright Springer-Verlag.)

becomes constricted by the matrix, forming Tomes's process. Then the ameloblasts move away from the newly elaborated enamel, and the constricted region expands to its previous size. The cyclic nature of Tomes's process formation continues until enamel formation ceases. As dentin matrix becomes calcified to form dentin, the process of calcification spreads into the enamel matrix, which becomes known as enamel.

Once all of the enamel and coronal dentin (dentin of the crown) are manufactured, the tooth germ enters the next stage of odontogenesis, **root formation.** The outer and inner enamel epithelia of the cervical loop elongate, forming a sleeve-like structure known as **Hertwig's epithelial root sheath (HERS),** and encompass ectomesenchymal cells located deep to the developing crown, forming an elongation of the dental papilla.

The absence of the stratum intermedium prevents the cells of the inner enamel epithelium from differentiating into ameloblasts; thus enamel will not be formed on the de-

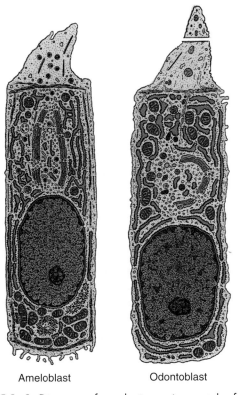

Ameloblast   Odontoblast

Figure 16–6. Diagram of an electron micrograph of an ameloblast and an odontoblast. (From Lentz, T.L.: Cell Fine Structure. An Atlas of Drawings of Whole-Cell Structure. Philadelphia, W.B. Saunders Company, 1971.)

veloping root surface. However, the peripheral-most cells of the root dental papilla differentiate into odontoblasts and begin to elaborate root dentin. As the HERS elongates, more and more of the root continues to be manufactured, and the region of HERS closer to the cervical loop begins to disintegrate, forming perforations in this sleeve-like structure. Ectomesenchymal cells from the dental sac migrate through the openings in the HERS, approximate the newly formed dentin, and differentiate into **cementoblasts.** These newly differentiated cells manufacture cementum matrix, which will become calcified **cementum.**

The elongation of the root is a consequence of the lengthening of the HERS. As the root becomes longer the crown approaches and eventually erupts into the oral cavity. It is interesting to note that although the two processes are simultaneous, the root is not "pushing" on the tissue apical to it; instead, it is believed that specialized fibroblasts, **myofibroblasts,** of the dental sac pull the forming tooth into the proper position.

Structures Associated with Teeth

Periodontal Ligament

The **periodontal ligament** is located in the periodontal ligament space, defined as the region between the cementum of the root and the bony alveolus (see Figs. 16–1, 16–2). The periodontal ligament space is less than 0.5 mm wide. Although this richly vascularized connective tissue is classified as dense irregular, it has **principal fiber groups,** composed of type I collagen fibers, that are arranged in specific, predetermined patterns to absorb and counteract masticatory forces. The ends of the principal fiber groups are embedded in the alveolus and cementum as **Sharpey's fibers,** which permit the periodontal ligament to suspend the tooth in its socket.

Nerves of the periodontal ligament include autonomic, pain, and proprioceptive fibers. The autonomic fibers regulate the luminal diameter of the arterioles, pain fibers mediate pain sensation, and **proprioceptive fibers** are responsible for the perception of spatial orientation.

CLINICAL CORRELATIONS

Proprioceptive fibers in the periodontal ligament are responsible for the **jaw-jerk reflex,** an involuntary opening of the jaw when one unexpectedly bites down on something hard. This reflex causes relaxation of the muscles of mastication and contraction of muscles responsible for opening the jaw, thus protecting the teeth from fracture.

Alveolus

The alveolar process, a bony continuation of the mandible and maxilla, is divided into compartments, each known as an **alveolus,** that house the root or, in the case of multirooted teeth, roots of a tooth. Adjacent alveoli are separated from each other by a bony interalveolar septum. The alveolus has three regions, the cortical plates, the spongiosa, and the alveolar bone proper (see Figs. 16–1, 16–2).

The **cortical plates,** disposed lingually and labially, form a firm supporting ledge of compact bone, lined by cancellous bone, the **spongiosa.** The spongiosa surrounds a thin layer of compact bone, the **alveolar bone proper,** whose morphology mirrors the shape of the root suspended in it.

Nutrient arteries travel in canals within the spongiosa, supplying the bony alveolus. The alveolar bone proper, said to be supported by the cortical plate and the spongiosa, has numerous perforations. Branches of the nutrient artery pass from the spongiosa into the periodontal ligament, contributing to its vascularization.

Gingiva (Gums)

Because the **gingiva,** a tough mucous membrane, is exposed to strenuous frictional forces, its stratified squamous epithelium is either fully keratinized or partially keratinized **(parakeratinized)** (see Figs. 16–1, 16–2). Deep to the epithelium is a dense, irregular collagenous connective tissue, whose type I collagen fibers form principal fiber groups that resemble those of the periodontal ligament.

As the epithelium of the gingiva approaches the tooth, it forms a hairpin turn, proceeds apically (toward the root tip) for 2 to 3 mm, and then attaches to the enamel surface by the formation of hemidesmosomes. The 2- to 3-mm-deep space between the gingiva and the tooth is the gingival sulcus.

The region of the gingival epithelium that attaches to the enamel surface is known as the **junctional epithelium,** which forms a collar around the neck of the tooth. The junctional epithelium forms a robust barrier between the bacteria-laden oral cavity and the gingival connective tissue. The principal fiber groups of the gingiva assist in the adherence of the junctional epithelium to the tooth surface, maintaining the integrity of the epithelial barrier.

Palate

The oral and nasal cavities are separated from each other by the **hard** and **soft palates.** The hard palate, positioned anteriorly, is immovable and receives its name from the bony shelf contained within it. In contrast, the soft palate is movable, and its core is occupied by skeletal muscle responsible for its movements.

The mucosa on the oral aspect of the hard palate is composed of a stratified squamous keratinized (or parakeratinized) epithelium underlain by dense, irregular collagenous connective tissue. The connective tissue of the anterior region of the hard palate displays clusters of adipose cells, whereas posteriorly it exhibits acini of mucous minor salivary glands. The nasal aspect of the hard palate is covered by respiratory epithelium with occasional patches of stratified squamous nonkeratinized epithelium.

The soft palate is covered by a stratified squamous nonkeratinized epithelium on its oral surface. The subjacent dense, irregular collagenous connective tissue has mucous minor salivary glands that are continuous with those of the hard palate. The epithelium of its nasal aspect, as that of the hard palate, is pseudostratified ciliated columnar. The posterior-most extension of the soft palate is the uvula, whose histological appearance is similar to that of the soft palate, except that its epithelium is composed solely of stratified squamous nonkeratinized epithelium.

Tongue

The **tongue** is the largest structure in the oral cavity. Its extreme mobility is due to the large intertwined mass of skeletal muscle fibers that compose its bulk (Fig. 16–8). The muscle fibers may be classified into two groups: those that originate outside the tongue, the **extrinsic muscles,** and those that originate in and insert into the tongue, the **intrinsic muscles.** The extrinsic muscles are responsible for moving the tongue, whereas the intrinsic muscles alter the shape of the tongue. The intrinsic muscles are arranged in four groups: superior and inferior longitudinal, vertical, and transverse.

The tongue has a dorsal surface, a ventral surface, and two lateral surfaces. Observation of its dorsal surface clearly delineates the tongue into two unequal regions, the larger **anterior two thirds** and the smaller **posterior one third.** The two regions are separated from one another by a shallow, V-shaped groove, the **sulcus terminalis,** whose apex points posteriorly and contains a deep concavity, the **foramen cecum.**

The dorsal surface of the posterior one third of the tongue is uneven because of the presence of the lingual tonsils (see Chapter 12). Lingual papillae, most of which project above the surface, cover the anterior two thirds of the tongue's dorsal surface.

Lingual Papillae

Based on their structure and function, the lingual papillae are classified into four types: filiform, fungiform, foliate,

Figure 16–8. Schematic diagram of the tongue and its lingual papillae.

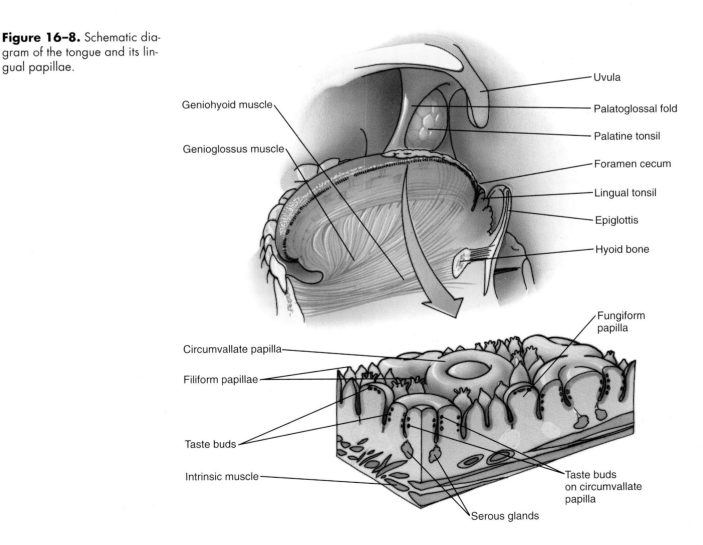

and circumvallate (see Fig. 16–8; Fig. 16–9). They are all located anterior to the sulcus terminalis on the dorsal or lateral aspect of the tongue.

Filiform papillae are numerous slender structures that impart a velvety appearance to the dorsal surface (see Figs. 16–8, 16–9). These papillae are covered by stratified squamous keratinized epithelium and function in scraping food off a surface. The high degree of keratinization is especially apparent in the sandpaper-like quality of the cat tongue. Filiform papillae do not have taste buds.

Each **fungiform papilla** resembles a mushroom, whose slender stalk connects a broad cap to the tongue surface (see Figs. 16–8, 16–9). The epithelial covering of these papillae are stratified squamous nonkeratinized; thus the blood coursing through the subepithelial capillary loops is evident as red dots distributed randomly among the filiform papillae on the dorsum of the tongue. Fungiform papillae have taste buds on the dorsal aspect of their cap.

Foliate papillae are located along the posterolateral aspect of the tongue. They appear as vertical furrows, reminiscent of pages of a book. These papillae have functional taste buds in the neonate, but these taste buds degenerate by the second or third year of life. Slender ducts of serous minor

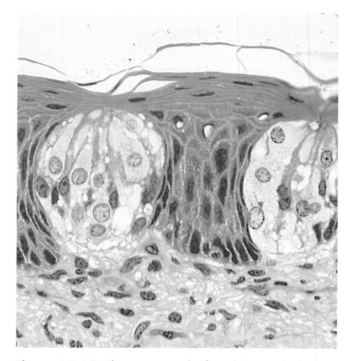

Figure 16–10. Photomicrograph of monkey taste buds (× 540).

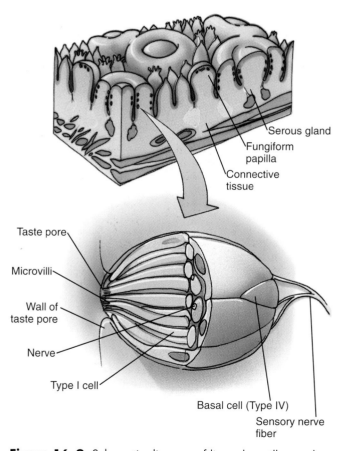

Figure 16–9. Schematic diagram of lingual papillae and a taste bud.

Labels: Serous gland; Fungiform papilla; Connective tissue; Taste pore; Microvilli; Wall of taste pore; Nerve; Type I cell; Basal cell (Type IV); Sensory nerve fiber

salivary **glands of von Ebner,** located in the core of the tongue, empty into the base of the furrows.

There are 8 to 12 large **circumvallate papillae** in a V-shaped arrangement just anterior to the sulcus terminalis. These papillae are submerged into the surface of the tongue so that they are surrounded by an epithelially lined groove, whose base is pierced by slender ducts of glands of von Ebner (see Figs. 16–8, 16–9). The epithelial lining of the groove and the side (but not the dorsum) of these papillae have taste buds.

TASTE BUDS. Taste buds are intraepithelial sensory organs that function in the perception of taste. The surface of the tongue and the posterior aspect of the oral cavity have approximately 3000 taste buds. Each taste bud, composed of 60 to 80 spindle-shaped cells, is an oval structure, 70 to 80 μm long and 30 to 40 μm wide, and is distinctly paler than the epithelium surrounding it (see Fig. 16–9; Figs. 16–10, 16–11). The narrow end of the taste bud, located at the free surface of the epithelium, projects into an opening, the **taste pore,** formed by the squamous epithelial cells that overlie the taste bud (see Fig. 16–11).

Four types of cells constitute the taste bud: basal cells (type IV cells), dark cells (type I cells), light cells (type II cells), and intermediate cells (type III cells). The relationship among the various cell types is not clear, although researchers agree that basal cells function as reserve cells and regenerate the cells of the taste buds, which have an average lifespan of 10 days. Most investigators believe in the follow-

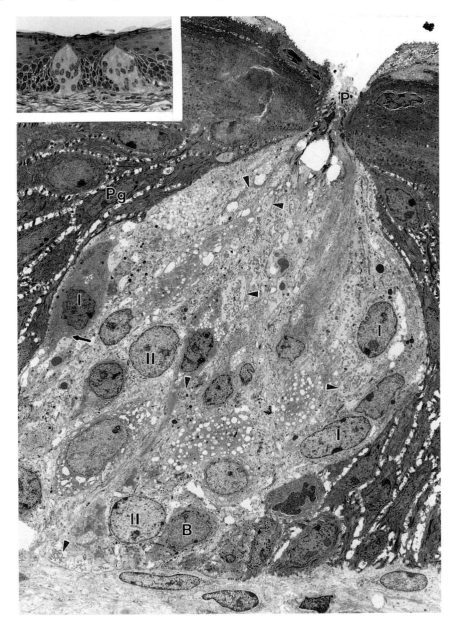

Figure 16–11. Low-power electron micrograph of a taste bud from the lamb epiglottis (× 2600). B, basal cell; I, type I cell; II, type II cell; P, taste pore; Pg, perigemmal cell; arrowheads, nerve fibers; arrow, synapse-like structure between a type I cell and a nerve fiber. (From Sweazy, R.D., Edwards, C.A., and Kapp, B.M.: Fine structure of taste buds located on the lamb epiglottis. Anat. Rec. **238:**517–527, 1994. Copyright © 1994. Reprinted by permission of John Wiley & Sons, Inc.)

ing progression: basal cells give rise to dark cells, which mature into light cells, which become intermediate cells and die.

Nerve fibers enter the taste bud and form synaptic junctions with type I, type II, and type III cells, indicating that probably all three cell types function in the discernment of taste. Each of these cell types has long, slender microvilli that protrude from the taste pore (see Fig. 16–11). In the past these microvilli were noted with the light microscope and were called **taste hairs.**

There are four primary taste sensations: salty, sweet, sour,

and bitter. It is believed that although every taste bud can discern each of the four sensations, each taste bud specializes in two of the four tastes. The reaction to these taste modalities is due to the presence of specific ion channels (salty and sour) and membrane receptors (bitter and sweet) in the plasmalemma of the cells of the taste bud.

The process of complex taste perception is due more to the olfactory apparatus than to the taste buds, as evidenced by the decreased taste ability of persons suffering from nasal congestion from colds.

Digestive System II— Alimentary Canal

17

The **alimentary canal,** the continuation of the oral cavity, is the tubular portion of the digestive tract. It is here that food is churned, liquefied, and digested; its nutritional elements and water are absorbed; and its indigestible components are eliminated. The alimentary canal, which is about 9 meters long, is subdivided into morphologically recognizable regions: the esophagus, stomach, small intestine (duodenum, jejunum, and ileum), and large intestine (cecum, colon, rectum, anal canal, and appendix).

Before discussing the individual regions of the alimentary canal, it is preferable to describe the entire tract as a whole and note its general plan. Once the conceptual design of the alimentary canal is understood, variations on that common theme are easier to assimilate.

General Plan of the Alimentary Canal

The alimentary canal is composed of several histological layers, which are schematically illustrated in Figure 17–1. These layers are innervated by parasympathetic and sympathetic nerves as well as by sensory fibers.

Histological Layers

The histology of the alimentary canal often is discussed in terms of four broad layers: the mucosa, submucosa, muscularis externa, and serosa (or adventitia). These layers are similar throughout the length of the digestive tract but display regional modifications and specializations.

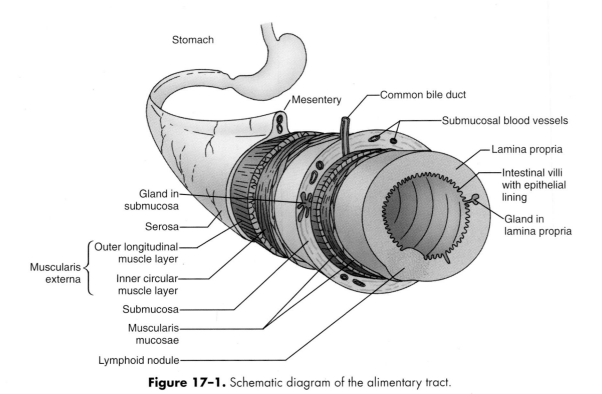

Figure 17–1. Schematic diagram of the alimentary tract.

Mucosa

The lumen of the alimentary canal is lined by an **epithelium,** deep to which is a loose connective tissue known as the **lamina propria.** This richly vascularized connective tissue houses glands as well as lymph vessels and occasional lymphoid nodules. Surrounding this connective tissue coat is the **muscularis mucosae,** composed of an inner circular and an outer longitudinal layer of smooth muscle. The epithelium, lamina propria, and muscularis mucosae are collectively called the **mucosa.**

Submucosa

The mucosa is surrounded by a dense, irregular fibroelastic connective tissue layer, the **submucosa** (see Fig. 17–1); this layer houses glands in the esophagus and duodenum. The submucosa also contains blood and lymph vessels as well as a parasympathetic neural plexus, **Meissner's submucosal plexus,** which controls the motility of the mucosa (and, to a limited extent, motility of the submucosa) and secretory activities of its glands.

Muscularis Externa

The submucosa is invested by a thick muscular layer, the **muscularis externa,** responsible for **peristaltic activity,** which moves the contents of the lumen along the alimentary tract. The muscularis externa is composed of smooth muscle (except in the esophagus) and is usually organized in an inner circular and an outer longitudinal layer. A parasympathetic nerve plexus, **Auerbach's myenteric plexus,** is situated between the two layers and regulates the activity of the muscularis externa (and, to a limited extent, the activity of the mucosa).

Three-dimensional reconstruction of the muscularis mucosae and of the muscularis externa shows that both the inner circular and the outer longitudinal layers are arranged helically. However, the pitch of the helices differs; the inner circular layer displays a tight helix, whereas the outer longitudinal presents a loose helix.

Serosa or Adventitia

The muscularis externa is enveloped by a thin connective tissue layer that may or may not be surrounded by the simple squamous epithelium of the visceral peritoneum. If the region of the alimentary canal is intraperitoneal, it is invested by peritoneum, and the covering is known as the **serosa;** however, if the organ is retroperitoneal, it adheres to the body wall by its **adventitia.**

Innervation of the Digestive Tract

The digestive tract receives its parasympathetic nerve supply from the vagus nerve, except for the descending colon and rectum, which are innervated by the craniosacral outflow. The sympathetic innervation is from the splanchnic nerves. The parasympathetic innervation is responsible for inducing secretions from the glands of the digestive tract as well as for smooth muscle contraction. Sympathetic fibers are vasomotor, controlling blood flow to the alimentary canal. Additionally, sensory fibers from the digestive tract travel with the sympathetic fibers to the central nervous system.

The parasympathetic fibers synapse with nerve cell bodies in the myenteric plexus. Nerve fibers originating in this plexus pierce the inner circular smooth muscle layer and assist in the formation of the submucosal plexus. Thus, neurons of the myenteric plexus communicate with neurons of the submucosal plexus.

The following may be stated as generalizations concerning the innervation of the alimentary canal:

1. Sympathetic nerves **inhibit peristalsis** and **activate sphincter muscles**
2. Parasympathetic innervation **stimulates peristalsis, inhibits sphincter muscles,** and **triggers secretory activity**
3. Both **Auerbach's myenteric** and **Meissner's submucosal plexuses** are part of the **parasympathetic** nerve supply, *but* they also have an **intrinsic nervous component** that is autonomous and is responsible for the coordinated functioning of the muscular components of the alimentary canal
4. Nerve fibers of the myenteric plexus control motility of the muscularis externa; therefore, the **myenteric plexus** is responsible for **peristalsis**
5. Nerve fibers from the submucosal plexus control motility of the muscularis mucosae; therefore, the **submucosal plexus** controls **movement** of the **mucosa** and **secretory activity** of the epithelial cells lining the lumen of the gut and the **glands** of the **lamina propria**
6. Sympathetic and parasympathetic fibers to the alimentary canal may be severed without compromising digestive functions, indicating that the **intrinsic nervous components** are primarily responsible for control of digestive activities

The remainder of this chapter discusses the various regions of the alimentary canal and examines how they differ from the general plan.

Esophagus

The **esophagus** is a muscular tube, approximately 25 cm in length, that conveys the bolus (masticated food) from the oral pharynx to the stomach.

Esophageal Histology

Mucosa

The lumen of the esophagus, lined by a stratified squamous nonkeratinized epithelium, almost 0.5 mm thick, is usually collapsed and opens only during the process of swallowing. Interspersed among the epithelial cells are **Langerhans cells,** which function as antigen-presenting cells; they phagocytose antigens, migrate to lymph nodes, and present the epitopes to lymphocytes (see Chapter 12). The lamina propria is unremarkable. It houses **esophageal cardiac glands,** which are located in two regions of the esophagus, a cluster near the pharynx and another one near its juncture with the stomach. The **muscularis mucosae** is unusual in that it consists of a single layer of longitudinally oriented smooth muscle fibers that become thicker closer to the stomach.

The esophageal cardiac glands produce mucus that coats the lining of the esophagus, lubricating it to protect the epithelium as the bolus is passed into the stomach. Because these glands resemble glands from the cardiac region of the stomach, some investigators suggest that they are ectopic patches of gastric tissue.

Submucosa

The **submucosa** of the esophagus is composed of a dense fibroelastic connective tissue, which houses the **esophageal glands proper.** The esophagus and the duodenum are the only two regions of the alimentary canal with glands in the submucosa. Electron micrographs of these tubuloacinar glands indicate that their secretory units are composed of two types of cells, mucous cells and serous cells.

Mucous cells have basally located flattened nuclei and apical accumulations of mucus-filled secretory granules. The second cell type appears to be **serous cells,** with round, centrally placed nuclei. The secretory granules of these cells have been shown to contain the proenzyme **pepsinogen** and the antibacterial agent **lysozyme.** The ducts of these glands deliver their secretions into the lumen of the esophagus.

The submucosal plexus is in its customary location within the submucosa, in the vicinity of the inner circular layer of the muscularis externa.

Muscularis Externa and Adventitia

The **muscularis externa** of the esophagus is arranged in two layers, inner circular and outer longitudinal. However, these muscle layers are unusual in that they are composed of both skeletal and smooth muscle fibers. The muscularis externa of the upper third of the esophagus has mostly skeletal muscle; the middle third has both skeletal and smooth muscle; and the lowest third has only smooth muscle fibers. Auerbach's plexus occupies its usual position between the inner circular and outer longitudinal smooth muscle layers of the muscularis externa.

The esophagus is covered by an **adventitia** until it pierces the diaphragm, when it is covered by a **serosa.**

Histophysiology of the Esophagus

The esophagus does not have an anatomical sphincter but has two physiological sphincters, the **pharyngoesophageal** and the **gastroesophageal sphincters,** which prevent reflux into the pharynx from the esophagus and into the esophagus from the stomach, respectively. A bolus entering the esophagus is conveyed, via peristaltic action of the muscularis externa, into the stomach at a rate of about 50 mm/sec.

CLINICAL CORRELATIONS

As the esophagus passes through the diaphragm, it is reinforced by fibers of that muscular structure. In some persons development is abnormal, causing a gap in the diaphragm around the wall of the esophagus, which permits herniation of the stomach into the thoracic cage. This condition, known as **hiatal hernia,** weakens the gastroesophageal sphincter, which allows reflux of the stomach contents into the esophagus.

Stomach

The **stomach,** the most dilated region of the alimentary canal, is a sac-like structure that in the average adult can accommodate approximately 1500 ml of food and gastric juices at maximal distention. The bolus passes through gastroesophageal junction into the stomach, where it is processed into a viscous fluid known as **chyme.** Intermittently, the stomach empties small aliquots of its contents through the **pyloric valve** into the duodenum. The stomach liquefies the food, continuing its digestion via the production of hydrochloric acid and the enzymes **pepsin, rennin,** and **gastric lipase** and via production of paracrine hormones.

Anatomically, the stomach has a concave lesser curvature and a convex greater curvature. Gross observations disclose that the stomach has four regions:

Cardia is a narrow region at the gastroesophageal junction, 2 to 3 cm wide

Fundus is a dome-shaped region to the left of the esophagus, frequently filled with gas

Body (corpus) is the largest portion, responsible for the formation of chyme

Pylorus is a funnel-shaped constricted portion, equipped with a thick pyloric sphincter, that controls the intermittent release of chyme into the duodenum

Histologically, the fundus and body are identical. All the gastric regions display **rugae,** longitudinal folds of the mucosa and submucosa, which disappear in the distended stomach. Rugae permit expansion of the stomach as it fills with food and gastric juices. Additionally, the epithelial lining of the stomach invaginates into the mucosa, forming **gastric pits (foveolae),** that are shallowest in the cardiac region and deepest in the pyloric region. Gastric pits increase the surface area of the gastric lining. Five to seven **gastric glands** of the lamina propria empty into the bottom of each gastric pit.

Gastric Histology

The ensuing discussion of the stomach details the fundic region, because the microscopic anatomy of the remaining regions are variations of the fundic region's histology. Figure 17–2 schematically depicts the major histological elements of the fundic region.

Fundic Mucosa

The **mucosa** of the fundic stomach is composed of the usual three components: an epithelium lining the lumen; an under-lying connective tissue, the lamina propria; and the smooth muscle layers forming the muscularis mucosae.

EPITHELIUM. The lumen of the fundic stomach is lined by a simple columnar epithelium composed of **surface lining cells,** which manufacture a thick **mucus** layer (Fig. 17–3A). The mucus lubricates the lining of the stomach and protects it from autodigestion. These cells continue into the gastric pits, forming their epithelial lining. **Regenerative cells** are also present in the base of these pits, but because they are more numerous in the neck of the gastric glands, they will be discussed along with the glands.

Electron micrographs of surface lining cells display glycocalyx-covered, short, stubby microvilli on their apical surfaces. Their apical cytoplasm houses secretory granules containing a homogeneous substance, the precursor of

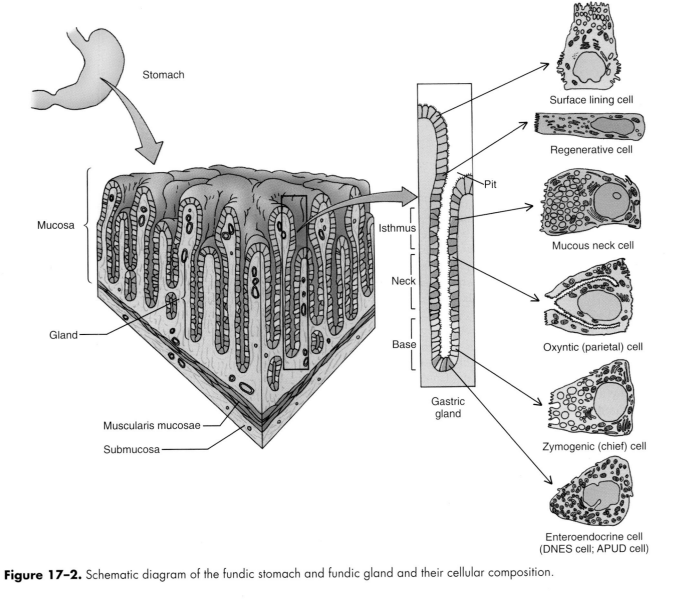

Figure 17–2. Schematic diagram of the fundic stomach and fundic gland and their cellular composition.

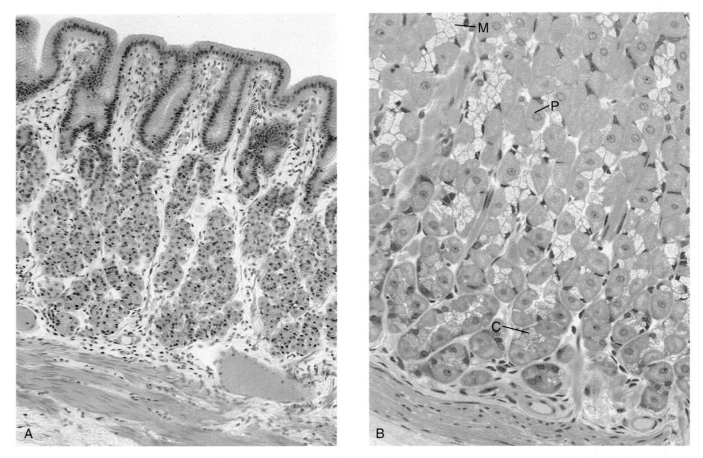

Figure 17–3. A, Photomicrograph of the mucosa of the fundic stomach (× 132). **B,** Photomicrograph of fundic glands. Parietal cell (P); mucous neck cell (M); chief cell (C) (× 270).

mucus (Fig. 17–4). The lateral cell membranes of these surface lining cells form intricate zonulae occludentes and adherentes with those of neighboring cells. The cytoplasm between their basally placed nuclei and apical secretory granules is occupied chiefly by mitochondria and the protein synthetic and packaging apparatus of the cell.

LAMINA PROPRIA. The loose, highly vascularized connective tissue of the lamina propria has a rich population of plasma cells, lymphocytes, mast cells, fibroblasts, and occasional smooth muscle cells. Much of the lamina propria is occupied by the 15 million closely packed gastric glands, known as **fundic (oxyntic) glands** in the fundic region (Fig. 17–3B).

Fundic Glands. Each fundic gland extends from the muscularis mucosae to the base of the gastric pit and is subdivided into three regions, the isthmus, neck, and base, of which the base is the longest (see Fig. 17–2). The simple columnar epithelium constituting the fundic gland is composed of six cell types: surface lining cells, parietal (oxyntic) cells, regenerative (stem) cells, mucous neck cells, chief (zymogenic) cells, and enteroendocrine (APUD; DNES) cells. The

distribution of these cells within the three regions of the gland is presented in Table 17–1.

The surface lining cells in the isthmus region are similar to those in the epithelium described earlier. The structure and function of the other five cell types are discussed in the following sections.

Mucous Neck Cells. **Mucous neck cells** are columnar and resemble surface lining cells, except that they are distorted by pressures from neighboring cells. Thus, they also have short microvilli, basally located nuclei, and a well-developed Golgi apparatus and rough endoplasmic reticulum (RER) (Fig. 17–5). Their mitochondria are located mostly in the basal region of the cell. The apical cytoplasm is filled with secretory granules containing a homogeneous secretory product that apparently differs from the mucus synthesized by surface lining cells. The lateral membranes of mucous neck cells form zonula occludentes and zonula adherentes with the surrounding cells.

Regenerative (Stem) Cells. A relatively few, thin **regenerative cells** are interspersed among the mucous neck cells of fundic glands (see Fig. 17–2). These columnar-shaped stem

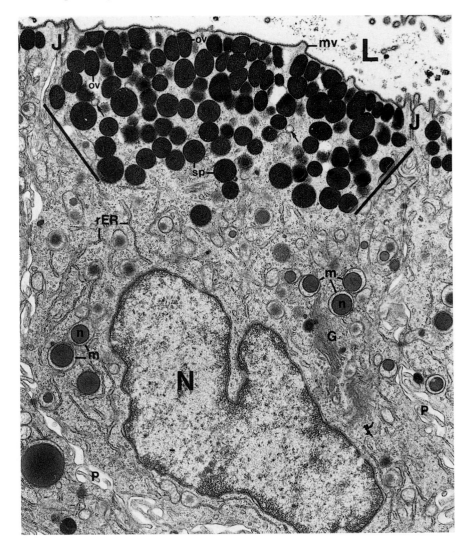

Figure 17–4. Electron micrograph of a surface lining cell from the body of a mouse stomach (× **13,000**). J, junctional complex; L, lumen; mv, microvillus; ov, oval secretory granules; sp, spherical granules; rER, rough endoplasmic reticulum; m, mitochondria exhibiting large spherical densities known as nodules (n); G, Golgi apparatus; N, nucleus; P, intercellular projections. (From Karam, S.F., and Leblond, C.P.: Identifying and counting epithelial cell types in the "corpus" of the mouse stomach. Anat. Rec. **232:**231–246, 1992. Copyright © 1992. Reprinted by permission of John Wiley & Sons, Inc.)

cells do not have many organelles but have a rich supply of ribosomes. Their nuclei are basally located, have little heterochromatin, and display a large nucleolus. The lateral cell membranes of these cells also form zonulae occludentes and adherentes with those of neighboring cells.

Regenerative cells proliferate to replace (with the exception of enteroendocrine cells) all of the specialized cells lining the fundic glands, gastric pits, and luminal surface. Newly formed cells migrate to their new locations either deep into the gland or up into the gastric pit and gastric lining. Surface lining cells and mucous neck cells are replaced every 5 to 7 days; thus regenerative cells have a high proliferative rate.

Parietal (Oxyntic) Cells. Large, round to pyramid-shaped **parietal cells** are located mainly in the upper half of the fundic glands and only occasionally in the base (see Figs. 17–2, 17–3). They are about 20 to 25 μm in diameter and are situated at the periphery of the gland. These cells produce **hydrochloric acid** and **gastric intrinsic factor.**

CLINICAL CORRELATIONS

Gastric intrinsic factor, a glycoprotein, is necessary for vitamin B_{12} absorption from the ileum. Absence of this factor results in deficiency of this vitamin with the consequent development of **pernicious anemia.** Because the liver stores high quantities of vitamin B_{12}, a deficiency of this vitamin may take several months to develop after production of gastric intrinsic factor ceases.

Parietal cells have round, basally located nuclei, and their cytoplasm is eosinophilic. Their most remarkable characteristic is the invaginations of their apical plasmalemma to form deep **intracellular canaliculi** lined by microvilli (Fig. 17–6). The cytoplasm bordering these canaliculi is richly endowed by round and tubular vesicles, the **tubulovesicular system.** Additionally, the cell is rich in mitochondria, whose combined volume constitutes almost half of that of the cytoplasm. RER is limited, and the Golgi apparatus is small.

Table 17-1. Distribution of Cell Type in Fundic Glands

Region	Cell Types
Isthmus	Surface-lining cells and few enteroendocrine cells
Neck	Mucous neck cells, regenerative cells, some parietal cells, and few enteroendocrine cells
Base	Chief cells, occasional parietal cells, and few enteroendocrine cells

The number of microvilli and the abundance of vesicles of the tubulovesicular system are indirectly related and vary with the HCl secretory activity of the cell. During active HCl production the number of microvilli increases and the amount of tubulovesicular system decreases. Thus it appears that the membrane, being stored as tubules and vesicles, is probably used for microvillar assembly, thus increasing the surface area of the cell by four to five times in preparation for HCl production.

The process of microvillus formation requires energy and involves polymerization of soluble forms of actin and myosin into filaments, which then interact to transport membranes from the tubulovesicular system to that of the intracellular canaliculus. The stored membranes have a high content of H^+,K^+-ATPase (a protein that pumps protons from the cytoplasm into the intracellular canaliculus). The process of HCl formation is described later in this chapter.

Chief (Zymogenic) Cells. Most of the cells in the base of fundic gland are **chief cells** (see Figs. 17–2, 17–3). These columnar cells display a basophilic cytoplasm, basally located nuclei, and apically situated secretory granules containing the proenzyme **pepsinogen** (and rennin and gastric lipase). Electron micrographs of chief cells exhibit a rich supply of rough ER, an extensive Golgi apparatus, and numerous apical secretory granules interspersed with a few lysosomes (Fig. 17–7). Short, blunt, glycocalyx-covered microvilli project from the apical aspect of the cell into the lumen of the gland.

Exocytosis of pepsinogen from chief cells is induced both by neural and by hormonal stimulation. Neural stimulation by the vagus nerve is the main contributor to pepsinogen release. Binding of **secretin** to receptors in the basal plasma membrane of chief cells triggers a second-messenger system that also leads to exocytosis of pepsinogen.

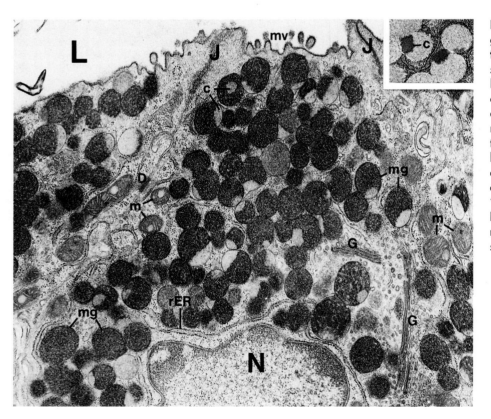

Figure 17–5. Electron micrograph of a mucous neck cell from the body of a mouse stomach. *Inset:* secretory granule. L, lumen; J, junctional complex; mv, microvillus; c, dense-cored granule; D, desmosome; m, mitochondria; mg, mucous granules; G, Golgi apparatus; rER, rough endoplasmic reticulum; N, nucleus. (From Karam, S.F., and Leblond, C.P.: Identifying and counting epithelial cell types in the "corpus" of the mouse stomach. Anat. Rec. **232**:231–246, 1992. Copyright © 1992. Reprinted by permission of John Wiley & Sons, Inc.)

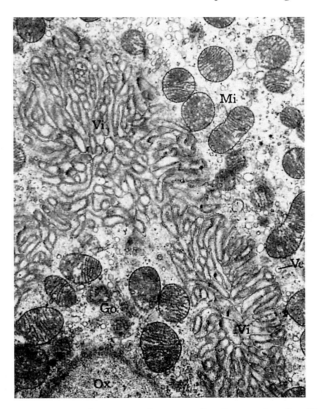

Figure 17–6. Electron micrograph of a parietal cell from the body of a mouse stomach (× 14,000). Vi, microvilli; Ve, tubulovesicular apparatus; Mi, mitochondria; Go, Golgi apparatus; Ox, nucleus of oxyphil cell. (From Rhodin, J.A.G.: An Atlas of Ultrastructure. W.B. Saunders, Philadelphia, 1963.)

Enteroendocrine Cells (APUD or DNES Cells). A group of small cells that are individually dispersed among the other epithelial cells of the gastric mucosa are known collectively by several names: argentaffine and argyrophilic cells, because they stain with silver stains; APUD cells, because some of them can take up the precursors of amines and decarboxylate them (**a**mine **p**recursor **u**ptake and **d**ecarboxylation); DNES cells, because they are members of the **d**iffuse **n**euro**e**ndocrine **s**ystem; and enteroendocrine cells, because they secrete hormones and are located in the enteric (alimentary) canal. Some of these cells are individually designated according to the hormone that they produce. Generally, a single type of enteroendocrine cell secretes only one hormone, although occasional cell types may secrete two different hormones. There are at least 13 different enteroendocrine cell types, only some of which are located in the mucosa of the stomach. Table 17–2 lists most of the better known cells; their locations, granule size, and hormone secretion; and the action of the released hormones. It is interesting to note that cells of the DNES have been localized not only in the digestive tract but also in the respiratory system and in the endocrine pancreas. Additionally, some of the hormones produced by these enteroendocrine cells are iden-

tical with neurosecretions localized in the central nervous system. The significance of their diverse location and hormone production is not understood.

Electron micrographs of enteroendocrine cells reveal that these small cells that sit on the basal lamina are of two types: those that reach the lumen of the gut, the **open type,** and those that do not, the **closed type.** The open type reach the lumen via long, thin apical processes with microvilli, which may function to monitor the lumenal contents. The cytoplasm of enteroendocrine cells has a well-developed RER and Golgi apparatus and numerous mitochondria. Additionally, small secretory granules are evident, disposed basally in most cells (Fig. 17–8).

All of these cells release the contents of their granules basally into the lamina propria. The hormones that these cells release either act on target cells in the immediate vicinity of the signaling cell (paracrine effect) or they enter the circulation and travel a distance to reach their target cell (endocrine effect).

MUSCULARIS MUCOSAE OF THE STOMACH. The smooth muscle cells that compose the **muscularis mucosae** are arranged in three layers. The inner circular and outer longitudinal layers are well defined; however, an occasional third layer, whose fibers are disposed circularly (**outermost circular),** is not always evident.

Differences in the Mucosa of the Cardiac and Pyloric Regions

The mucosa of the **cardiac region** of the stomach differs from that of the fundic region in that the gastric pits are shallower and the base of its glands is highly coiled. The cell population of these cardiac glands is composed mostly of surface lining cells, some mucous neck cells, a few enteroendocrine cells and parietal cells, and no chief cells (Table 17–3).

The glands of the **pyloric region** contain the same cell types as those in cardiac glands, but the predominant cell type in the pylorus is the mucous neck cell. In addition to producing mucus, these cells secrete **lysozyme,** a bactericidal enzyme. Pyloric glands are highly convoluted and tend to branch. Additionally, the gastric pits of the pyloric region are deeper than in both cardiac and pyloric regions, extending approximately half way down into the lamina propria (Fig. 17–9; see Table 17–3).

Submucosa of the Stomach

The dense, irregular collagenous connective tissue of the gastric **submucosa** has a rich vascular and lymphatic network that supplies and drains the vessels of the lamina propria. The cell population of the submucosa resembles that of any connective tissue proper. The submucosal plexus is in its accustomed location, within the submucosa in the vicinity of the muscularis externa.

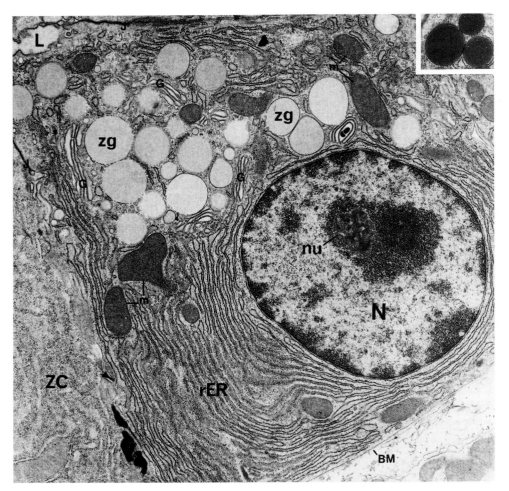

Figure 17–7. Electron micrograph of a chief cell from the fundus of a mouse stomach (× 13,000). L, lumen; BM, basement membrane; N, nucleus; nu, nucleolus; zg, zymogen granules; G, Golgi apparatus; rER, rough endoplasmic reticulum; m, mitochondria; ZC, zymogenic (chief) cell. (From Karam, S.F., and Leblond, C.P.: Identifying and counting epithelial cell types in the "corpus" of the mouse stomach. Anat. Rec. **232:**231–246, 1992. Copyright © 1992. Reprinted by permission of John Wiley & Sons, Inc.)

Muscularis Externa of the Stomach

The smooth muscle cells of the gastric **muscularis externa** are arranged in three layers. The **innermost oblique layer** is not well defined except in the cardiac region. The **middle circular layer** is clearly evident along the entire stomach and is especially pronounced in the pyloric region, where it forms the **pyloric sphincter.** The **outer longitudinal muscle layer** is most evident in the cardiac region and the body of the stomach but is poorly developed in the pylorus. The myenteric plexus is located between the middle circular and outer longitudinal layers of smooth muscle.

Figure 17–8. Electron micrograph of an enteroendocrine cell from the body of a mouse stomach. N, nucleus; nu, nucleolus; m, mitochondria; rER, rough endoplasmic reticulum; G, Golgi apparatus; g, secretory granules. (From Karam, S.F., and Leblond, C.P.: Identifying and counting epithelial cell types in the "corpus" of the mouse stomach. Anat. Rec. **232:**231–246, 1992. Copyright © 1992. Reprinted by permission of John Wiley & Sons, Inc.)

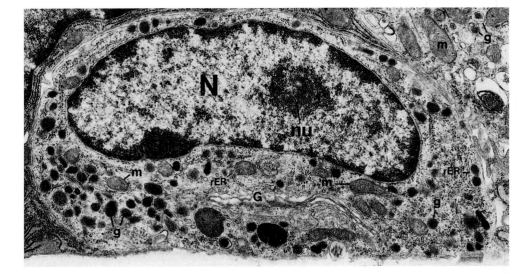

Table 17–2. Enteroendocrine Cells and Hormones of the Gastrointestinal Tract

Cell	Location	Hormone Produced	Granule Size (nm)	Hormonal Action
A	Stomach and small intestine	Glucagon (entero-glucagon)	250	Stimulates glycogenolysis by hepatocytes, thus elevating blood glucose levels
D	Stomach, small and large intestines	Somatostatin	350	Inhibits release of hormones by enteroendocrine cells in its vicinity
EC	Stomach, small and large intestines	Serotonin Substance P	300	Increases peristaltic movement
ECL	Stomach	Histamine	450	Stimulates HCl secretion
G	Stomach and small intestine	Gastrin	300	Stimulates HCl secretion, gastric motility (especially contraction of the pyloric region and relaxation of pyloric sphincter to regulate stomach emptying), and proliferation of regenerative cells in the body of the stomach
GL	Stomach, small and large intestines	Glicentin	400	Stimulates hepatocyte glycogenolysis, thus elevating blood glucose levels
I	Small intestine	Cholecystokinin	250	Stimulates the release of pancreatic hormone and contraction of the gall bladder.
K	Small intestine	Gastric inhibitory peptide	350	Inhibits HCl secretion
Mo	Small intestine	Motilin		Increases intestinal peristalsis
N	Small intestine	Neurotensin	300	Increases blood flow to ileum and decreases peristaltic action of small and large intestines
PP (F)	Stomach and large intestine	Pancreatic polypeptide	180	Unknown
S	Small intestine	Secretin	200	Stimulates release of bicarbonate-rich fluid from pancreas
VIP	Stomach, small and large intestines	Vasoactive intestinal peptide		Increases peristaltic action of small and large intestines and stimulates elimination of water and ions by GI tract

The entire stomach is invested by a **serosa** composed of a thin, loose, subserous connective tissue covered by a smooth, wet, simple squamous epithelium. This external covering provides an almost friction-free environment during the churning movements of the stomach.

Histophysiology of the Stomach

The gastric glands of the stomach produce approximately 2 to 3 L of gastric juices a day. These secretions are composed of water; **hydrochloric acid** (manufactured by parietal cells); the enzymes **pepsinogen, rennin,** and **gastric lipase** (manufactured by chief cells); and a protective glycoprotein, **mucus** (manufactured by surface lining cells and mucous neck cells), which forms a mucous coat that lines the epithelium of the stomach. Little absorption of food products occurs in the stomach, although some substances, such as alcohol, can be absorbed by the gastric mucosa.

The three muscle layers of the muscularis externa interact such that during the contraction, the contents of the stomach are churned and the ingested food is liquefied to form chyme, a viscous fluid resembling split pea soup in consistency. Independent contraction of the muscularis mucosae exposes the chyme to the entire surface area of the gastric mucosa.

Table 17–3. Histology of the Alimentary Canal

Organ	Epithelium	Cell Type of Epithelium	Lamina Propria	Cells of Glands	Muscularis Mucosae	Submucosa	Muscularis Externa	Serosa or Adventitia
Esophagus	Stratified squamous nonkeratinized		Esophageal cardiac glands	Mucus-secreting	Longitudinal layer only	Esophageal glands proper	Inner circular and outer longitudinal	Adventitia (except serosa in abdominal cavity)
Cardiac stomach	Simple columnar	Surface lining cells (no goblet cells)	Cardiac glands; shallow gastric pits	Surface lining cells, mucous neck cells, regenerative cells, enteroendocrine cells, parietal cells	Inner circular, outer longitudinal and, in places, outermost circular	No glands	Inner oblique, middle circular, outermost longitudinal	Serosa
Fundic stomach	Simple columnar	Surface lining cells (no goblet cells)	Fundic glands	Surface lining cells, mucous neck cells, parietal cells, regenerative cells, chief cells, enteroendocrine cells	Inner circular, outer longitudinal and, in places, outermost circular	No glands	Inner oblique, middle circular, outermost longitudinal	Serosa
Pyloric stomach	Simple columnar	Surface lining cells (no goblet cells)	Pyloric glands; deep gastric pits	Mucous neck cells, surface lining cells, parietal cells, regenerative cells, enteroendocrine cells	Inner circular, outer longitudinal and, in places, outermost circular	No glands	Inner oblique, middle circular (well developed to form pyloric sphincter), outermost longitudinal	Serosa
Duodenum	Simple columnar (goblet cells)	Surface absorptive cells, goblet cells, enteroendocrine cells	Crypts of Lieberkühn	Surface absorptive cells, goblet cells, regenerative cells, enteroendocrine cells, Paneth cells	Inner circular, outer longitudinal	Brunner's glands	Inner circular, outer longitudinal	Serosa and adventitia
Jejunum	Simple columnar (goblet cells)	Surface absorptive cells, goblet cells, enteroendocrine cells	Crypts of Lieberkühn	Surface absorptive cells, goblet cells, regenerative cells, enteroendocrine cells, Paneth cells	Inner circular, outer longitudinal	No glands	Inner circular, outer longitudinal	Serosa

Table 17–3. Histology of the Alimentary Canal (continued)

Organ	Epithelium	Cell Type of Epithelium	Lamina Propria	Cells of Glands	Muscularis Mucosae	Submucosa	Muscularis Externa	Serosa or Adventitia
Ileum	Simple columnar (goblet cells)	Surface absorptive cells, goblet cells, enteroendocrine cells	Crypts of Lieberkühn; Peyer patches	Surface absorptive cells, goblet cells, regenerative cells, enteroendocrine cells, Paneth cells	Inner circular, outer longitudinal	No glands (Peyer patches may extend into this layer)	Inner circular, outer longitudinal	Serosa
Colon*	Simple columnar (goblet cells)	Surface absorptive cells, goblet cells, enteroendocrine cells	Crypts of Lieberkühn	Surface absorptive cells, goblet cells, regenerative cells, enteroendocrine cells	Inner circular, outer longitudinal	No glands	Inner circular, outer longitudinal modified to form taeniae coli	Serosa and adventitia
Rectum	Simple columnar (goblet cells)	Surface absorptive cells, goblet cells, enteroendocrine cells	Shallow crypts of Lieberkühn	Surface absorptive cells, goblet cells, regenerative cells, enteroendocrine cells	Inner circular, outer longitudinal	No glands	Inner circular, outer longitudinal	Adventitia
Anal canal	Simple cuboidal; stratified squamous nonkeratinized; stratified squamous keratinized		Rectal columns; circumanal glands; *at anus:* hair follicles and sebaceous glands		Inner circular, outer longitudinal	No glands; internal and external hemorrhoidal plexuses	Inner circular (forms internal anal sphincter), outer longitudinal (becomes fibroelastic sheet)	Adventitia
Appendix	Simple columnar (goblet cells)	Surface absorptive cells, goblet cells, enteroendocrine cells	Shallow crypts of Lieberkühn; lymphoid nodules	Surface absorptive cells, goblet cells, regenerative cells, enteroendocrine cells, Paneth cells	Inner circular, outer longitudinal	No glands; occasional lymphoid nodules; possible fatty infiltration	Inner circular, outer longitudinal	Serosa

*Includes cecum.

Emptying of Gastric Contents

Interaction between neurons of the myenteric and submucosal plexuses maintains a constant intraluminal pressure, irrespective of the degree of distention of the stomach. Coordinated contraction of the muscularis externa and momentary relaxation of the pyloric sphincter permit emptying of the stomach by intermittently delivering small aliquots of the chyme into the duodenum. The rate at which the stomach releases its chyme into the duodenum is a function of the acidity, the caloric and fat content, and the osmolality of the chyme.

The factors that facilitate emptying are degree of distention of the stomach and the action of gastrin, a hormone that stimulates contraction of the muscularis externa of the py-

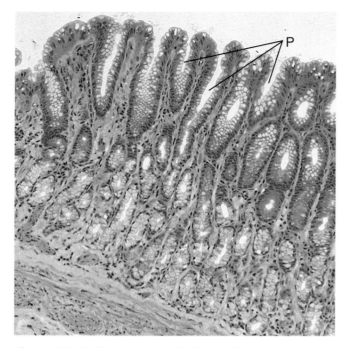

Figure 17–9. Photomicrograph of the pyloric stomach. Gastric pits (P) (× 132).

loric region and relaxation of the pyloric sphincter. Factors that inhibit emptying include distension of the duodenum; overabundance of fat, proteins, or carbohydrates; and increased osmolarity and excessive acidity of the chyme in the duodenum. These factors activate a neural feedback mechanism by stimulating release of cholecystokinin, which counteracts gastrin, and release of gastric inhibitory peptide, which also inhibits gastric contractions.

Gastric HCl Production

Hydrochloric acid not only breaks down food material but also activates the proenzyme pepsinogen to become the ac-

tive proteolytic enzyme **pepsin.** Because pepsin requires a low pH for its acidity, the presence of HCl also provides the necessary acidic conditions (pH 1 to pH 2).

HCl secretion occurs in three phases as a result of different stimuli:

1. **Cephalic:** secretion due to psychological factors (e.g., the thought, smell, or sight of food; stress) is elicited by parasympathetic impulses from the vagus nerve, which cause the release of **acetylcholine.**

2. **Gastric:** secretion due to the presence of certain food substances in the stomach as well as to the stretching of the stomach wall is elicited by the paracrine hormones **gastrin** and **histamine,** which are released by the enteroendocrine cells (G cells and ECL cells) of the stomach, respectively.

3. **Intestinal:** secretion due to the presence of food in the small intestine is elicited by the endocrine hormone **gastrin,** released by G cells of the small intestine.

Parietal cells have receptors for gastrin, histamine, and acetylcholine on their basal plasmalemma. Binding of any of these signaling molecules to the appropriate receptor causes the cell to manufacture and release hydrochloric acid into the intracellular canaliculus. The process occurs as follows (Fig. 17–10):

1. The enzyme **carbonic anhydrase** facilitates the dissociation of H_2CO_3 to H^+ and HCO_3^- in the cytoplasm of the parietal cell.

2. An H^+,K^+-ATPase, using adenosine triphosphate as an energy source, pumps intracellular H^+ ions out of the cell into the intracellular canaliculi and transfers extracellular K^+ into the cell.

3. Conductive channels, utilizing ATP as an energy source, pump K^+ and Cl^- out of the cell and into the intracellular canaliculus. Thus Cl^- and H^+ **enter the lumen of the intracellular canaliculus separately to combine into HCl.**

4. Water enters the canaliculus because of the osmotic forces generated by the movement of ions.

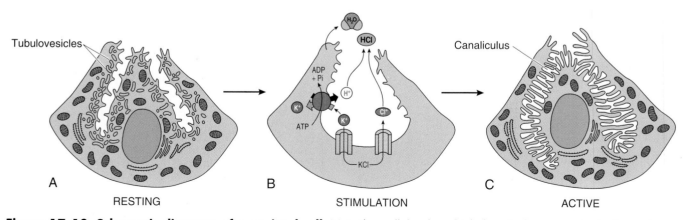

Figure 17–10. Schematic diagram of a parietal cell. Note the well-developed tubulovesicular apparatus in the resting cell (**A**) and the numerous microvilli in the active cell (**C**). The mechanism of HCl release is indicated in (**B**).

The lining of the stomach is protected from the high acid content by the buffering activity of the HCO_3^- present in the layer of mucus manufactured by the mucous lining cells and the surface lining cells. Additionally, the zonulae occludentes of the epithelial cells prevent the influx of HCl into the lamina propria, thus protecting the mucosa from damage. Moreover, recent evidence suggests that **prostaglandins** not only protect the cells lining the gastric lumen but also increase local circulation, especially when the integrity of the epithelial barrier is compromised. This increased blood flow removes the H^+ ions from the lamina propria.

The hormones **somatostatin, prostaglandin,** and **gastric inhibitory peptide (GIP)** inhibit gastric HCl production. Somatostatin acts on G cells and ECL cells, inhibiting their release of gastrin and histamine, respectively. Prostaglandins and GIP act directly on parietal cells and inhibit their ability to produce HCl.

CLINICAL CORRELATIONS

Possibly the most common cause of **ulcers** in the United States is the prevalent use of **ibuprofen** and **aspirin** for the relief of inflammation. Both of these drugs inhibit the manufacture of prostaglandins, thus precluding their protective effects on the stomach lining.

The bacterium *Helicobacter pylori,* which is localized in the mucus layer protecting the gastric epithelium, has also been implicated as a possible factor in ulcer formation.

Small Intestine

Digestion begins in the oral cavity and continues in the stomach and in the **small intestine,** which at 7 m of length is the longest region of the alimentary tract. It is divided into three regions, the duodenum, jejunum, and ileum. Although these regions are similar histologically, their minor differences permit their identification.

The small intestine digests food material and absorbs end-products of the digestive process. In order to perform its digestive functions, the first region of the small intestine, the duodenum, receives enzymes and an alkaline buffer from the pancreas and bile from the liver. Additionally, epithelial cells and glands of the mucosa contribute buffers and enzymes to facilitate digestion.

Common Histological Features

Because the three regions of the small intestine are similar histologically, the common features are described first. Following this discussion, variations from this plan are described for each segment (Table 17–3), and then functional aspects are considered.

Modifications of the Luminal Surface

The luminal surface of the small intestine is modified to increase its surface area. Three types of modifications have been noted: plicae circulares (valves of Kerckring), villi, and microvilli.

Plicae circulares are transverse folds of the submucosa and mucosa, forming semicircular to helical elevations, some as large as 8 mm tall and 5 cm long. Unlike rugae of the stomach, these are permanent fixtures of the duodenum and jejunum and end in the proximal half of the ileum. They increase the surface area by a factor of 2 to 3.

Villi are epithelially covered, finger-like or oak-leaf-like protrusions of the lamina propria. The core of each villus contains capillary loops, a blindly ending lymphatic channel **(lacteal),** and a few smooth muscle fibers, embedded in loose connective tissue and rich in lymphoid cells. Villi are permanent structures (Figs. 17–11, 17–12, 17–13). Their numbers are greater in the duodenum than in the jejunum or the ileum. Also, their height decreases from 1.5 mm in the duodenum to about 0.5 mm in the ileum. These delicate structures confer a velvety appearance to the lining of the living organ. Villi increase the surface area of the small intestine by a factor of 10.

Microvilli, modifications of the apical plasmalemma of the epithelial cells covering the intestinal villi, increase the surface area of the small intestine by a factor of 20. Thus, the three types of intestinal surface modifications increase the total surface area available for absorption of nutrients by a factor of 400 to 600.

Invaginations of the epithelium into the lamina propria between the villi form intestinal glands, **crypts of Lieberkühn,** which also augment the surface area of the small intestine.

Intestinal Mucosa

The mucosa of the small intestine is composed of the usual three layers: a simple columnar epithelium, the lamina propria, and the muscularis mucosae.

EPITHELIUM. The simple columnar epithelium covering the villi and the surface of the intervillar spaces is composed of surface absorptive cells, goblet cells, and enteroendocrine cells.

Surface Absorptive Cells. The most numerous cells of the epithelium are **surface absorptive cells** (see Figs. 17–11, 17–13; Fig. 17–14). They are tall cells, about 25 μm in length, with basally located oval nuclei. Their apical surface presents a **brush border,** and in good preparations, terminal bars are also evident. The principal functions of these cells are terminal digestion and absorption of water and nutrients. Additionally, these cells reesterify fatty acids into triglycerides, form chylomicrons, and transport the bulk of the ab-

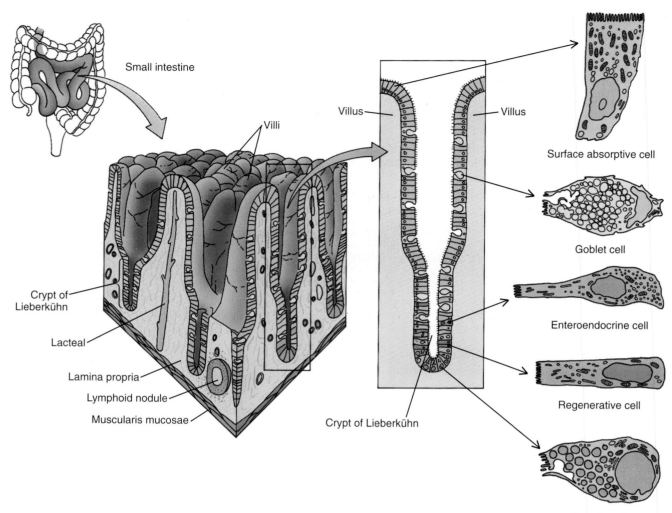

Small intestine

Villi

Villus — — Villus

Surface absorptive cell

Goblet cell

Enteroendocrine cell

Crypt of
Lieberkühn

Lacteal

Lamina propria

Lymphoid nodule

Muscularis mucosae

Crypt of Lieberkühn

Regenerative cell

Paneth cell

Figure 17–11. Schematic diagram of the mucosa, villi, crypts of Lieberkühn, and component cells of the small intestine.

sorbed nutrients into the lamina propria for distribution to the rest of the body. The process of absorption is discussed later in this chapter.

Electron micrographs of these cells display numerous **microvilli,** approximately 1 μm long, whose tips are covered with a thick **glycocalyx** layer. The glycocalyx coat not only protects the microvilli from autodigestion, but its enzymatic components function in terminal digestion of dipeptides and disaccharides into their monomers. The actin core of the microvilli is anchored into the actin and intermediate filaments of the cell web. The cytoplasm of surface absorptive cells is rich in organelles, especially endosomes, smooth endoplasmic reticulum, RER and Golgi apparatus.

The lateral cell membranes of these cells form zonulae occludentes, zonulae adherentes, desmosomes, and gap junctions with adjacent cells. The tight junctions prevent the passage of material via a paracellular route to or from the lumen of the gut.

Goblet Cells. Goblet cells are unicellular glands (see Figs. 17–11, 17–13), whose structure and function were detailed in Chapter 5 on epithelium and glands. The duodenum has the smallest number of goblet cells, and their number increases toward the ileum. These cells manufacture **mucinogen,** whose hydrated form is **mucin,** a component of mucus, a protective layer lining the lumen.

Enteroendocrine Cells. The small intestine has various types of enteroendocrine cells that produce paracrine and endocrine hormones. These cells were described in the earlier section on the stomach and are listed in Table 17–2. Approximately 1% of the cells covering the villi and intervillar surface of the small intestine are composed of enteroendocrine cells.

M Cells (Microfold Cells). The simple columnar epithelial lining of the small intestine is replaced by squamous-like

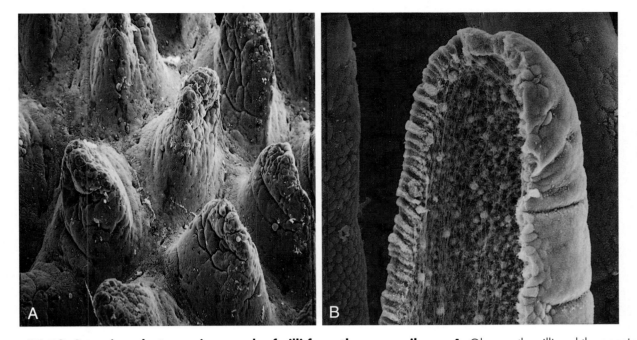

Figure 17–12. Scanning electron micrograph of villi from the mouse ileum. A, Observe the villi and the openings of the crypts of Lieberkühn in the intervillar spaces (x 160). **B,** Note that the villus is fractured, revealing its core of connective tissue and migrating cells (x 500). (From Magney, J.E., Erlandsen, S.L., Bjerknes, M.L., and Cheng, H.: Scanning electron microscopy of isolated epithelium of the murine gastrointestinal tract: Morphology of the basal surface and evidence for paracrine-like cells. Am. J. Anat. **177:**43–53, 1986. Copyright © 1986. Reprinted with permission of John Wiley & Sons, Inc.)

M cells in regions where lymphoid nodules abut the epithelium. These M cells are believed to belong to the mononuclear phagocyte system of cells, and they sample, phagocytose, and transport antigens present in the intestinal lumen.

LAMINA PROPRIA. The loose connective tissue of the **lamina propria** forms the core of the villi, which like trees of a forest rise above the surface of the small intestine (see Fig. 17–12; Fig. 17–15). The rest of the lamina propria, extending down to the muscularis mucosae, is compressed into thin sheets of highly vascularized connective tissue by the numerous tubular intestinal glands, the crypts of Lieberkühn. The lamina propria also is rich in lymphoid cells, which help protect the intestinal lining from invasion by microorganisms, as discussed later.

Crypts of Lieberkühn. **Crypts of Lieberkühn** are simple tubular (or branched tubular) glands (see Fig. 17–11). These glands open into the intervillar spaces as perforations of the epithelial lining. Scanning electron micrographs indicate that the base of each villus is surrounded by the openings of numerous crypts. These tubular glands are composed of surface absorptive cells, goblet cells, regenerative cells, enteroendocrine cells, and Paneth cells.

Surface absorptive and goblet cells occupy the upper half of the gland. These goblet cells have a short lifespan; it is

believed that after they disgorge their mucinogen, they die and are desquamated. The basal half of the gland has no surface absorptive and only a few goblet cells; instead, most of the cells are regenerative cells (and their progeny), enteroendocrine cells, and Paneth cells. Only regenerative and Paneth cells are described here, because the others were discussed earlier.

Regenerative Cells. The **regenerative cells** of the small intestine are stem cells that extensively proliferate to repopulate the epithelium of the crypts, mucosal surface, and villi. They are narrow cells that appear to be wedged into limited spaces among the newly formed cells (see Figs. 17–11, 17–14). Their rate of cell division is high, with a relatively short cell cycle of 24 hours. It has been suggested that 5 to 7 days after the appearance of the new cell, that cell has progressed to the tip of the villus and has been exfoliated. Electron micrographs of these undifferentiated cells display few organelles but many free ribosomes. Their single, basally located, oval nuclei are electron-lucent, indicating the presence of a large amount of euchromatin.

Paneth Cells. **Paneth cells** are clearly distinguishable because of the presence of large, eosinophilic, apical secretory granules (see Fig. 17–11; Fig. 17–16). These pyramid-shaped cells occupy the bottom of the crypts of Lieberkühn and manufacture the antibacterial agent **lysozyme.** Unlike

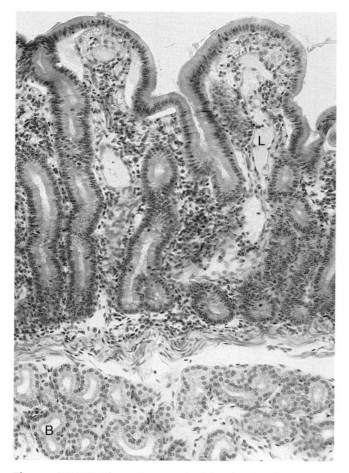

Figure 17–13. Photomicrograph of the duodenal mucosa. Brunner's glands (B); lacteals of villus (L) (× 132).

the other cells of the intestinal epithelium, Paneth cells have a long lifespan and secrete lysozyme continuously. Electron micrographs of these cells display a well-developed Golgi apparatus, a large complement of RER, numerous mitochondria, and large apical secretory granules housing a homogeneous secretory product.

MUSCULARIS MUCOSAE. The muscularis mucosae of the small intestine is composed of an inner circular and outer longitudinal layer of smooth muscle cells (see Fig. 17–15). Muscle fibers from the inner circular layer enter the villus and extend through its core to the tip of the connective tissue, as far as the basement membrane. During digestion, these muscle fibers rhythmically contract, shortening the villus several times a minute.

Submucosa

The **submucosa** of the small intestine is composed of dense, irregular fibroelastic connective tissue with a rich lymphatic and vascular supply. The intrinsic innervation of the submucosa is from the parasympathetic **submucosal (Meissner's)**

plexus. The submucosa of the **duodenum** is unusual because it houses glands, known as Brunner's glands (duodenal glands).

BRUNNER'S GLANDS. Brunner's glands are branched, tubuloalveolar glands, whose secretory portions resemble mucous acini (see Fig. 17–13). The ducts of these glands penetrate the muscularis mucosae and usually pierce the base of the crypts of Lieberkühn to deliver their secretory product into the lumen of the duodenum. Occasionally, their ducts open into the intervillar spaces. Electron micrographs of the acinar cells display a well-developed RER and Golgi apparatus, numerous mitochondria, and flattened to round nuclei.

Brunner's glands secrete a mucous, alkaline fluid in response to parasympathetic stimulation. This fluid helps neutralize the acidic chyme that enters the duodenum from the pyloric stomach. This gland also manufactures the polypeptide hormone **urogastrone** (now known to be human epidermal growth factor), which is released into the duodenal lumen along with the alkaline buffer. Urogastrone inhibits production of HCl and amplifies the rate of mitotic activity in epithelial cells.

Muscularis Externa and Serosa

The **muscularis externa** of the small intestine is composed of an inner circular and an outer longitudinal smooth muscle layer. Auerbach's **myenteric plexus** is located between the two muscle layers and is the intrinsic neural supply of the external muscle coat. The muscularis externa is responsible for the peristaltic activity of the small intestine.

With the exception of the second and third parts of the duodenum, the entire small intestine is invested by a **serosa.**

Lymphatic and Vascular Supply of the Small Intestine

The small intestine has a well-developed lymphatic and vascular system. Blindly ending lymph capillaries called **lacteals,** which are located in the cores of villi, deliver their contents into the **submucosal lymphatic plexus.** From here lymph passes through a series of lymph nodes to be delivered to the thoracic duct, the largest lymph vessel in the body. The thoracic duct empties its content into the circulatory system at the junction of the left internal jugular and subclavian veins.

Capillary loops adjacent to the lacteals are drained by blood vessels that are tributaries of the **submucosal vascular plexus.** Blood from here is delivered to the portal vein to enter the liver for processing.

Regional Differences

The **duodenum** is the shortest segment of the small intestine, being only 25 cm in length. It receives bile from the

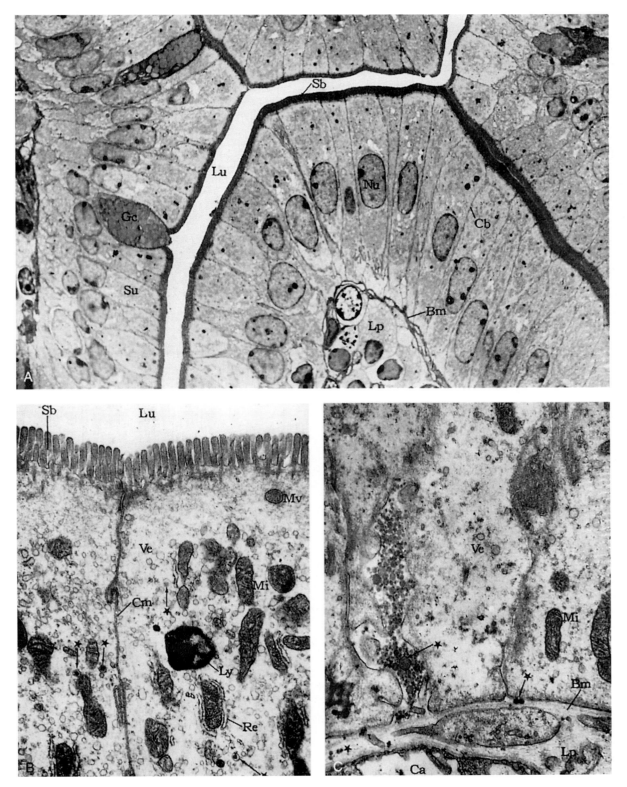

Figure 17–14. Surface absorptive cells from a villus of the mouse jejunum. A, Low-magnification electron micrograph displaying two goblet cells (Gc) and numerous surface absorptive cells (Su) (× 2500). Note the striated border (Sb) facing the lumen (Lu). Nuclei (Nu) and cell boundaries (Cb) are clearly evident. Observe also that the epithelium is separated from the lamina propria by a well-defined basement membrane (Bm). **B,** A higher-magnification electron micrograph of two adjoining surface absorptive cells (× 15,000). The striated border (Sb) is clearly composed of numerous microvilli that project into the lumen (Lu). The adjoining cell membranes (Cm) are close to each other. Mi, mitochondria; Ly, lysosomes; Re, rough endoplasmic reticulum; Ve, vesicles; *, membrane-bounded lipid droplets. **C,** Electron micrograph of the basal aspect of the surface absorptive cells (× 16,000). Ve, vesicles; Mi, mitochondria; Bm, basement membrane; Lp, lamina propria; *, chylomicrons. (From Rhodin, J.A.G.: An Atlas of Ultrastructure. W.B. Saunders, Philadelphia, 1963.)

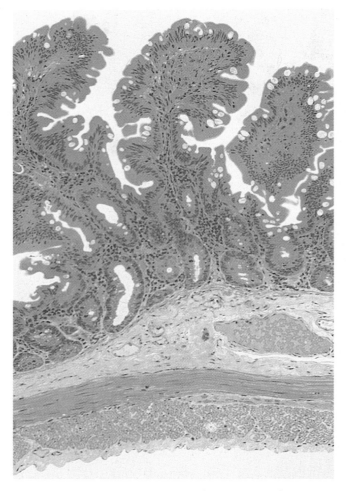

Figure 17–15. Photomicrograph of the mucosa of a monkey jejunum (× 132).

liver and digestive juices from the pancreas via the common bile ducts and pancreatic ducts respectively, which open into its lumen at the **duodenal papilla (of Vater).** The duodenum differs from the jejunum and ileum in that its villi are broader, taller, and more numerous per unit area. It has fewer goblet cells per unit area than the other segments, and it has **Brunner's glands** in its submucosa.

The villi of the **jejunum** are narrower, shorter, and sparser than those of the duodenum. The number of goblet cells per unit area is greater in the jejunum than in the duodenum.

The villi of the ileum are the sparsest, shortest, and narrowest of the three regions of the small intestine. The lamina propria of the ileum houses permanent clusters of lymphoid nodules, known as **Peyer's patches.** These structures are located in the wall of the ileum that is opposite the attachment of the mesentery.

Histophysiology of the Small Intestine

In addition to its roles in digestion and absorption, the small intestine exhibits immunological and secretory activity. These activities are considered first, after which the primary function of the small intestine is described.

Immunological Activity of the Lamina Propria

The lamina propria is rich in plasma cells, lymphocytes, mast cells, extravasated leukocytes, and fibroblasts. Additionally, solitary lymphoid nodules are frequently present in the lamina propria, adjacent the epithelial lining of the mucosa. Moreover, the ileum has permanent clusters of lymphoid nodules collectively known as **Peyer's patches.**

Where these lymphoid nodules come into contact with the epithelium, the columnar cells are replaced by M cells, which phagocytose lumenal antigens (Figs. 17–17, 17–18). Endocytosed antigens enter the endosomal system of these cells, but instead of being processed, they are packaged in clathrin-coated vesicles, transferred to the basal aspect of the cell, and released into the lamina propria. Antigen-presenting cells and dendritic cells of the lymphoid nodule endocytose the transferred antigens, process them, and present the epitopes to lymphocytes for the initiation of an immune response.

Activated lymphocytes migrate to mesenteric lymph nodes, where they form germinal centers. The resultant B cells return to the lamina propria, where they differentiate into IgA-producing plasma cells.

Some of the released antibodies bind to IgA receptors of epithelial cells and are complexed to **secretory component** (proteins manufactured by these cells) within the epithelial cells. The IgA–protein complex is transported into the lumen, a process known as **transcytosis,** and bound to the glycocalyx to defend the body against antigenic onslaught.

Most of the IgA produced in the lamina propria enters the circulatory system, is transported to the liver where hepatocytes complex it with secretory component, and is released as a complex into bile. Thus, much of the luminal IgA enters the intestine through the common bile duct, accompanying bile.

Secretory Activity of the Small Intestine

Glands of the small intestine secrete mucus and a watery fluid in response to neural and hormonal stimulation. Neural stimulation, originating in the submucosal plexus, is the principal trigger, but the hormones secretin and cholecystokinin also play a minor part in regulating the secretory activities of Brunner's glands in the duodenum and of the crypts of Lieberkühn, which produce almost 2 L of slightly alkaline fluid per day.

The enteroendocrine cells of the small intestine produce numerous hormones that affect movement of the small intestine and help regulate gastric HCl secretion and release of pancreatic secretions (see Table 17–2).

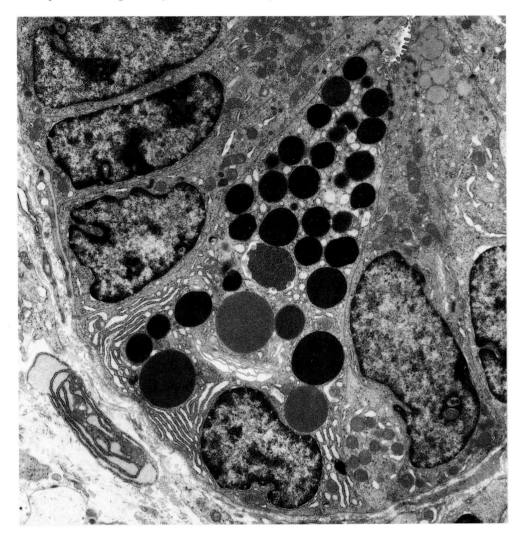

Figure 17-16. Electron micrograph of a Paneth cell from the rabbit ileum (× 7600). Note the large, round granules in the cytoplasm of the Paneth cell. (From Satoh, Y., Yamano, M., Matsuda, M., and Ono, K.: Ultrastructure of Paneth cell in the intestine of various mammals. J. Electron Microsc. Tech. **16:**69–80, 1990. Copyright © 1990. Reprinted by permission of John Wiley & Sons, Inc.)

CLINICAL CORRELATIONS

The rate of fluid secretion into the small intestine is greatly increased in response to **cholera toxin.** The amount of fluid loss as diarrhea may amount to as much as 10 L per day, and, if not replaced, may lead to circulatory shock and death within a few hours. The fluid loss is accompanied by electrolyte imbalance, a contributory factor to the lethal effect of cholera.

Movement of the Small Intestine

Movement of the small intestine may be subdivided into two interrelated phases, mixing and propulsive.

Mixing contractions are more localized and sequentially redistribute the chyme to expose it to the digestive juices.

Propulsive contractions occur as **peristaltic waves** that facilitate the movement of the chyme along the small intestine. Because the chyme moves at an average of 1 to 2 cm per minute, it thus spends several hours in the small intestine. The rate of peristalsis is controlled by neural impulses

and hormonal factors. In response to gastric distension, a **gastroenteric reflex** mediated by the **myenteric** plexus provides the neural impetus for peristalsis in the small intestine. The hormones cholecystokinin, gastrin, motilin, substance P, and serotonin increase intestinal motility, whereas secretin and glucagon decrease it.

CLINICAL CORRELATIONS

If the intestinal mucosa is exposed to profound irritation by toxic substances, the muscularis externa can undergo intense, swift contractions of long durations, known as **peristaltic rush.** These strong contractions propel the chyme into the colon within minutes for elimination as diarrhea.

Digestion

The chyme that enters the duodenum is in the process of being digested by enzymes produced by glands of the oral

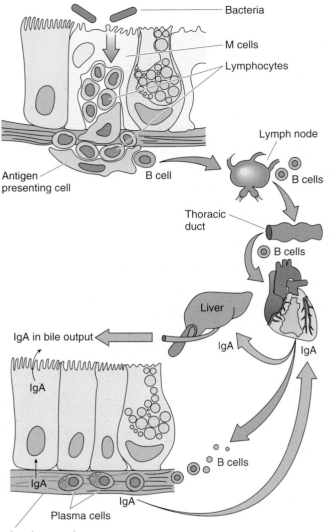

Figure 17–17. Schematic diagram of an M cell and its immunological relationship to the alimentary canal.

cavity and glands of the stomach. The process of digestion is intensified in the duodenum by enzymes derived from the exocrine pancreas. The final breakdown of proteins and carbohydrates occurs at the microvilli, where **dipeptidases** and **disaccharidases,** adherent to the glycocalyx, liberate individual amino acids and monosaccharides. These monomers are transported into the surface absorptive cells by specific carrier proteins. Lipids are **emulsified** by bile salts into small fat globules that are split into monoglycerides and fatty acids. Bile salts segregate monoglycerides and free fatty acids into micelles, 2 nm in diameter, which diffuse into the surface absorptive cells through their plasmalemma.

Absorption

Approximately 6 to 7 L of fluid, 30 to 35 g of sodium, 0.5 kg of carbohydrates and proteins, and 1 kg of fat are absorbed by the surface absorptive cells of the small intestine each day. Water, amino acids, ions, and monosaccharides enter the surface absorptive cells and are released into the intercellular space at the basolateral membrane. These nutrients then enter the capillary bed of the villi and are transported to the liver for processing.

As diagrammed in Figure 17–19, long-chain fatty acids and monoglycerides enter the smooth endoplasmic reticulum of the surface absorptive cell, where they are reesterified to triglycerides. The triglycerides are transferred to the Golgi apparatus, where they are combined with a β-lipoprotein coat, manufactured on the RER, to form **chylomicrons.** These large lipoprotein droplets, packaged and released from the Golgi apparatus, are transported to the basolateral cell membrane to be released into the lamina propria. The chylomicrons enter the lacteals, filling these blindly ending lymphatic vessels with a lipid-rich substance known as **chyle.** Rhythmic contractions of the smooth muscle cells located in the cores of the villi cause shortening of each villus, which acts as a syringe, injecting the chyle from the lacteal into the submucosal plexus of lymph vessels.

Short-chain fatty acids (less than 12 carbons in length) do not enter the smooth endoplasmic reticulum for reesterification. These free fatty acids, which are short enough to be somewhat water-soluble, progress to the basolateral membrane of the surface absorptive cell, diffuse into the lamina propria, and enter the capillary loops to be delivered to the liver for processing.

CLINICAL CORRELATIONS

Malabsorption in the small intestine may occur even though the pancreas delivers its normal complement of enzymes. The various diseases that result in malabsorption are called **sprue.** An interesting form of sprue, **gluten enteropathy (nontropical sprue),** is caused by **gluten,** a substance present in rye and wheat, which destroys microvilli and even villi of susceptible persons. These effects may result from an allergic response to gluten. Persons suffering from this disorder have a reduced surface area available for absorption of nutrients. Treatment involves elimination of gluten-containing grains from the diet.

Large Intestine

The **large intestine,** composed of the cecum, colon (ascending, transverse, descending, and sigmoid), rectum, and anus, is approximately 1.5 m long (see Table 17–3). Its function is to absorb most of the water and ions from the chyme it receives from the small intestine and to compact it into feces for elimination. The cecum and the colon are indistinguishable histologically and are discussed as a single entity, called the colon. The **appendix,** a blind outpocketing of the cecum, is described separately.

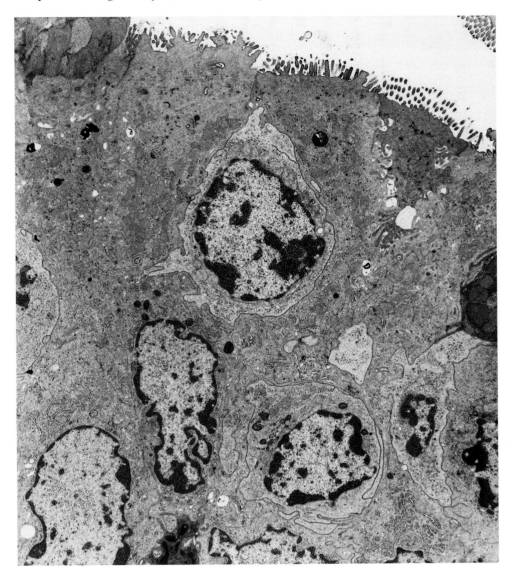

Figure 17–18. Electron micrograph of M cells of the mouse colon (× 7250). Observe the electron-dense M cells surrounding the electron-lucent lymphocytes. (From Owen, R.L., Piazza, A.J., and Ermak, T.H.: Ultrastructural and cytoarchitectural features of lymphoreticular organs in the colon and rectum of adult BALB/c mice. Am. J. Anat. **190:**10–18, 1991. Copyright © 1991. Reprinted by permission of John Wiley & Sons, Inc.)

Colon

The **colon** accounts for almost the entire length of the large intestine. It receives chyme from the ileum at the **ileocecal valve,** an anatomical as well as a physiological sphincter that prevents backflow of the cecal content into the ileum.

Histology of the Colon

The colon has no villi but is richly endowed with **crypts of Lieberkühn** that are similar in composition to those of the small intestine, except for the absence of Paneth cells (Figs. 17–20 to 17–23). The number of goblet cells increases from the cecum to the sigmoid colon, but the surface absorptive cells are the most numerous cell type. Enteroendocrine cells are also present, although they are few. Rapid mitotic activity of the regenerative cells replaces the epithelial lining of the crypts and of the mucosal surface every 6 to 7 days.

The lamina propria, muscularis mucosae, and submucosa

of the colon resemble those of the small intestine. The **muscularis externa** is unusual in that the outer longitudinal layer is not continuous along the surface but is gathered into three narrow ribbons of muscle fascicles, known as **taenia coli.** The constant tonus maintained by the taenia coli puckers the large intestine into sacculations, called **haustra coli.** The **serosa** displays numerous fat-filled pouches, called **appendices epiploicae.**

Histophysiology of the Colon

The colon absorbs water and electrolytes (approximately 1400 ml per day) and compacts and eliminates feces (about 100 ml per day).

Feces are composed of water (75%), dead bacteria (7%), roughage (7%), fat (5%), inorganic substances (5%), and undigested protein, dead cells, and bile pigment (1%). The odor of feces varies with the individual and is a function of the diet and bacterial flora, which produce varied amounts of **in-**

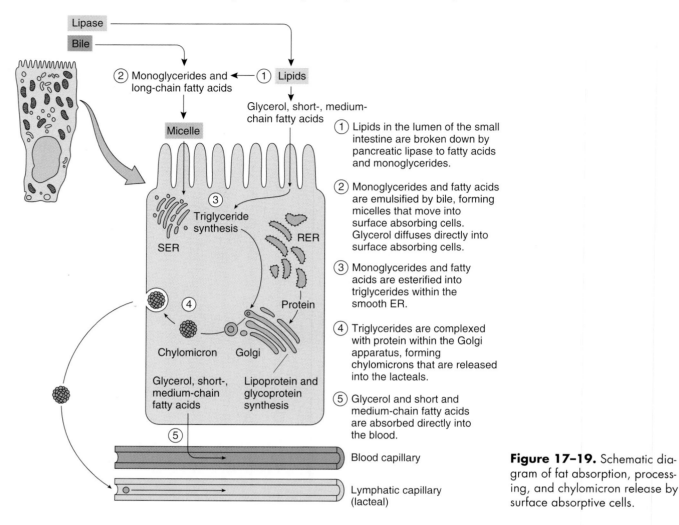

Figure 17–19. Schematic diagram of fat absorption, processing, and chylomicron release by surface absorptive cells.

Within the figure:

Lipase

Bile

② Monoglycerides and ◄— ① Lipids
long-chain fatty acids

Glycerol, short-, medium-chain fatty acids

Micelle

③ Triglyceride synthesis

SER

RER

Protein

④ Chylomicron   Golgi

Glycerol, short-, medium-chain fatty acids

Lipoprotein and glycoprotein synthesis

⑤

Blood capillary

Lymphatic capillary (lacteal)

① Lipids in the lumen of the small intestine are broken down by pancreatic lipase to fatty acids and monoglycerides.

② Monoglycerides and fatty acids are emulsified by bile, forming micelles that move into surface absorbing cells. Glycerol diffuses directly into surface absorbing cells.

③ Monoglycerides and fatty acids are esterified into triglycerides within the smooth ER.

④ Triglycerides are complexed with protein within the Golgi apparatus, forming chylomicrons that are released into the lacteals.

⑤ Glycerol and short and medium-chain fatty acids are absorbed directly into the blood.

---

dole, **hydrogen sulfide,** and **mercaptans.** Bacterial byproducts include riboflavin, thiamin, vitamin B_{12}, and vitamin K.

Bacterial action in the colon produces gases, released as **flatus,** composed of carbon dioxide, methane, and hydrogen, which then is mixed with the nitrogen and oxygen from swallowed air. The gas is combustible and may explode during sigmoidoscopy with the use of electrical cauterization. The large intestine holds 7 to 10 L of gases each day, of which only $\frac{1}{2}$ L is expelled as flatus; the rest is absorbed through the lining of the colon.

The colon also secretes mucus and bicarbonate ions. Mucus not only protects the mucosa of the colon but also facilitates the compaction of feces, because it is the mucus that permits adherence of the solid wastes into a compact mass. The bicarbonate ions adhere to the mucus and act as a buffer, protecting the mucosa from the acid byproducts of bacterial metabolism within the feces.

CLINICAL CORRELATIONS

Intense irritation of the colonic mucosa, as in **enteritis,** results in the secretion of large quantities of mucus, water, and electrolytes. Voiding of copious quantities of liquid stool, known as **diarrhea,** protects the body by diluting and eliminating the irritant. Long-term diarrhea and loss of a large amount of fluid and electrolytes, without a regimen of replacement therapy, may result in circulatory shock and even death.

Rectum and Anal Canal

The histology of the **rectum** resembles that of the colon, except that its crypts of Lieberkühn are deeper but fewer per unit area (see Table 17–3).

The **anal canal,** the constricted continuation of the rectum, is about 3 to 4 cm long. Its crypts of Lieberkühn are short, few, and no longer present in the distal half of the canal. The mucosa also displays longitudinal folds, the **anal columns (rectal columns of Morgagni).** These meet one another to form pouch-like outpocketings, the **anal valves** with intervening **anal sinuses.** The anal valves assist the anus in supporting the column of feces.

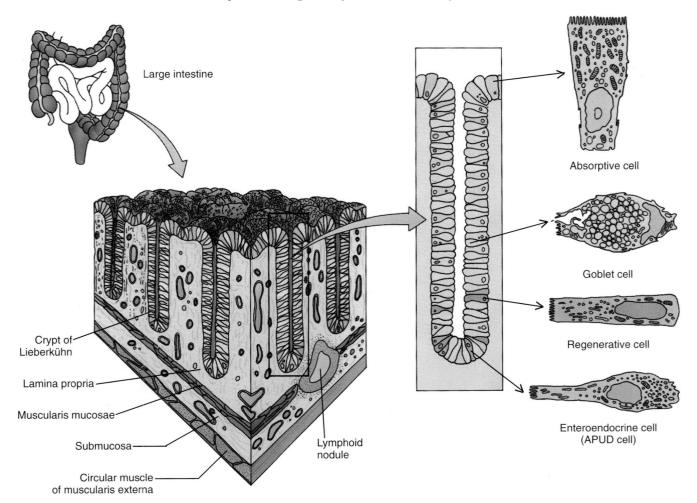

Large intestine

Crypt of Lieberkühn

Lamina propria

Muscularis mucosae

Submucosa

Circular muscle of muscularis externa

Lymphoid nodule

Absorptive cell

Goblet cell

Regenerative cell

Enteroendocrine cell (APUD cell)

Figure 17–20. Schematic diagram of the colon, crypts of Lieberkühn, and associated cells.

Anal Mucosa

The **epithelium** of the anal mucosa is simple cuboidal from the rectum to the **pectinate line** (at the level of the anal valves), stratified squamous nonkeratinized from the pectinate line to the external anal orifice, and stratified squamous keratinized (epidermis) at the anus. The **lamina propria,** a fibroelastic connective tissue, houses **anal glands** at the rectoanal junction and **circumanal glands** at the distal end of the anal canal. Additionally, hair follicles and sebaceous glands are present at the anus. The **muscularis mucosae** is composed of an inner circular and an outer longitudinal layer of smooth muscle. These muscular layers do not extend beyond the pectinate line.

Anal Submucosa and Muscularis Externa

The **submucosa** of the anal canal is composed of fibroelastic connective tissue. It houses two venous plexuses, the **internal hemorrhoidal plexus,** situated above the pectinate line, and the **external hemorrhoidal plexus,** located at the junction of the anal canal with its external orifice, the **anus.**

The **muscularis externa** consists of an inner circular and an outer longitudinal smooth muscle layer. The inner circular layer becomes thickened as it encircles the region of the pectinate line to form the **internal anal sphincter** muscle. The smooth muscle cells of the outer longitudinal layer continue as a fibroelastic sheet surrounding the internal sphincter.

Skeletal muscles of the floor of the pelvis form an **external anal sphincter muscle** that surrounds the fibroelastic sheet and the internal anal sphincter. The external sphincter is under voluntary control and exhibits a constant tonus.

CLINICAL CORRELATIONS

Increase in the size of the vessels of the submucosal venous plexuses of the anal canal results in the formation of **hemorrhoids,** a condition common in pregnancy and in persons over 50 years of age. This condition may manifest itself in painful defecation, appearance of fresh blood with defecation, and anal itching.

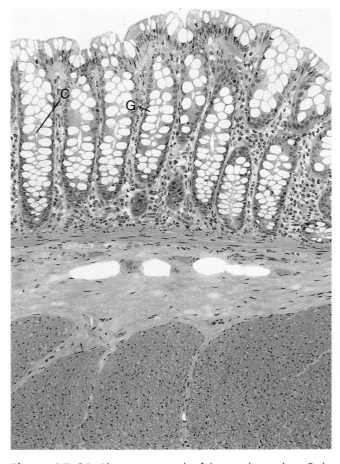

Figure 17-21. Photomicrograph of the monkey colon. Goblet cells (G); crypts of Lieberkühn (C) (× 132).

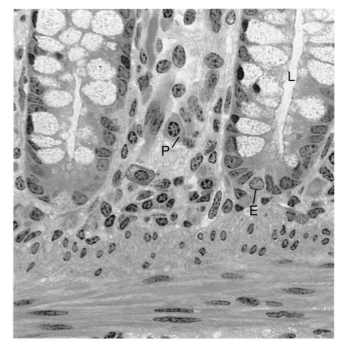

Figure 17-22. Photomicrograph of the crypts of Lieberkühn of the monkey colon. Lumen of crypt (L); plasma cell (P); enteroendocrine cell (E) (× 270).

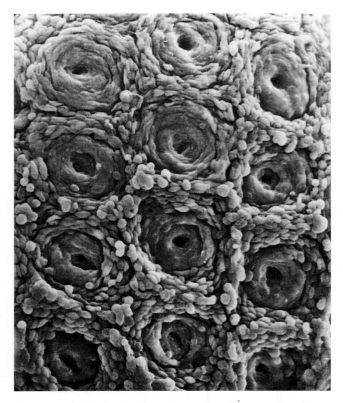

Figure 17-23. Scanning electron micrograph of a monkey colon (× 580). Observe the opening of the crypts. (From Specian, R.D., and Neutra, M.R.: The surface topography of the colonic crypt in rabbit and monkey. Am. J. Anat. **160:**461–472, 1981. Copyright © 1981. Reprinted by permission of John Wiley & Sons, Inc.

As a **rectal examination** is performed by inserting the index finger through the external anal orifice, the external anal sphincter tightens around the finger. Continued penetration results in activation of the internal anal sphincter, which also tightens around the finger. In males, structures that may be palpated through the anal canal include the bulb of the penis, the prostate, enlarged seminal vesicles, the inferior aspect of the distended bladder, and enlarged iliac lymph nodes; in females, these structures include the cervix of the uterus and, in pathological conditions, the ovaries and broad ligament.

Appendix

The **vermiform appendix** is a 5- to 6-cm-long diverticulum of the cecum with a stellate-shaped lumen that usually is occupied by debris. The mucosa of the appendix is composed of a simple columnar epithelium, consisting of surface absorptive cells, goblet cells, and M cells where lymphoid nodules adjoin the epithelium (see Table 17–3). The lamina propria is a loose connective tissue with numerous lymphoid nodules and shallow crypts of Lieberkühn. The cells composing these crypts are surface absorptive cells, goblet cells,

Chapter 17 ■ **Digestive System II—Alimentary Canal**   337

regenerative cells, numerous enteroendocrine cells, and infrequent Paneth cells. The muscularis mucosae, submucosa, and muscularis externa do not deviate from the general plan of the alimentary canal, although lymphoid nodules and occasional fatty infiltration are present in the submucosa. The appendix is invested by a serosa.

CLINICAL CORRELATIONS

The incidence of inflammation of the appendix, **appendicitis,** is greater in teenagers and young adults than in older persons; it also occurs more frequently in males than in females. Appendicitis usually is caused by obstruction of the lumen, which results in inflammation accompanied by swelling and an unremittent, severe pain in the lower right quadrant of the abdomen. Additional clinical signs are nausea and vomiting, fever (usually below 102° F), tense abdomen, and elevated leukocyte count. If the condition is not treated within 1 to 2 days, the appendix may rupture, leading to the onset of peritonitis, which may result in death if untreated.

Digestive System III—Glands

18

Extramural glands of the digestive system include the major salivary glands associated with the oral cavity (parotid, submandibular, and sublingual glands), the pancreas, and the liver and gallbladder. Each of these glands has numerous functions aiding the digestive process. The secretory products of these glands are delivered to the lumen of the alimentary tract by a system of ducts.

By producing saliva, the salivary glands facilitate the process of tasting food, initiate its digestion, and permit its deglutition (swallowing). These glands also protect the body by secreting the antibacterial agents lysozyme and lactoferrin, as well as the secretory immunoglobulin, IgA.

The pancreas manufactures a bicarbonate-rich fluid that buffers the acid chyme and produces enzymes necessary for the digestion of fats, proteins, and carbohydrates. The exocrine secretions of the pancreas are released into the lumen of the duodenum as necessary. Additionally, the pancreas synthesizes and releases endocrine hormones, including insulin, glucagon, somatostatin, gastrin, and pancreatic polypeptide.

Bile, the exocrine secretion of the liver, is required for proper absorption of lipids, whereas many of the liver's endocrine functions are essential for life. These include metabolism of proteins, lipids, and carbohydrates, synthesis of blood proteins and factors, manufacture of vitamins, and detoxification of bloodborne toxins. The gallbladder concentrates and stores bile until its release into the lumen of the duodenum.

Major Salivary Glands

The major salivary glands are the paired parotid, submandibular, and sublingual glands. They are branched **tubuloalveolar glands** whose connective tissue capsule provides septa that subdivide the glands into lobes and lobules. Individual acini are also invested by thin connective tissue elements. The vascular and neural components of the glands reach the secretory units via the connective tissue framework.

Regions of the Salivary Gland

Each of the major salivary glands has a secretory and a duct portion as diagrammed in Figure 18–1.

Secretory Portions

The **secretory portions,** arranged in tubules and acini, are composed of three types of cells: serous, mucous, and myoepithelial cells.

Serous cells are really seromucous cells because they secrete both proteins and a considerable amount of polysaccharides. These cells resemble truncated pyramids and have single, round, basally located nuclei, a well-developed rough endoplasmic reticulum (RER) and Golgi complex, numerous basal mitochondria, and abundant apically situated secretory granules rich in ptyalin. The basal aspects of the lateral cell membranes form tight junctions with each other. Apical to the tight junctions, intercellular canaliculi communicate with the lumen. The plasmalemma basal to the tight junctions forms many processes that interdigitate with those of neighboring cells.

Mucous cells are similar in shape to the serous cells. Their nuclei also are basally located but are flattened instead of being round (Fig. 18–2). The organelle population of these cells differs from those of the serous cells in that mucous cells have fewer mitochondria, a less extensive RER, and a considerably greater Golgi apparatus, indicative of the greater carbohydrate component of their secretory product (Fig. 18–3). The apical region of the cytoplasm is occupied by abundant secretory granules. The intercellular canaliculi and processes of the basal cell membranes are much less extensive than those of serous cells.

Myoepithelial cells (basket cells) share the basal laminae of the acinar cells. They have a cell body, housing the nucleus and several long processes that envelop the secretory acinus and intercalated ducts (see Fig. 18–1). The cell body houses a small complement of organelles in addition to the nucleus and makes hemidesmosomal attachments with

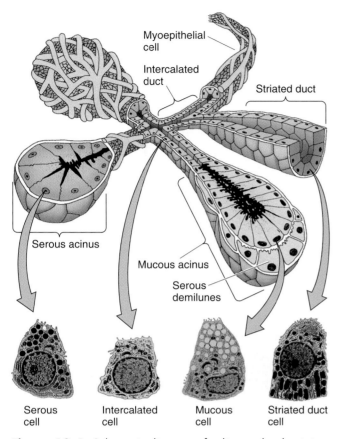

Figure 18-1. Schematic diagram of salivary gland acini, ducts, and cell types.

Striated ducts join with each other, forming **intralobular ducts** of increasing caliber, which are surrounded by more abundant connective tissue elements. Ducts arising from lobules unite to form **interlobular ducts,** which in turn form **interlobar ducts. The terminal (principal) duct** of the gland delivers saliva into the oral cavity.

Histophysiology of the Salivary Glands

The major salivary glands produce approximately 700 to 1100 ml of saliva a day. Additionally, minor salivary glands are located in the mucosa and submucosa of the oral cavity, but they contribute only 5% to the total daily salivary output.

Saliva has numerous functions: lubricating and cleansing of the oral cavity; antibacterial activity; participating in the taste sensation by dissolving food material; initial digestion via the action of ptyalin (salivary amylase) and salivary lipase; aiding swallowing by moistening the food and permitting the formation of bolus; and participating in the clotting process and wound healing because of the clotting factors and epidermal growth factor in saliva.

The saliva manufactured by the acinar cells, called **primary saliva,** is modified by the cells of the striated ducts. These ducts remove sodium and chloride ions from the primary saliva and replace them with potassium and bicarbonate ions. Thereafter, the altered secretion is called **secondary saliva.**

The secretory component required to transfer IgA from the connective tissue into the lumen of the secretory acinus

the basal lamina. The cytoplasmic processes, which form desmosomal contacts with the acinar and duct cells, are rich in actin and myosin; in electron micrographs these processes resemble smooth muscle cells. It has been shown that as the processes of myoepithelial cells contract, they press on the acinus, facilitating release of the secretory product into the duct of the gland.

Duct Portions

The duct portions of the major salivary glands are highly branched structures. The smallest branches of the system of ducts are the **intercalated ducts,** to which the secretory acini (and tubules) are attached. These small ducts are composed of a single layer of small cuboidal cells. Several intercalated ducts merge with each other to form **striated ducts,** composed of a single layer of cuboidal to low columnar cells (see Fig. 18–1). The basolateral membranes of these cells are highly folded, subdividing the cytoplasm into longitudinal compartments that are occupied by elongated mitochondria. The basolateral cell membranes of these cells have Na$^+$-ATPase that pumps sodium out of the cell into the connective tissue, conserving sodium.

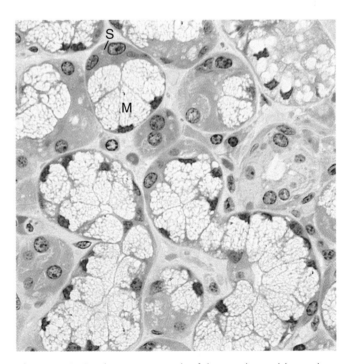

Figure 18-2. Photomicrograph of the monkey sublingual gland, displaying mucous acini (M) with serous demilunes (S) (× 540).

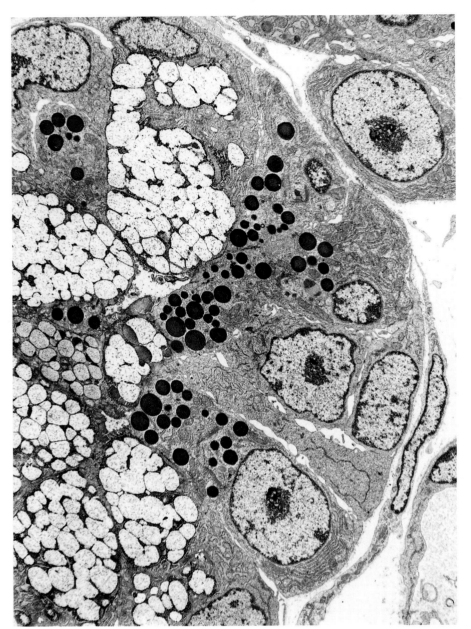

Figure 18–3. Electron micrograph of the rat sublingual gland, displaying serous and mucous granules in the cytoplasm of their acinar cells (× 6300). (From Redman, R.S., and Ball, W.D.: Cytodifferentiation of secretory cells in the sublingual glands of the prenatal rat: A histological, histochemical, and ultrastructural study. Am. J. Anat. **153:**367–390, 1978.)

(or duct) is manufactured by the acinar cells and duct cells. **Secretory IgA** complexes with antigens in the saliva, debilitating their deleterious affects. Saliva also contains lactoferrin, lysozyme, and thiocyanate ions. **Lactoferrin** binds iron, an element essential for bacterial metabolism; **lysozyme** breaks down bacterial capsules, permitting the entry of **thiocyanate ions,** a bactericidal agent, into the bacteria.

The major salivary glands do not secrete continuously. Secretory activity is stimulated via **parasympathetic innervation.** Innervation may be intraepithelial (i.e., formation of synaptic contact between the end-foot and acinar cell) or subepithelial. In subepithelial innervation the end-feet of axons do not make synaptic contact with the acinar cells; instead they release their acetylcholine in the vicinity of the secretory cell, at a distance of approximately 100 to 200 nm

from its basal plasmalemma. The cell thus activated stimulates neighboring cells via **gap junctions** to release their secretory products and serous fluid into the lumen of the acinus. **Sympathetic innervation** is responsible for the release of the mucous component of saliva. This component is responsible for the adhesion of food particles into the bolus as well as for the creation of a slippery surface, facilitating swallowing.

Properties of Individual Glands

Parotid Gland

The **parotid gland,** the largest salivary gland, weighs about 20 to 30 g but produces only approximately 30% of the total output of saliva. Although this gland is said to produce a purely **serous secretion,** the secretory product has some mucous component. The saliva produced by this gland has high levels of the enzyme **ptyalin** and secretory IgA. Electron micrographs of the apical regions of serous cells display numerous secretory granules filled with an electron-dense product that has an even more electron-dense core of unknown composition.

The connective tissue capsule of the parotid gland is well developed and forms numerous septa, which subdivide the gland into lobes and lobules. The duct system follows the distribution detailed earlier. By the 40th year of age, the gland becomes invaded by adipose tissue, which spreads from the connective tissue into the glandular parenchyma.

CLINICAL CORRELATIONS

Benign pleomorphic adenoma, a noncancerous salivary gland tumor, usually affects the parotid and the submandibular glands. Surgical removal of the parotid gland must be performed with care because of the presence of the facial nerve plexus within the substance of the gland.

The parotid gland (and occasionally the other major salivary glands) is also affected by viral infections, causing **mumps,** a painful disease in children that may result in sterility when affecting adults.

Submandibular Gland

The **submandibular gland,** although only 12 to 15 g in weight, produces approximately 60% of the total salivary output. About 90% of the acini are serous-producing; the remainder of the acini manufacture mucous saliva. Electron micrographs of the apical aspects of the serous cells display electron-dense secretory products, with a denser core, within membrane-bounded secretory granules. The number of serous demilunes is limited. The striated ducts of the submandibular gland are much longer than those of the parotid or sublingual glands; therefore, histological sections of this gland display many cross-sectional profiles of these ducts, a characteristic feature of the submandibular gland.

The connective tissue capsule of the submandibular gland is extensive and forms abundant septa, which subdivide the gland into lobes and lobules. Fatty infiltration of the connective tissue elements into the parenchyma is evident by mid-life.

Sublingual Gland

The **sublingual gland,** the smallest of the three major salivary glands, is almond-shaped, weighs only 2 to 3 g, and produces approximately 5% of the total salivary output. The gland is composed of mucous tubular secretory units capped by serous demilunes (see Fig. 18–2). The sublingual gland produces a mixed, but mostly mucous, saliva. The intercel-

lular canaliculi are well developed between the mucous cells of the secretory units. Electron micrographs of the cells of the serous demilunes display apical accumulations of secretory vesicles; however, unlike the cells of the parotid and submandibular glands, these vesicles do not have an electron-dense core (see Fig. 18–3).

The sublingual gland has a scanty connective tissue capsule, and its duct system does not form a terminal duct. Instead, several ducts open into the floor of the mouth and into the duct of the submandibular gland. Because of the organization of the ducts, some authors consider the sublingual gland to be composed of several smaller glandular subunits.

Pancreas

The **pancreas,** situated on the posterior body wall, deep to the peritoneum, has four regions: the uncinate process, head, body, and tail. It is about 25 cm long, 5 cm wide, and 1 to 2 cm thick, and it weighs approximately 150 g. Its flimsy connective tissue capsule forms septa, which subdivide the gland into lobules. The vascular and nerve supply of the pancreas, as well as its system of ducts, travels in these connective tissue compartments. The pancreas produces exocrine and endocrine secretions. The endocrine components of the pancreas, **islets of Langerhans,** are scattered among the exocrine secretory acini.

Exocrine Pancreas

The exocrine pancreas is a compound tubuloacinar gland that produces daily about 1200 ml of a bicarbonate-rich fluid containing digestive proenzymes. Forty to fifty acinar cells form a round to oval **acinus** whose lumen is occupied by three or four **centroacinar cells,** the beginning of the duct system of the pancreas (Fig. 18–4). The presence of centroacinar cells in the center of the acinus is a distinguishing characteristic of this gland.

Secretory and Duct Portions

Each **acinar cell** is shaped like a truncated pyramid, with its base positioned on the basal lamina separating the acinar cells from the connective tissue compartment. The round nucleus of the cell is basally located and is surrounded by basophylic cytoplasm (Fig. 18–5). The apex of the cell, facing the lumen of the acinus, is filled with proenzyme-containing **secretory granules (zymogen granules),** whose number diminishes after a meal. The Golgi region, located between the nucleus and the zymogen granules, varies in size in inverse relation to the zymogen granule concentration.

The basal cell membranes of acinar cells have receptors for the hormone **cholecystokinin.** Electron micrographs of acinar cells display an abundance of basally located RER, a rich supply of polysomes, and numerous mitochondria exhibiting matrix granules. The Golgi apparatus is well devel-

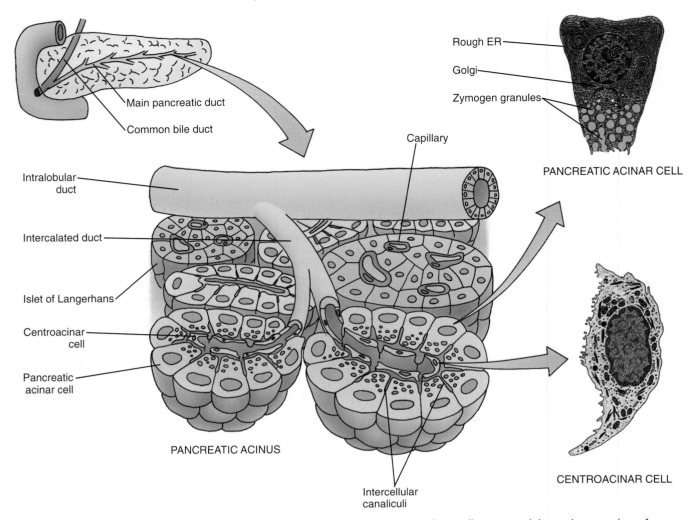

Figure 18–4. Schematic diagram of the pancreas, displaying secretory acini, their cell types, and the endocrine islets of Langerhans.

oped but fluctuates in size, being smaller when the zymogen granules are numerous and larger after the granules release their contents.

The zymogen granules may release their contents individually, or several secretory vesicles may fuse with each other, forming a channel to the lumen of the acinus from the apical cytoplasm.

The **duct system** of the pancreas begins within the center of the acinus, with the terminus of the **intercalated ducts,** composed of pale, low cuboidal **centroacinar cells** (see Fig. 18–4, 18–5). Centroacinar cells and intercalated ducts both have receptors on their basal plasmalemma for the hormone **secretin.** Intercalated ducts join each other to form larger **intralobular ducts,** several of which converge to form **interlobular ducts.** These ducts are surrounded by a considerable amount of connective tissue and deliver their contents into the **main pancreatic duct,** which joins the **common bile duct** before opening in the duodenum at the **papilla of Vater.**

Histophysiology of the Exocrine Pancreas

The acinar cells of the exocrine pancreas manufacture, store, and release a large number of enzymes: pancreatic amylase, pancreatic lipase, ribonuclease, DNase, and the proenzymes trypsinogen, chymotrypsinogen, procarboxypeptidase, and elastase. The cells also manufacture **trypsin inhibitor,** a protein that protects the cell from accidental intracellular activation of trypsin.

Release of the pancreatic enzymes is effected by the hormone **cholecystokinin** (pancreozymin) manufactured by enteroendocrine cells of the small intestine, especially the duodenum.

The centroacinar cells and intercalated ducts manufacture a serous, bicarbonate-rich alkaline fluid, which neutralizes and buffers the acid chyme that enters the duodenum. This fluid is enzyme-poor, and its release is effected by the hormone **secretin,** produced by enteroendocrine cells of the small intestine. Thus the enzyme-rich and enzyme-poor se-

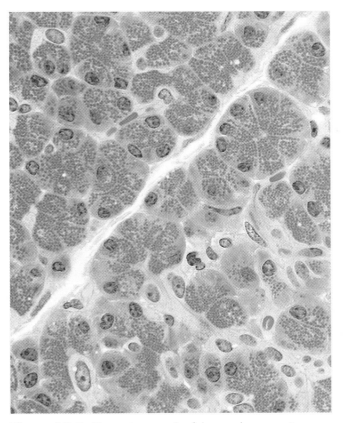

Figure 18–5. Photomicrograph of the monkey exocrine pancreas (× 540).

cretions are regulated separately, and the two secretions may be released at different times or concomitantly.

CLINICAL CORRELATIONS

Occasionally, the pancreatic digestive enzymes become active within the cytoplasm of the acinar cells, resulting in **acute pancreatitis,** which is often fatal. The histological changes involve: inflammatory reaction, necrosis of the blood vessels, proteolysis of the pancreatic parenchyma, and enzymatic destruction of adipose cells not only within the pancreas but also in the surrounding region of the abdominal cavity.

Pancreatic cancer is the fifth leading cause of mortality from all cancers, killing about 25,000 people in the United States per year. Less than 50% of those diagnosed with it survive more than 1 year, and fewer than 5% survive 5 years. Men are more susceptible to this disease than are women. It is interesting to note that cigarette smokers have a 70% greater risk of developing pancreatic cancers than nonsmokers.

Endocrine Pancreas

Each **islet of Langerhans** is a richly vascularized spherical conglomeration of approximately 3000 cells. The approxi-

mately 1 million islets distributed throughout the human pancreas constitute the endocrine pancreas. A somewhat greater number of islets are present in the tail than in the remaining regions. Each islet is surrounded by reticular fibers, which also enter the substance of the islet to encircle the network of capillaries that pervade it (see Fig. 18–4; Fig. 18–6).

Cells Composing the Islets of Langerhans

Five types of cells compose the parenchyma of each islet of Langerhans: β-cells, α-cells, δ-cells, PP cells, and G cells. However, these cells cannot be differentiated from one another by routine histology, but immunocytochemical procedures are available that permit them to be recognized. Electron micrographs also display the features that distinguish the various cells, especially the size and electron density of their granules (Fig. 18–7). Otherwise the cells do not exhibit any unusual morphologies but resemble cells that specialize in protein synthesis. The characteristic features, locations, and hormones synthesized by these cells are presented in Table 18–1.

Histophysiology of the Endocrine Pancreas

The two hormones produced in the greatest amounts by the endocrine pancreas, insulin and glucagon, act to decrease and increase blood glucose levels, respectively.

Insulin production begins with synthesis of a single

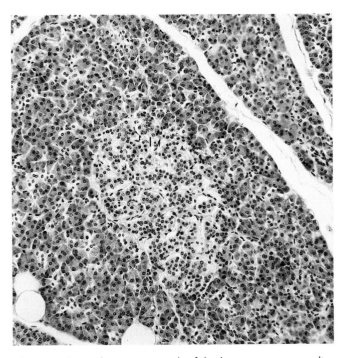

Figure 18–6. Photomicrograph of the human pancreas, displaying secretory acini and an islet of Langerhans (I) (× 132).

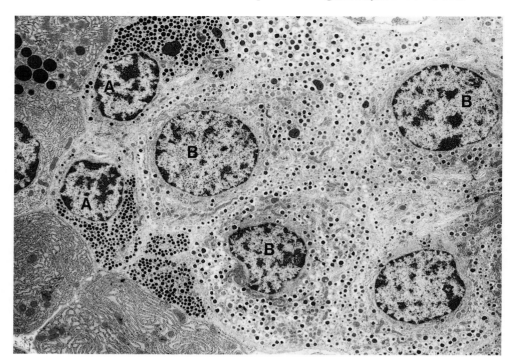

Figure 18–7. Electron micrograph of α-cells (A) and β-cells (B) of the rabbit islet of Langerhans (x 5040). (From Jorns, A., and Grube, D.: The endocrine pancreas of glucagon- and somatostatin-immunized rabbits. Cell Tissue Res. **265:**261–273, 1991.)

polypeptide chain, **pre-proinsulin,** on the RER of β-cells. Within the RER cisternae, this initial product is converted to **proinsulin** by enzymatic cleavage of a polypeptide fragment. Within the trans-Golgi network, proinsulin is packaged into clathrin-coated vesicles, which lose their clathrin coat as they travel toward the plasmalemma. A segment of the proinsulin molecule near its center is removed by self-excision, thus forming insulin, which is composed of two short polypeptide chains linked by disulfide bonds. Insulin is released into the intercellular space in response to increased blood glucose levels, as occurs after consumption of a carbohydrate-rich meal.

The released insulin binds to cell-surface insulin receptors on many cells, especially skeletal muscle, liver, and adipose cells. The plasma membranes of these cells also have glucose transport proteins, **glucose permease (glucose transport units),** which are activated to take up glucose, thus decreasing blood glucose levels. It is interesting to note that subplasmalemmal vesicles, rich in glucose permease, are added to the cell membrane during insulin stimulation and returned to their intracellular position when insulin levels are reduced.

Glucagon, a peptide hormone produced by α-cells, is released in response to low blood glucose levels. As in insulin production, a prohormone is produced first; this undergoes proteolytic cleavage to yield the active hormone. Glucagon acts mainly on hepatocytes, causing these cells to activate glycogenolytic enzymes. These enzymes break glycogen down to glucose, which is released into the bloodstream, increasing blood glucose levels. Glucagon also activates the hepatic enzymes responsible for **gluconeogenesis** (the syn-

thesis of glucose from noncarbohydrate sources) if the intracellular glycogen depot of the hepatocytes is depleted.

Somatostatin, manufactured by δ-cells, has both paracrine and endocrine effects. The hormone's paracrine effects are to inhibit the release of endocrine hormones by nearby α-cells and β-cells. Its endocrine effects are on smooth muscle cells of the alimentary tract and gallbladder, reducing the motility of these organs. Somatostatin is released in response to the increased levels of blood glucose, amino acids, or chylomicrons that occur subsequent to a meal.

Gastrin, released by G cells, stimulates gastric release of HCl, gastric motility and emptying, and the rate of cell division in gastric regenerative cells. **Pancreatic polypeptide,** a hormone produced by PP cells inhibits the exocrine secretions of the pancreas.

CLINICAL CORRELATIONS

Diabetes mellitus is a hyperglycemic metabolic disorder that results from (1) lack of insulin production by β-cells of the islets of Langerhans or (2) defective insulin receptors on the target cells. There are two major forms of diabetes mellitus, type I and type II (Table 18–2). The incidence of type II is about five to six times that of type I. If uncontrolled, both types of diabetes may have debilitating sequalae, including circulatory disorders, renal failure, blindness, gangrene, stroke, and myocardial infarcts. The most significant laboratory result indicative of diabetes is elevated blood-glucose levels after an overnight fast.

Type I diabetes (insulin-dependent; juvenile-onset diabetes) usually affects persons under 20 years of age. It

Table 18–1. Cells and Hormones of the Islets of Langerhans

Cell	% of Total	Location	Fine Structure of Granules	Hormone and Molecular Weight	Function
β-cell	70%	Scattered throughout the islet (but concentrated in the center)	300 nm in diameter; dense core granule surrounded by a wide electron-lucent halo	Insulin 6000 D	Decreases blood sugar levels
α-cell	20%	Islet periphery	250 nm in diameter; dense core granule with a narrow electron-lucent halo	Glucagon 3500 D	Increases blood sugar levels
δ-cell	5%	Scattered throughout the islet	350 nm in diameter; electron-lucent homogeneous granule	Somatostatin 1640 D	*Paracrine:* inhibits hormone release; *Endocrine:* reduces contractions of alimentary tract and gall bladder smooth muscles
G cell	1%	Scattered throughout the islet	300 nm in diameter	Gastrin 2000 D	Stimulates HCl production by parietal cells of stomach
PP cell (F cell)	1%	Scattered throughout the islet	180 nm in diameter	Pancreatic polypeptide 4200 D	Inhibits exocrine secretions of pancreas

Table 18–2. A Comparison of Type I and Type II Diabetes Mellitus

Type	Common Synonyms	Clinical Characteristics	Patient Weight	Hereditary Component	Islets of Langerhans
Type I (insulin-dependent)	Juvenile-onset diabetes; juvenile diabetes; idiopathic diabetes	Abrupt onset of symptoms; age under 20 years; decreased blood insulin level; ketoacidosis is common; antibodies present against β-cells; possible autoimmune disease; reacts to insulin; polyphagia, polydipsia, polyuria	Normal (or weight loss in spite of increase in food intake)	About 50% concordance in identical twins; environmental factors important in the development of the disease	Decrease in the size and number of β-cells; islets are atrophied and fibrotic
Type II (non–insulin-dependent)	Adult-onset diabetes; ketosis-resistant diabetes	Onset after 40 years of age; mild decrease in blood insulin levels; ketoacidosis is rare; no antibodies against β-cells; impaired insulin release; insulin-resistant; decrease in number of insulin receptors; impaired postreceptor signaling	80% of the affected individuals are obese	About 90–100% concordance in identical twins	Some decrease in β-cell number; **amylin** present in the tissue surrounding β-cells

is characterized by the three cardinal signs of **polydipsia** (constant thirst), **polyphagia** (undiminished hunger), and **polyuria** (excessive urination). **Type II diabetes** (non–insulin-dependent diabetes) is the *most common* and usually affects persons over 40 years of age.

Liver

The **liver,** weighing approximately 1500 g, is the largest gland in the body. It is located in the upper right-hand quadrant of the abdominal cavity, just inferior to the diaphragm. The liver is subdivided into four lobes—right, left, quadrate, and caudate—of which the first two constitute its bulk (Fig. 18–8A).

Similar to the pancreas, the liver has both endocrine and exocrine functions. But unlike the pancreas, the same cell—the **hepatocyte**—is responsible for the formation of the liver's exocrine secretion, **bile,** and its numerous endocrine products. Additionally, hepatocytes convert noxious substances into nontoxic materials that are excreted in bile.

General Hepatic Structure and Vascular Supply

With the exception of the bare area, the liver is completely enveloped by peritoneum, which forms a simple squamous epithelium covering over the dense, irregular connective tissue **capsule (Glisson's capsule)** of the gland. Glisson's capsule is loosely attached over the entire circumference of the liver, except at the porta hepatis, where it enters the liver, forming a conduit for the blood and lymph vessels and bile ducts. The liver is unusual in that its connective tissue elements are sparse, so that the bulk of the liver is composed of uniform parenchymal cells, the **hepatocytes.**

The superior aspect of the liver is convex, whereas its inferior region presents a hilum-like indentation, the **porta hepatis.** The liver has a dual blood supply, receiving oxygenated blood from the **left** and **right hepatic arteries** (25%) and nutrient-rich blood via the **portal vein** (75%). Both of these vessels enter the liver at the porta hepatis. Blood leaves the liver at the posterior aspect of the organ through the **hepatic veins,** which deliver their contents into the inferior vena cava. Bile also leaves the liver at the porta hepatis, by way of the right and left hepatic ducts, to be delivered to the **gallbladder** for concentration and storage.

Because the liver occupies a central position in metabolism, all nutrients (except for chylomicrons) absorbed in the alimentary canal are transported directly to the liver via the portal vein. Additionally, iron-rich blood from the spleen is also routed, by way of the portal vein, directly to the liver for processing. Much of the nutritive materials delivered to the liver are converted by the **hepatocytes** into storage products, such as glycogen, to be released as glucose when required by the body.

Hepatocytes are arranged in hexagonal-shaped lobules (**classical lobules**) about 2 mm in length and 700 μm in diameter. These lobules are clearly demarkated by slender connective tissue elements in animals such as the pig and the camel. However, in humans, their boundaries can only be approximated because of the scarcity of connective tissue and the closely packed arrangement of the lobules.

Where three classical lobules contact each other, the connective tissue elements are increased, and these regions are known as **portal areas (triads).** Portal areas house slender branches of the hepatic artery, tributaries of the relatively large portal vein, interlobular bile ducts (recognized by their simple cuboidal epithelium), and lymph vessels. These vessels and ducts follow the longitudinal axis of each lobule (Fig. 18–8B).

The portal areas are isolated from the liver parenchyma by the **limiting plate,** a sleeve of modified hepatocytes. A narrow space, the **space of Möll,** separates the limiting plate from the connective tissue of the portal area.

Although one would expect six portal areas around each classical lobule, usually only *three,* equally distributed portal areas are present at a random section. Along the length of each vessel and bile duct within the portal area, fine branches, known as **distributing arterioles,** arise; like outstretched arms, they reach toward their counterparts in the neighboring portal areas. Smaller vessels, known as **inlet arterioles,** branch from the distributing arterioles (or from the parent vessel). Additionally, the interlobular bile ducts are vascularized by a **peribiliary capillary plexus.** Venules are also of two sizes: the larger **distributing veins** and the smaller **inlet venules.**

The longitudinal axis of each classical lobule is occupied by the **central vein,** the initial branch of the hepatic vein. Hepatocytes radiate, like spokes of a wheel, from the central vein, forming anastomosing, fenestrated plates of liver cells, separated from each other by large vascular spaces, known as **hepatic sinusoids** (see Fig. 18–8C; Fig. 18–9). **Inlet arterioles, inlet venules,** and branches from the **peribiliary capillary plexus** pierce the limiting plate (of modified hepatocytes) to join the hepatic sinusoids (Fig. 18–9). As blood enters the sinusoids, its flow slows considerably, and it slowly percolates into the central vein.

Because there is only one central vein in each lobule, it receives blood from every sinusoid of that lobule, and its diameter increases as it progresses through that structure. As the central vein leaves the lobule, it terminates in the **sublobular vein.** Numerous central veins deliver their blood into a single sublobular vein; sublobular veins join each other to form **collecting veins,** which in turn form the right and left hepatic veins.

Three Concepts of Liver Lobules

There are three basic conceptualizations of the liver lobule (Fig. 18–10). The **classical liver lobule** was the first to be defined histologically, because the connective tissue arrange-

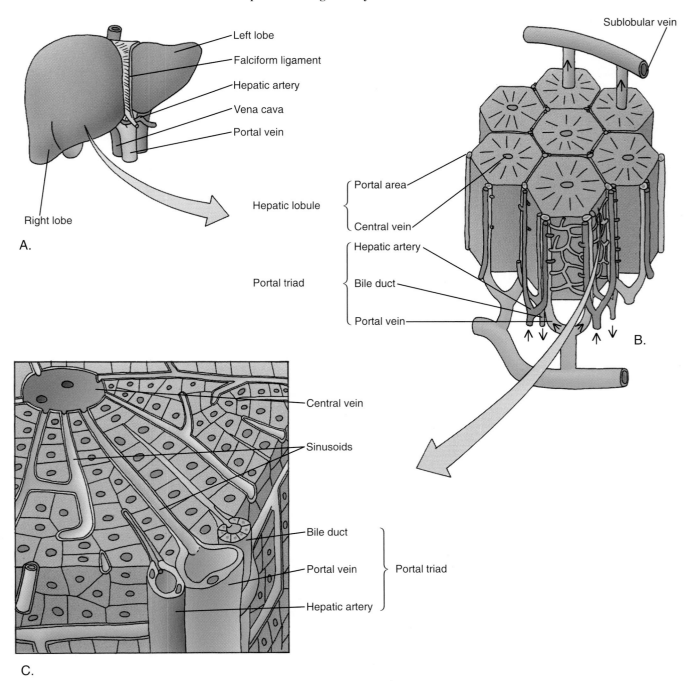

Figure 18–8. Schematic diagram of the liver. A, Gross anatomy of the liver. **B,** Liver lobules, displaying the portal areas and the central vein. **C,** Portion of the liver lobule, displaying the portal area, liver plates, sinusoids, and bile canaliculi.

ment in the pig liver afforded an obvious rationale. In this concept blood flows from the periphery to the *center of the lobule* into the central vein. Bile, manufactured by liver cells, enters into small intercellular spaces, **bile canaliculi,** located between hepatocytes and flows to the *periphery of the lobule* to the interlobular bile ducts of the portal areas.

The concept of an exocrine secretion flowing to the periphery of a lobule was not consistent with the situation in most glands, where the secretion enters a central lumen (as in an acinus). Therefore, histologists suggested that all hepatocytes that deliver their bile to a particular interlobular bile duct constitute a lobule, called the **portal lobule.** In histological sections, the portal lobule is defined as that triangular region whose center is the portal area and whose periphery is bounded by imaginary straight lines connecting the three surrounding central veins that form the three apices of the triangle.

A third conceptualization of hepatic lobules is based on

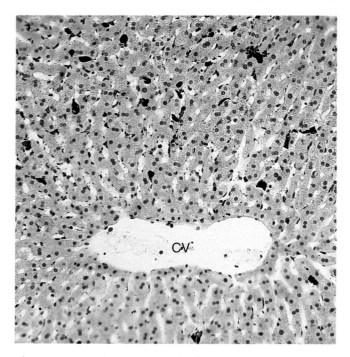

Figure 18-9. Photomicrograph of a dog liver, displaying the central vein (CV), liver plates, and sinusoids (× 270).

blood flow from the distributing arteriole and, consequently, on the order in which hepatocytes degenerate subsequent to toxic or hypoxic insults. This ovoid to diamond-shaped lobule is known as the hepatic acinus (portal acinus of Rappaport). This is viewed as three poorly defined, concentric regions of hepatic parenchyma surrounding a distributing

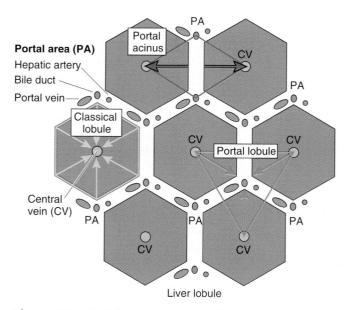

Figure 18-10. Schematic diagram of the three types of lobules in the liver: classical lobule, portal lobule, and liver acinus.

artery in the center. The outermost layer, zone 3, extends as far as the central vein and is the most oxygen-poor of the three zones. The remaining region is equally divided into two zones (1 and 2), with zone 1 being the richest in oxygen.

Hepatic Sinusoids and Hepatocyte Plates

Anastomosing plates of hepatocytes, no more than two cells thick, radiate from the central vein toward the periphery of the classical lobule (see Fig. 18–8C). The spaces between the plates of hepatocytes are occupied by hepatic sinusoids, and the blood flowing in these wide vessels is prevented from contacting the hepatocytes by the presence of an endothelial lining composed of **sinusoidal lining cells.** Often, the cells of this endothelial lining do not contact each other, leaving gaps of up to 0.5 μm between them. The sinusoidal lining cells also have fenestrae that are present in clusters, known as **sieve plates.** Thus, particulate matter of less than 0.5 μm in diameter may leave the lumen of the sinusoid with relative ease.

Resident macrophages, known as **Kupffer cells,** are associated with the sinusoidal lining cells in the sinusoids (Figs. 18–11, 18–12). Frequently, phagosomes of Kupffer cells contain endocytosed particulate matter and cellular debris, especially defunct erythrocytes that are being destroyed by these cells. Electron micrographs of Kupffer cells display numerous filopodia-like projections, mitochondria, some RER, a small Golgi apparatus, and an abundance of lysosomes and late endosomes. Because these cells do not make

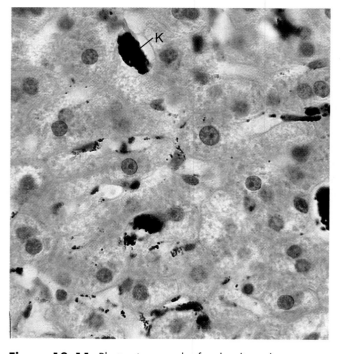

Figure 18-11. Photomicrograph of a dog liver demonstrating plates of hepatocytes, sinusoids, and india ink containing Kupffer cells (K) (× 540).

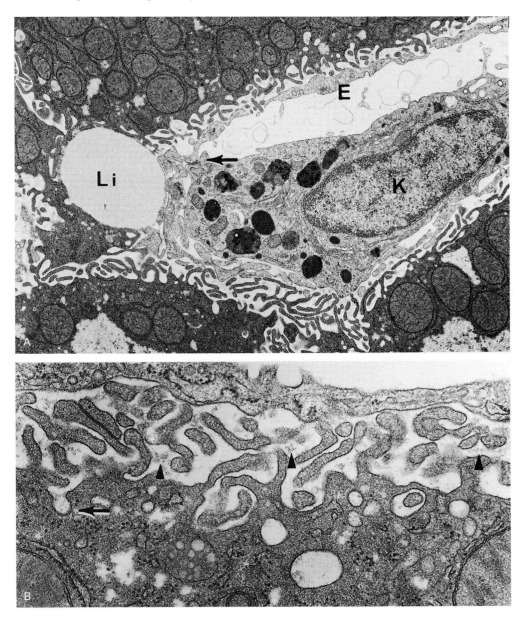

Figure 18–12. Electron micrograph of the shrew liver. A, Observe the sinusoid, with its sinusoidal lining cell (E), Kupffer cell (K), and a small region of a lipid-droplet (Li) containing Ito cell (× 10,500). **B,** A higher magnification of the hepatocyte displays its numerous microvilli (arrowheads) protruding into the space of Disse (× 34,500). The arrow indicates the process of pinocytosis. (From Matsumoto, E., and Hirosawa, K.: Some observations on the structure of *Suncus* liver with special reference to the Vitamin A–storing cell. Am. J. Anat. **167:**193–204, 1983.)

intercellular junctions with the neighboring cells, it has been suggested that they may be migratory scavengers.

Perisinusoidal Space of Disse

The sinusoidal lining cells are separated from the hepatocytes by a narrow, **perisinusoidal space (space of Disse),** and plasma escaping from the sinusoids has free access to this space (see Fig. 18–12; Fig. 18–13). Microvilli of the hepatocytes occupy much of the space of Disse; the extensive surface area of the microvilli facilitates exchange of materials between the bloodstream and the hepatocytes. It is important to realize that hepatocytes do not come into contact with the bloodstream; instead the space of Disse acts as an intermediate compartment between them.

Although the perisinusoidal space contains type III collagen fibers (reticular fibers) that support the sinusoids, basal lamina is absent. Occasionally, nonmyelinated nerve fibers and stellate-shaped **fat-storing cells** (Ito cells) have been noted in this space (see Fig. 18–12). It is believed that Ito cells store vitamin A. Additionally, **pit cells,** which display short pseudopodia and cytoplasmic granules, have been noted in the perisinusoidal space of mice and rats. These cells, believed to be natural killer cells, are also assumed to be in the human liver.

Hepatic Ducts

Bile canaliculi anastomose with one another, forming labyrinthine tunnels among the hepatocytes. As these bile canaliculi reach the periphery of the classic lobules, they merge with **cholangioles,** short tubules composed of a combination of hepatocytes and low cuboidal cells. Bile from cholangioles enters **canals of Herring,** slender branches of the **interlobular bile ducts,** that radiate parallel to the inlet arterioles and inlet venules. Interlobular bile ducts merge to form increasingly larger conduits, which eventually unite to form the **right** and **left hepatic ducts.** The extrahepatic system of bile ducts is described later.

Epithelial cells of the cholangioles, canals of Herring, and interlobular bile ducts secrete a bicarbonate-rich fluid, similar to that produced by the duct system of the pancreas. The formation and release of this alkaline buffer is controlled by the hormone secretin, produced by enteroendocrine cells of the duodenum. This fluid acts, with fluid from the pancreas, to neutralize the acidic chyme that enters the duodenum.

Hepatocytes

Hepatocytes are polygonal cells, approximately 20 to 30 μm in diameter, that are closely packed together to form anastomosing plates of liver cells, one to two cells in thickness. They exhibit variations in their structural, histochemical, and biochemical properties, depending on their location within liver lobules.

Domains of Hepatocyte Plasmalemma

Hepatocytes are arranged such that each cell not only contacts other cells but also borders a space of Disse. Thus the

plasmalemma of hepatocytes is said to have lateral domains and sinusoidal domains.

LATERAL DOMAINS. The **lateral domains** of the hepatocyte membrane form elaborate, labyrinthine intercellular spaces, 1 to 2 μm in diameter, known as **bile canaliculi,** which conduct bile between hepatocytes to the periphery of the classic lobules (see Fig. 18–8C). Leakage is prevented by the formation of fasciae occludentes between adjoining liver cells, isolating the bile canaliculi from the remaining extracellular space.

Short, blunt microvilli project from the hepatocyte plasmalemma into the bile canaliculi, thus increasing the surface areas through which bile is secreted (see Fig. 18–13). The actin cores of these microvilli mingle with the thickened network of actin and intermediate filaments that reinforce the region of the hepatocyte plasmalemma, which participates in the formation of bile canaliculi.

The cell membranes that form the walls of bile canaliculi display high levels of **Na⁺-K⁺ ATPase** and **adenylate cyclase.** The lateral domains also have isolated gap junctions, whereby hepatocytes communicate with each other.

SINUSOIDAL DOMAINS. The **sinusoidal domains** of hepatocyte plasma membranes also have microvilli, which project into the space of Disse (see Figs. 18–12, 18–13). It has been calculated that these microvilli increase the surface area of the sinusoidal domain by a factor of six, facilitating the exchange of material between the hepatocyte and the plasma in the perisinusoidal space. This cell membrane is

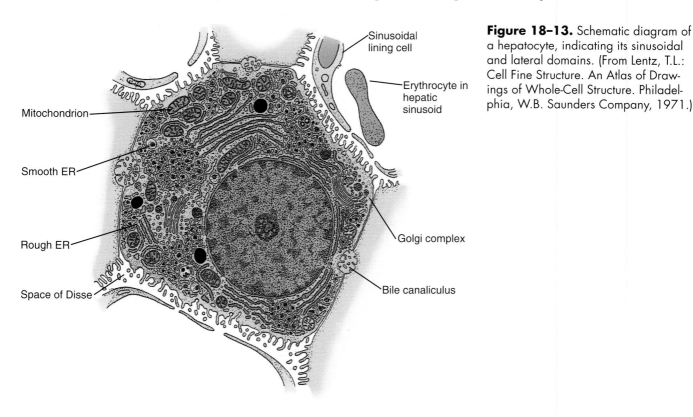

Figure 18–13. Schematic diagram of a hepatocyte, indicating its sinusoidal and lateral domains. (From Lentz, T.L.: Cell Fine Structure. An Atlas of Drawings of Whole-Cell Structure. Philadelphia, W.B. Saunders Company, 1971.)

rich in mannose-6-phosphate receptors, Na+-K+-ATPase, and adenylate cyclase, because it is here that the endocrine secretions of the hepatocyte are released and enter the sinusoidal blood, and material carried by the bloodstream is transported into the hepatocyte cytoplasm.

Hepatocyte Organelles and Inclusions

Approximately 75% of the hepatocytes have a single nucleus, and the remainder have two nuclei. The nuclei vary in size, the smallest ones (about 50% of the nuclei) being diploid, the larger ones being polyploid, with the largest nuclei reaching 64 N.

Hepatocytes actively synthesize proteins for their own use as well as for export. Thus they have an abundance of free ribosomes, RER, and Golgi apparatus (Figs. 18–14, 18–15). Each cell houses several sets of Golgi apparatuses, located preferentially in the vicinity of bile canaliculi.

Because of the high energy requirements of hepatocytes, each cell contains as many as 2000 mitochondria. Cells near the central vein (zone 3 of the liver acinus) have nearly twice as many, but considerably smaller, mitochondria than hepatocytes in the periportal area (zone 1 of the liver acinus). Liver cells also have a rich complement of endosomes, lysosomes, and peroxisomes.

The complement of smooth endoplasmic reticulum (SER)

of hepatocytes varies not only by region but also by function. Cells in zone 3 of the liver acinus have a much richer endowment of SER than those in the periportal area. Moreover, the presence of certain drugs and toxins in the blood induces an increase in the SER content of liver cells because detoxification occurs within the cisternae of this organelle.

Hepatocytes contain varying amounts of inclusions in the form of lipid droplets and glycogen (Fig. 18–16). The lipid droplets are mostly **very-low-density lipoprotein** and are especially prominent after the consumption of a fatty meal.

Glycogen deposits are present as accumulations of electron-dense granules 20 to 30 μm, known as β-**particles,** in the vicinity of SER. The distribution of glycogen varies with hepatocyte location. Liver cells in the vicinity of the portal area (zone 2 of liver acinus) display large clumps of β-particles surrounded by SER, whereas pericentral hepatocytes (zone 3 of liver acinus) exhibit diffuse glycogen deposits (Figure 18–16). The number of these particles varies with the dietary state of the individual. They are abundant subsequent to feeding and fewer after fasting.

CLINICAL CORRELATIONS

Persons who have consumed hepatotoxic substances, such as alcohol, display an increased number of lipid deposits in their zone-3 hepatocytes. Additionally, persons

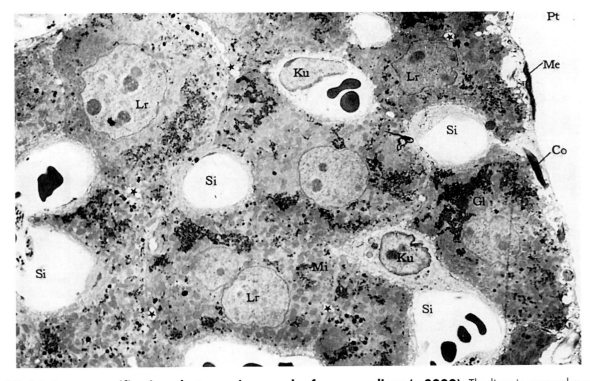

Figure 18–14. Low-magnification electron micrograph of a mouse liver (× 3000). The liver is covered over most of its surface by peritoneum (Me), which overlies the collagenous capsule (Co) of the liver. Observe the sinusoids (Si), Kupffer cells (Ku), and glycogen deposits (Gl) in the hepatocyte (Lr) cytoplasm. Bile canaliculi are denoted by asterisks (*). (From Rhodin, J.A.G.: An Atlas of Ultrastructure. Philadelphia, W.B. Saunders Company, 1963.)

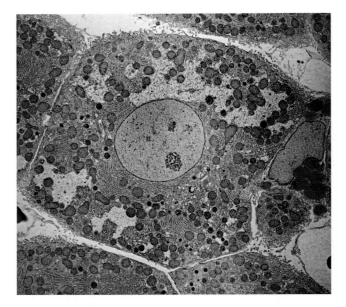

Figure 18–15. Electron micrograph of a rat hepatocyte (×2500). (From Tandler, B., Krahenbuhl, S., and Brass, E.P.: Unusual mitochondria in the hepatocytes of rats treated with a vitamin B$_{12}$ analogue. *Anat. Rec.* **231:**1–6, 1991.)

who are taking barbiturates display an increase in the SER content of zone-3 liver cells.

Alcoholics and people who suffer from obstruction of the biliary tract or chronic poisoning are prone to develop **cirrhosis,** a disease characterized by fibrosis, degeneration of hepatocytes, and disintegration of the normal organization of the liver.

Histophysiology of the Liver

The liver may have as many as 100 different functions, most of which are performed by the hepatocytes. Each of these liver cells produces not only the exocrine secretion bile but also various endocrine secretions. Hepatocytes metabolize the end-products of absorption from the alimentary canal, store them as inclusion products, and release them in response to hormonal and nervous signals. Additionally, liver cells detoxify drugs and toxins (protecting the body from their deleterious effects) and transfer secretory IgA from the space of Disse into bile. In addition, Kupffer cells phagocytose bloodborne foreign particulate matter and defunct erythrocytes.

Bile Manufacture

The liver produces approximately 600 to 1200 ml of bile per day. This fluid, which is mostly water, contains bile salts (bile acids), bilirubin glucuronide, phospholipids, lecithin, cholesterol, plasma electrolytes (especially sodium and bicarbonate), and IgA. It absorbs fat, eliminates approxi-

mately 80% of the cholesterol synthesized by the liver, and excretes bloodborne waste products such as bilirubin.

Most of the **bile salts** are resorbed from the lumen of the small intestine, enter the liver via the portal vein, are endocytosed by hepatocytes, and are transported into the bile canaliculi for subsequent re-release back into the duodenum (enterohepatic recirculation of bile salts). The remaining 10% of bile salts are manufactured *de novo* in the SER of hepatocytes by the conjugation of cholic acid, a metabolic byproduct of cholesterol, to either taurine (tauricholic acid) or glycine (glycocholic acid).

CLINICAL CORRELATIONS

Bile salts emulsify fats in the small intestine to facilitate their digestion. Absence of bile salts prevents fat digestion and absorption, resulting in **fatty stool.**

Bilirubin, a water-insoluble, yellowish-green pigment, is the toxic degradation product of hemoglobin. As defunct erythrocytes are destroyed by macrophages in the spleen and by Kupffer cells in the liver, bilirubin is released into the bloodstream and is bound to plasma albumin. In this form, known as **free bilirubin,** it is endocytosed by hepatocytes. The enzyme **glucuronyltransferase,** located in the SER of the hepatocyte, catalyzes the conjugation of bilirubin with glucuronide to form the water-soluble **bilirubin glucuronide (conjugated bilirubin).** Some of the bilirubin glucuronide is released into the bloodstream, but most of it is excreted into the bile canaliculi for delivery into the alimentary canal for subsequent elimination with the feces (Fig. 18–17).

CLINICAL CORRELATIONS

The yellowish discoloration of the skin that is the hallmark of **jaundice** results from excessively high levels of free or conjugated bilirubin (which are yellowish-green) in the bloodstream. The two primary types of jaundice have different causes. A decrease in bilirubin conjugation, either because of hepatocyte malfunction (as in hepatitis) or, more commonly, obstruction of the bile ducts, causes **obstructive jaundice.** Increased hemolysis of erythrocytes, producing so much free bilirubin that hepatocytes, even though unimpaired, cannot eliminate bilirubin rapidly enough, causes **hemolytic jaundice.**

Lipid Metabolism

Chylomicrons released by surface absorbing cells of the small intestine enter the lymphatic system and reach the liver through branches of the hepatic artery. Within hepatocytes they are degraded into fatty acids and glycerol. The fatty acids are subsequently desaturated and are used to synthesize phospholipids and cholesterol or are degraded into acetyl-CoA. Two molecules of acetyl-CoA are combined to

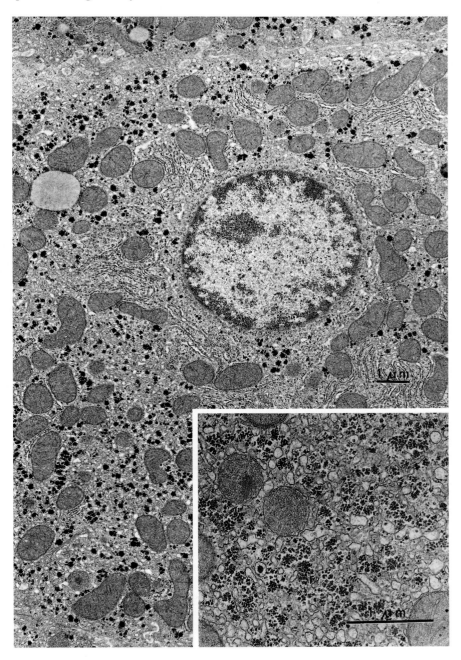

Figure 18–16. Electron micrograph of glycogen and lipid deposits in the pericentral hepatocyte of a rat. The inset shows the presence of glycogen particles at a higher magnification. (From Cardell, R.R., and Cardell, E.L.: Heterogeneity of glycogen distribution in hepatocytes. J. Electron Microsc. Techn. **14:**126–139, 1987).

form acetoacetic acid. Much of the acetoacetic acid is converted into β-hydroxybutyric acid and some into acetone. These three compounds are known as **ketone bodies.** Phospholipids, cholesterol, and ketone bodies are stored in hepatocytes until their release into the space of Disse. Additionally, the liver manufactures **very-low-density lipoproteins (VLDL),** which are also released into the space of Disse as droplets 30 to 100 nm in diameter.

CLINICAL CORRELATIONS

Ketosis occurs when the concentration of ketone bodies in the blood becomes too high (as in persons suffering from diabetes or starvation). It is recognizable by the typical acetone breath of affected persons. If untreated, ketosis results in decreased blood pH **(acidosis),** possibly leading to death.

Carbohydrate and Protein Metabolism

The liver maintains normal levels of glucose in the blood. It performs this function by transporting glucose from the blood into the hepatocytes and storing it in the form of glycogen. If blood glucose levels drop below normal, hepatocytes hydrolyze glycogen **(glycogenolysis)** into glucose and transport it out of the cells into the space of Disse (Fig.

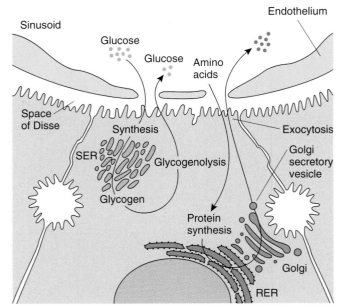

A Protein synthesis and carbohydrate storage in the liver

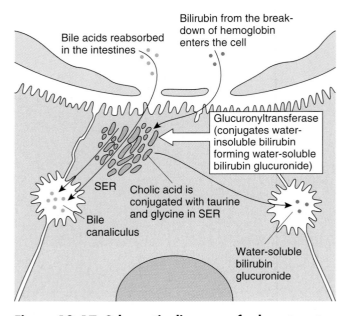

B Secretion of bile acids and bilirubin

Figure 18–17. Schematic diagram of a hepatocyte function. A, Protein synthesis and carbohydrate storage. **B,** Secretion of bile acids and bilirubin.

18–17). Hepatocytes also can synthesize glucose from other sugars (such as fructose and galactose) or from noncarbohydrate sources (such as amino acids), a process known as **gluconeogenesis.**

One of the most essential roles of the liver is the elimination of bloodborne ammonia by converting it into **urea.**

There are two major sources of ammonia in the body, the deamination of amino acids by hepatocytes and the synthesis of ammonia by bacterial action in the alimentary canal.

CLINICAL CORRELATIONS

Excessive blood ammonia levels, indicative of impaired liver function or drastic reduction in blood flow to the liver, may lead to **hepatic coma,** a condition that is incompatible with life.

Approximately 90% of the blood proteins are manufactured by the liver (see Fig. 18–17). These include factors necessary for coagulation (such as fibrinogen, factor III, accelerator globulin, and prothrombin), proteins required for the complement reactions, proteins that function in transport of metabolites, and albumins. All of the globulins, with the exception of γ-globulins, also are synthesized by the liver. Additionally, hepatocytes can synthesize all of the nonessential amino acids that the body requires.

Vitamin Storage

Vitamin A is stored in the greatest amount in the liver, but vitamins D and B_{12} also are present in substantial quantities. It has been estimated that the liver contains enough vitamin stores to prevent deficiency of vitamin A for 10 months, vitamin D for 4 months, and vitamin B_{12} for over 12 months.

Degradation of Hormones and Detoxification of Drugs and Toxins

The liver endocytoses and degrades hormones of the endocrine glands. The endocytosed hormones are either transported into the bile canaliculi in their native form to be digested in the lumen of the alimentary canal, or they are delivered into late endosomes for degradation by lysosomal enzymes.

Drugs, such as barbiturates and antibiotics, and toxins are inactivated by **microsomal mixed-function oxidases** in hepatocytes. These drugs and toxins usually are inactivated in the cisterna of the SER by methylation, conjugation, or oxidation. Occasionally, detoxification occurs in peroxisomes rather than in the SER.

CLINICAL CORRELATIONS

Continued long-term use of certain drugs, such as barbiturates, decreases their effectiveness, requiring the prescription of increased doses. This drug **tolerance** is due to the hypertrophy of the SER complement of hepatocytes and a concomitant increase in their mixed-function oxidases. The increase in the organelle size and the enzyme concentration is **induced** by the barbiturate, which is detoxified via oxidative demethylation. Additionally, these hepatocytes concurrently become more efficient in detoxifying other drugs and toxins.

Immune Function

Most of the IgA antibodies formed by plasma cells in the mucosa of the alimentary canal enter the circulatory system and are transported to the liver. Hepatocytes complex the IgA with secretory component and release the complex into bile, which then enters the lumen of the duodenum. Thus much of the lumenal IgA enters the intestine through the common bile duct, accompanying bile. The remainder of the lumenal IgA is transported from the intestinal mucosa into the lumen by surface absorptive cells.

Kupffer cells, which are derived from monocyte precursors, have Fc receptors as well as receptors for complement and thus can phagocytose foreign particulate matter. The importance of these cells is appreciable, because blood from the portal vein contains a considerable number of microorganisms that enter the bloodstream from the lumen of the alimentary canal. These bacteria become opsonized in the lumen or mucosa of the gut or in the bloodstream. Kupffer cells recognize and endocytose at least 99% of these microorganisms. Kupffer cells also remove cellular debris and defunct erythrocytes from the blood.

Liver Regeneration

Hepatocytes are long-lived cells with a lifespan of approximately 150 days; thus mitotic figures are present only infrequently. However, if hepatoxic drugs are administered or a portion of the liver is excised, hepatocytes proliferate and the liver regenerates its normal architecture and previous size.

The regenerative ability of the liver of rodents is so enormous that if 75% of the organ is excised, it will regenerate itself to its normal size within 4 weeks. The human liver's regenerative capacity is much less than that of mice and rats. It has been demonstrated that the mechanism of regeneration is controlled by transforming growth factor-α, transforming growth factor-β, and hepatopoietin.

Gallbladder

The **gallbladder** is a small, pear-shaped organ situated on the inferior aspect of the liver. It is about 10 cm in length and 4 cm in cross-section, and it can store about 70 ml of bile. This organ resembles a sack with a single opening. The bulk of the organ forms the **body,** and the opening, which is continuous with the **cystic duct,** is called the **neck.** The function of the gallbladder is to store and concentrate bile and to release it into the duodenum as required.

Structure of the Gallbladder

The four layers composing the gallbladder are, from the lumen outward, epithelium, lamina propria, smooth muscle, and serosa/adventitia. The mucosa of the empty gallbladder is highly folded into tall, parallel ridges (Fig. 18–18). As it is distended with bile, the plication is reduced to a few short folds, and the mucosa becomes relatively smooth.

The lumen of the gallbladder is lined by a **simple columnar epithelium,** whose cells are composed of two cell types: the more common **clear cells** and the infrequent **brush cells** (Fig. 18–19). The oval nuclei of these cells are basally positioned and the supranuclear cytoplasm displays occasional secretory granules containing mucinogen. In electron micrographs, their luminal surface displays short microvilli, coated by a thin layer of glycocalyx. The basal region of the cytoplasm is particularly rich in mitochondria, providing abundant energy for the Na^+-K^+ ATPase pump present in the basolateral cell membrane.

The lamina propria is composed of a vascularized loose connective tissue well endowed with elastic and collagen fibers. In the neck of the gallbladder the lamina propria houses simple tubuloalveolar glands, which produce a small amount of mucus to lubricate the lumen of this constricted region. The thin smooth muscle layer of the gallbladder is composed mostly of **obliquely** oriented fibers, whereas oth-

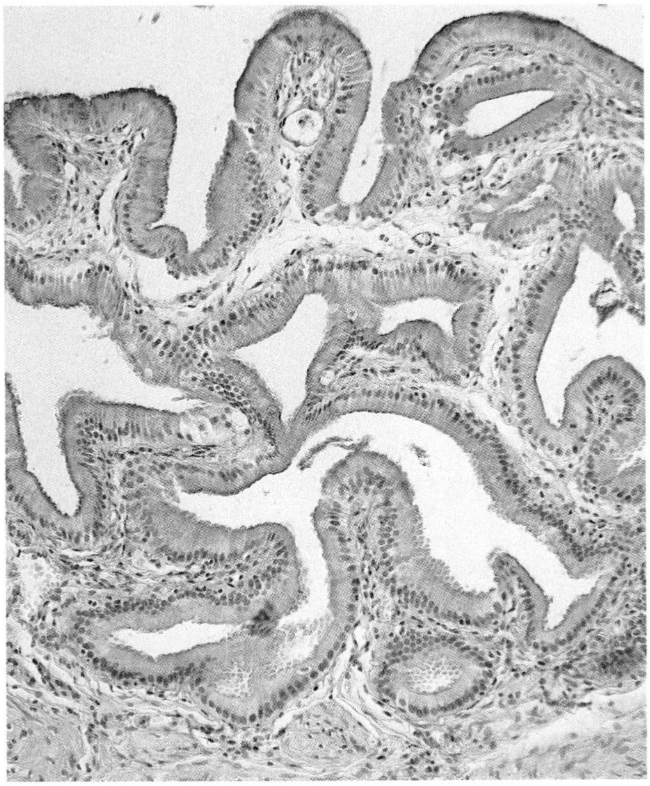

Figure 18–18. Photomicrograph of an empty gallbladder (× 132).

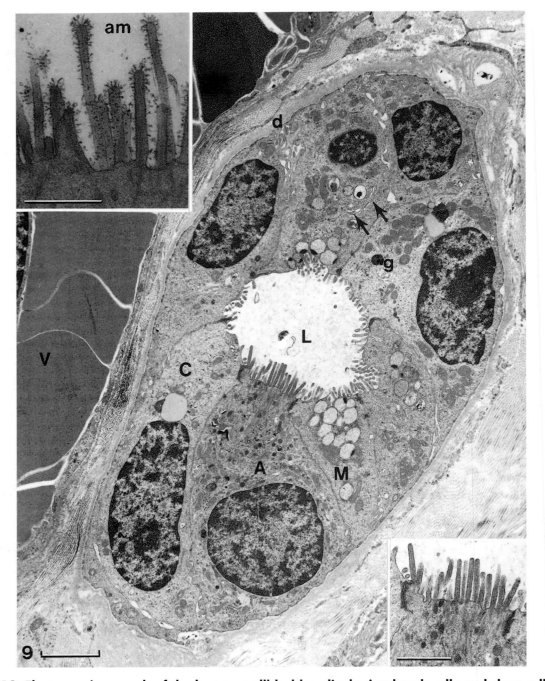

Figure 18–19. Electron micrograph of the human gallbladder, displaying brush cells and clear cells of the epithelium. L, lumen; A, brush cell; C, clear cells; d, interdigitations; g, granules; M, clear cells with mucoid granules; g, Golgi complex, bar = 2 μm. *Upper inset:* Clear cell microvilli (am), bar = 0.5 μm. *Lower inset:* Brush cell microvilli, bar = 1.0 μm. (From Gilloteaux, J., Pomerants, B., and Kelly, T.: Human gallbladder mucosa ultrastructure: Evidence of intraepithelial nerve structures. Am. J. Anat. **184:**321–333, 1989.)

ers are oriented longitudinally. The connective tissue adventitia is attached to Glisson's capsule of the liver but may be separated from it with relative ease. The nonattached surface of the gallbladder is invested by peritoneum, providing it with a smooth, simple squamous epithelial serosa.

Extrahepatic Ducts

The right and left **hepatic ducts** unite to form the **common hepatic duct,** which is joined by the **cystic duct,** arising from the gallbladder. The merger of these two ducts forms the **common bile duct,** 7 to 8 cm long, which fuses with the pancreatic duct to form the **ampulla of Vater** that opens at the duodenal papilla into the lumen of the duodenum.

The opening of the common bile duct and the pancreatic duct is controlled by a complex of four sphincter muscles, collectively called the **sphincter of Oddi.** The locations and functions of these muscles are summarized in Table 18–3.

Histophysiology of the Gallbladder

The primary functions of the gallbladder are to store, concentrate, and release bile. Bile is constantly manufactured by the liver and must make its way to the gall bladder. This requires that the sphincters choledecus, pancreaticus, and ampullae be maintained in a closed position, so that the bile backs up the common bile duct and the cystic duct to enter the gallbladder.

Na^+ is actively transported from the basolateral region of the simple columnar epithelium of the gallbladder into the extracellular space and is passively followed by Cl^- and water. In order to compensate for the loss of intracellular ions, apical ion channels permit sodium and chloride to enter the simple columnar cells, reducing the salt concentration of bile. The requirement for osmotic equilibrium drives water from the bile into the simple columnar cell, thus concentrating bile.

The signaling molecule **cholecystokinin** is released by I cells (enteroendocrine cells) of the duodenum in response to a fatty meal. This molecule contacts cholecystokinin receptors on the smooth muscle cells of the gallbladder and causes them to contract intermittently. Concurrently, contact of cholecystokinin receptors on the smooth muscle cells of the sphincter of Oddi causes the sphincter muscles to relax. The result is that the rhythmic contractile forces of the gallbladder inject the bile into the lumen of the duodenum.

CLINICAL CORRELATIONS

Gallstones (cholelithiasis) are more common in women than in men, occurring most frequently in the fourth decade in life. Approximately 20% of all women and 8% of all men have gallstones. Usually, the person is unaware of their presence, because gallstones are either small enough to be eliminated with normal bile flow or too large to leave the gallbladder. Once they enter and become entrapped in the cystic or common hepatic ducts, gallstones obstruct bile flow and cause excruciating pain. Approximately 80% of gallstones are composed of cholesterol **(cholesterol stones);** most of the remainder are formed from the calcium salt of bile, calcium bilirubinate **(pigment stones).** Cholesterol stones are large (1 to 3 cm) and pale yellow, have numerous facets, and are few in number. Pigment stones are smaller (1 cm), black, and ovoid, and they occur in large numbers. Usually, both types of stones are radiolucent.

Table 18–3. The Sphincter of Oddi and Its Component Parts

Sphincter Muscle	Location and Function
Sphincter choledochus	Surrounds and controls the terminal region of the common bile duct to stop bile flow into the duodenum
Sphincter pancreaticus	Surrounds and controls the terminal portion of the pancreatic duct to stop pancreatic juices from entering the duodenum and prevents the entry of bile into the pancreatic duct
Sphincter ampullae	Surrounds and controls the ampulla of Vater and prevents the entry of bile and pancreatic juices into the duodenum
Fasciculus longitudinalis	Located in the triangular interval delineated by the ampulla of Vater, pancreatic duct, and common bile duct; facilitate the entry of bile into the lumen of the duodenum

19

Urinary System

The urinary system removes toxic byproducts of metabolism from the bloodstream and disposes **urine** from the body. These actions are performed by the two kidneys, which not only remove the toxins from the bloodstream but also conserve salts, glucose, proteins, and water, as well as additional materials essential for proper health. Because of these eliminating and conserving functions, the kidneys also help to regulate blood pressure, hemodynamics, and the acid–base balance of the body. Urine is delivered from the kidneys into the two **ureters,** from where it passes to a storage organ, the **urinary bladder.** During voiding, the urinary bladder is emptied via the **urethra,** which delivers the urine to outside of the body. Additionally, the kidneys have an endocrine function in that they produce renin, erythropoietin, and prostaglandins and convert a circulating precursor of vitamin D, to the active vitamin.

Kidney

The **kidneys** are large, reddish, bean-shaped organs, situated retroperitoneally on the posterior abdominal wall. Because of the position of the liver, the right kidney is approximately 1 to 2 cm lower than the left. Each kidney is about 11 cm long, 4 to 5 cm wide, and 2 to 3 cm thick. The kidney, embedded in perirenal fat, lies with its convex border situated laterally and its concave **hilum** facing medially. Branches of the renal artery and vein, lymph vessels, and ureter pierce the kidney at its hilum. The ureter is expanded at this region, forming the **renal pelvis.** A fat-filled extension of the hilum deeper into the kidney is called the **renal sinus.**

The kidney is invested by a thin, loosely adhering **capsule,** consisting mainly of dense, irregular collagenous connective tissue, with occasional elastic fibers and smooth muscle cells.

Overview of Kidney Structure

A hemisected view of the kidney shows that it is separated into a cortex and a medulla (Fig. 19–1). The cortical region appears dark brown and granular, whereas the medulla contains 6 to 12 discrete, pyramid-shaped, pale, striated regions, the **renal pyramids.** The base of each pyramid is oriented toward the cortex, constituting the corticomedullary border, whereas its apex, known as the **renal papilla,** is pointing toward the hilum. The apex is perforated by 20 or so openings of the **ducts of Bellini;** this sieve-like region is known as the **area cribrosa.** The apex is surrounded by a cup-like **minor calyx,** which, joining two or three neighboring minor calyces, forms a **major calyx.** The three or four major calyces are larger subdivisions that empty into the **renal pelvis,** the expanded continuation of the proximal portion of the ureter. Neighboring pyramids are separated from each other by material resembling the cortex, the **cortical columns** (of Bertin).

The portion of the cortex overlying the base of each pyramid is known as a cortical arch. Macroscopically, three types of substances may be observed in the cortex: red, dot-like granules, **renal corpuscles;** convoluted tubules, the **cortical labyrinth;** and longitudinal striations, **medullary rays,** which are cortical continuations of material located in the renal pyramids.

A renal pyramid, with its associated cortical arch and cortical columns, represents a **lobe** of the kidney. Hence, the kidney is a multilobar organ. Each medullary ray and part of the cortical labyrinth surrounding it is considered a kidney **lobule,** which continues into the medulla as a cone-shaped structure.

CLINICAL CORRELATIONS

During fetal development, the lobes of the kidney are accentuated by deep clefts, but this characteristic is normally obliterated in the adult. When the lobation is retained subsequent to infancy, the condition is known as **lobated kidney.**

Another anomalous kidney development is known as **polycystic kidney disease,** which presents varied mor-

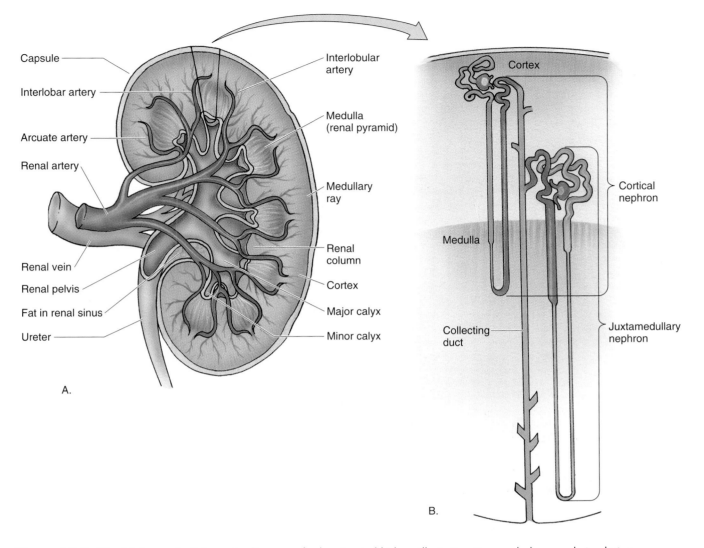

Figure 19–1. The kidney. A, Schematic diagram of a hemisected kidney illustrating its morphology and circulation.
B, Arrangement of cortical and juxtamedullary nephrons.

Illustration continued on following page

phologies depending on the severity of the affliction but involves the appearance of thin-walled cysts on and in the kidneys.

Uriniferous Tubules

The functional unit of the kidney is the **uriniferous tubule,** a highly convoluted structure that modifies the fluid passing through it to form **urine** as its final output. The uriniferous tubule consists of two parts, each with a different embryological origin, the **nephron** and the **collecting tubule** (see Fig. 19–1). There are approximately 1.3 million nephrons in each kidney. Several nephrons are drained by a single collecting tubule, and multiple collecting tubules join in the deeper aspect of the medulla to form larger and larger ducts. The largest of these ducts, the ducts of Bellini, perforate the renal papilla at the area cribrosa.

Uriniferous tubules are densely packed so that the connective tissue stroma of the kidney is scant. Much of the connective tissue is occupied by the rich vascular supply of the kidney. The functional relationship between the vascular supply and the uriniferous tubules is discussed later in this chapter.

Nephron

Two types of nephrons are found in the human kidney: shorter **cortical nephrons** and longer **juxtamedullary nephrons,** whose renal corpuscle is located in the cortex and tubular parts are located in the medulla (see Fig. 19–1). The specific locations of the two types of nephrons, the cellular composition of their various regions, and the specific alignments of these regions in register with one another permit the subdivision of the medulla into an **outer zone** and an

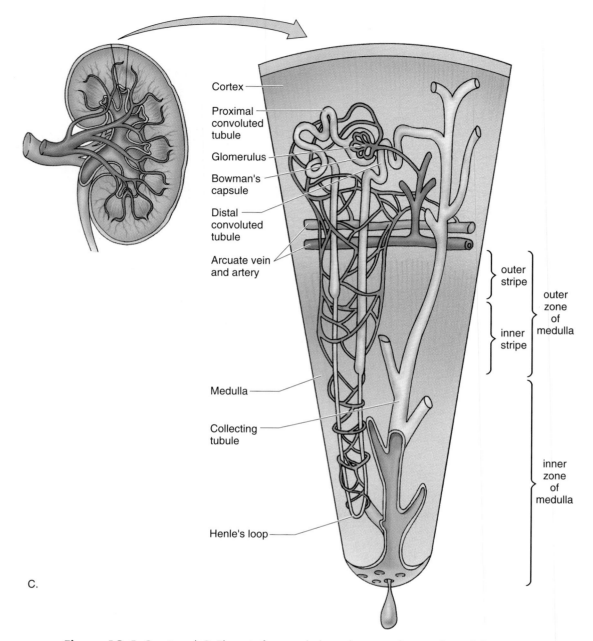

Cortex

Proximal convoluted tubule

Glomerulus

Bowman's capsule

Distal convoluted tubule

Arcuate vein and artery

outer stripe

inner stripe

outer zone of medulla

Medulla

Collecting tubule

inner zone of medulla

Henle's loop

C.

Figure 19–1 *Continued* **C,** The uriniferous tubule and its vascular supply and drainage.

inner zone. The outer zone of the medulla is further subdivided into an **outer stripe** and an **inner stripe.** Unless otherwise noted, all of the descriptions in this textbook refer to juxtamedullary nephrons, even though they constitute only 15% of all nephrons.

Each juxtamedullary nephron is about 40 mm long. The constituent parts of the nephron are modified to perform specific physiological functions. The renal corpuscle, with its attendant glomerulus, filters the fluid expressed from the bloodstream. The subsequent tubular portions of the nephron—namely the proximal tubule, the thin limb of the Henle loop, and the distal tubule—modify the filtrate to form urine.

RENAL CORPUSCLE. The renal corpuscle, an oval to round structure, about 200 to 250 μm in diameter, is composed of a tuft of capillaries, the **glomerulus,** which is invaginated into **Bowman's capsule,** the dilated, pouchlike, proximal end of the nephron (see Fig. 19–1; Figs. 19–2, 19–3, 19–4). During development, the capillaries become invested by the blind end of the tubular nephron, almost as if a hand were to push into the end of an expanded balloon. Hence, the space inside Bowman's capsule, known as **Bowman's space (urinary space),** is decreased in volume. The glomerulus is in intimate contact with the **visceral layer of Bowman's capsule,** composed of modified epithelial cells called **podocytes.** The outer wall surrounding Bow-

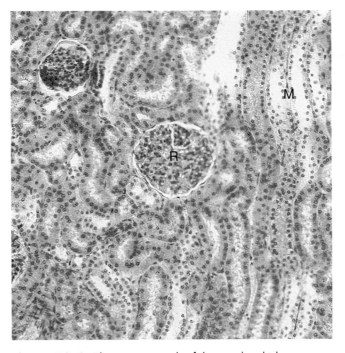

Figure 19–2. Photomicrograph of the monkey kidney cortex, illustrating renal corpuscles (R), medullary rays (M), and cross-sectional profiles of the uriniferous tubules (× 132).

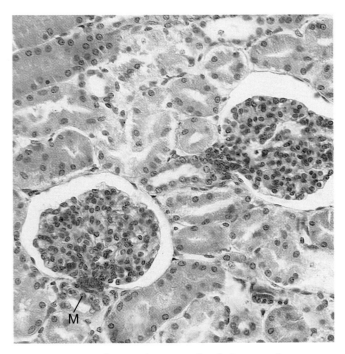

Figure 19–3. Photomicrograph of the monkey renal corpuscle surrounded by cross-sectional profiles of proximal and distal tubules (× 270). Note the presence of the macula densa (M).

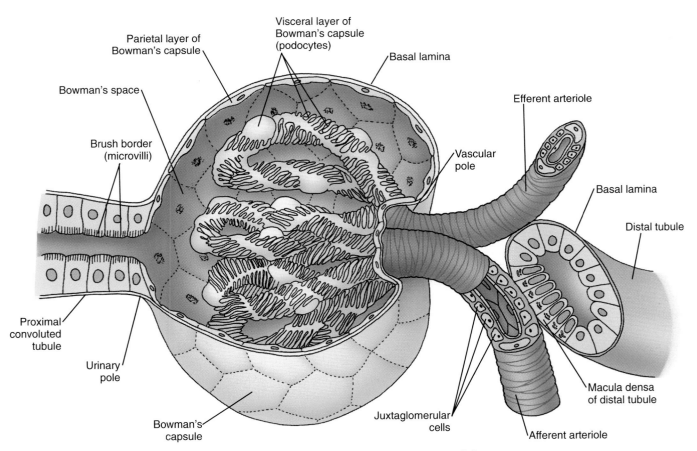

Figure 19–4. Diagram of a renal corpuscle and its juxtamedullary apparatus.

man's space, composed of simple squamous epithelial cells (sitting on a thin basal lamina), is the **parietal layer** (see Fig. 19–4).

The region where the vessels supplying and draining the glomerulus enter and exit Bowman's capsule is known as the **vascular pole.** The region of continuation between the renal corpuscle and the proximal tubule, which drains Bowman's space, is called the **urinary pole.** The glomerulus is supplied by the short, straight **afferent glomerular arteriole** and drained by the **efferent glomerular arteriole.** Hence, the glomerulus is a completely arterial capillary bed. Although the outer diameter of the afferent arteriole is greater than that of the efferent arteriole, their luminal diameters are approximately equal.

The efferent glomerular arteriole presents greater resistance to blood flow, resulting in higher capillary pressures in the glomerulus than in other capillary beds. Filtrate leaking out of the glomerulus enters Bowman's space through a complex **filtration barrier** composed of the endothelial wall of the capillary, the basal lamina, and the visceral layer of Bowman's capsule.

Glomerulus. The **glomerulus** is formed as several tufts of anastomosing capillaries that arise from branches of the afferent glomerular arteriole. The connective tissue component of the afferent arteriole does not enter Bowman's capsule, and the normal connective tissue cells are replaced by a specialized cell type known as **mesangial cells.** There are two groups of mesangial cells, the **extraglomerular mesangial cells** located at the vascular pole and pericyte-like **intraglomerular mesangial** cells situated within the renal corpuscle (Figs. 19–5, 19–6).

Intraglomerular mesangial cells are probably phagocytic and function in resorption of the basal lamina. Mesangial cells also may be contractile, because they have receptors for vasoconstrictors such as angiotensin II and thus reduce blood flow through the glomerulus. Moreover, they may support the capillaries of the glomerulus in regions where the visceral layer of Bowman's capsule does not come into contact with the capillaries.

The capillaries constituting the glomerulus are similar to the fenestrated type of capillaries (see Figs. 19–5, 19–6; Fig. 19–7). Their endothelial cells are highly attenuated, with the exception of the region containing the nucleus, but the pores are usually not covered by a diaphragm. The pores are large, ranging between 70 and 90 nm in diameter; hence these capillaries act as a barrier only to formed elements of the blood and to macromolecules whose effective diameter exceeds the size of the fenestrae (e.g., albumin, 69,000 Da).

Basal Lamina. Investing the glomerulus is a basal lamina, approximately 300 nm thick, consisting of three layers (see Figs. 19–6, 19–7). The middle dense layer, the **lamina densa,** is about 100 nm in thickness and consists of type IV collagen. Less electron-dense layers, the **laminae rarae,**

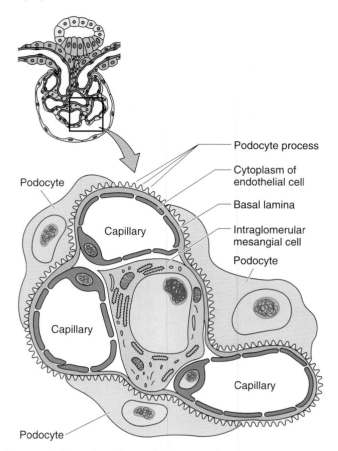

Figure 19–5. The relationship among the intraglomerular mesangial cell, podocytes, and glomerulus.

which contain **laminin, fibronectin,** and a polyanionic proteoglycan rich in **heparan sulfate,** are located on either side of the lamina densa. Some refer to a lamina rara interna, between the endothelial cells of the capillary and the lamina densa, and the lamina rara externa, between the lamina densa and the visceral layer of Bowman's capsule. Fibronectin and laminin help pedicels and endothelial cells to maintain their attachment to the lamina densa.

Visceral Layer of Bowman's Capsule. The visceral layer of Bowman's capsule is composed of epithelial cells that are highly modified to perform a filtering function. These large cells, called **podocytes,** bear numerous long, tentacle-like cytoplasmic extensions, **primary (major) processes,** which follow, but usually do not come in close contact with, the longitudinal axes of the glomerular capillaries (see Fig. 19–7). Each primary process bears many secondary processes, **pedicels,** arranged in an orderly fashion. These completely envelop most of the glomerular capillaries by interdigitating with pedicels from neighboring major processes of different podocytes (Figs. 19–8, 19–9).

Pedicels have a well-developed glycocalyx composed of a negatively charged sialoprotein, **podocalyxin.** Pedicels rest

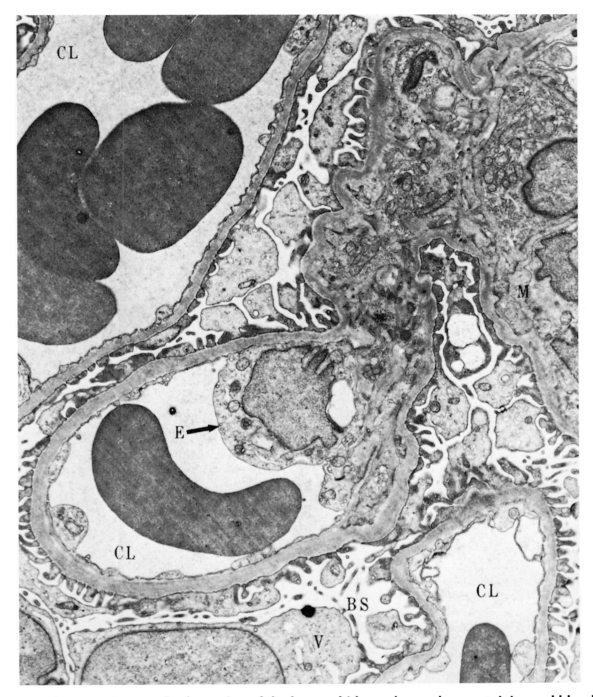

Figure 19–6. Electron micrograph of a region of the human kidney glomerulus, containing red blood cells (× 6700). Note the association between the intraglomerular mesangial cell and the podocytes around the glomerular capillaries. CL, capillary lumen; BS, Bowman's space; M, mesangial cells; E, endothelial cells; V, podocyte. (From Brenner, B.M., and Rector, F.C.: The Kidney, 4th ed., vol. 1. W.B. Saunders, Philadelphia, 1991).

on the lamina rara externa of the basal lamina. Their cytoplasm is devoid of organelles but does house microtubules and microfilaments. Interdigitation occurs such that narrow clefts (20 to 40 nm), known as **filtration slits,** remain between adjacent pedicels. Filtration slits are not completely open; rather, they are covered by a thin (6-nm-thick) **slit di-aphragm,** which extends between neighboring pedicels and acts as a part of the filtration barrier (see Fig. 19–7; Fig. 19–10). The slit diaphragm has circular pores bridged by spoke-like configurations that radiate from a central density. These spokes are separated from one another by 3- to 5-nm spaces.

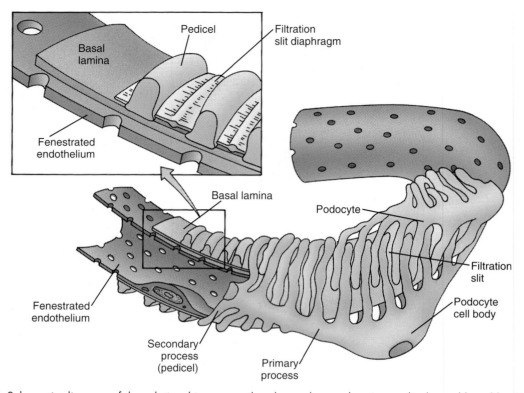

Figure 19–7. Schematic diagram of the relationship among the glomerulus, podocytes, pedicels, and basal laminae.

The cell body of the podocyte is not at all unusual in organelle content. It houses the irregularly shaped nucleus as well as rough endoplasmic reticulum, Golgi apparatus, and numerous free ribosomes.

Filtration Process. Fluid leaving the glomerular capillaries through the fenestrae is filtered by the basal lamina. The lamina densa traps larger molecules (> 69,000 Da), whereas the polyanions of the laminae rarae impede the passage of negatively charged molecules and molecules that are incapable of deformation. The fluid that penetrates the lamina densa, passing through the pores in the diaphragm of the filtration slits and entering Bowman's space, is known as the glomerular **ultrafiltrate.**

Because the basal lamina traps larger macromolecules, it would become clogged were it not continuously resorbed by intraglomerular mesangial cells and replenished by both the visceral layer of Bowman's capsule and glomerular endothelial cells.

CLINICAL CORRELATIONS

The presence of albumin in the urine, **albuminuria,** is the result of increased permeability of the glomerular endothelium. Among the causes of this condition are vascular injury, hypertension, mercury poisoning, and exposure to bacterial toxins.

The basal lamina may also become impaired because of the deposition of antigen–antibody complexes that are filtered from the glomeruli or from the reaction of antibasement membrane antibody with the basal lamina itself. Both of these instances produce types of **glomerulonephritis.**

In cases of **lipoid nephrosis** the basal laminae are not congested with antibodies, but adjacent pedicels appear to fuse with one another. This disease is one of the most prevalent of kidney disorders in children.

PROXIMAL TUBULE. Bowman's space drains into the **proximal tubule** at the urinary pole. In this junctional region, sometimes called the **neck** of the proximal tubule (negligible in humans), the simple squamous epithelium of the parietal layer of Bowman's capsule joins the simple cuboidal epithelium of the tubule (see Fig. 19–4). The proximal tubule, constituting much of the renal cortex, is approximately 60 μm in diameter and about 14 mm long. The tubule consists of a highly tortuous region, the **pars convoluta (proximal convoluted tubule),** located near renal corpuscles, and a straighter portion, the **pars recta,** which descends in medullary rays within the cortex and then in the medulla to become continuous with Henle's loop at the junction of the outer and inner stripes. The pars recta is also called the **descending thick limb of Henle's loop.**

Viewed with the light microscope, the convoluted portion of the proximal tubule is noted to be composed of a simple cuboidal type of epithelium with an eosinophilic, granular

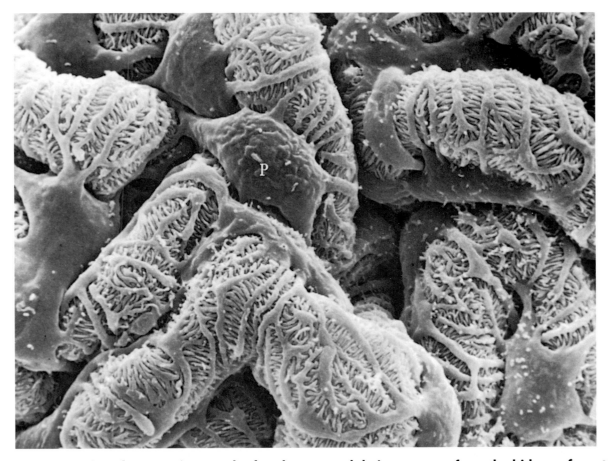

Figure 19–8. Scanning electron micrograph of podocytes and their processes from the kidney of a rat (× 6000). PP, podocytes. (From Brenner, B.M., and Rector, F.C.: The Kidney, 4th ed., vol. 1. Philadelphia, W.B. Saunders Company, 1991).

cytoplasm (see Fig. 19–3; Fig. 19–11). The cells have an elaborate striated border and an intricate system of interlocking and interwoven lateral cell processes. Thus the lateral cell membranes are usually indistinguishable with the light microscope. The height of the cells varies with functional state from a low cuboidal to an almost high cuboidal epithelium.

The method and rapidity of fixation modify the microscopic morphology of the proximal convoluted tubule because its lumen is kept open by fluid pressure. Ideal fixation demonstrates wide open, empty lumina and no clumping of the striated border. However, paraffin sections usually display mostly occluded lumina; fluted and ragged-appearing striated borders; few, basally placed nuclei per cross-section of the tubule; and a lack of distinct lateral cell membranes. The cuboidal cells sit on a well-defined basement membrane, easily demonstrated by the periodic acid–Schiff reaction. Each cross-section is composed of approximately 10 to 20 cells, but because these cells are large, usually only 6 to 8 nuclei are included in the plane of section (see Fig. 19–3).

Based on the ultrastructural features of its component cells, the proximal tubule can be subdivided into three regions. The first two thirds of the pars convoluta is designated

S_1; the remainder of the pars convoluta and much of the pars recta, S_2; and the remainder of the pars recta, S_3.

Cells of the S_1 region have long (1.3 to 1.6 μm), closely packed microvilli and a system of intermicrovillar caveolae, **apical canaliculi,** which extend into the apical cytoplasm (Fig. 19–12). This system is more extensive during active diuresis, suggesting that it functions in resorption of proteins during tubular clearing of the glomerular filtrate. Mitochondria, Golgi apparatus, and other normal cellular components are present in these cells. Elaborate lateral and basal processes may extend almost the entire height of the cell. These processes are long and narrow and usually accommodate elongated, tubular mitochondria.

Cells composing the S_2 region of the proximal tubule are similar to those of the S_1 region, but they have fewer mitochondria and apical canaliculi, have less elaborate intercellular processes, and are lower in height. Cells of the S_3 region are low cuboidal with few mitochondria. These cells have only infrequent intercellular processes and no apical canaliculi.

About 80% of sodium, chloride, and water are resorbed from the glomerular ultrafiltrate and transported into the

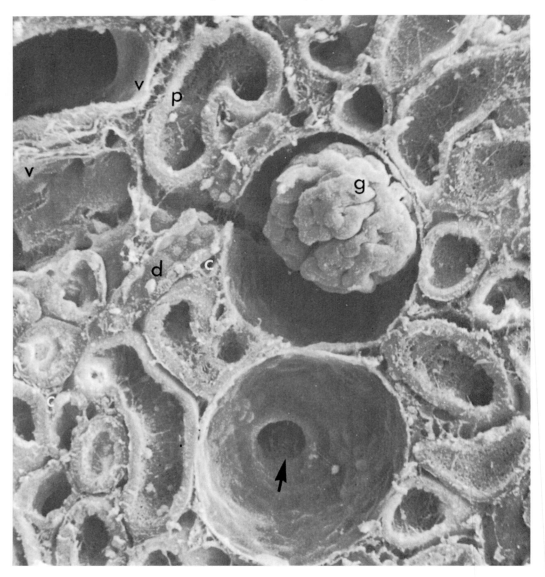

Figure 19–9. Scanning electron micrograph of the rat renal cortex displaying a renal corpuscle with its glomerulus (g) (× 750). The renal corpuscle below it does not have its glomerulus, so the urinary pole (arrow) is evident. P, proximal convoluted tubule; d, distal convoluted tubule; c, capillaries; v, blood vessels. (From Leeson, T.S., Leeson, C.R., and Paparo, A.A.: Text/Atlas of Histology. Philadelphia, W.B. Saunders Company, 1988.)

connective tissue stroma by cells of the proximal tubule. Sodium is actively pumped out of the cell at the basolateral cell membranes by a sodium pump associated with Na^+-K^+ ATPase. The sodium is followed by Cl^- to maintain electrical neutrality and by water to maintain osmotic equilibrium. Additionally, all of the glucose, amino acids, and protein in the glomerular ultrafiltrate are resorbed by cells of the proximal tubule.

THIN LIMBS OF HENLE'S LOOP. The pars recta of the proximal tubule continues as the **thin limb of Henle's loop** (see Fig. 19–11). This thin tubule, whose overall diameter is about 15 to 20 μm, is composed of squamous epithelial cells whose average height ranges between 1.5 and 2 μm. The

length of the thin segments varies with the location of the nephron (see Fig. 19–1). In cortical nephrons the thin segment is only 1 to 2 mm long or may be completely absent. Juxtamedullary nephrons have much longer thin segments, 9 to 10 mm in length, and they form a hairpin-like loop that extends deep into the medulla as far down as the renal papilla. The region of the loop continuous with the pars recta of the proximal tubule is called the **descending thin limb (of Henle's loop);** the hairpin-like bend is **Henle's loop;** and the region that connects Henle's loop to the pars recta of the **distal tubule** is known as the **ascending thin limb (of Henle's loop).**

The nuclei of the cells composing the thin limbs bulge into the lumen of the tubule; hence, in paraffin section, these

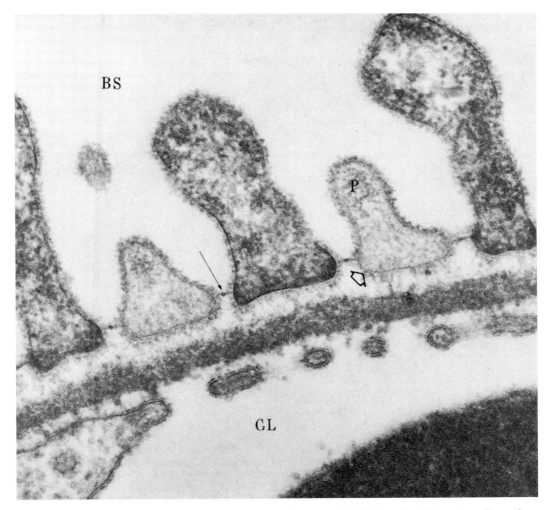

Figure 19–10. Electron micrograph of pedicels and diaphragms bridging the filtration slits of a rat glomerulus (× 120,000). BS, Bowman's space; CL, capillary lumen; hollow arrow, lamina rara externa; arrow, filtration slit diaphragm. (From Brenner, B.M., and Rector, F.C.: The Kidney, 4th ed., vol. 1. Philadelphia, W.B. Saunders Company, 1991).

limbs resemble capillaries in cross-section (see Fig. 19–11). However, they may be distinguished from capillaries in that their epithelial lining cells are slightly thicker, their nuclei stain less densely, and their lumina contain no blood cells.

The fine structure of the epithelial cells constituting the thin segments is not unusual. They present a few short, stubby microvilli on their luminal surfaces and a few mitochondria in the cytoplasm surrounding the nucleus. Numerous processes project from the basal portion of the cell to interdigitate with those of neighboring cells.

It is possible to differentiate among four types of epithelial cells composing differing regions of Henle's loop according to their fine structural features. The locations and fine structural features of the four cell types are listed in Table 19–1.

The descending thin limb is highly permeable to water and reasonably permeable to urea, sodium, chloride, and other ions. The major difference between the ascending and descending thin limbs is that the ascending thin limb is only moderately permeable to water. The significance of this difference in water permeability is discussed later in this chapter.

DISTAL TUBULE. The distal tubule is subdivided into the **pars recta** which, as the continuation of the ascending thin limb of Henle's loop, is also known as the **ascending thick limb of Henle's loop** and the **pars convoluta (distal convoluted tubule).** Interposed between the ascending thick limb and the distal convoluted tubule is a modified region of the distal tubule known as the **macula densa.**

The ascending thick limb of Henle's loop is 9 to 10 mm in length and 30 to 40 μm in diameter. It joins the ascending thin limb at the junction of the inner stripe with the inner zone of the medulla and ascends straight up through the medulla to reach the cortex. The low cuboidal epithelial cells composing the ascending thick segment have centrally placed, round to slightly oval nuclei and a few club-shaped, short microvilli. Although the lateral aspects of these cells

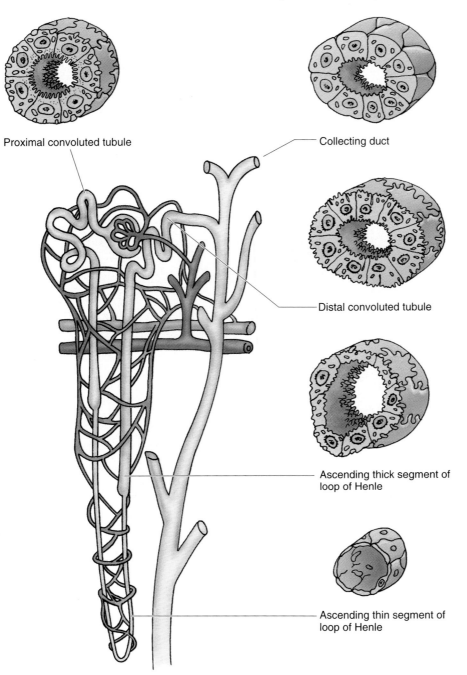

Proximal convoluted tubule

Collecting duct

Distal convoluted tubule

Ascending thick segment of
loop of Henle

Ascending thin segment of
loop of Henle

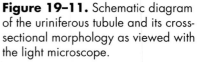

Figure 19–11. Schematic diagram
of the uriniferous tubule and its cross-
sectional morphology as viewed with
the light microscope.

interdigitate with each other, the interrelationships between neighboring cells are not nearly as elaborate as in the proximal convoluted tubules. However, basal interdigitations are much more extensive and the number of mitochondria is greater in these cells than in those of the proximal convoluted tubules. Moreover, these cells form highly efficient zonulae occludentes with their neighboring cells.

The thick ascending limb is not permeable to water or urea. Additionally, its cells have chloride (and perhaps sodium) pumps that function in the active transport of chloride (and sodium) from the lumen of the tubule. Thus, as the filtrate reaches the cortex of the kidney within the lumen of the distal tubule, its salt concentration is low and its urea concentration remains high.

As the ascending thick limb of the Henle loop passes near its own renal corpuscle, it lies between the afferent and efferent glomerular arterioles. This region of the distal tubule is called the **macula densa.** Because the cells of the macula densa are tall and narrow, the nuclei of these cells appear to be much closer together than those of the remainder of the distal tubule.

Distal convoluted tubules are short (4 to 5 mm) with an

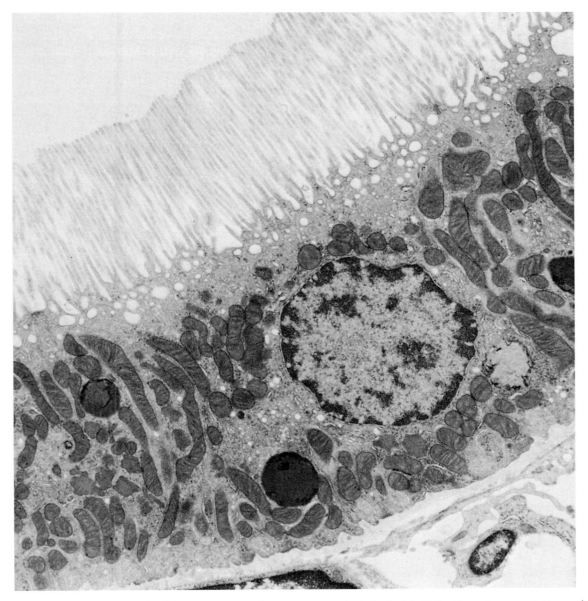

Figure 19–12. Electron micrograph of the S₁ segment of the rat proximal tubule (× 10,600). (From Brenner, B.M., and Rector, F.C.: The Kidney, 4th ed., vol. 1. Philadelphia, W.B. Saunders Company, 1991).

overall diameter of 25 to 45 μm. In paraffin sections the lumina of these tubules are wide open, the granular cytoplasm of the low cuboidal lining epithelium is paler than those of proximal convoluted tubules, and because the cells are narrower, more nuclei are apparent in tubular cross-section. The ultrastructure of these cells demonstrates a clear, pale cytoplasm with a few, blunt apical microvilli (Fig. 19–13). Nuclei are more or less round and apically located, having one or two dense nucleoli. Mitochondria are not as numerous, nor are the basal interdigitations as extensive as those of the ascending thick limb of Henle's loop.

Because distal convoluted tubules are much shorter than proximal convoluted tubules, any section of the kidney cortex will present many more cross-sections of proximal convoluted tubules than cross-sections of distal convoluted tubules. Indeed, the ratio of cross-sections of proximal to distal convoluted tubules surrounding any renal corpuscle is usually seven to one.

Distal convoluted tubules usually ascend slightly above their renal corpuscles and drain into the arched portion of the collecting tubules.

Similar to the thick ascending limbs the distal convoluted tubule is impermeable to water and urea. However, in the basolateral plasmalemma of its cells, high Na⁺-K⁺ ATPase activity powers sodium pumps. Thus, in response to the hormone **aldosterone**, these cells can actively resorb all of the remaining sodium (and, passively, chloride) from the lumen of the tubule into the renal interstitium. Additionally, potas-

Table 19-1. Cell Types Composing the Thin Limbs of Henle's Loop

Cell Type	Location	Fine Structural Features
Type I	Cortical nephrons	Squamous cells with no lateral processes and no interdigitations
Type II	Juxtamedullary nephrons; descending thin limb of the outer zone of the medulla	Squamous cells with numerous, long radiating processes that interdigitate with those of neighboring cells; fascia occludentes between cells; infoldings of the basal plasmalemma
Type III	Juxtamedullary nephrons; descending thin limb of the inner zone of the medulla	Squamous cells with fewer processes and interdigitations than those of type II
Type IV	Juxtamedullary nephrons; ascending thin limb	Squamous cells with numerous, long radiating processes that interdigitate with those of neighboring cells as in type II cells; no infoldings of the basal plasmalemma

sium and hydrogen ions are actively secreted *into* the lumen, thus controlling the body's extracellular fluid potassium level and the acidity of urine, respectively.

JUXTAGLOMERULAR APPARATUS. The **juxtaglomerular apparatus** consists of the macula densa of the distal tubule, juxtaglomerular cells of the adjacent afferent (and, occasionally, efferent) glomerular arteriole, and the extraglomerular mesangial cells (also known as polkissen, lacis cells, and polar cushions). The details of these structures are shown schematically in Figure 19-14.

The cells of the **macula densa** are tall, narrow, pale cells with centrally placed nuclei (see Figs. 19-2, 19-3, 19-4, 19-14; Fig. 19-15). Because of the narrowness of these cells, the densely staining nuclei are near to each other; collectively, viewed with the light microscope, they appear as a

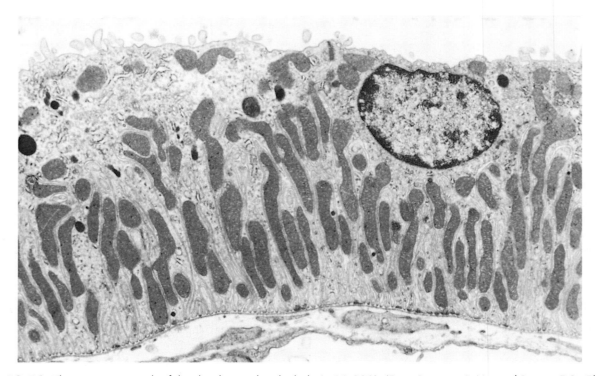

Figure 19-13. Electron micrograph of the distal convoluted tubule (× 10,000). (From Brenner, B.M., and Rector, F.C.: The Kidney, 4th ed., vol. 1. Philadelphia, W.B. Saunders Company, 1991).

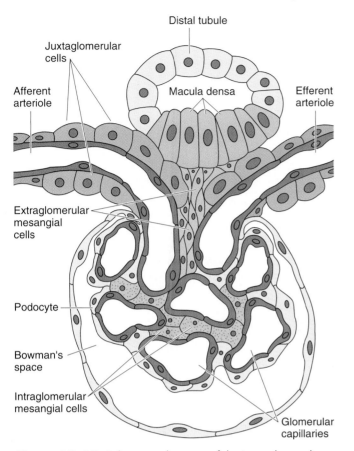

Figure 19–14. Schematic diagram of the juxtaglomerular apparatus.

dense spot. With the electron microscope, these cells have been shown to have numerous microvilli, small mitochondria, and an infranuclearly located Golgi apparatus (see Fig. 19–15).

The **juxtaglomerular cells (JG cells)** are modified smooth muscle cells located in the tunica media of afferent (and, infrequently, efferent) glomerular arterioles. The nuclei of these cells are round instead of elongated. JG cells contain specific granules demonstrated to be the proteolytic enzyme **renin** (see Fig. 19–15). Additionally, converting enzyme, angiotensin I, and angiotensin II have also been noted in these cells.

JG cells and the cells of the macula densa have a special geographical relationship because the basal lamina, normally present in epithelium and other tissues, is absent at this point, permitting intimate contact between the macula densa and the juxtaglomerular cells.

The third member of the juxtaglomerular apparatus, the extraglomerular mesangial cells, occupies the space bounded by the afferent arteriole, macula densa, efferent arteriole, and vascular pole of the renal corpuscle. These extraglomerular mesangial cells may contain occasional granules and are probably contiguous with the intraglomerular mesangial

cells. The functional significance of the juxtaglomerular apparatus will be discussed later in this chapter.

Collecting Tubules

Collecting tubules are not part of the nephron. They have different embryological origins, and it is only later in development that they meet the nephron and join it to form a continuous structure. The distal convoluted tubules of several nephrons join to form a short connecting tubule that leads into the collecting tubule (see Fig. 19–11). The glomerular ultrafiltrate that enters the collecting tubule will be modified and delivered to the medullary papillae. Collecting tubules are about 20 mm in length and have three recognized regions: cortical, medullary, and papillary (see Fig. 19–1).

Cortical collecting tubules are located in the medullary rays and are composed of two types of cuboidal cells—principal cells and intercalated cells (see Figs. 19–2, 19–11). **Principal cells** have oval, centrally located nuclei, a few small mitochondria, and short, sparse microvilli. The basal membranes of these cells display numerous infoldings. Because the lateral cell membranes are not plicated, they are clearly evident with the light microscope. **Intercalated cells** display numerous apical vesicles 50 to 200 nm in diameter, microplicae on their apical plasmalemma, and an abundance of mitochondria. The nuclei of these cells are round and centrally located. The functions of principal cells are not known, but intercalated cells actively transport and secrete hydrogen ions against high concentration gradients, thus modulating the acid–base balance of the body.

Medullary collecting tubules are of larger caliber, because they are formed by the union of several cortical collecting tubules (see Fig. 19–11). Those in the outer zone of the medulla display both principal and intercalated cells, whereas tubules of the inner zone of the medulla have principal cells only (Fig. 19–16).

Papillary collecting tubules (ducts of Bellini) are each formed by the confluence of several medullary collecting tubules. These are large ducts, 200 to 300 μm in diameter, and they open at the area cribrosa of the renal papilla to deliver the urine that they convey into the minor calyx of the kidney. These ducts are lined by tall columnar principal cells only.

Collecting tubules are impermeable to water. However, in the presence of antidiuretic hormone (ADH) they become permeable to water (and, to a certain extent, urea). Thus, in the absence of ADH, urine is copious and hypotonic, and in the presence of ADH the volume of urine is low and concentrated.

Renal Interstitium

The kidney is invested by a dense, irregular collagenous type of connective tissue, with some elastic fibers interspersed among the bundles of collagen. This capsule is not

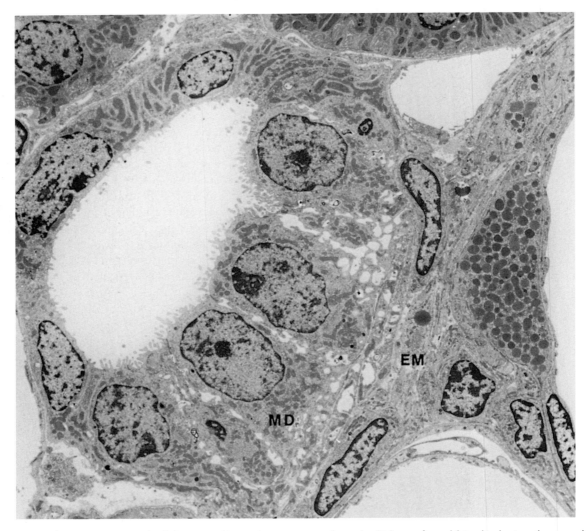

Figure 19–15. Electron micrograph of the juxtaglomerular apparatus from the kidney of a rabbit, displaying the macula densa (MD), juxtaglomerular cell (containing electron-dense granules), and extraglomerular mesangial cells (EM) (× 3700). (From Brenner, B.M., and Rector, F.C.: The Kidney, 4th ed., vol. 1. Philadelphia, W.B. Saunders Company, 1991).

attached firmly to the underlying cortex. As blood vessels enter the hilum, they travel in a thin connective tissue cover, some of which is derived from the capsule. The cortical region has only delicate connective tissue elements, mostly associated with the basement membranes investing the uriniferous tubules and their vascular supply. The two cellular components of the cortical connective tissue are fibroblasts and cells that are probably macrophages.

The medullary interstitial connective tissue component is more extensive than that found in the cortex. Embedded in this connective tissue are the various components of the uriniferous tubules as well as the extensive vascular network located in the medulla. The cell population of this connective tissue consists of three cell types—fibroblasts, macrophages, and interstitial cells. **Interstitial cells** appear to be placed like rungs of a ladder, one on top of the other, and are most numerous between straight collecting ducts

and between the ducts of Bellini. Interstitial cells have elongated nuclei and numerous lipid droplets. It is believed that these cells synthesize **medullipin I,** a substance that is converted in the liver to **medullipin II,** a potent vasodilator that lowers blood pressure.

Renal Circulation: Arterial Supply

The kidney receives an extremely extensive blood supply via the large **renal artery,** a direct branch of the abdominal aorta (see Fig. 19–1). Before entering the hilum of the kidney, the renal artery bifurcates into an anterior and a posterior division, which in turn subdivide to form a total of five **segmental arteries.** The branches of any one segmental artery do not form anastomoses with the branches of other segmental arteries. Hence, if blood flow through one of these arteries is arrested, circulation to the region of the kid-

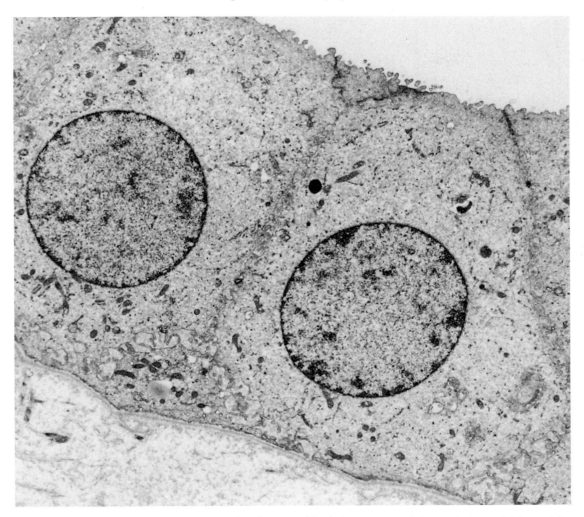

Figure 19-18. Electron micrograph of a collecting duct from a rabbit kidney (× 7000). (From Brenner, B.M., and Rector, F.C.: The Kidney, 4th ed., vol. 1. Philadelphia, W.B. Saunders Company, 1991).

ney supplied by the affected vessel will be interrupted. Therefore, the kidney is said to be subdivided into vascular segments, with each segment supplied by a specific artery.

The first subdivisions of the segmental arteries are called **lobar arteries,** one for each lobe of the kidney. These in turn branch to form two or three **interlobar arteries,** which travel between the renal pyramids to the corticomedullary junction. At the corticomedullary junction these arteries form a series of vessels (perpendicular to the parent vessel) which, to a large extent, remain at that junction, occupying the same curved plane. Because these arteries describe a slight arc over the base of the renal pyramid, they are named **arcuate arteries.**

Although arcuate arteries once were believed to anastomose with each other, recent studies suggest that terminal branches of these arteries do not join each other. Instead terminal branches, as do all other branches of the arcuate arteries, ascend into the cortex, forming **interlobular arteries.**

Interlobular arteries ascend within the cortical labyrinth

approximately halfway between neighboring medullary rays. Hence, they travel in the interstices between any two lobules. Many branches arise from the interlobular arteries. These branches supply the glomeruli of renal corpuscles and are known as **afferent glomerular arterioles.** Some of the interlobular arteries ascend through the cortex to perforate the kidney capsule. Here they contribute to the formation of the capsular plexus. Most of the interlobular arteries, however, terminate as afferent glomerular arterioles.

Each glomerulus is drained by another arteriole, the **efferent glomerular arteriole.** There are two types of efferent glomerular arterioles, those draining glomeruli of cortical nephrons and those draining glomeruli of juxtamedullary nephrons.

Efferent glomerular arterioles from cortical nephrons are short and branch to form a system of capillaries, the **peritubular capillary network.** This capillary bed supplies the entire cortical labyrinth, with the obvious exception of the glomeruli. It is believed that the endothelial cells of the peritubular capillary network manufacture and release the hormone **erythropoietin.**

The efferent glomerular arterioles, derived from glomeruli of juxtamedullary nephrons as well as from glomeruli located in the lower quadrant of the cortex, each give rise to 10 to 25 long, hairpin-like capillaries that dip deep into the medulla (Fig. 19–17). Their descending limbs are called **arteriolae rectae,** and their ascending limbs are **venae rectae.** Frequently these vessels are simply called **vasa recta.** The hairpin-like shape of the vasa recta, which closely follows the two limbs of Henle's loop, is essential in the physiology of urine concentration, which is discussed later in this chapter.

Renal Circulation: Venous Drainage

Venae rectae deliver their blood to **arcuate veins,** vessels that follow the paths of the same-named arteries. Blood is thus drained from the medulla. Cortical blood is collected into a star-shaped system of subcapsular veins named **stellate veins,** which are tributaries of the **interlobular veins.** The interlobular veins, paralleling the same-named arteries, deliver their blood to the **arcuate veins.** Hence, arcuate veins drain both the medulla and the cortex. Arcuate veins are tributaries of **interlobar veins** that unite, near the hilum,

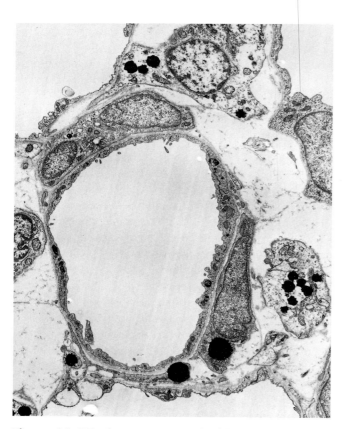

Figure 19–17. Electron micrograph of the arteria recta of a rat kidney. (From Takahashi-Iwanaga, H.: The three-dimensional cytoarchitecture of the interstitial tissue in the rat kidney. Cell Tissue Res. **264:**269–281, 1991.)

to form the **renal vein.** This large vein delivers the blood to the inferior vena cava. Note the absence of lobar and segmental veins in contrast with the arterial system of the kidney.

Lymphatic Supply of the Kidney

The **lymphatic supply** of the kidney is not completely understood. It is believed that most lymphatic vessels follow the larger arteries. According to most investigators, the lymphatic supply of the kidney may be subdivided into superficial and deep aspects located in the subcapsular region and the medulla, respectively. The two systems may or may not join each other near the hilum, where they form several large lymphatic trunks. Lymph nodes in the vicinity of the vena cava and the abdominal aorta receive lymph from the kidneys. Recently it has been demonstrated that there are lymph vessels in the cortex that do not follow the larger arteries, but they do drain their lymph into a plexus of lymph vessels at the hilum.

Renal Innervation

Most nerve fibers that reach the kidney are unmyelinated, sympathetic fibers that form the renal plexus, traveling along the renal artery. The cell bodies of these fibers are probably located in the aortic and celiac plexuses. Sympathetic fibers are distributed by branches of the renal arterial tree, and these vessels are modulated by some of these fibers. Additional sympathetic fibers reach the epithelium of the renal tubules, the juxtaglomerular and interstitial cells, and the capsule of the kidney. Sensory fibers and parasympathetic fibers (probably from the vagus nerve) have also been described in the kidney.

General Functions of the Kidney

The kidneys function in excretion as well as in the regulation of body fluid composition and volume. Specifically, they regulate solute components (e.g., Na+, K+, Cl−, glucose, amino acids) and acid–base balance. Thus, during the summer, when a lot of fluid is lost through perspiration, the urinary output is reduced in volume and increased in osmolarity. During the winter months, when fluid loss due to perspiration is minimal, the urinary output is increased in volume and the urine is dilute.

In addition, the kidneys excrete detoxified end-products, regulate the osmolality of urine, and secrete substances such as erythropoietin, medullipin I, renin, and prostaglandins. Finally, they regulate blood pressure and aid in the conversion of vitamin D to dihydroxycholecalciferol, which apparently controls calcium transport. Although all of these functions are important aspects of kidney histophysiology, only the mechanism of urine formation is discussed in this chapter.

Mechanism of Urine Formation

The two kidneys receive a large volume of circulating blood because the renal arteries are large and they are direct branches of the abdominal aorta. Inulin, a fructose polymer, can be used to measure the **glomerular filtration rate.** Such studies have shown that the entire blood supply circulates through the two kidneys every 5 minutes. Thus, approximately 1220 ml of blood enters the two kidneys per minute, from which 125 ml/min of glomerular filtrate is formed in the average male. Thus, 180 L of glomerular filtrate is formed per day, of which only 1.5 to 2.0 L is excreted as urine. Therefore, every day at least 178 L is resorbed by the kidneys, and only about 1% of the total glomerular filtrate is excreted.

Filtration in the Renal Corpuscle

As blood passes from the afferent glomerular arteriole into the glomerulus, it encounters a region of differential pressure, where the intracapillary blood pressure is greater than the opposing fluid pressure in Bowman's space, forcing fluid from the capillary into that space. An additional factor, colloid osmotic pressure of the blood proteins, opposes the entry of fluid into the Bowman space, but the net effect, the **filtration force,** is high (25 mm Hg). The fluid entering Bowman's space is called the **(glomerular) ultrafiltrate.**

Because of the tripartite **filtration barrier** (endothelial cell, basal lamina, filtration slit/diaphragm), cellular material and large macromolecules cannot leave the glomerulus; thus, the ultrafiltrate is similar to plasma (without its constituent macromolecules). Molecules greater than 69,000 Da (e.g., albumin) are trapped by the basal lamina. In addition to molecular weight, the molecular shape and charge of a molecule and the functional state of the filtration barrier all influence the ability of a molecule to traverse the filtration barrier. Because the filtration barrier has negatively charged components, macromolecules that are negatively charged are less able to cross the filtration barrier than are positively charged or neutral macromolecules.

Resorption in the Proximal Tubule

The ultrafiltrate leaves Bowman's space via the urinary pole to enter the proximal convoluted tubule, where modification of this fluid begins. Materials resorbed from the tubular lumina enter the tubular epithelial cells, from where they are excreted into the interstitial connective tissue. Here, the resorbed substances gain entrance to the rich capillary network and thus are returned to the body via the bloodstream.

Most resorption of materials from the ultrafiltrate occurs in the proximal tubule. Normally, 100% of proteins, glucose, amino acids, and creatine, almost 100% of bicarbonate ions, 80% of Na^+ and Cl^- ions, and 80% of the water are resorbed in the proximal tubule.

As the Na^+-K^+ ATPase powered **sodium pumps** in the basolateral plasma membrane of the proximal tubule cell pump sodium into the renal interstitium, sodium leaves the ultrafiltrate and enters the cell. In this fashion the net sodium flow is from the ultrafiltrate into the renal connective tissue. To maintain electrical neutrality, Cl^- ions passively follow sodium. Also, to maintain osmotic equilibrium, water passively follows sodium (by osmosis).

Additional energy-requiring pumps, located in the apical plasmalemma of proximal tubule cells, cotransport amino acids and glucose with sodium into the cell to be released into the renal interstitium. Proteins, brought into the cell by pinocytotic vesicles, are degraded by lysosomal enzymes within late endosomes.

Each day, 140 g of glucose, 430 g of Na^+, 500 g of Cl^-, 300 g of bicarbonate, 18 g of K^+ ions, and approximately 142 L of H_2O are conserved by the proximal tubules of the kidney.

The proximal tubule also releases certain substances into the tubular lumen. These include H^+, ammonia, phenol red, hippuric acid, uric acid, organic bases, and ethylene diamine tetraacetate, as well as certain drugs, such as penicillin.

Henle's Loop and the Countercurrent Multiplier System

The osmolality of the glomerular ultrafiltrate is the same as that of circulating blood. This osmolality has not been altered by the proximal tubule, because water left its lumen in response to the movement of ions. However, the osmotic pressure of formed urine is different from that of blood. The osmotic pressure differential is established by the remaining regions of the uriniferous tubule. Interestingly, the osmolarity and volume of urine varies, indicating that the kidneys can modulate these factors.

A gradient of osmolarity, increasing from the corticomedullary junction deep into the medulla, is maintained in the renal medullary interstitium. The long loops of Henle of **juxtamedullary nephrons** aid the creation and the maintenance of this osmotic gradient via a **countercurrent multiplier system** (Fig. 19–18). The cells of the thin descending limb of Henle's loop are freely permeable to water and salts. Therefore, the movement of water reacts to the osmotic forces in its microenvironment. The thin ascending limb is relatively impermeable to water, but salts can enter or leave the tubule depending on conditions in the interstitium. It is important to note at this point (to be explained later in this chapter) that *urea enters* the lumina of the thin limbs of Henle's loop.

The thick ascending limb of Henle's loop is completely impermeable to water; however, a chloride pump actively removes chloride ions from the lumen of the tubules and these ions enter the interstitium. Sodium follows passively (although some suggest the presence of a sodium pump) to preserve electrical neutrality. As the filtrate ascends it contains fewer and fewer ions; hence the amount of salts that

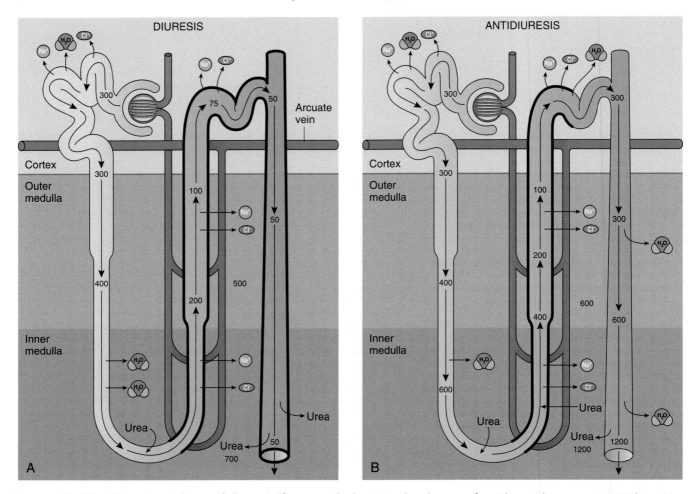

Figure 19–18. Histophysiology of the uriniferous tubule. A, In the absence of antidiuretic hormone (ADH) (diuresis). **B,** In the presence of ADH (antidiuresis). Numbers indicate milliosmoles per liter. Areas outlined by thick line indicate that the tubule is impermeable to water. Note that in the presence of ADH, not only does the collecting tubule change so that it becomes permeable to water, but the concentration in the interstitium of the inner medulla increases. The vasa recta was simplified in this drawing, because it encompasses the entire uriniferous tubule (see Fig. 19–1).

may be transferred out into the interstitium decreases. Thus, a gradient of salt concentration is established, in which the highest interstitial osmolarity is deep in the medulla, and the osmolarity of the interstitium decreases toward the cortex.

Because the medulla is tightly packed with thick and thin (ascending and descending) limbs of Henle's loop and collecting tubules, the gradient of osmolarity that is established is pervasive and affects all the tubules equally (see Fig. 19–18). Therefore, as the filtrate descends, water leaves the thin descending limb of Henle's loop *(reducing volume and increasing osmolarity),* reacting to the osmotic gradient of the interstitium, so that the intraluminal filtrate more or less becomes equilibrated with that of the surrounding connective tissue. This fluid of high osmolarity now ascends in the thin ascending limb of Henle's loop, which is mostly impermeable to water but not to salts. Thus the volume will not change, but the osmolarity of the ultrafiltrate inside the tubule will adjust to the osmolarity of the interstitium.

The fluid entering the ascending thick limb of Henle's loop passes a region that is impermeable to water but has a chloride pump, which removes Cl⁻ ions from the lumen, followed passively (or perhaps also actively) by Na⁺ ions. Because water cannot leave the lumen, the ultrafiltrate becomes *hypotonic but its volume remains constant* as it ascends to the cortex in the ascending thick limb. The chloride and sodium that were transferred from the lumen of the ascending thick limb into the connective tissue are responsible for the establishment of a concentration gradient in the renal interstitium of the outer medulla.

Monitoring the Filtrate in the Juxtaglomerular Apparatus

The cells of the macula densa probably monitor the filtrate volume and Na⁺ concentration. If these levels exceed a specific threshold, macula densa cells instruct the JG cells to release the enzyme renin into circulation. Renin converts **angiotensinogen,** normally present in the bloodstream, into the decapeptide **angiotensin I,** a mild vasoconstrictor. In the capillaries of the lungs, but also to a lesser extent in those of the kidneys and other organs of the body, **converting enzyme** converts angiotensin I to **angiotensin II,** an octapeptide hormone with numerous biological effects (Table 19–2). As a potent vasoconstrictor, angiotensin II reduces the luminal diameter of blood vessels, thus increasing the systemic blood pressure. Angiotensin II also influences the adrenal cortex to release **aldosterone,** a hormone that acts primarily on cells of the distal convoluted tubules, increasing their resorption of sodium and chloride ions.

CLINICAL CORRELATIONS

One of the contributing causes to **chronic essential hypertension** is the presence of elevated levels of angiotensin II. Elevated blood levels of angiotensin II once were believed to be due to the excessive release of renin from the juxtaglomerular cells of the juxtaglomerular apparatus. However, it is now realized that the increased activity of converting enzyme is directly responsible for elevating the concentration of angiotensin II rather than the renal release of renin.

Loss of Water and Urea from Filtrate in Collecting Tubules

The filtrate that leaves the distal convoluted tubule to enter the collecting tubule is hypotonic. As the collecting tubule passes through the medulla to reach the area cribrosa, it is also subject to the same osmotic gradients as the ascending and descending limbs of Henle's loop. In the absence of **ADH (vasopressin),** the cells of the collecting tubule and, to a lesser extent, of the distal convoluted tubule are completely impermeable to water (see Fig. 19–18). Therefore, the filtrate, or urine, is not modified in the collecting tubule and the urine remains dilute (hypotonic).

However, under the influence of ADH, the cells of the collecting tubule (and in animals other than humans and monkeys, also the distal convoluted tubules) become freely permeable to water and urea. As the filtrate descends through the renal medulla in the collecting tubule, it is subject to the osmotic pressure gradients established by the hairpin-like loops of Henle and the vasa recta, and water leaves the lumina of the collecting tubules to enter the interstitium. Hence, the urine, in the presence of ADH, becomes concentrated and hypertonic.

Additionally, the concentration of urea becomes extremely high in the lumen of the collecting tubule, and in the presence of ADH, it passively enters the interstitium of the inner medulla. Thus, much of the concentration gradient of the renal interstitium in the inner medulla is due to the presence of urea rather than sodium and chloride.

Vasa Recta and Countercurrent Exchange System

The vasa recta helps maintain the osmotic gradient in the medulla, because both arterial and venous limbs are freely permeable to water and salts (Fig. 19–19). Moreover, the luminal diameter of the arterial limb is smaller than that of the venous limb. Therefore, as the blood courses down the arterial limb, it loses water and gains salts, and as it returns via the venous limb, it loses salts and gains water, thus acting as a **countercurrent exchange system.**

Table 19–2. Functions of Angiotensin II

Function	Result
Potent vasoconstriction	increases blood pressure
Facilitates synthesis and release of aldosterone	resorption of sodium and chloride from lumen of distal convoluted tubule
Facilitates release of ADH	resorption of water from lumen of collecting tubule
Increases thirst	increases tissue fluid volume
Inhibits renin release	feedback inhibition
Facilitates release of prostaglandins	vasodilation of afferent glomerular arteriole thus maintaining glomerular filtration rate

ADH, antidiuretic hormone.

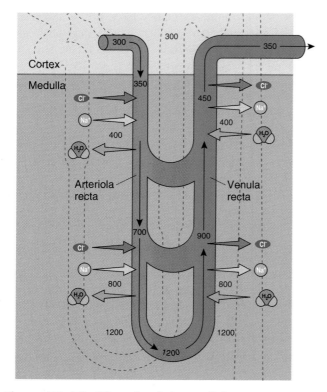

Figure 19–19. Histophysiology of the vasa recta. The numbers represent milliosmoles per liter. Note that the arteriola recta is smaller in diameter than the venula recta.

This mechanism ensures that the system of osmotic gradients remains undisturbed, because the osmolarity of the blood in the vessels will be more or less equilibrated with that of the interstitium. However, the volume of salts and fluid being brought in by the arterial limb is less than that being taken away by the venous limb. This exchange system causes salt and water to be resorbed (returned back to the body) because of the concentration gradient in the renal medulla.

The structure and function of the various regions of the uriniferous tubule are presented in Table 19–3.

Excretory Passages

The excretory passages of the urinary system consist of the minor and major calyces, the pelvis of the kidney, the ureter, the single urinary bladder, and the single urethra.

Calyces

The renal papilla of each renal pyramid fits into a **minor calyx,** a funnel-shaped chamber that accepts the urine leaving the ducts of Bellini at the area cribrosa (see Fig. 19–1). The portion of the apex of the pyramid that projects into the minor calyx is covered by **transitional epithelium,** which acts as a barrier, separating the urine from the underlying

connective tissue lamina propria. Deep to the lamina propria is a thin muscular coat, composed entirely of smooth muscle. This muscular layer propels the urine into a **major calyx,** one of three or four larger funnel-shaped chambers, each of which collects urine from two to four minor calyces. The major calyces are similar in structure to the minor calyces as well as to the expanded proximal region of the ureters, the **renal pelvis.** The walls of the excretory passages thicken from the minor calyces to the urinary bladder.

Ureter

Each **ureter** is about 3 to 4 mm in diameter, is approximately 25 to 30 cm long, and pierces the base of the urinary bladder. The ureters are hollow, cylindrical tubes, consisting of a mucosa, which lines the lumen, a muscular coat, and a fibrous, connective tissue covering.

The **mucosa** of the ureter presents several folds, which project into the lumen when the ureter is empty but that are absent when the ureter is distended. The **transitional epithelial lining,** three to five cell layers in thickness, overlies a layer of dense, irregular fibroelastic connective tissue, which constitutes the **lamina propria.** As always, the epithelium is separated from the underlying lamina propria by a basal lamina.

The **muscularis** of the ureter is composed of two predominantly inseparable layers of smooth muscle cells. The arrangement of the layers is opposite that found in the digestive tract, because the outer layer is arranged circularly and the inner layer is longitudinally disposed. This arrangement is true for the proximal two thirds of the ureter, but in the lower third, near the urinary bladder, a third muscle layer, whose fibers are oriented longitudinally, is added onto the existing surface of the existing muscle coat. Hence the muscular fiber orientation in the lower one third of the ureter is **outer longitudinal, middle circular,** and **inner longitudinal.**

The fibrous outer coat of the ureter is unremarkable and, at its proximal and distal terminals, blends with the capsule of the kidney and the connective tissue of the bladder wall, respectively. Contrary to expectation, urine does not pass down the ureter because of gravitational forces; instead, muscular contraction of the ureteric wall establishes peristaltic-like waves that convey urine to the urinary bladder. As the ureters pierce the posterior aspect of the base of the bladder, a valve-like flap of mucosa hangs over each ureteric orifice, preventing regurgitation of urine from the bladder back into the ureters.

Urinary Bladder

The **urinary bladder** is essentially an organ for storing urine until the pressure becomes sufficient to induce the urge for micturition, or voiding. Its mucosa also acts as an osmotic barrier between the urine and the lamina propria

Table 19–3. Structure and Function of the Uriniferous Tubule

Region of Uriniferous Tubule	Major Functions	Miscellaneous Comments
Renal Corpuscle: Simple squamous epithelium, fused basal laminae podocytes	Filtration	Filtration barrier: endothelial cell, fused basal laminae, filtration slits
Proximal Tubule: Simple cuboidal epithelium	Resorption of 80% of water, sodium, and chloride (reducing volume of ultrafiltrate); resorption of 100% of protein, amino acids, glucose, and bicarbonate	Sodium pump in basolateral membrane; ultrafiltrate is isotonic with blood
Descending Thin Limb of Henle's Loop: Simple squamous epithelium	Completely permeable to water and salts (reducing volume of ultrafiltrate)	Ultrafiltrate is hypotonic with respect to blood; urea enters lumen of tubule
Ascending Thin Limb of Henle's Loop: Simple squamous epithelium	Impermeable to water, permeable to salts; sodium and chloride leave tubule to enter renal interstitium	Ultrafiltrate is hypertonic with respect to blood; urea leaves renal interstitium and enters the lumen of tubule
Ascending Thick Limb of Henle's Loop: Simple cuboidal epithelium	Impermeable to water; chloride and sodium leave tubule to enter renal interstitium	Ultrafiltrate becomes hypotonic with respect to blood; chloride pump in basolateral cell membrane is responsible for the establishment of osmotic gradient in interstitium of outer medulla
Macula Densa: Simple columnar cells	Monitors sodium level and volume of ultrafiltrate in lumen of distal tubule	Contacts and communicates with juxtaglomerular cells
Juxtaglomerular Cells: Modified smooth muscle cells	Synthesize and release renin into bloodstream	Renin initiates the reaction for the eventual formation of angiotensin II (see Table 19–2)
Distal Convoluted Tubule: Simple cuboidal epithelium	Responds to aldosterone by resorbing sodium and chloride from lumen	Ultrafiltrate becomes more hypotonic (in the presence of aldosterone); sodium pump in basolateral membrane; potassium is secreted into the lumen
Collecting Tubule: Simple cuboidal epithelium	In the presence of ADH, water and urea leave the lumen to enter the renal interstitium	Urine becomes hypertonic in the presence of ADH; urea in interstitium is responsible for gradient of concentration in interstitium of the inner medulla

ADH, antidiuretic hormone.

(Fig. 19–20). The mucosa of the bladder is arranged in numerous folds, which disappear when the bladder becomes distended with urine. During distension, the large, round, **dome-shaped cells** of the transitional epithelium become stretched and change their morphology to become flattened.

The accommodation of cell shape is performed by a unique feature of the **transitional epithelial cell** plasmalemma, which is composed of a mosaic of specialized, rigid, thickened regions, **plaques,** interspersed by normal cell membrane, **interplaque regions.** When the bladder is empty, the plaque regions are folded into irregular, angular contours, which disappear when the cell becomes stretched. These rigid plaque regions, anchored to intracytoplasmic filaments, resemble gap junctions, but this similarity is only superficial.

Plaques appear to be impermeable to water and salts; thus these cells act as osmotic barriers between the urine and the underlying lamina propria. The superficial cells of the tran-

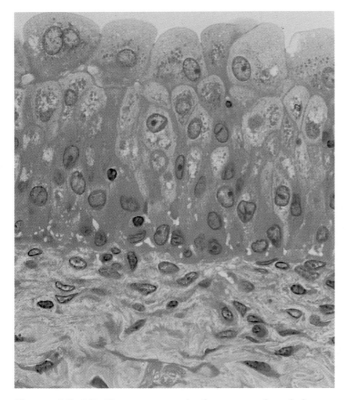

Figure 19–20. Photomicrograph of transitional epithelium from the bladder of a monkey (× 540).

sitional epithelium are held together by desmosomes and, possibly, by tight junctions, which also aid the establishment of the osmotic barrier by preventing the passage of fluid between the cells.

The triangular region of the bladder, whose apices are the orifices of the two ureters and the urethra, is known as the **trigone** of the bladder. The mucosa of the trigone is always smooth and is never thrown into folds. The embryonic origin of the trigone differs from that of the remainder of the bladder.

The lamina propria of the bladder may be subdivided into two layers: a more superficial, dense, irregular collagenous connective tissue and a deeper, looser layer of connective tissue composed of a mixture of collagen and elastic fibers. The lamina propria contains no glands except at the region surrounding the urethral orifice, where **mucous glands** may be found. Usually, these glands extend only into the superficial layer of the lamina propria. They secrete a clear viscous fluid that apparently lubricates the urethral orifice.

The muscular coat of the urinary bladder is composed of three interlaced layers of smooth muscle, which can be separated only in the region of the neck of the bladder. Here, they are arranged as a thin, inner longitudinal layer, a thick middle circular layer, and a thin outer longitudinal layer. The middle circular layer forms the **internal sphincter muscle** around the internal orifice of the urethra.

The adventitia of the bladder is composed of a dense, irregular collagenous type of connective tissue, containing a generous amount of elastic fibers. Certain regions of the adventitia are covered by a serosa, a peritoneal reflection onto the wall of the bladder, whereas other regions may be surrounded by fat.

Urethra

The urinary bladder is drained by a single tubular structure, the **urethra,** which communicates with the outside, permitting elimination of urine from the body. As the urethra pierces the perineum, skeletal muscle fibers form the **external sphincter muscle** surrounding the urethra. This muscle permits voluntary control of micturition. The urethra of the male is longer than that of the female and has a dual function in that it acts as a route for urine as well as for semen.

CLINICAL CORRELATIONS

Loss of voluntary control over the **external sphincter muscle** of the urethra causes **urinary incontinence,** a condition affecting primarily older women.

Female Urethra

The female urethra is about 4 to 5 cm in length and 5 to 6 mm in diameter. It extends from the urinary bladder to the external urethral orifice just above and anterior to the opening of the vagina. Normally, the lumen is collapsed, except during micturition. It is lined by a **transitional epithelium** near the bladder and by a **stratified squamous nonkeratinized epithelium** along the remainder of its length. Interspersed in the epithelium are patches of pseudostratified columnar epithelium. The mucosa is arranged in elongated folds because of the organization of the fibroelastic **lamina propria.** Along the entire length of the urethra are numerous clear, mucus-secreting **glands of Littre.**

A thin, vascular, erectile coat surrounds the mucosa, resembling the corpus spongiosum of the male. The muscular layer of the urethra is continuous with that of the bladder but is composed of two layers only, an inner longitudinal and an outer circular smooth muscle layer. As the urethra pierces the perineum (urogenital diaphragm), a sphincter of skeletal muscle surrounds it and permits voluntary control of micturition.

Male Urethra

The male urethra is 15 to 20 cm long, and its three regions are named according to the structures through which it passes. The segments are the prostatic, membranous, and penile urethra.

The **prostatic urethra,** 3 to 4 cm long, lies entirely in the prostate gland. It is lined by a transitional epithelium and receives the openings of many tiny ducts of the prostate, the prostatic utricle (a rudimentary homologue of the uterus), and the paired ejaculatory ducts.

The second segment of the male urethra is only 1 to 2 cm long and is known as the **membranous urethra,** because it passes through the perineal membrane (urogenital diaphragm). The membranous urethra is lined by stratified columnar epithelium, interspersed with patches of pseudostratified columnar epithelium.

The final segment is the longest portion of the urethra (15 cm in length). It passes through the length of the penis, terminating at the tip of the glans penis as the external urethral orifice. This segment is known as the **spongiose urethra (penile urethra)** because it is located in the corpus spongiosum. The spongiose urethra is lined by stratified columnar epithelium interspersed with patches of pseudostratified columnar and stratified squamous nonkeratinized epithelia. The enlarged terminal portion of the urethra in the glans penis is known as the **navicular fossa;** it is lined by stratified squamous, nonkeratinized epithelium.

The **lamina propria** of all three regions is composed of a loose fibroelastic connective tissue with a rich vascular supply. It houses numerous **glands of Littre,** whose mucous secretion lubricates the epithelial lining of the urethra.

Female Reproductive System

20

The **female reproductive system** consists of the internal reproductive organs—the paired ovaries and oviducts, the uterus, and the vagina (Fig. 20–1)—and the external genitalia, which include the clitoris, labia majora, and labia minora.

The reproductive organs are incompletely developed and lie in a state of rest until **gonadotropic hormones** secreted by the pituitary gland signal the initiation of puberty. Thereafter, many changes take place in the entire reproductive system, including further differentiation of the reproductive organs, culminating in **menarche,** the first menstrual flow, at about 13 years of age. After the first menstrual flow, the menstrual cycle, which involves many hormonal, histological, and psychological changes, is repeated each month (28 days) throughout the entire reproductive years, unless interrupted by pregnancy. As a woman nears the end of her reproductive years, her menstrual cycles become less regular as hormonal and neurological signals begin to change, initiating **menopause.** Eventually, the menstrual cycles cease; after menopause limited involution of the reproductive organs occurs. Thus the female reproductive system is controlled by complex orchestrations of hormonal, neurological, and psychological factors.

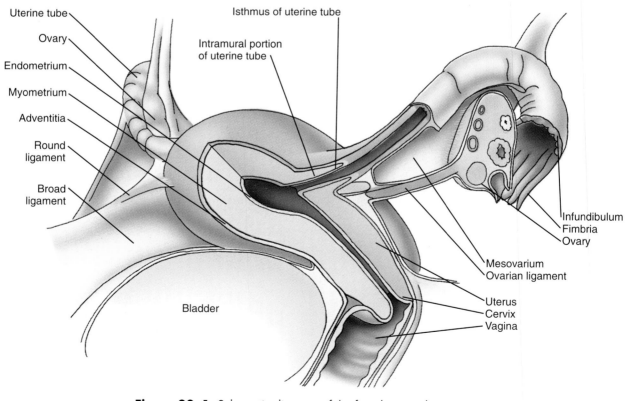

Figure 20–1. Schematic diagram of the female reproductive tract.

Although the mammary glands are not considered part of the female reproductive system, their physiology and function are so closely associated with the reproductive system that they are discussed in this chapter.

Ovaries

The paired **ovaries,** located within the pelvis, are almond-shaped bodies 3 cm long, 1.5 to 2 cm wide, and 1 cm thick. The ovaries are suspended in the **broad ligament of the uterus** by an attachment called the **mesovarium,** a special fold of the peritoneum that conveys blood vessels to the ovaries (see Fig. 20–1).

The surface epithelium covering the ovaries is a modified peritoneum, called the **germinal epithelium.** This low cuboidal epithelium was originally thought to give rise to

the germ cells; although this is now known to be untrue, the name persists. Directly beneath this epithelium is the **tunica albuginea,** a poorly vascularized, dense, irregular collagenous connective tissue capsule whose collagen fibers are oriented parallel to the ovary surface. Each ovary is subdivided into the highly cellular **cortex** and a **medulla,** which consists mostly of a richly vascularized loose connective tissue. The blood vessels of the medulla are derived from the ovarian arteries. Histologically, however, the division between the cortex and the medulla is indistinct.

Ovarian Cortex

The cortex is composed of a connective tissue framework, the **stroma, ovarian follicles** in various stages of development, and fibroblast-like **stromal cells** (Fig. 20–2A).

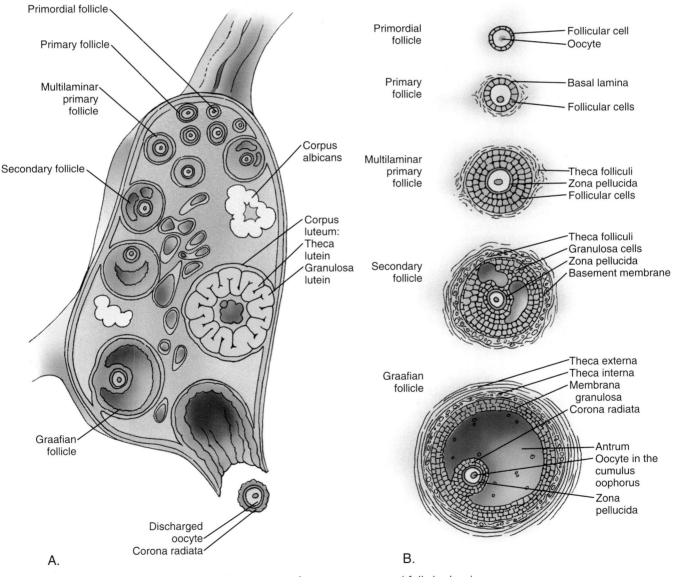

Figure 20–2. Diagram of ovary structure and follicle development.

Primordial germ cells, called **oogonia,** develop in the yolk sac shortly after the first month of gestation. They undergo several mitotic divisions and migrate to the germinal ridges to populate the cortex of the developing ovaries. Here they continue to undergo mitotic divisions until near the end of the fifth fetal month. At this point in time, each ovary contains about 3 million oogonia, but most of them undergo **atresia** (i.e., they degenerate and die).

Those oogonia that survive undergo their final mitotic division to become **primary oocytes** (Fig. 20–3). These cells enter the **prophase of meiosis I,** and then meiosis is arrested. Primary oocytes remain in that phase until just before ovulation, when they are triggered to complete their first meiotic division.

At menarche a young woman has about 400,000 follicles and usually ovulates one oocyte each 28 days for the next 30 to 40 years, thus ovulating about 450 oocytes over this period. The remaining follicles degenerate and die over the same period of time.

Ovarian Follicles

Ovarian follicles are surrounded by stromal tissue and consist of a **primary oocyte** and its associated **follicular cells** arranged in a single spherical layer or several concentric layers around the primary oocyte. There are four identifiable stages of follicular development based on the growth of the follicle and the development of the oocyte (Fig. 20–2B).

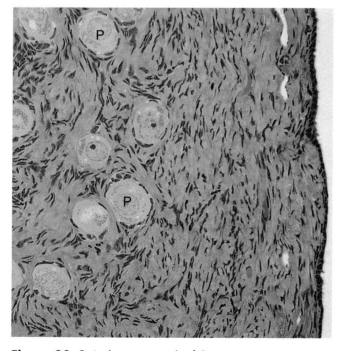

Figure 20–3. Light micrograph of the ovarian cortex demonstrating mostly primordial follicles (P), which are primary oocytes surrounded by follicular cells (× 270).

Follicular development usually culminates in the release of a single oocyte (ovulation).

PRIMORDIAL FOLLICLES. Primordial follicles, the most primitive follicles, are most abundant before birth, after which they become fewer. The primordial follicle is composed of a **primary oocyte** surrounded by a single layer of flattened **follicular cells** (see Fig. 20–3; Fig. 20–4).

The **primary oocyte** (arrested in the **prophase stage** of **meiosis I)** is a spherical cell about 25 μm in diameter. It has a large, acentric nucleus containing a single nucleolus. The nucleoplasm appears vesicular because of the uncoiled chromosomes. The organelles include numerous mitochondria, abundant Golgi regions, a rough endoplasmic reticulum (RER) containing only a few ribosomes, and some annulate lamellae.

The squamous **follicular cells** completely surround the primary oocyte and are attached to each other by desmosomes. They are separated from the stromal cells by a basal lamina.

PRIMARY FOLLICLES. Primordial follicles develop into **primary follicles** (see Fig. 20–3) distinguished as a result of changes in the primary oocyte, the follicular cells, and the surrounding stromal tissue.

The **primary oocyte** grows to about 100 to 150 μm in diameter with an enlarged nucleus (which some authors call the **germinal vesicle**). Several Golgi complexes are scattered throughout the cell, the RER becomes rich with ribosomes, free ribosomes are abundant, and mitochondria are numerous and dispersed throughout the cell.

Follicular cells become cuboidal in shape. As long as only a single layer of follicular cells encircles the oocyte, the follicle is called a **unilaminar primary follicle.** When the follicular cells proliferate, forming several layers of cells around the primary oocyte, the follicle is called a **multilaminar primary follicle,** and the follicular cells become known as **granulosa cells.**

During this stage an amorphous substance appears, the **zona pellucida,** separating the oocyte from the surrounding follicular cells. The zonula pellucida is composed of three different glycoproteins ZP_1, ZP_2, and ZP_3, secreted by the oocyte. Microvilli of the oocyte and filopodia of the follicular cells invade the zonula pellucida, contact each other, and form gap junctions through which they communicate throughout follicular development.

Stromal cells begin to be organized around the multilaminar primary follicle, forming an inner **theca interna,** composed mostly of a richly vascularized cellular layer, and an outer **theca externa,** composed mostly of fibrous connective tissue. The cells composing the theca interna assume the ultrastructural characteristics of steroid-producing cells. Their cytoplasm accumulates numerous lipid droplets and has abundant smooth endoplasmic reticulum; the cristae of their mitochondria are tubular. These theca interna cells produce

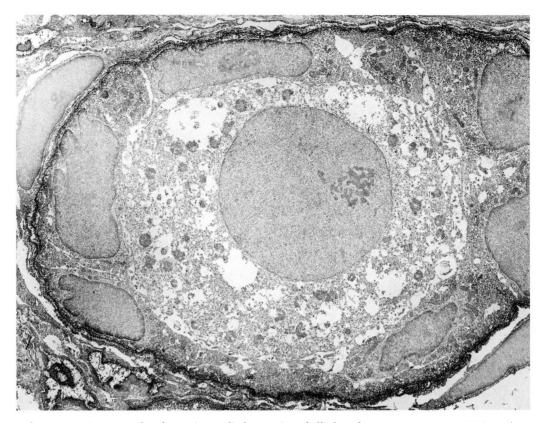

Figure 20–4. Electron micrograph of a primordial ovarian follicle of a rat ovary (× 7000). Observe the oocyte surrounded by follicular cells. (From Leardkamolkarn, V., and Abrahamson, D.R.: Immunoelectron microscopic localization of laminin in rat ovarian follicles. Anat. Rec. **233:**41–52, 1992. Reprinted by permission of John Wiley & Sons, Inc.)

the male sex hormone **androstenedione,** which enters the granulosa cells, where it is converted into **estradiol.** The granulosa cells are still separated from the theca interna by a thickened basal lamina.

SECONDARY (ANTRAL) FOLLICLES. The multilaminar primary follicle continues to develop and increase in size, reaching up to 200 μm in diameter. Continued proliferation of the granulosa cells depends on **follicle-stimulating hormone (FSH)** released by the basophil cells of the anterior pituitary. A large spherical follicle is formed with numerous layers of granulosa cells around the primary oocyte (whose size remains constant). Several intercellular spaces develop within the mass of granulosa cells and become filled with a fluid known as **liquor folliculi.** This fluid, an exudate of plasma, contains glycoaminoglycans and steroid binding proteins produced by the granulosa cells. Moreover, it contains the hormones **progesterone, estradiol, inhibin, folliostatin,** and **activin,** which regulate the release of luteinizing hormone and FSH. Additionally, FSH induces the granulosa cells to manufacture receptors for **luteinizing hormone (LH),** which become incorporated into their plasmalemma.

Once the multilaminar primary follicle displays the presence of liquor folliculi, it is known as a **secondary follicle** (see Fig. 20–2B; Fig. 20–5). As more fluid is produced, individual droplets of liquor folliculi coalesce to form a single, fluid-filled chamber, the **antrum.**

The granulosa cells become rearranged, so that the primary oocyte is now surrounded by a small group of granulosa cells that project out from the wall into the fluid-filled antrum. This structure is called the **cumulus oophorus.** The loosely arranged low cuboidal granulosa cells immediately adjacent to the zona pellucida move slightly away from the oocyte, but their filopodia remain within the zona pellucida, maintaining contact with the primary oocyte. This single layer of granulosa cells that is immediately surrounding the primary oocyte is called the **corona radiata.**

Toward the end of this stage, stromal cells become enlarged and the theca interna is invaded by capillaries that nourish them as well as the avascular granulosa cells. Most of the follicles that reach this stage of development will undergo atresia, but some of the granulosa cells associated with the atretic follicles do not degenerate and die. Rather, they form **interstitial glands,** which secrete small amounts of androgens until menopause is concluded. A few secondary follicles continue to develop into mature follicles.

MATURE (GRAAFIAN) FOLLICLES. Continued proliferation of the granulosa cells and continued formation of liquor folliculi results in the formation of a **mature**

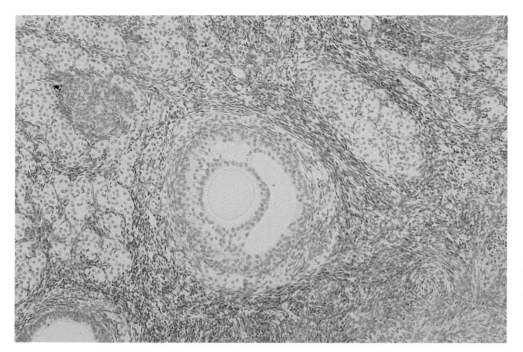

Figure 20-5. Light micrograph of a secondary follicle. Observe the primary oocyte and the follicular fluid surrounded by membrana granulosa (× 132).

(graafian) follicle whose diameter reaches 2.5 cm by the time of ovulation. The mature follicle may be observed as a transparent bulge on the surface of the ovary, nearly as large as the ovary itself.

The follicular cells of the wall of the follicle are called the **membrana granulosa.** Continued formation of liquor folliculi causes the cumulus oophorus—composed of the primary oocyte, the corona radiata, and associated follicular cells—to become detached from its base to float freely within the liquor folliculi (see Fig. 20-2B).

Ovulation. By the 14th day of the menstrual cycle, estrogen produced mostly by the developing graafian but also by secondary follicles causes elevation of blood estrogen to levels high enough to cause the following:

1. Negative feedback inhibition shuts off FSH release by the anterior pituitary
2. A sudden surge of LH is released by basophils of the anterior pituitary

The surge in **luteinizing hormone** levels results in increased blood flow to the ovaries, and capillaries within the theca external begin leaking plasma, resulting in edema. Concomitant with edema formation, histamine, prostaglandins, and collagenase are released in the vicinity of the graafian follicle.

Additionally, the LH surge is responsible for the following events:

1. The primary oocyte of the graafian follicle resumes and completes its first meiotic division, resulting in the formation of two daughter cells, the **secondary oocyte** and the

first polar body. Because of the uneven distribution of the cytoplasm, the first polar body is composed of a nucleus surrounded by only a narrow rim of cytoplasm.

2. The newly formed secondary oocyte enters the **second meiotic division** and is arrested in the **metaphase** stage.

3. The secondary oocyte and its attendant follicular cells are ovulated.

4. The remnants of the graafian follicle are converted into the corpus hemorrhagicus and then corpus luteum.

Just prior to ovulation, the surface of the ovary, where the graafian follicle is pressing against the tunica albuginea, loses its blood supply. This avascular region becomes blanched and is known as the **stigma.** The connective tissue at the stigma degenerates, as does the wall of the graafian follicle contacting the stigma, forming an opening between the peritoneal cavity and the antrum of the graafian follicle. It is through this opening that the oocyte is released from the ovary, resulting in **ovulation,** an event that takes place at about day 14 of the 28-day menstrual cycle.

The distal, fimbriated end of the oviduct, which presses against the ovary, whisks the secondary oocyte and follicular cells into the **infundibulum** of the **oviduct** to begin its journey into the ampulla, where it may be fertilized (see Fig. 20-1). If it is not fertilized within approximately 24 hours, the secondary oocyte degenerates and is phagocytosed. The process of fertilization is discussed later in the chapter.

Corpus Luteum

After the secondary oocyte and its associated cells are ovulated, the remainder of the graafian follicle collapses and becomes folded; some of the ruptured blood vessels leak blood into the follicular cavity, forming a central clot. The resulting structure is known as the **corpus hemorrhagicus.** As the clot is removed by phagocytes, continued high levels of **LH** convert the corpus hemorrhagicus into a temporary structure known as the **corpus luteum,** which functions as an endocrine gland (Fig. 20–6). This highly vascularized structure is composed of granulosa lutein cells (modified granulosa cells) and theca lutein cells (modified theca interna cells).

GRANULOSA LUTEIN CELLS. The granulosa cells remaining in the central region of the follicle account for about 80% of the cell population of the corpus luteum. They become modified into large, pale-staining cells (30 to 50 μm in diameter) called **granulosa lutein cells.** These cells have many long microvilli and develop all of the necessary organelles for steroid production, including abundant smooth endoplasmic reticulum and RER, abundant mitochondria, several well-developed Golgi complexes, and some lipid droplets scattered throughout the cytoplasm (Fig. 20–7). The granulosa lutein cells produce **progesterone** and convert androgens produced by the theca lutein cells into **estrogens.**

THECA LUTEIN CELLS. The **theca interna cells** at the periphery of the corpus luteum account for about 20% of the luteal cell population. These dark-staining cells remain small (15 μm in diameter) but become modified into hormone-

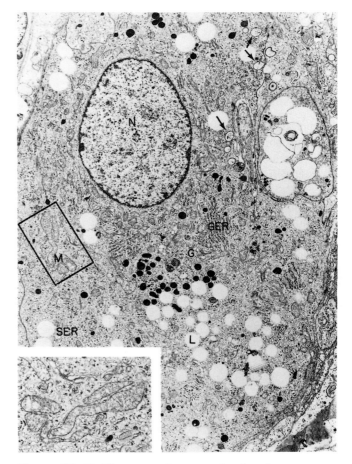

Figure 20–7. Electron micrograph of a rhesus monkey granulosa lutein cell with its large acentric nucleus and numerous organelles. GER, rough endoplasmic reticulum; G, Golgi apparatus; M, mitochondria (displayed at a higher magnification in the inset, lower left) (× 7090). (From Booher, C., Enders, A.C., Hendrick, X., and Hess, D.L.: Structural characteristics of the corpus luteum during implantation in the rhesus monkey *(Macaca mulatta).* Am. J. Anat. **160:**17–36, 1981. Reprinted by permission of John Wiley & Sons, Inc.)

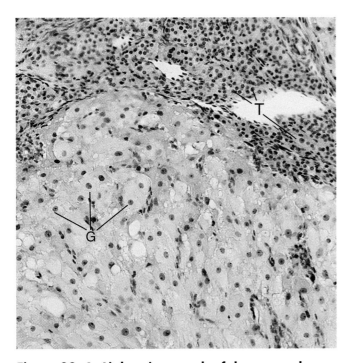

Figure 20–6. Light micrograph of the corpus luteum. Note the difference between the large granulosa lutein (G) and small theca lutein (T) cells (× 132).

secreting cells known as **theca lutein cells.** They specialize in the production of **progesterone,** some estrogens, and **androgens.**

Progesterone and estrogens secreted by granulosa and theca lutein cells inhibit the secretion of LH and FSH, respectively. The absence of FSH prevents the development of new follicles, thus preventing a second ovulation. If pregnancy does not occur, the absence of LH leads to degeneration of the corpus luteum, forming the **corpus luteum of menstruation.** If pregnancy occurs, **human chorionic gonadotropin** secreted by the placenta maintains the corpus luteum for 3 months. Now called the **corpus luteum of pregnancy,** it grows to a diameter of 5 cm and continues to secrete hormones necessary for the maintenance of pregnancy. Although the placenta becomes the main site for production of the various hormones involved in maintaining pregnancy 2 to 3 months after its formation, the corpus luteum continues to form these hormones for several months (see later discussion).

Corpus Albicans

The corpus luteum of menstruation (or of pregnancy) is invaded by fibroblasts, becomes fibrotic, and ceases to function. Its remnants undergo autolysis and are phagocytized by macrophages. The fibrous connective tissue that forms in its place is known as the **corpus albicans,** which persists for some time before being resorbed. The remnants of the corpus albicans persist as a scar on the surface of the ovary.

Atretic Follicles

The ovaries contain many follicles in various stages of development. Most follicles degenerate before reaching the mature stage, but multiple graafian follicles develop during each menstrual cycle. Nevertheless, once a single mature follicle ruptures and releases its secondary oocyte and associated cells, the remaining maturing follicles undergo atresia; the resulting **atretic follicles** eventually are phagocytized by macrophages. Thus, normally, only a single follicle ovulates during each menstrual cycle. Occasionally, two separate follicles develop to maturity and ovulate, leading to fraternal twins if both oocytes are fertilized. Although about 2% of all follicles reach the mature stage and are primed to ovulate, only 5% to 6% of these actually are ovulated. Of all the follicles present in the ovaries at menarche, just 0.1% to 0.2% develop to maturity and are ovulated.

Ovarian Medulla

The central region of the ovary, the **medulla,** is composed of fibroblasts loosely embedded in a collagen-rich meshwork containing elastic fibers (see Fig. 20–2A). The medulla also contains large blood vessels, lymph vessels, and nerve fibers. The medulla of the premenstrual human ovary has a few clusters of epithelioid **interstitial cells** that secrete estrogens. In mammals having large litters, the ovaries contain many clusters of these interstitial cells, which collectively are called the **interstitial gland.** In humans, most of these interstitial cells involute during the first menstrual cycle and have little, if any, function.

   Hilus cells constitute another group of epithelioid cells in the ovarian medulla. These cells have a similar configuration of organelles and contain the same substances in their cytoplasm as Leydig cells of the testes. Evidence has shown that these cells secrete androgens.

Hormonal Regulation of Ovarian Function

As mentioned previously, **FSH** and **LH** regulate maturation of ovarian follicles and ovulation. The secretion of these go-

nadotrophic hormones, which are produced in the pars distalis of the anterior pituitary, is in turn controlled by **gonadotropin-releasing hormone** produced by neurons in the hypothalamus (Fig. 20–8). Although it is unclear what signal stimulates primordial and early (unilaminar) primary follicles to develop, their development appears to be independent of FSH. However, continued development of multilaminar primary follicles into secondary follicles depends on FSH.

   Binding of gonadotropin-releasing hormone (GnRH) to receptors on the cells of the pars distalis induces the release of stored FSH and stimulates continued FSH synthesis. Subsequent binding of FSH to specific receptors on the granulosa cells of multilaminar primary follicles stimulates their development into secondary follicles. FSH also induces the theca interna cells of developing follicles to begin producing androgens, which are converted to **estrogens** by the granulosa cells. The granulosa cells of secondary follicles also produce several other hormones, including **inhibin, folliostatin,** and **activin,** which help to regulate release of FSH (see Fig. 20–8).

   As the blood levels of estrogen and other hormones produced by the granulosa cells rise, they stimulate production of LH by gonadotrophs in the anterior pituitary. When estrogen blood concentration reaches a threshold level, it restricts secretion of FSH in two ways: indirectly by suppressing gonadotropin-releasing hormone release from the hypothalamus and directly by inhibiting FSH release from the anterior pituitary. Just before the midpoint of the menstrual cycle (about day 14), the high estrogen level in the blood causes a surge of LH to be released by gonadotrophs of the pituitary. The sudden high blood-LH level stimulates the primary oocyte to complete meiosis I, becoming a secondary oocyte, which enters meiosis II and proceeds to metaphase. Meiosis II is interrupted in metaphase until fertilization triggers its completion.

   This surge of **LH** also launches the process of ovulation, whereby the secondary oocyte is expelled from the mature follicle. The granulosa cells and theca interna cells of the remaining ovulated follicle, which have **LH receptors,** are activated by **LH** to form the **corpus luteum.** The granulosa cells and the theca interna cells are converted into granulosa lutein cells and theca lutein cells, respectively. Both of these luteal cell types now actively produce **progesterone,** although most of it is produced by the granulosa lutein cell. Additionally, inhibin, folliostatin, and activin, feedback regulators of FSH release, continue to be produced by the corpus luteum. If fertilization and implantation do not occur, the secretory activity of the corpus luteum continues for about 14 days, and the organ is called the **corpus luteum of menstruation.** When fertilization and implantation occur, the corpus luteum increases in size and is known as the **corpus luteum of pregnancy.** This organ continues its secretory function even though the placenta assumes the primary responsibility for hormonal regulation (see Fig. 20–8).

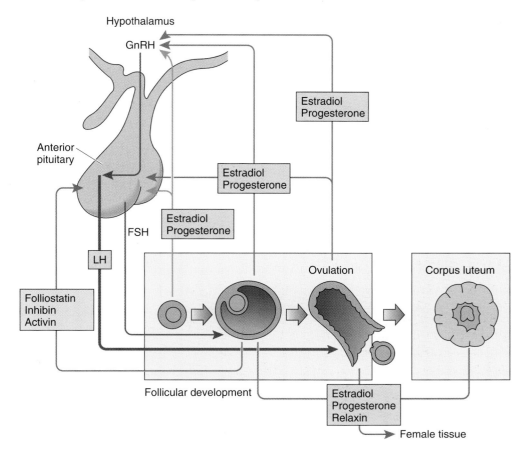

Figure 20–8. Schematic diagram illustrating the hormonal interactions between the hypothalamo-pituitary axis and the female reproductive system.

Progesterone stimulates development of the uterine endometrium during each menstrual cycle and inhibits the production of LH directly and indirectly (acting on both the hypothalamus and the pituitary gonadotrophs). In the absence of pregnancy, LH soon falls below the level required to maintain the corpus luteum, and the process of corpus luteum degeneration begins. If pregnancy occurs, **human chorionic gonadotropin** produced by the placenta provides positive feedback to the corpus luteum of pregnancy, thereby maintaining the production of progesterone early in pregnancy. By the fourth month of pregnancy, much of the hormonal control is assumed by the placenta. Another hormone, **relaxin,** produced by the placenta, facilitates parturition by softening of the fibrocartilage of the pubic symphysis to ease the widening of the pelvic outlet.

Oviducts (Fallopian Tubes)

The **oviducts,** or **fallopian tubes,** are paired, muscular-walled tubular structures approximately 12 cm long, each with an open end and an attached end (see Fig. 20–1). The oviducts become continuous with the wall of the uterus at their attached ends, where they traverse the uterine wall to open into its lumen. The free ends open into the peritoneal cavity close to the ovaries.

The oviducts are divided into four anatomical regions. Beginning at the open end is the **infundibulum,** whose open end is fringed with projections called **fimbriae,** which help to capture the secondary oocyte. The second region is the expanded **ampulla,** where fertilization usually takes place. The third region is the **isthmus,** the narrowed portion between the ampulla and the fourth region, the **intramural region,** which passes through the uterine wall to open into the lumen of the uterus. The oviducts are covered by visceral peritoneum. Their walls are composed of three layers: **mucosa, muscularis,** and **serosa** (Fig. 20–9).

The **mucosa** is characterized by many longitudinal folds. These folds are present in all four regions of the oviduct but are most pronounced in the ampulla, where they branch; in the other regions, the mucosal folds are reduced to low elevations. The **simple columnar epithelium** that lines the lumen is tallest in the infundibulum and shortens as the oviduct approaches the uterus. Two different cell types constitute this epithelium: nonciliated **peg cells** and **ciliated cells.**

Peg cells have no cilia. They have a secretory function, providing a nutritive and protective environment for maintaining spermatozoa on their migration route to reach the secondary oocyte. Products within the secretions of the peg cells facilitate **capacitation** of spermatozoa, a process

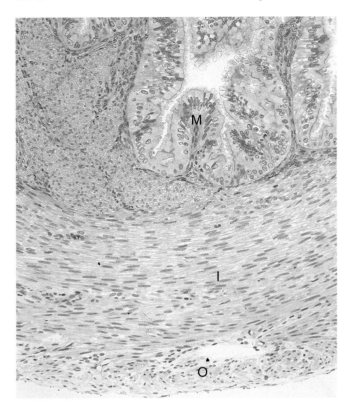

Figure 20-9. Light micrograph of the oviduct in cross-section. Observe the outer longitudinal (O) and inner circular (I) muscle layers and the mucosa (M) (× 132).

whereby spermatozoa become fully mature and capable of fertilizing the ovum. Secretory products also provide nutrition and protection to the ovum and, if the ovum is fertilized, these same secretions provide nutrients to the embryo during the initial phases of its development. The secretions of peg cells coupled with the movement of the fluid toward the uterus inhibit microorganisms from the uterus, moving to the oviduct and into the peritoneal cavity.

The **cilia** of **ciliated cells** beat in unison toward the uterus. As a result, the fertilized ovum, spermatozoa, and the viscous liquid produced by the peg cells all are propelled toward the uterus (Fig. 20-10).

The **lamina propria** of the oviduct mucosa is unremarkable because it is composed of loose connective tissue containing fibroblasts, mast cells, lymphoid cells, collagen, and reticular fibers. The **muscularis** consists of poorly defined inner circular and outer longitudinal layers of smooth muscles. Loose connective tissue also fills spaces between the bundles of muscles. A simple squamous epithelium provides the **serosal covering** of the oviduct. The loose connective tissue between the serosa and the muscularis contains many blood vessels and autonomic nerve fibers.

Because the oviducts are so richly vascularized with mostly large veins, contractions of the muscularis during ovulation constricts the engorged veins. This causes disten-

tion of the entire oviduct and brings the fimbriae into contact with the ovary, thereby aiding the capture of the released secondary oocyte. Continued rhythmic contractions of the layers of the muscularis, coupled with the beating of the cilia within, help to propel the captured oocyte to the uterus.

Uterus

The **uterus,** a single, thick, pear-shaped structure located in the midline of the pelvis, receives at its broad, closed end the terminals of the paired oviducts. The uterus is a robust muscular organ measuring about 7 cm long, 4 cm wide, and 2.5 cm thick. It is divided into three regions: the **body,** the broad portion into which the oviducts open; the **fundus,** the rounded base located superior to the exit ports of the oviducts in the body; and the **cervix,** the narrow circular portion that protrudes and opens into the vagina (see Fig. 20-1).

Body and Fundus

The uterine wall of the body and the fundus is composed of an **endometrium, myometrium,** and either an **adventitia** or a **serosa.**

Endometrium

The **endometrium,** or mucosal lining of the uterus, is composed of a simple columnar epithelium and a lamina propria. The epithelium is composed of nonciliated secretory columnar cells and ciliated cells, whereas the lamina propria houses simple branched tubular glands that extend as far as the myometrium (Fig. 20-11). Although the glandular cells resemble those of the surface epithelium, there are no ciliated cells in the glands. The dense, irregular collagenous connective tissue of the **lamina propria** is highly cellular and contains stellate–shaped cells, macrophages, leukocytes, and an abundance of reticular fibers. The morphological and physiological alterations that occur in the endometrium during the phases of the menstrual cycle are controlled by various hormones and are described later.

The endometrium consists of two layers: a thick, superficial layer called the **functionalis** (sloughed at menstruation) and a deep, narrow layer called the **basalis,** whose glands and connective tissue elements proliferate and thereby regenerate the functionalis during each menstrual cycle (see Fig. 20-11).

The **functionalis** is vascularized by numerous **coiled helical arteries,** which originate from the **arcuate arteries** of the stratum vasculare, located in the middle layer of the myometrium. The coiled arteries give rise to a rich capillary network that supplies the glands and connective tissue of the functionalis. Another set of arteries, the **straight arteries,** also originate from the arcuate arteries but are much shorter and supply only the basalis.

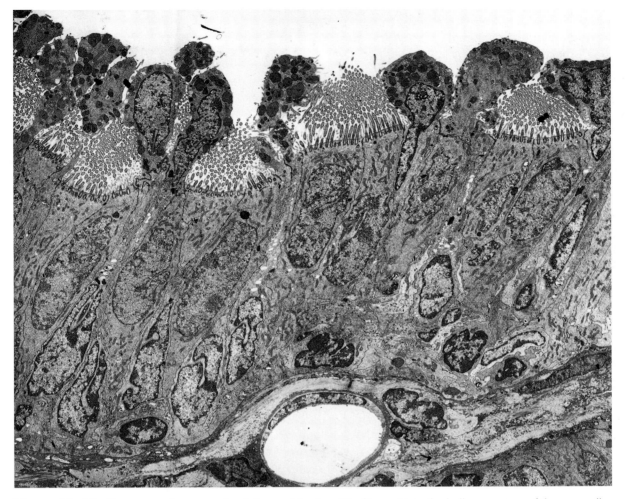

Figure 20-10. Electron micrograph of the oviduct epithelium. Note the bulbous apices of the peg cells as well as the cilia of the ciliated cells (× 40,000). (From Hollis, D.E., Frith, P.A., Vaughan, J.D., Chapman, R.E., and Nancarrow, C.D.: Ultrastructural changes in the oviductal epithelium of merino ewes during the estrous cycle. Am. J. Anat. **171**:441–456, 1984. Reprinted by permission of John Wiley & Sons, Inc.)

Myometrium

The thick muscular wall of the uterus, the **myometrium,** is composed of three layers of smooth muscle. **Longitudinal muscle** makes up the inner and outer layers, whereas the richly vascularized middle layer contains mostly **circularly** arranged smooth muscle bundles. This richly vascularized region houses the **arcuate arteries** and is called the **stratum vasculare.** As the uterus narrows toward the cervix, muscle tissue diminishes and is replaced by fibrous connective tissue. At the cervix, the myometrium is composed of dense, irregular connective tissue containing elastic fibers and only a small number of scattered smooth muscle cells.

The size and number of the myometrial muscle cells is related to estrogen levels. The muscle cells are largest and most numerous during pregnancy, when much estrogen is produced, and smallest after the conclusion of menstruation, when little estrogen is being produced. When estrogen is absent, the myometrial muscle atrophies, with some cells suc-

cumbing to programmed cell death. Although most of the increase in uterine size during pregnancy is related to hypertrophy of the smooth muscle cells, the smooth muscle cell population also increases, suggesting that hyperplasia also occurs. However, it is unclear if the increase in cell number results only from division of smooth muscle cells or also from differentiation of undifferentiated cells into smooth muscle fibers.

Sexual stimulation causes moderate uterine contractions. During menstruation, the contraction may be painful in certain persons. Powerful, rhythmic contractions of the pregnant uterus during delivery expel the fetus and later the placenta from the uterus. The process of uterine contractions during parturition is due to hormonal actions:

1. Under the influence of **corticotropic hormone,** the myometrium and the fetal membranes produce **prostaglandins**
2. The pituitary gland releases the hormone **oxytocin**

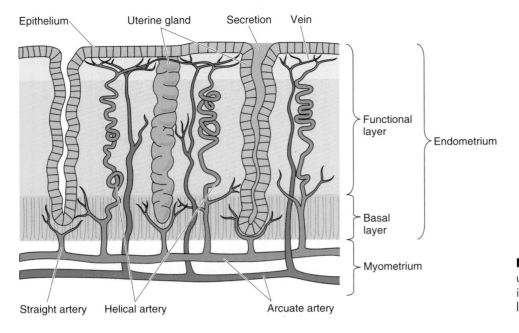

Epithelium   Uterine gland   Secretion   Vein

Functional layer
Endometrium

Basal layer

Myometrium

Straight artery   Helical artery   Arcuate artery

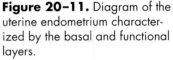

Figure 20–11. Diagram of the uterine endometrium characterized by the basal and functional layers.

3. Prostaglandins and oxytocin stimulate uterine contractions

4. After delivery, oxytocin continues to stimulate uterine contractions, which inhibit excessive blood loss from the detachment site of the placenta

Uterine Serosa or Adventitia

Because the uterus is tipped anteriorly and is lying against the bladder, much of its anterior portion is covered by **adventitia** (connective tissue without an epithelial covering); thus, this area is retroperitoneal. The fundus and posterior portion of the body is covered by a **serosa,** composed of a layer of squamous mesothelial cells resting on areolar connective tissue.

CLINICAL CORRELATIONS

The presence of endometrial tissue in the pelvis or in the peritoneal cavity is known as **endometriosis.** This often painful condition may cause dysmenorrhea and even infertility. The origin of endometrial tissue outside of the uterus is not known, but three theories have been proposed: regurgitation theory, metaplastic theory, and vascular and lymphatic dissemination theory. The regurgitation theory proposes that menstrual flow escapes from the uterus via the fallopian tubes to enter the peritoneal cavity. The metaplastic theory suggests that the epithelial cells of the peritoneum differentiate into endometrial cells. The vascular (lymphatic) dissemination theory proposes that endometrial cells enter vascular (or lymphatic) channels during menstruation and are distributed by the blood (or lymph)

vascular system. It has been demonstrated that these extrauterine endometrial tissues also undergo cyclic changes. Hemorrhaging of this tissue may cause adhesions and extreme pain. If not corrected, the pelvic viscera may be embroiled in a fibrotic mass, possibly resulting in sterility.

Cervix

The **cervix** is the terminal end of the uterus that protrudes into the vagina (see Fig. 20–1). The lumen of the cervix is lined by a **mucus-secreting simple columnar epithelium;** however, its external surface, where the cervix protrudes into the vagina, is covered by a **stratified squamous nonkeratinized epithelium,** like that of the vagina. The wall of the cervix consists mostly of dense collagenous connective tissue containing many elastic fibers and only a few smooth muscle fibers. Cervical mucosa contains branched **cervical glands.** Although the cervical mucosa changes during the menstrual cycle, it does not slough during menstruation.

At the midpoint in the menstrual cycle, around the time of ovulation, the cervical glands secrete a serous fluid that facilitates entry of the spermatozoa into the uterus. At other times, and during pregnancy, the secretions of the cervical glands become more viscous, forming a mucus plug in the orifice of the cervix, thus preventing the entry of sperm and microorganisms into the uterus. The hormone **progesterone** regulates the changes in the viscosity of the cervical gland secretions.

At the time of parturition, another luteal hormone, **relaxin,** induces lysis of collagen in the cervical walls. This results in a softening of the cervix, thus facilitating cervical dilation.

CLINICAL CORRELATIONS

The **Papanicolaou** or **"Pap smear" technique** is a diagnostic tool for detecting cervical cancer. It is performed by aspirating cervicular fluid from the vagina or taking scrapings directly from the cervix. The tissue or fluid is prepared and stained on a microscope slide, then examined for variations in the cell populations to detect anaplasia, dysplasia, and carcinoma.

Cervical carcinoma is one of the most common cancers in women, although it is rare in virgins and in nulliparous women (women who have not given birth). The incidence increases in women with multiple sex partners and herpes infections. It develops from the stratified squamous nonkeratinized epithelium of the cervix, where it is called **carcinoma in situ.** If detected by Pap smear in this stage, it usually can be successfully treated with surgery. If undetected early, however, it may invade other areas and metastasize, thus changing to **invasive carcinoma,** which carries a poor prognosis.

Menstrual Cycle

Normally the average menstrual cycle is a 28-day cycle. Although the successive events constituting the cycle occur continuously, they can be described in three phases: **menstrual phase, proliferative (follicular) phase,** and **secretory (luteal) phase** (Fig. 20–12).

Menstrual Phase (Days 1 to 4)

Menstruation, which begins on the day bleeding from the uterus starts, occurs when fertilization does not take place. In this case, the corpus luteum becomes nonfunctional about 14 days after ovulation, thus *reducing* the levels of **progesterone** and **estrogen.**

A couple of days before bleeding begins, the functionalis layer of the endometrium becomes deprived of blood as the coiled (helical) arteries are intermittently constricted. After 2 days or so, the coiled arteries become permanently constricted, which reduces oxygen to the functionalis. This

Figure 20–12. Diagram correlating the events in follicular development, ovulation, hormonal interrelationships, and the menstrual cycle.

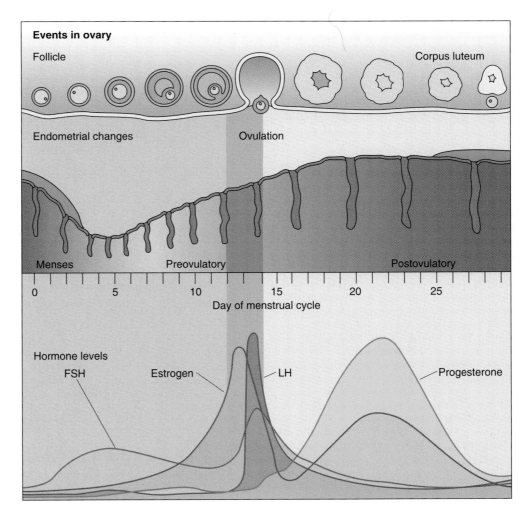

leads to a shutdown of the glands, invasion by leukocytes, ischemia, and eventual **necrosis** of the **functionalis.** Shortly thereafter the coiled arteries dilate once again; however, because these coiled arteries have been weakened by the previous events, they rupture. The disgorged blood removes patches of the functionalis to be discharged as a **hemorrhagic discharge (menses),** initiating menstruation on day 1.

Although the entire functionalis layer of the endometrium is sloughed, it is not completely released from the wall immediately; rather, this process continues for 3 to 4 days. In a normal menstruation the approximate blood loss is only 35 ml, although in some women it may be greater.

Prior to and during the menstrual phase, the basalis continues to be vascularized by its own straight arteries and thus remains viable. The basal cells of the glands of the basalis begin to proliferate and the newly formed cells migrate to the surface to begin reepithelialization of the connective tissue wound of the uterine lumen. These events commence the proliferative phase.

Proliferative (Follicular) Phase (Days 4 to 14)

The **proliferative phase** (also known as the follicular phase because it occurs at the same time as the development of the ovarian follicles) begins when the menstrual flow ceases, on about day 4, and continues through day 14. The proliferative phase is characterized by a re-epithelization of the lining of the endometrium; reconstruction of the glands, connective tissue, and the coiled arteries of the lamina propria; and renewal of the functionalis.

During this phase the functional layer becomes much thicker (up to 2 to 3 mm) because of the proliferation of the cells in the base of the glands that remained unaffected during the menstrual phase because their blood supply was intact. As stated before, it is these cells that are responsible for the formation of the epithelial lining of the uterus as well as for the establishment of new glands in the functionalis. These tubular glands are straight, not yet coiled, but their cells begin to accumulate glycogen, as do the cells of the stroma that proliferated to renew the stroma of the functionalis. The coiled arteries that were lost in the menstrual phase are replaced but are not tightly coiled and reach only two thirds of the way into the functionalis. By the 14th day of the menstrual cycle (ovulation), the functionalis layer of the endometrium has been fully restored to its previous status with a full complement of epithelium, glands, stroma, and coiled arteries.

Secretory (Luteal) Phase (Days 15 to 28)

The **secretory phase** (also known as the **luteal phase)** commences after ovulation. During this phase the endometrium continues to thicken as a result of edema and accumulated glycogen secretions of the endometrial glands, which become highly convoluted and branched. The secretory prod-

ucts first accumulate in the basal region of the cytoplasm of the cells constituting the endometrial glands. As more secretory product is manufactured, the secretory granules move apically and are released into the lumen of the gland. This glycogen-rich material will nourish the conceptus before the formation of the placenta. Most of the changes that result in the thickening of the endometrium are attributed to the functionalis, although the lumina of the glands located in the basalis are also filled with secretory product (Fig. 20–13). The coiled arteries of the functionalis attain full development, becoming more coiled and extending fully into the functional layer by the 22nd day. Thus at this point in the secretory phase, the endometrium is about 5 mm thick.

The secretory phase completes the cycle as the 28th day approaches, presaging the menstrual phase of a new menstrual cycle.

Fertilization and Implantation and Placental Development

Fertilization

The oocyte and its attendant follicular cells are transported down the oviduct by the beating of the cilia of the ciliated cells of the epithelial lining and by rhythmic contractions of the smooth muscle of the oviduct (Fig. 20–14). The nutrient-rich fluid produced by peg cells of the mucosal epithelium nourishes the oocyte on its way to the uterus.

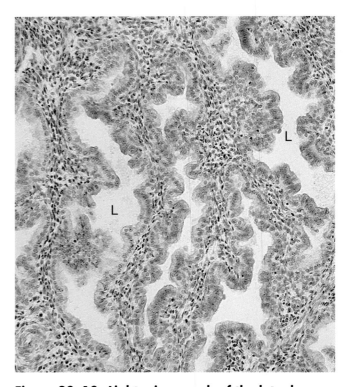

Figure 20–13. Light micrograph of the luteal phase uterus. Note the lumina (L) of the glands surrounded by stromal cells (× 132).

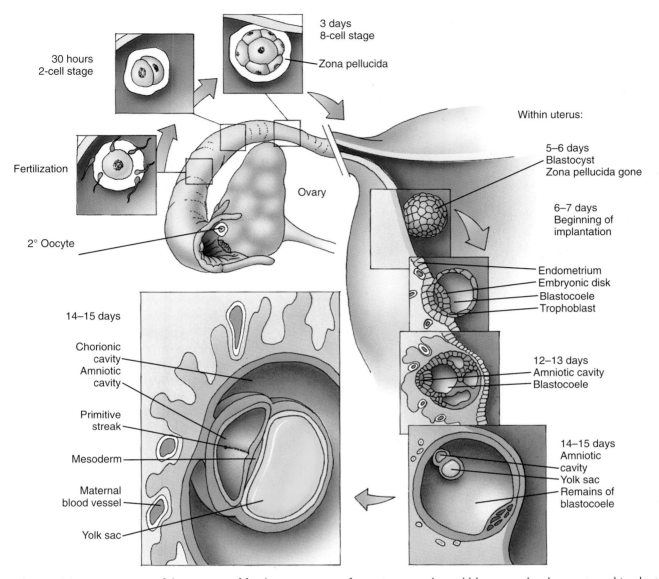

Figure 20-14. Diagram of the process of fertilization, zygote formation, morula and blastocyst development, and implantation.

Spermatozoa introduced into the vagina during sexual intercourse swim through the cervix, the uterine lumen, and up the oviduct to the ampulla to encounter the secondary oocyte. Fertilization usually occurs in the ampulla (Fig. 20–15). At this time the cells of the corona radiata still surround the **zona pellucida** and the secondary oocyte. Specific oligosaccharides attached to proteins of the zona pellucida bind to receptor proteins located in the head of the sperm, triggering the **acrosome reaction.** This reaction results in fusion of the plasmalemma of the sperm head and ooctye, thus permitting the sperm nucleus to enter the oocyte's cytoplasm.

The contact between the sperm and the oocyte is responsible for the **cortical reaction,** which is the release of numerous cortical granules located in the oocyte's cytoplasm into the perivitelline space. Enzymes within the cortical granules act to destroy sperm receptors in the zona pellucida, thus preventing additional spermatozoa from reaching the oocyte.

Also at this time, entry of the sperm nucleus triggers the secondary oocyte to resume and complete its second meiotic division. This results in an unequal division of the cytoplasm, forming two haploid cells, the **ovum** and the **second polar body.** The nucleus of the ovum (**female pronucleus**) fuses with the nucleus of the spermatozoa (**male pronucleus**), forming a **zygote** with the diploid number of chromosomes and thus completing the event of fertilization. It is interesting to note that the window of time between ovulation and fertilization is about 24 hours. If fertilization does not occur during this period, the ovum degenerates and is phagocytized by macrophages.

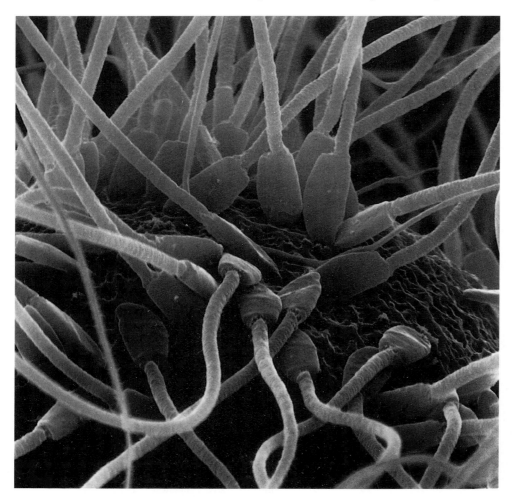

Figure 20–15. Scanning electron micrograph of fertilization (× 6500). (From Phillips, D.M., Shalgi, R., and Dekel, N.: Mammalian fertilization as seen with the scanning electron microscope. Am. J. Anat. **174:**357–372, 1985. Reprinted by permission of John Wiley & Sons, Inc.)

Implantation

As the **zygote** continues its journey through the oviduct on its way to the uterus, it undergoes numerous mitotic divisions, becoming the spherical clump of cells known as the **morula** (see Fig. 20–14). With further divisions and modifications, the morula is transformed into the **blastocyst,** composed of a hollow ball of cells. The lumen of the blastocyst contains a fluid and a few cells at one pole. The peripheral cells are known as **trophoblasts,** whereas the cells trapped inside the blastocyst are the **embryoblasts.** The blastocyst enters the uterine cavity about 4 days after fertilization and begins to embed itself into the uterine wall, a process known as **implantation.** The trophoblasts of the blastocyst stimulate the transformation of the stellate **stromal cells** of the uterine endometrium into pale-staining **decidual cells,** whose stored glycogen probably provides nourishment for the developing embryo.

The embryoblasts are predestined to develop into the embryo, whereas the **trophoblast cells** give rise to the embryonic portion of the placenta and to the amniotic sac. Trophoblastic cells rapidly proliferate, forming an inner conglomeration of individual cells, which are mitotically ac-

tive and known as the **cytotrophoblast,** and a thicker outer syncytium of cells that do not undergo mitosis, called the **syncytiotrophoblasts.**

The **cytotrophoblasts** proliferate, with the new cells joining the syncytiotrophoblasts. As the syncytiotrophoblasts increase in number they form vacuoles that coalesce into large, labyrinthine spaces known as **lacunae.** Continued growth of the syncytium erodes the endometrium. This process permits deep penetration of the blastocyst into the wall of the endometrium, and by the 11th day of gestation the endometrial epithelium seals over the implantation site.

Placenta Development

Continued erosion of the highly vascular endometrium by the **syncytiotrophoblasts** also erodes the maternal blood vessels. The blood from these vessels empties into the lacunae of the syncytiotrophoblasts that surround the embryo. Thus the maternal blood provides nourishment for the developing embryo. With further growth and development, the **placenta** begins to be formed with the resultant separation between the blood of the developing embryo and that of the mother (maternal blood). From the remainder of the trophoblastic cells the **chorion** develops and evolves into the **chorionic plate,** which gives rise to the **chorionic villi** (Fig. 20–16).

The developing trophoblasts induce changes in the endometrium in their vicinity, altering it to begin the formation of the maternal portion of the placenta. This altered maternal tissue, called the **decidua,** is subdivided into three regions: **decidua capsularis, decidua basalis,** and **decidua parietalis.**

- Decidua capsularis is interposed between the uterine lumen and the developing embryo

- Decidua basalis is interposed between the developing embryo and the myometrium
- Decidua parietalis composes the balance of the decidua

Initially the entire embryo is surrounded by decidua in order to nourish it. The region of the chorion in contact with the decidua capsularis will form short, insubstantial villi, thus remaining smooth-surfaced; that region of the chorion is known as the **chorion laeve.** The region of the decidua capsularis, however, will become highly vascularized by maternal blood vessels; in this region the placenta will develop. The region of the chorionic plate in contact with the decidua basalis will form extensive chorionic villi, **primary**

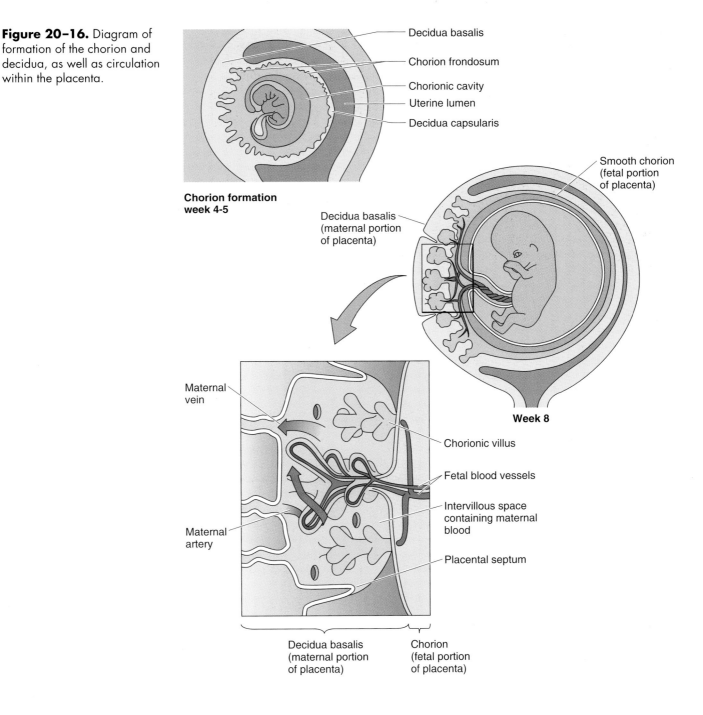

Figure 20–16. Diagram of formation of the chorion and decidua, as well as circulation within the placenta.

Decidua basalis
Chorion frondosum
Chorionic cavity
Uterine lumen
Decidua capsularis

Chorion formation week 4-5

Smooth chorion (fetal portion of placenta)

Decidua basalis (maternal portion of placenta)

Week 8

Maternal vein

Chorionic villus

Fetal blood vessels

Intervillous space containing maternal blood

Maternal artery

Placental septum

Decidua basalis (maternal portion of placenta)

Chorion (fetal portion of placenta)

villi; thus, this region of the chorion is known as the **chorion frondosum.** The primary villi are composed of both syncytiotrophoblasts and cytotrophoblasts. With further development, extraembryonic mesenchymal cells enter the core of the primary villi, converting them into **secondary villi** (Fig. 20–17). The connective tissue of the secondary villi will become vascularized by extensive capillary beds, which will be linked to the developing vascular supply of the embryo. As development continues, the cytotrophoblast population will decrease because these cells will join the syncytium and contribute to its growth. The decidua basalis forms large vascular spaces, **lacunae,** that are compartmentalized into smaller regions by **placental septa,** extensions of the decidua. Secondary villi project into these vascular spaces and are surrounded by maternal blood that is delivered and drained from the lacunae by maternal blood vessels of the decidua basalis.

Most of the villi are not anchored to the decidua basalis but are suspended in maternal blood of the lacunae like roots of vegetables grown in hydroponic environments and are known as **free villi.** The villi anchored to the decidua basalis are called anchoring villi. Capillaries of free and anchoring villi are near the surface of the villi and are separated from the maternal blood by a slight amount of connective tissue and the syncytiotrophoblasts covering the secondary villus. Thus, maternal blood and fetal blood do not intermix; instead, nutrients and oxygen from the maternal blood diffuse through the syncytiotrophoblasts, connective tissue, and endothelial cells of the capillaries of the villi to reach the fetal blood. These structures form the **placental barrier.** Certain substances, such as water, oxygen, CO_2, small molecules, some proteins, lipids, hormones, drugs, and some antibodies (especially IgG) can penetrate the placental barrier, whereas most macromolecules cannot.

Not only is the placenta where nutritious substances, waste, and gases are exchanged between maternal and fetal blood, the placenta, specifically the syncytiotrophoblast, also serves as an endocrine organ secreting **human chorionic gonadotropin, chorionic thyrotropin, progesterone, estrogen,** and **chorionic somatomammotropin** (a growth-promoting and lactogenic hormone). Additionally, stromal connective tissue cells of the decidua form the **decidual cells,** which enlarge and synthesize **prolactin** and **prostaglandins.**

Vagina

The **vagina** is a fibromuscular tubular structure 8 to 9 cm in length connected to the uterus proximally and the vestibule of the external genitalia distally. The vagina consists of three layers: a **mucosa,** a **muscularis,** and an **adventitia.**

The lumen of the vagina is lined by a thick **stratified squamous nonkeratinized epithelium** (150 to 200 μm thick), although some of the superficial cells may contain some keratohyalin. Langerhans cells in the epithelium are thought to participate in antigen presentation to T lymphocytes housed in the lymph nodes. The epithelial cells are stimulated by estrogen to synthesize and store large deposits of **glycogen,** which is released into the lumen as the vaginal epithelial cells are sloughed. Naturally occurring vaginal bacterial flora metabolize the glycogen, forming **lactic acid,** which is responsible for the low pH in the lumen of the vagina, especially at the midpoint of the menstrual cycle. The lowered pH also helps to restrict pathogenic invasion.

The **lamina propria** of the mucosa is composed of a loose fibroelastic connective tissue containing a rich vascular supply in its deeper regions. It also contains numerous lymphocytes and neutrophils that reach the lumen by passing through intercellular spaces during certain periods in the menstrual cycle, where they participate in immunity. Although the vagina does not contain glands, there is an increase in vaginal fluid during sexual stimulation, arousal, and intercourse that serves to lubricate its lining. The fluid is derived from transudate from the lamina propria combined with secretions from glands of the cervix.

The **muscularis** layer of the vagina is composed of smooth muscle cells arranged so that the mostly longitudinal bundles of the external surface intermingle with the more circularly arranged bundles near the lumen. A sphincter muscle, composed of skeletal muscle fibers, encircles the vagina at its external opening.

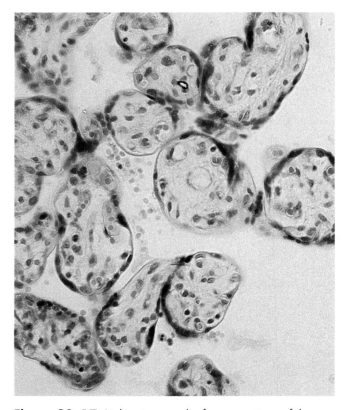

Figure 20–17. Light micrograph of cross-sections of the chorionic villi of the placenta (× 270).

Dense, fibroelastic connective tissue constitutes the **adventitia** of the vagina, attaching it to surrounding structures. Contained within the adventitia is a rich vascular supply with a vast venous plexus and nerve bundles derived from the pelvic splanchnic nerves.

External Genitalia

The **external genitalia (vulva)** is composed of the **labia majora, labia minora, vestibule,** and **clitoris.**

The **labia majora** are two folds of skin heavily endowed with adipose tissue and a thin layer of smooth muscle. The homologue of these structures in the male is the scrotum, with the smooth muscle layer corresponding to the dartos muscle of the scrotum. The labia majora are covered with coarse hair on their external surface but are devoid of hair on their smooth inner surface. Numerous sweat and sebaceous glands open on both surfaces.

The **labia minora,** located medial to and slightly deep to the labia majora, are the homologues of the urethral surface of the penis in the male. The labia minora are two smaller folds of skin devoid of hair follicles and adipose tissue. Their core is composed of a spongy connective tissue containing elastic fibers arranged in networks. They contain numerous sebaceous glands and are richly supplied with blood vessels and nerve endings.

The cleft situated between the labia minora is the **vestibule,** a space that receives secretions of the **glands of Bartholin,** paired mucus-secreting glands, and many small **minor vestibular glands.** Also located in the vestibule are the orifices of the urethra and the vagina. The orifice of the vagina is narrowed in the virgin by a fold of epithelially enclosed fibrovascular tissue called the **hymen.**

The **clitoris** is located between the two folds of the labia minora superiorly, where they unite to form the prepuce over the top of the **glans clitoridis.** The **clitoris,** the female homologue of the penis, is covered by stratified squamous epithelium and is composed of two **erectile bodies** containing numerous blood vessels and sensory nerves, including Meissner's and pacinian corpuscles, which are sensitive during sexual arousal.

Mammary Glands

Mammary glands secrete milk, a fluid containing proteins, lipids, and lactose as well as lymphocytes and monocytes, antibodies, minerals, and fat-soluble vitamins, to provide the proper nourishment for the newborn.

The mammary glands develop in the same manner and are of the same structure in both sexes until puberty, when changes in the hormonal secretions in females cause further development and structural changes within the glands. Secretions of **estrogen** and **progesterone** from the ovary (and later from the placenta) and **prolactin** from the acidophils of the anterior pituitary initiate development of **lobules** and

terminal ductules. Full development of the ductal portion of the breast requires **glucocorticoids** and further activation by **somatotropin.** Concomitant with these events is an increase in connective tissue and adipose tissue within the stroma, causing the gland to enlarge. Full development occurs at about age 20 with minor cyclic changes during each menstrual period, whereas major changes occur during pregnancy and in lactation. After about the age of 40, the secretory portions as well as some of the ducts and connective tissue elements of the breasts begin to atrophy and continue this process through menopause.

The glands within the breasts are classified as **compound tubuloalveolar glands,** consisting of 15 to 20 lobes radiating out from the nipple and separated from each other by adipose and collagenous connective tissue. Each lobe is drained by its own **lactiferous duct** leading directly to the **nipple,** where it opens onto its surface. Before reaching the nipple, each of the ducts is dilated to form a **lactiferous sinus** for milk storage, then narrows before reaching the nipple.

Resting Mammary Glands

Resting or **nonsecreting mammary glands** of nonpregnant women have the same basic architecture as the lactating (active) mammary gland, except that they are smaller and without developed alveoli, which occur only during pregnancy. Near the opening at the nipple, lactiferous ducts are lined by a stratified squamous (keratinized) epithelium. The lactiferous sinus and the lactiferous duct leading to it are lined by stratified cuboidal epithelium, whereas the smaller ducts leading to the lactiferous duct are lined by a simple columnar epithelium. Stellate myoepithelial cells located between the epithelium and the basal lamina also wrap around the developing alveoli and become functional during pregnancy.

Lactating (Active) Mammary Glands

Mammary glands are activated by elevated surges of **estrogen** and **progesterone** during pregnancy to become lactating glands to provide milk for the newborn. At this time the terminal portions of the ducts branch and grow, and the alveoli develop and mature (Fig. 20–18). As pregnancy progresses, the breasts enlarge as a result of hypertrophy of the glandular parenchyma and engorgement with **colostrum,** a protein-rich fluid, in preparation for the newborn. Within a few days after birth, when estrogen and progesterone secretions have subsided, **prolactin,** secreted by acidophils of the anterior pituitary, activates the secretion of **milk,** which replaces the colostrum.

The **alveoli** of the lactating (active) mammary glands are composed of cuboidal cells partially surrounded by a meshwork of myoepithelial cells. These secretory cells possess abundant RER and mitochondria, several Golgi complexes, many lipid droplets, and numerous vesicles (Fig. 20–19)

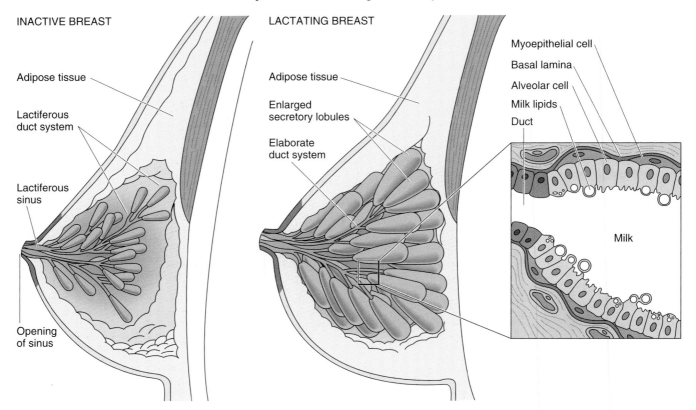

Figure 20–18. Diagram comparing the glandular differences between an inactive and a lactating breast.

containing caseins (milk proteins) and lactose. It should be noted, however, that not all regions of the alveolus are in the same stage of production, because different acini display various degrees of preparation for synthesis of milk substances (Fig. 20–20).

The secretions of the alveolar cells are of two kinds: **lipids** and **proteins.**

Lipids that are stored in droplets within the cytoplasm are released from the secretory cells, possibly by the **apocrine** mode of exocytosis, whereby small droplets coalesce to form larger and larger droplets that move to the periphery of the cell projecting into the lumen, surrounded by plasmalemma. Eventually these lipid droplets are pinched off and surrounded by a narrow rim of cytoplasm and enclosed by a plasmalemma.

Proteins synthesized within these secretory cells are liberated from the cells by the **merocrine** mode of exocytosis in much the same manner as would be expected of other cells that synthesize and release proteins into the extracellular space.

Areola and Nipple

The circular, heavily pigmented skin in the center of the breast is the **areola,** containing sweat and sebaceous glands at its margin as well as **areolar glands (of Montgomery)** that resemble both sweat and mammary glands. In the center of the areola is the **nipple,** a protuberance covered by stratified squamous epithelium containing the terminal openings of the lactiferous ducts. In fair-skinned persons, a pinkish color is imparted to the nipple as a result of the color of blood in the rich vascular supply within the long dermal papillae that extend near its surface. During pregnancy, however, the color becomes darker because of increased pigmentation of the areola and the nipple. The core of the nipple is composed of dense collagenous connective tissue with abundant elastic fibers connected to the surrounding skin or interlaced within the connective tissue. The wrinkling of the skin on the nipple results from the attachments of the elastic fibers. The abundant smooth muscle fibers are arranged in two ways: circularly around the nipple and radiating longitudinally along the long axis of the nipple. The contraction of these muscle fibers is responsible for erection of the nipple.

Most of the sebaceous glands located around the lactiferous ducts open onto the surface or sides of the nipple, although some open into the lactiferous ducts just before those ducts open onto the surface.

Mammary Gland Secretions

Although the mammary gland is prepared to secrete milk even before birth, certain hormones prohibit this. However,

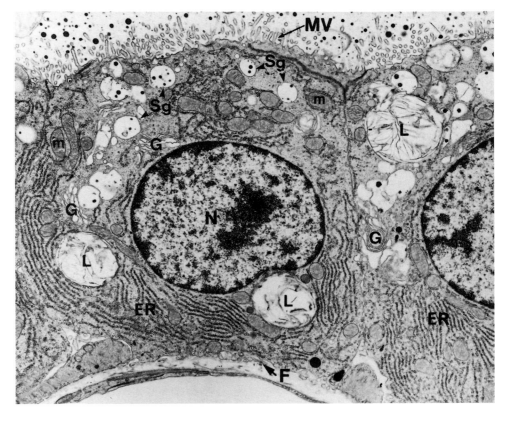

Figure 20-19. Electron micrograph of an acinar cell from the lactating mammary gland of the rat. Note the large lipid droplets (L), abundant rough endoplasmic reticulum (ER), and the Golgi apparatus (G). Sg, secretory granules; m, mitochondria; MV, microvilli; F, folds of the basal plasmalemma (× 10,000). (From Clermont, Y., Xia, I., Rambourg, A., Turner, J.D., and Hermo, L.: Structure of the Golgi apparatus in stimulated and nonstimulated acinar cells of mammary glands of the rat. Anat. Rec. **237:**308–317, 1993. Reprinted by permission of John Wiley & Sons, Inc.)

when the placenta is detached in the adult female, **prolactin** from the anterior pituitary stimulates the production of milk, which reaches full capacity in a few days. Before that, for the first 2 or 3 days after birth, a protein-rich thick fluid called **colostrum** is secreted. This high-protein secretion, rich in vitamin A, sodium, and chloride, also contains lymphocytes and monocytes, minerals, lactalbumin, and antibodies (IgA) to nourish and protect the newborn.

Milk, usually produced by the 4th day after parturition, is a fluid that contains minerals, electrolytes, carbohydrates (including lactose), immunoglobulins (mostly IgA), proteins (including caseins), and lipids. Production of milk results from the stimuli of sight, touch, handling of the newborn, and anticipation of nursing, events that create a surge in **prolactin** release. Once initiated, milk production is continuous with the milk being stored within the duct system. Concomitant with the production of prolactin, **oxytocin** is released from the posterior lobe of the pituitary, which initiates the **milk ejection reflex** by inducing contractions of the myoepithelial cells around the alveoli and the ducts, thus expelling the milk.

CLINICAL CORRELATIONS

Mothers who cannot **breast feed** their baby on a regular feeding schedule are inclined to suffer from poor lactation. This may motivate a decision to discontinue nursing alto-

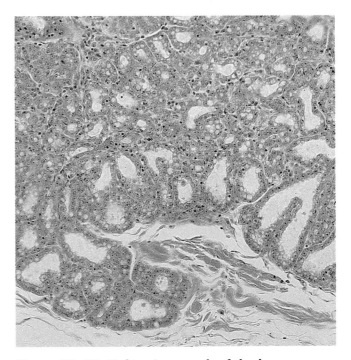

Figure 20-20. Light micrograph of the human mammary gland. Observe the crowded alveoli and note that various regions of the gland are in different stages of the secretory process (× 132).

gether, with the result that the infant is deprived of the passive immunity conferred by ingesting antibodies from the mother.

Breast cancer, one of the major cancers in women, may be of two different types: **ductal carcinoma** of the ductal cells or **lobular carcinoma** of the terminal ductules. De-tection must be early or prognosis is poor because the carcinoma may **metastasize** to the axillary lymph nodes and from there to the lungs, bone, and brain. At the recommendation of the medical profession in recent years, early detection through self-examination and mammography have helped to reduce the breast cancer mortality rates.

Male Reproductive System

21

The male reproductive system consists of the two **testes** suspended in the scrotum, a system of intratesticular and extratesticular **genital ducts,** associated **glands,** and the male copulatory organ, the **penis** (Fig. 21–1). The testes are responsible for the formation of the male gametes, known as **spermatozoa,** as well as the synthesis, storage, and release of the male sex hormone, **testosterone.** The glands associated with the male reproductive tract are the paired **seminal vesicles,** the single **prostate gland,** and the two **bulbourethral glands (of Cowper).** These glands form the noncellular portion of semen, which not only nourishes the spermatozoa but also provides a fluid vehicle for their delivery into the female reproductive tract. The **penis** has a dual function: it delivers **semen** (spermatozoa suspended in the secretions of the accessory glands) to the female reproductive tract during copulation and serves as the conduit of urine from the urinary bladder to outside the body.

Testes

Each testis of a mature man is an oval-shaped organ, approximately 4 cm long, 2 to 3 cm wide, and 3 cm thick. During embryogenesis the testes develop retroperitoneally on the posterior wall of the abdominal cavity, and as they descend into the scrotum they carry with them a portion of the peritoneum. This peritoneal outpocketing, the **tunica vagi-**

Figure 21–1. Schematic diagram of the male reproductive system.

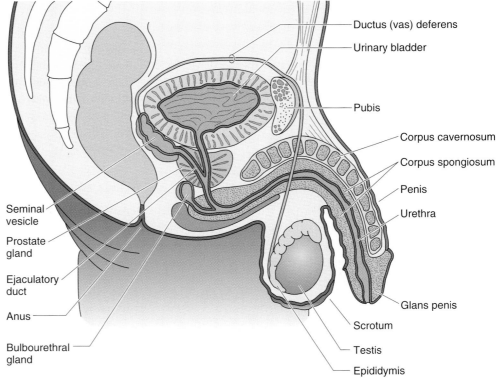

- Ductus (vas) deferens
- Urinary bladder
- Pubis
- Corpus cavernosum
- Corpus spongiosum
- Penis
- Urethra
- Glans penis
- Scrotum
- Testis
- Epididymis
- Seminal vesicle
- Prostate gland
- Ejaculatory duct
- Anus
- Bulbourethral gland

nalis, forms a serous cavity that partially surrounds the anterolateral aspect of each testis, permitting it some degree of mobility within its compartment in the scrotum.

General Structure and Vascular Supply of the Testes

Each testis is surrounded by a capsule of dense, irregular collagenous connective tissue known as the **tunica albuginea.** Immediately deep to this layer is a highly vascularized loose connective tissue, the **tunica vasculosa,** that forms a vascular capsule of the testis. The posterior aspect of the tunica albuginea is somewhat thickened, forming the **mediastinum testis,** from which connective tissue septa radiate to subdivide each testis into approximately 250 pyramid-shaped intercommunicating compartments, the **lobuli testis** (Fig. 21–2).

Each lobule has one to four blindly ending **seminiferous tubules,** surrounded by a richly innervated and highly vascularized loose connective tissue, derived from the tunica vasculosa. Dispersed throughout this connective tissue are small conglomerations of endocrine cells, the **interstitial cells (of Leydig)** that are responsible for the synthesis of testosterone.

Spermatozoa are produced in the **seminiferous epithelium** of the seminiferous tubules. They enter short straight ducts, **tubuli recti,** that connect the open end of each seminiferous tubule to the **rete testis,** a system of labyrinthine spaces housed within the mediastinum testis. The spermatozoa leave the rete testis through 10 to 20 short tubules, the **ductuli efferentes,** to enter the **ductus epididymis.** Together, the ductuli efferentes and the ductus epididymis constitute the **epididymis.**

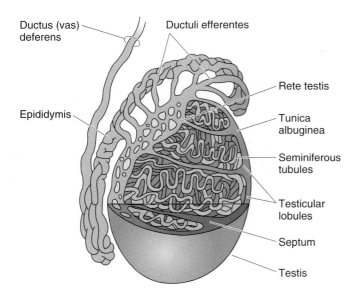

Figure 21–2. Schematic diagram of the testis and epididymis.

The vascular supply of each testis is derived from the **testicular artery** that descends with the testis into the scrotum along with the **ductus deferens (vas deferens).** The testicular artery forms several branches before it pierces the capsule of the testis to form the intratesticular vascular elements. The capillary beds of the testes are collected into several veins, the **pampiniform plexus of veins,** which are wrapped around the testicular artery. The artery, veins, and ductus deferens together form the **spermatic cord,** which passes through the inguinal canal, passing from the abdominal cavity to the scrotum. Blood in the pampiniform plexus of veins is cooler than that in the testicular artery, and acts to reduce the temperature of the arterial blood, thus forming a **countercurrent heat exchange system.** In this fashion it helps to keep the temperature of the testes a few degrees lower than that of the remainder of the body. At this cooler temperature (35° C) spermatozoa develop normally, whereas spermatozoa that develop at body temperature are sterile.

Seminiferous Tubules

Seminiferous tubules are highly convoluted hollow tubules, 30 to 70 cm long and 150 to 250 μm in diameter, surrounded by extensive capillary beds. About 1000 seminiferous tubules are in the two testes, for a total length of nearly 0.5 km (0.3 miles), dedicated to the production of spermatozoa.

The wall of the seminiferous tubule is composed of a slender connective tissue layer, the **tunica propria,** and a thick seminiferous epithelium. The tunica propria and the seminiferous epithelium are separated from one another by a well-developed **basal lamina.** The connective tissue comprises mostly interlaced slender type I collagen fiber bundles housing several layers of fibroblasts. In some animals, but not in humans, smooth muscle–like **myoid cells** are also present; these impart contractility to the seminiferous tubules of those animals.

The seminiferous epithelium (also known as **germinal epithelium**) is several cell layers thick (Fig. 21–3) and is composed of two types of cells, Sertoli cells and spermatogenic cells (see Fig. 21–3; Fig. 21–4). The latter are in various stages of maturation.

Sertoli Cells

Sertoli cells are tall, columnar cells whose lateral cell membranes present complex infoldings, so that their lateral cell boundaries cannot be distinguished by light microscopy. Their apical cell membranes are also highly folded and project into the lumina of the seminiferous tubules. These cells have a basally located, clear, oval nucleus with a large centrally positioned nucleolus (see Fig. 21–4). The cytoplasm has been shown to house inclusion products known as **crystalloids of Charcot-Bottcher,** whose composition and function are not known.

Electron micrographs reveal that the cytoplasm of Sertoli

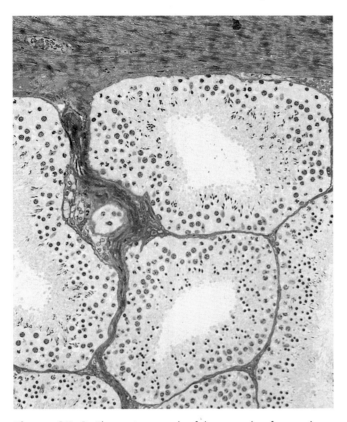

Figure 21–3. Photomicrograph of the capsule of a monkey testis and cross-sectional profiles of seminiferous tubules (× 132).

The Sertoli cells have the following functions:

- Physical and nutritional support of the developing germ cells
- Phagocytosis of cytoplasm eliminated during spermiogenesis
- Establishment of a blood–testis barrier by the formation of zonulae occludentes between adjacent Sertoli cells
- Synthesis and release of **androgen-binding protein (ABP),** a macromolecule that facilitates an increase in the concentration of testosterone in the seminiferous tubule by binding to it and preventing it from leaving the tubule
- Synthesis and release (during embryogenesis) of **anti-müllerian hormone,** which suppresses the formation of a müllerian duct (precursor of the female reproductive system) and thus establishes the "maleness" of the developing embryo
- Synthesis and secretion of **inhibin,** a hormone that inhibits the release of follicle-stimulating hormone by the anterior pituitary
- Secretion of a fructose-rich medium that nourishes and facilitates the transport of spermatozoa to the genital ducts
- Synthesis and secretion of **testicular transferrin,** an apoprotein that accepts iron from serum transferrin and conveys it to maturing gametes

cells is replete with profiles of smooth endoplasmic reticulum, but the amount of rough endoplasmic reticulum (RER) is limited. The cell also has numerous mitochondria, a well-developed Golgi apparatus, and numerous vesicles that belong to the endolysosomal complex. The cytoskeletal elements of Sertoli cells are also abundant, reflecting that one function of these cells is to provide structural support for the developing gametes.

The lateral cell membranes of adjacent Sertoli cells form occluding junctions with each other, thus subdividing the lumen of the seminiferous tubule into two isolated, concentric compartments (see Fig. 21–4; Fig. 21–5). The **basal compartment** is narrower, is located basal to the zonulae occludentes, and surrounds the wider **adluminal compartment.** Thus the zonulae occludentes of these cells establish a blood–testis barrier that isolates the adluminal compartment from connective tissue influences, thereby protecting the developing gametes from the immune system. Because spermatogenesis begins after puberty, the newly differentiating germ cells would be considered to be "foreign cells" by the immune system. Were it not for their isolation from the connective tissue compartments by the zonulae occludentes of the Sertoli cells, an immune response would be mounted against them.

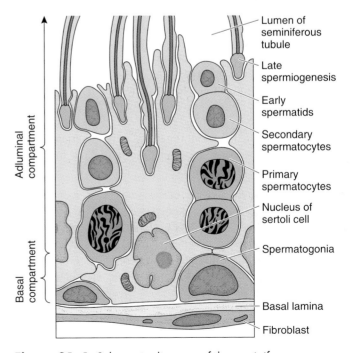

Figure 21–4. Schematic diagram of the seminiferous epithelium.

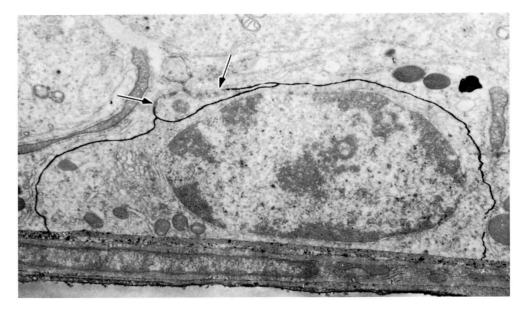

Figure 21–5. Electron micrograph of the basal compartment of the seminiferous epithelium (× 15,000). Observe that the testis was perfused with an electron-dense tracer, lanthanum nitrate, to demonstrate that the occluding junctions (arrows) between adjacent Sertoli cells prevent the lanthanum nitrate from entering the adluminal compartment. (From Leeson, T.S., Leeson, C.R., and Papparo, A.A.: Text/Atlas of Histology. Philadelphia, W.B. Saunders Company, 1988.)

Spermatogenic Cells

Most of the cells composing the thick seminiferous epithelium are **spermatogenic cells** in various stages of maturation (see Fig. 21–4). Some of these cells, **spermatogonia,** are located in the basal compartment, whereas the great majority of the developing cells—**primary spermatocytes, secondary spermatocytes, spermatids,** and **spermatozoa**—occupy the adluminal compartment. Spermatogonia are diploid cells that undergo mitotic division to form more spermatogonia as well as primary spermatocytes, which migrate from the basal into the adluminal compartment. Primary spermatocytes enter the first **meiotic division** to form secondary spermatocytes, which undergo the **second meiotic division** to form **haploid** cells known as **spermatids.** These haploid cells are transformed into spermatozoa (mature sperm) by shedding much of their cytoplasm, rearranging their organelles, and forming a flagellum.

The various cell types that result from this process of cell maturation, called **spermatogenesis,** are diagrammed in Figure 21–6. The maturation process is divided into three phases:

- **Spermatocytogenesis:** differentiation of spermatogonia into primary spermatocytes
- **Meiosis:** reduction division whereby diploid primary spermatocytes reduce their chromosome complement, forming haploid spermatids
- **Spermiogenesis:** transformation of spermatids into spermatozoa (sperm)

DIFFERENTIATION OF SPERMATOGONIA (SPERMATOCYTOGENESIS).
Spermatogonia are small, diploid germ cells located in the basal compartment of the seminiferous tubules (see Figs. 21–5 and 21–6). These cells lie on the basal lamina and, subsequent to puberty, become influenced by testosterone to enter the cell cycle. There are three categories of spermatogonia: dark type A, pale type A, and type B.

Dark type-A spermatogonia are small (12 μm in diameter), dome-shaped cells. These cells have oval (flattened) nuclei with abundant heterochromatin, imparting a dense appearance to the nucleus. Dark type-A spermatogonia are **reserve cells** that have *not* entered the cell cycle but may do so. Once they undergo mitosis, they form additional dark type-A spermatogonia as well as pale type-A spermatogonia.

Pale type-A spermatogonia are identical to the dark type-A cells except for the appearance of their nuclei. These nuclei have abundant euchromatin, imparting a pale coloration to the oval nuclei. These cells have only a few organelles, including mitochondria, a limited Golgi complex, some RER, and numerous free ribosomes. These cells are induced by testosterone to *proliferate* and give rise, by mitosis, to additional pale type-A spermatogonia and to type-B spermatogonia.

Type-B spermatogonia resemble pale type-A spermatogonia, but usually their nuclei are round rather than flattened. These cells also divide mitotically to give rise to primary spermatocytes.

MEIOTIC DIVISION OF SPERMATOCYTES.
As soon as **primary spermatocytes** are formed, they migrate from the basal into the adluminal compartment. As they migrate between adjacent Sertoli cells, they form zonulae occludentes with the Sertoli cells and thus help maintain the integrity of the blood–testis barrier. Primary spermatocytes are the largest cells of the seminiferous epithelium (see Fig. 21–4). They have large, vesicular-appearing nuclei whose chromosomes are in various stages of condensation. Shortly

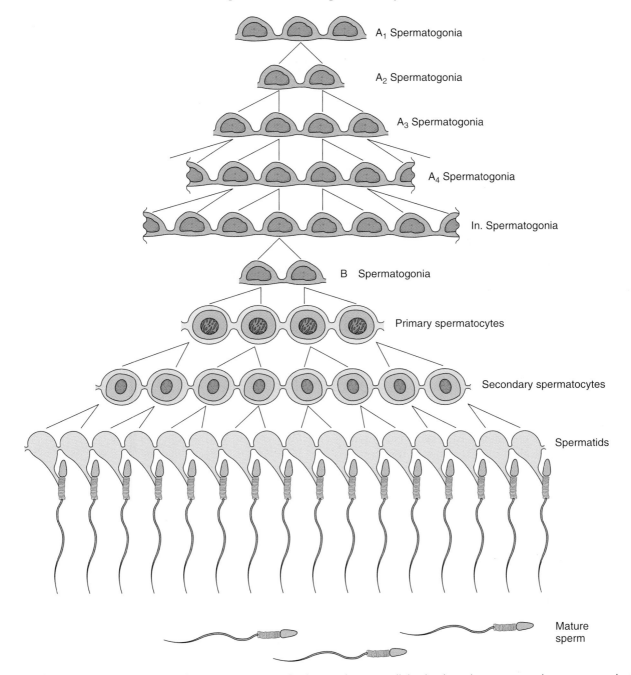

Figure 21–6. A schematic diagram of spermatogenesis, displaying the intercellular bridges that maintain the syncytium during differentiation and maturation. (Modified after Ren, X.-D., and Russell, L.: Clonal development of interconnected germ cells in the rat and its relationship to the segmental and subsegmental organization of spermatogenesis. Am. J. Anat. **192:**127, 1991. Reprinted with permission of John Wiley & Sons, Inc.)

after their formation, primary spermatocytes duplicate their chromosomes to obtain a 4N DNA content (and diploid chromosome number). During the **first meiotic division** the DNA content is halved (to 2N DNA) in each daughter cell, and the chromosome number is reduced to haploid. During the **second meiotic division** the DNA content of each new daughter cell is reduced to haploid (1N DNA), whereas the chromosome number remains unaltered (haploid).

Prophase I of the first meiotic division lasts for 22 days and involves four stages: leptotene, zygotene, pachytene, and diakinesis. The chromosomes of a primary spermatocyte begin to condense, forming long threads during **leptotene** and pair with their homologues during **zygotene.** Further condensation yields short, thick chromosomes, recognizable as tetrads, during **pachytene.** The exchange of segments **(crossing-over)** of homologous chromosomes occurs during **diakinesis;** this random genetic recombination results in the unique genome of each gamete and contributes to the variation of the gene pool.

During **metaphase I** the paired homologous chromosomes line up at the equatorial plate. The members of each pair then migrate to opposite poles of the cell in **anaphase I,** and the daughter cells separate (although a cytoplasmic bridge remains), forming 2 secondary spermatocytes during **telophase I.**

Because the homologous chromosomes are segregated during anaphase, the X and Y chromosomes are sorted into separate secondary spermatocytes, eventually forming spermatozoa that carry either X or Y chromosomes. Thus it is the spermatozoon that will determine the chromosomal sex of the future embryo.

Secondary spermatocytes are relatively small cells and, because they are short-lived, they are not readily seen in the seminiferous epithelium. These cells, which contain 2N DNA, do not replicate their chromosomes; they quickly enter the second meiotic division, forming two haploid (1N DNA) spermatids.

During mitosis of spermatogonia and meiosis of spermatocytes, nuclear division **(karyokinesis)** is accompanied by a **modified cytokinesis.** As each cell divides to form two cells, a **cytoplasmic bridge** remains between them, holding the newly formed cells tethered to each other (see Fig. 21–6). Because this incomplete division occurs over a number of mitotic and meiotic events, it results in the formation of a **syncytium,** a large number of spermatids that are connected to one another. Because of this connection, the spermatogenic cells can communicate with each other and thus can synchronize their activities.

CLINICAL CORRELATIONS

The most common abnormality due to nondisjunction of the XX homologues is known as **Klinefelter's syndrome.** Persons afflicted with this syndrome usually have XXY chromosomes (an extra X chromosome). They typically are infertile, are tall and thin, exhibit various degrees of masculine characteristics (including small testes), and are somewhat retarded mentally.

TRANSFORMATION OF SPERMATIDS (SPERMIO-GENESIS).

Spermatids are small, round haploid cells (8 μm in diameter). All the spermatids that arise from a single pale type-A spermatogonium are connected to each other by cytoplasmic bridges. They form small clusters and occupy a position near the lumen of the seminiferous tubule. These cells have abundant RER, numerous mitochondria, and a well-developed Golgi complex. During their transformation into spermatozoa they accumulate hydrolytic enzymes, rearrange and reduce the number of their organelles, form a flagellum and associated skeletal apparatus, and shed some of their cytoplasm. This process of **spermiogenesis** is

subdivided into four phases: Golgi phase, cap phase (Fig. 21–7), acrosomal phase, and maturation phase (Fig. 21–8).

Golgi Phase. During the **Golgi phase** of spermiogenesis hydrolytic enzymes are formed on the RER, modified in the Golgi apparatus, and packaged by the **trans-Golgi network** as small, membrane-bounded **pre-acrosomal granules.** These small vesicles fuse with each other, forming an **acrosomal vesicle.** The hydrolytic enzymes in this vesicle are visualized with the electron microscope as an electron-dense material known as the **acrosomal granule.** The acrosomal vesicle comes into contact with and becomes bound to the nuclear envelope.

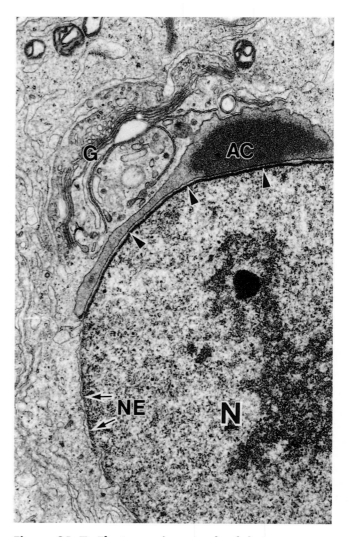

Figure 21–7. Electron micrograph of the cap stage of a rodent spermatid (× 18,000). AC, acrosome; G, Golgi apparatus; N, nucleus; NE, nuclear envelope. (From Oshako, S., Bunick, D., Hess, R.A., Nishida, T., Kurohmaru, M., and Hayashi, Y.: Characterization of a testis specific protein localized in the endoplasmic reticulum of spermatogenic cells. *Anat. Rec.* **238:**335–348, 1994. Reprinted with permission of John Wiley & Sons, Inc.)

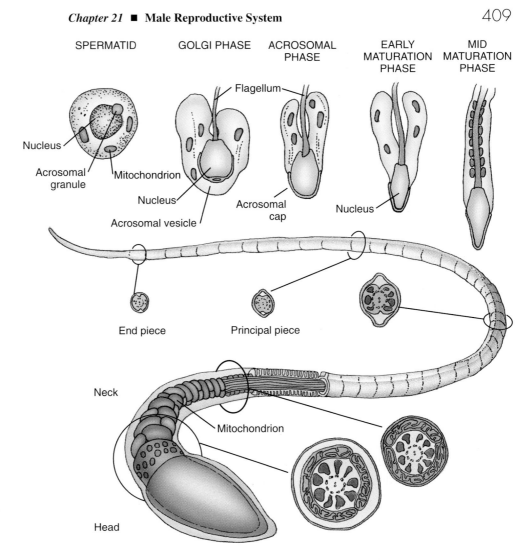

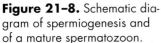

Figure 21–8. Schematic diagram of spermiogenesis and of a mature spermatozoon.

As the acrosomal vesicle is being formed, the centrioles leave the vicinity of the nucleus, and one of them participates in the formation of the **flagellar axoneme.** After the generation of the microtubules is initiated, the centrioles return to the nucleus and help form the **connecting piece,** a structure that will surround the centrioles and that is discussed later in the description of the spermatozoon.

Cap Phase. During the **cap phase** the acrosomal vesicle increases in size, and its membrane partially surrounds the nucleus (see Fig. 21–7). As this vesicle enlarges to its final size it becomes known as the **acrosome (acrosomal cap).**

Acrosomal Phase. The **acrosomal phase** is characterized by several alterations in the morphology of the spermatid. The nucleus becomes condensed, the cell elongates, and the mitochondria shift location.

The chromosomes become tightly condensed and become tightly packaged. As the chromosomal volume decreases, the volume of the entire nucleus is also reduced. Additionally, the nucleus becomes flattened and assumes its specific morphology.

Microtubules assemble to form a cylindrical structure, known as the **manchette,** which aid the elongation of the spermatid. As the elongating cytoplasm reaches the microtubules of the flagellar axoneme, the manchette microtubules disassemble. Their place is assumed by the **annulus,** an electron-dense, ring-like structure that will delineate the union of the spermatozoon tail's mid-piece with its principal piece (see Fig. 21–8).

As the spermatid elongates, its mitochondria become collected in the region just behind the nucleus. Here they form a cylindrical sheath of mitochondria surrounding the region of the axoneme that is located in the vicinity of the nucleus, thus establishing the **middle piece** of the tail of the spermatozoon.

During formation of the mitochondrial sheath and the elongation of the spermatid, nine columns of **outer dense fibers** form around the axoneme. These dense fibers are attached to the connecting piece formed during the Golgi phase. After their establishment, the dense fibers become surrounded by ribs, a series of ring-like, dense structures known as the **fibrous sheath.**

Maturation Phase. The **maturation phase** is characterized by the shedding of spermatid cytoplasm. As the excess cytoplasm is released, the syncytium is disrupted and individual spermatozoa are liberated from the large cellular mass. The cytoplasmic remnants are phagocytosed by Sertoli cells, and the disengaged spermatozoa are released (**spermiation**) into the lumen of the seminiferous tubule.

It is important to note that the newly formed spermatozoa are **immotile** and cannot fertilize an oocyte. Only after they enter the female reproductive system do spermatozoa become **capacitated** (i.e., they become motile and capable of fertilization).

STRUCTURE OF SPERMATOZOA. The **spermatozoa (sperm)** produced by spermatogenesis are long cells, about 65 μm in length. Each spermatozoon is composed of a **head,** housing the nucleus, and a tail, which accounts for most of its length (see Fig. 21–8; Fig. 21–9).

Head of the Spermatozoon. The flattened head of the spermatozoon is about 5 μm long and is surrounded by the plasmalemma (see Fig. 21–8). It is occupied by the condensed electron-dense nucleus, containing 23 chromosomes, and the **acrosome** that partially surrounds the anterior aspect of the nucleus. The acrosome comes into contact with the cell membrane of the spermatozoon anteriorly and houses various enzymes, including neuraminidase, hyaluronidase, acid phosphatase, aryl sulfatase, and acrosin (a trypsin-like protease). Binding of a spermatozoon to a secondary oocyte triggers release of these enzymes, which digest the extracel-

lular matrix of the oocyte, thereby facilitating access of the spermatozoon to the plasma membrane of the oocyte (see Fig. 20–15). This process is called the **acrosomal reaction.**

Tail of the Spermatozoon. The tail of the spermatozoon is subdivided into four regions: the neck, middle piece, principal piece, and the end-piece (see Fig. 21–8). The plasmalemma of the head is continuous with the tail's plasma membrane.

The **neck** is about 5 μm length and connects the head to the remainder of the tail. It is composed of the cylindrical arrangement of the nine columns of the **connecting piece** that encircles the two centrioles, one of which is usually fragmented. The posterior aspects of the columnar densities are continuous with the nine **outer dense fibers.**

The **middle piece,** also about 5 μm long, is located between the neck and the principal piece. It is characterized by the presence of the mitochondrial sheath, which encircles the **outer dense fibers** and the central-most **axoneme.** The middle piece stops at the **annulus,** a ring-like, dense structure to which the plasmalemma adheres, thus preventing the mitochondrial sheath from moving caudally into the tail. Also at the annulus, two of the nine outer dense fibers terminate; the remaining seven continue into the principal piece.

The **principal piece,** the longest segment of the tail, is approximately 45 μm in length and extends from the annulus to the end-piece. The axoneme of the principal piece is continuous with that of the middle piece. Surrounding the axoneme are the seven outer dense fibers that are continuous with those of the middle piece and are surrounded, in turn, by the **fibrous sheath.** The principal piece tapers near its caudal extent, where both the outer dense fibers and the fibrous sheath terminate, and is continuous with the end-piece.

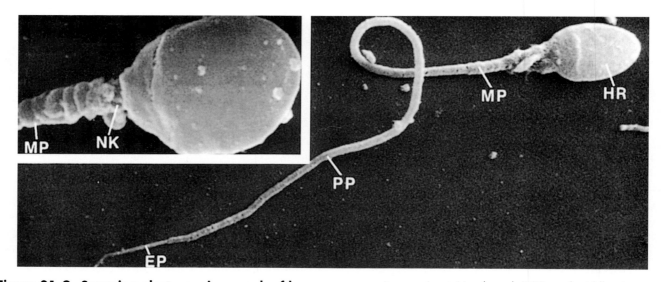

Figure 21–9. Scanning electron micrograph of human spermatozoa. Inset, Head, neck (NK), and middle piece (MP) (× 15,130). Figure, The entire spermatozoon. Head region (HR), middle piece (MP), principal piece (PP), and end-piece (EP) (× 6540). (From Kessel, R.G.: Tissue and Organs. A Text Atlas of Scanning Electron Microscopy. San Francisco, W.H. Freeman, 1979.)

The **end-piece,** which is only about 5 μm long, is composed of the central axoneme surrounded by plasmalemma. The axoneme is disorganized in the last 0.5 to 1.0 μm so that instead of the nine doublets and two singlets, 20 individual, haphazardly arranged microtubules are evident.

Cycle of the Seminiferous Epithelium

Because germ cells that arise from a single pale type-A spermatogonium are connected by cytoplasmic bridges and constitute a syncytium, they can communicate with each other

and synchronize their development. Careful examination of the human seminiferous epithelium reveals six possible characteristic associations of developing cell types, known as the six **stages of spermatogenesis,** as they are undergoing transformations to form spermatozoa (Fig. 21–10). Each cross-sectional profile of a seminiferous tubule may be subdivided into three or more wedge-shaped areas, each displaying a different stage of spermatogenesis.

Studies following the fate of ^{3}H-thymidine injected into the testes of human volunteers have demonstrated that radioactivity appears in 16-day intervals in the same stage of

Figure 21–10. Schematic diagram of the six stages of spermatogenesis in the human seminiferous tubule. (Redrawn from Clermont, Y.: The cycle of the seminiferous epithelium in man. Am. J. Anat. **112:** 35–52, 1963. Reprinted with permission of John Wiley & Sons, Inc.)

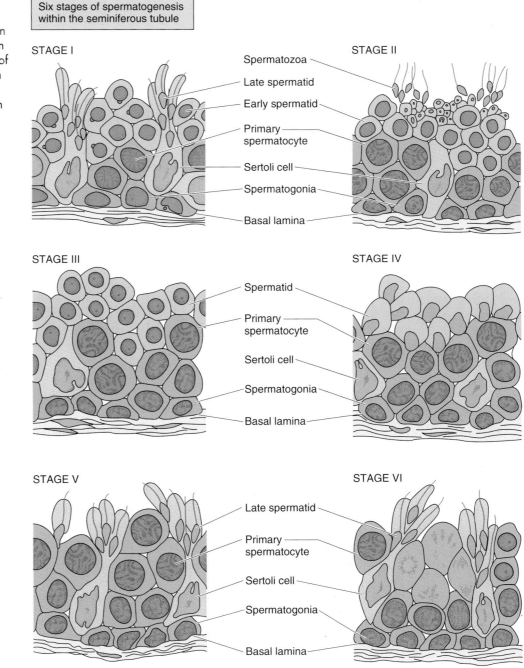

spermatogenesis. Each 16-day interval is known as a **cycle of the seminiferous epithelium,** and the process of spermatogenesis requires the passage of four cycles, or 64 days. Examination of serial cross-sections of a single seminiferous tubule reveals that the same stage of the seminiferous epithelium continues to reappear at specific distances along the length of the tubule. The distance between two identical stages of the seminiferous epithelium is known as the **wave of the seminiferous epithelium.** Thus in the human there are six repeating waves of the seminiferous epithelium, corresponding to the six stages.

Interstitial Cells of Leydig

The regions between coils of the seminiferous tubules are occupied by elements of the tunica vasculosa, a richly vascularized, loose connective tissue layer housing scattered fibroblasts, mast cells, and additional cellular constituents normally found in connective tissue. Also, dispersed throughout the tunica vasculosa are small collections of endocrine cells, the **interstitial cells (of Leydig),** which produce the hormone **testosterone.**

Interstitial cells of Leydig are polyhedral, are approximately 15 μm in diameter, and have a single nucleus (although occasionally they may be binucleate). They are typical steroid-producing cells that have mitochondria with tubular cristae, a large accumulation of smooth ER, and a well-developed Golgi apparatus (Fig. 21–11). These cells also house some RER and numerous lipid droplets, but they contain no secretory vesicles because testosterone is probably released as soon as its synthesis is complete. Lysosomes and peroxisomes are also evident, as are lipochrome pigments (especially in older men). The cytoplasm also contains crystallized proteins, the **crystals of Reinke,** a characteristic of human interstitial cells.

Histophysiology of the Testes

The major functions of the testes are the production of spermatozoa and the synthesis and release of testosterone.

The two testes form about 200 million spermatozoa per day by a process that may be considered to be a holocrine type of secretion. Sertoli cells of the seminiferous epithelium also produce a fluid that acts to nourish and transport the newly formed spermatozoa from the lumen of the seminiferous tubule to the extratesticular genital ducts.

Luteinizing hormone (LH), a gonadotropin released from the anterior pituitary, binds to LH receptors on the Leydig cells, activating adenylate cyclase to form cyclic adenosine monophosphate (cAMP). Activation of protein kinases of the Leydig cells by cAMP induces inactive cholesterol esterases to become active and cleave free cholesterol from intracellular lipid droplets. The free cholesterol is shuttled between the smooth endoplasmic reticulum and mitochon-

dria as it is converted into **testosterone,** the male hormone that is ultimately released by these cells (Fig. 21–12).

Because blood testosterone levels are not sufficient to initiate and maintain spermatogenesis, follicle stimulating hormone (FSH), another anterior pituitary gonadotropin, induces Sertoli cells to synthesize and release **androgen binding protein (ABP)** (Fig. 21–13). As its name implies, ABP binds testosterone, thereby preventing it from leaving the region of the seminiferous tubule and elevating the testosterone levels in the local environment sufficiently to sustain spermatogenesis.

Release of LH is inhibited by increased levels of testosterone, whereas FSH release is inhibited by the hormone **inhibin,** which is produced by Sertoli cells (see Fig. 21–13). It is interesting to note that estrogens, female sex hormones, are also bound by ABP and thus can reduce the levels of spermatogenesis.

Testosterone is also required for the normal functioning of the seminal vesicles, prostate, and bulbourethral glands, as well as for the appearance and maintenance of the male secondary sexual characteristics.

Genital Ducts

The genital ducts may be subdivided into two categories, those located within the testes (intratesticular genital ducts) and those located external to the testes (extratesticular genital) ducts.

Intratesticular Genital Ducts

The genital ducts located within the testis connect the seminiferous tubules to the epididymis. These intratesticular ducts are the tubuli recti and the rete testis (see Fig. 21–2).

Tubuli Recti

The **tubuli recti** are short, straight tubules that are continuous with the seminiferous tubules and deliver the spermatozoa, formed by the seminiferous epithelium, to the rete testis. These short tubules are lined by Sertoli cells in their first half, near the seminiferous tubule, and by a simple cuboidal epithelium in their second half, near the rete testis. The cuboidal cells have short, stubby microvilli and usually a single flagellum.

Rete Testis

The **rete testis** consists of labyrinthine spaces, lined by a simple cuboidal epithelium, within the mediastinum testis. These cuboidal cells, which resemble those of the tubuli recti, have numerous short microvilli with a single flagellum (Fig. 21–14).

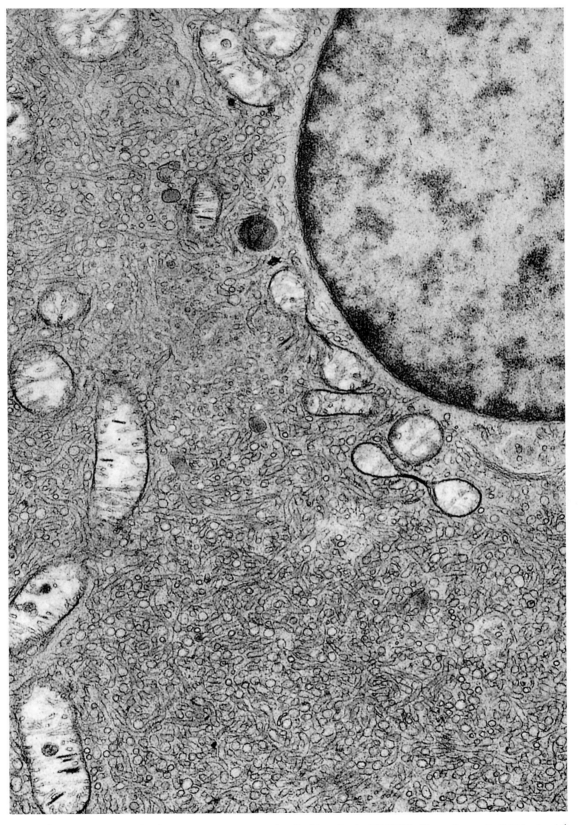

Figure 21-11. Electron micrograph of an opossum interstitial cell of Leydig (× 23,300). (From Fawcett, D.W.: An Atlas of Fine Structure. *The Cell*. Philadelphia, W.B. Saunders Company, 1966.)

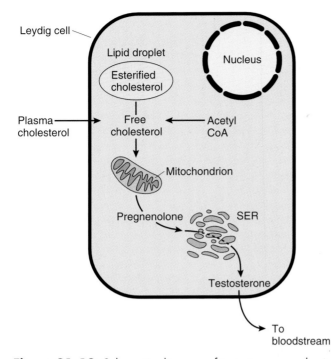

Figure 21-12. Schematic diagram of testosterone synthesis by interstitial cells of Leydig.

Extratesticular Genital Ducts

There are four types of extratesticular ducts associated with each testis: the ductuli efferentes and ductus epididymis, which together constitute the **epididymis,** and the ductus (vas) deferens and the ejaculatory duct (see Fig. 21–1). The epididymis secretes numerous factors that facilitate maturation of spermatozoa by an unknown mechanism. As noted previously, however, sperm cannot fertilize a secondary oocyte until they undergo **capacitation,** which is triggered by secretions produced in the female genital tract.

Ductuli Efferentes

The 10 to 20 **ductuli efferentes** are short tubules that drain spermatozoa from the rete testis and pierce the tunica albuginea of the testis to conduct the sperm to the ductus epididymis (see Fig. 21–2). The simple epithelial lining of the lumen of each ductule consists of patches of **nonciliated cuboidal cells** alternating with regions of **ciliated columnar cells.** The successive clusters of short and tall epithelial cells impart the characteristic festooned appearance to the lumina of the ductuli efferentes. The cuboidal cells are believed to resorb some of the luminal fluid elaborated by the Sertoli cells of the seminiferous tubule, whereas the cilia of the columnar cells probably move the spermatozoa toward the ductus epididymis.

The simple epithelium sits on a basal lamina that separates it from the thin, loose connective tissue wall of each ductule. The connective tissue is surrounded by a thin layer of smooth muscle whose cells are circularly arrayed.

Ductus Epididymis

Each **ductus epididymis** is a thin, long (approximately 4 to 6 m), highly convoluted tubule that is folded into a space only 7 cm long on the posterior aspect of the testis (see Fig. 21–2). The ductus epididymis may be subdivided into three regions, the head, body, and tail. The head, formed by the union of the 10 to 20 ductuli efferentes, becomes highly coiled and continues as the equally highly coiled body. The distal portion of the tail loses its convolutions as it becomes continuous with the ductus deferens. Spermatozoa are stored in the tail of the epididymis for a short period.

The lumen of the ductus epididymis is lined by a **pseudostratified epithelium** composed of two cell types: short basal cells and tall principal cells (Fig. 21–15).

The short **basal cells** of the ductus epididymis epithelium are pyramidal to polyhedral. They have round nuclei whose large accumulation of heterochromatin imparts a dense appearance to this structure. Their sparse cytoplasm is relatively clear with a scarcity of organelles. It is believed that these cells function as stem cells, regenerating the principal cells as the need arises.

The tall **principal cells** of the ductus epididymis epithelium have irregular, oval nuclei with one or two large nucleoli. The nuclei of these cells are much paler than those of the basal cells and are located basally within the cell. The cytoplasm of the principal cells houses abundant RER located between the nucleus and the basal plasmalemma. The cytoplasm also has a large, supranuclearly positioned Golgi complex, numerous profiles of apically located smooth ER, endolysosomes, and multivesicular bodies. The apical cell membranes of these cells display a profusion of pinocytotic and coated vesicles at the bases of the many **stereocilia** that project into the lumen of the epididymis. These long, branched, cellular extensions are clusters of nonmotile microvilli that appear to form clumps as they adhere to one another.

The principal cells resorb the luminal fluid, which is endocytosed by pinocytotic vesicles and delivered to the endolysosomes for disposal. Additionally, these cells phagocytose remnants of cytoplasm that were not removed by Sertoli cells. They also manufacture **glycerophosphocholine,** a glycoprotein that inhibits spermatozoon capacitation, thus preventing the spermatozoon from fertilizing a secondary oocyte until the sperm enters the female genital tract.

The epithelium of the ductus epididymis is separated by a basal lamina from the underlying loose connective tissue. A layer of circularly arranged smooth muscle cells surrounds the connective tissue layer. **Peristaltic contractions** of this layer help in conducting the spermatozoa to the ductus deferens.

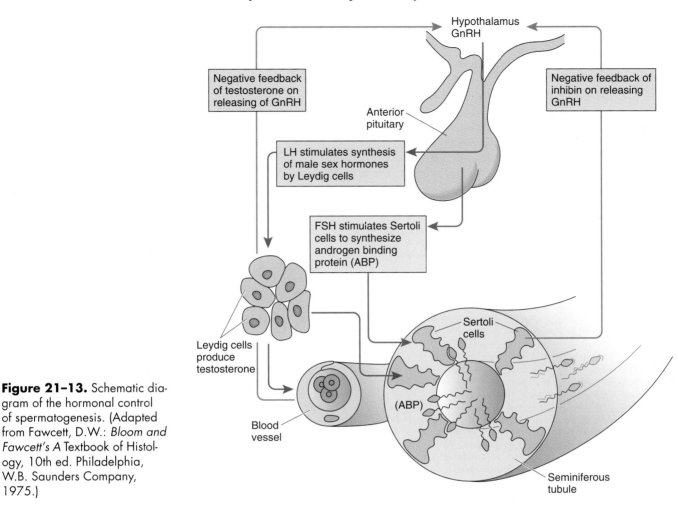

Figure 21-13. Schematic diagram of the hormonal control of spermatogenesis. (Adapted from Fawcett, D.W.: *Bloom and Fawcett's A* Textbook of Histology, 10th ed. Philadelphia, W.B. Saunders Company, 1975.)

Ductus (Vas) Deferens

Each **ductus deferens** (vas deferens) is a thick-walled muscular tube with a small, irregular lumen that conveys spermatozoa from the tail of the epididymis to the ejaculatory duct (see Figs. 21–1 and 21–2).

The stereociliated **pseudostratified columnar** epithelium of the ductus deferens is similar to that of the ductus epididymis, although the principal cells are shorter. A basal lamina separates the epithelium from the underlying loose fibroelastic connective tissue, which has numerous folds, thus making the lumen appear irregular. The thick smooth muscle coat surrounding the connective tissue is composed of three layers, inner and outer longitudinal layers with an intervening middle circular layer. The smooth muscle coat is invested by a thin layer of loose fibroelastic connective tissue.

CLINICAL CORRELATIONS

Because the ductus deferens has a 1-mm-thick muscular wall, it is easily perceptible through the skin of the scrotum as a dense, rolling tubule. **Vasectomy** is performed via a small slit through the scrotal sac, thus sterilizing the person.

The dilated terminus of each ductus deferens, known as the **ampulla,** has a highly folded, thickened epithelium. As the ampulla approaches the prostate gland, it is joined by the seminal vesicle. The continuation of the junction of the ampulla with the seminal vesicle is known as the ejaculatory duct.

Ejaculatory Duct

Each **ejaculatory duct** is a short, straight tubule that enters the substance of and is surrounded by the prostate gland (see Fig. 21–1). The duct ends as it pierces the posterior aspect of the prostatic urethra at the **colliculus seminalis.** The lumen of the ejaculatory duct is lined by a simple columnar epithelium. The subepithelial connective tissue is folded, which is responsible for the irregular appearance of its lumen. The ejaculatory duct has no smooth muscle in its wall.

Accessory Genital Glands

The male reproductive system has five **accessory glands,** the paired seminal vesicles, the single prostate gland, and the paired bulbourethral glands (see Fig. 21–1).

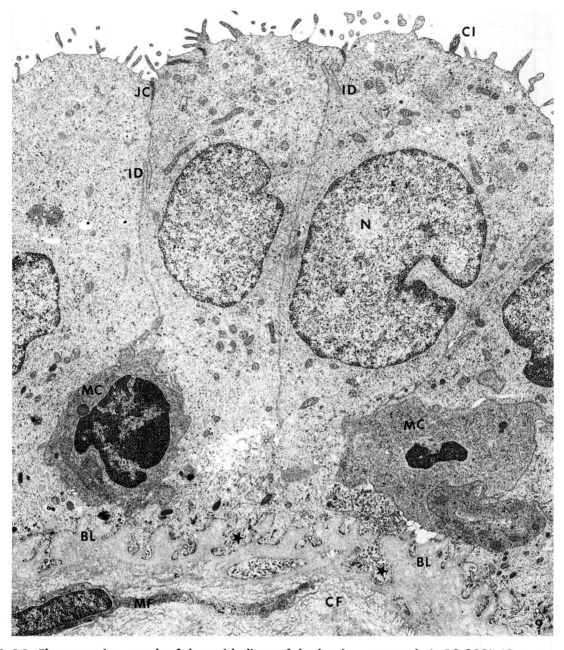

Figure 21–14. Electron micrograph of the epithelium of the bovine rete testis (× 19,900). JC, junctional complexes; N, nucleus; ID, interdigitation of the lateral plasmalemmae; BL, basal lamina; CF, collagen fibers; MF, myofibroblast; MC, mononuclear cell; CI, cilium. (From Hees, H., Wrobel, K. H., Elmagd, A.A., and Hees, I.: The mediastinum of the bovine testis. Cell Tissue Res. **255:**29–39, 1989. © Springer-Verlag.)

Seminal Vesicles

The paired seminal vesicles are highly coiled tubular structures about 15 cm long. They are located between the posterior aspect of the neck of the bladder and the prostate gland and join the ampulla of the ductus deferens just above the prostate gland.

The mucosa of the gland is highly convoluted, forming labyrinth-like cul-de-sacs that, in three dimensions, are ob-

served to open into a central lumen. The lumen is lined by a pseudostratified columnar epithelium composed of short basal cells and low columnar cells (Fig. 21–16).

The **columnar cells** have numerous short microvilli and a single flagellum projecting into the lumen of the gland. The cytoplasm of these cells displays RER, Golgi apparatus, numerous mitochondria, some lipid and lipochrome pigment droplets, and abundant secretory granules. The height of the cells varies directly with blood testosterone levels. The

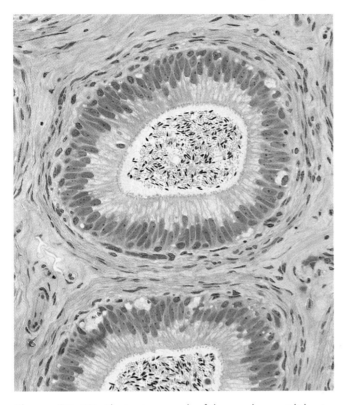

Figure 21–15. Photomicrograph of the monkey epididymis (× 270).

and main. Each tubuloalveolar gland has its own duct that delivers the secretory product of the secretory unit to the prostatic urethra. The **mucosal glands** are closest to the urethra and thus are the shortest of the glands. The **submucosal glands** are peripheral to the mucosal glands and are consequently larger than the mucosal glands. The largest and most numerous of the glands are the peripheral-most **main glands,** which compose the bulk of the prostate.

The glands of the prostate are lined by a simple to **pseudostratified columnar epithelium** (Fig. 21–18), whose cells are well endowed with organelles responsible for the synthesis and packaging of proteins. Hence there is abundant RER, a large Golgi apparatus, and numerous secretory granules (Fig. 21–19). These cells also have many lysosomes.

The lumina of the tubuloalveolar glands frequently house round to oval **prostatic concretions (corpora amylacia),** composed of calcified glycoproteins, whose numbers increase with the age of the person (see Fig. 21–18). The significance of these concretions, if any, is not understood.

The **prostatic secretion** constitutes a part of semen. It is a serous, white fluid rich in lipids, proteolytic enzymes, acid phosphatase, fibrinolysin, and citric acid. Its formation, synthesis, and release are regulated by the hormone **dihydrotestosterone.**

subepithelial connective tissue is **fibroelastic** and is surrounded by smooth muscle cells, arranged as an inner circular and an outer longitudinal layer. The **smooth muscle coat** is, in turn, surrounded by a flimsy layer of fibroelastic connective tissue.

The seminal vesicles once were believed to store spermatozoa, some of which are always present in the lumen of this gland. It is now known that these glands produce a viscous, yellow **fructose-rich fluid** that constitutes 70% of the volume of semen. The characteristic pale yellow color of semen is due to the lipochrome pigment released by the seminal vesicles.

Prostate Gland

The **prostate gland,** the largest of the accessory glands, is pierced by the urethra and the ejaculatory ducts (Fig. 21–17). The slender connective tissue **capsule** of the gland is composed of a richly vascularized, dense irregular collagenous connective tissue interspersed with **smooth muscle cells.** The connective tissue **stroma** of the gland is derived from the capsule and is therefore also enriched by smooth muscle fibers in addition to their normal connective tissue cells.

The prostate is actually a conglomeration of 30 to 50 individual **compound tubuloalveolar glands** that are arranged in three discrete, concentric layers: mucosal, submucosal,

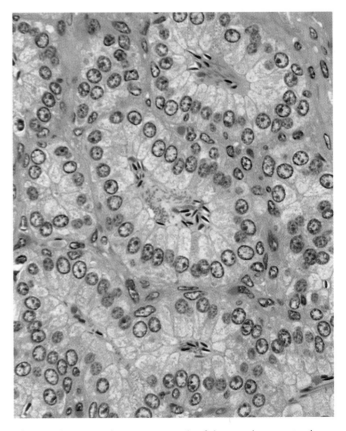

Figure 21–16. Photomicrograph of the monkey seminal vesicle (× 270).

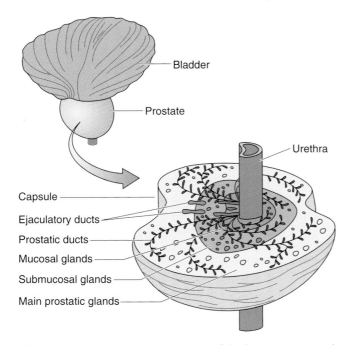

Figure 21-17. Schematic diagram of the human prostate illustrating the mucosal, submucosal, and main prostatic glands.

CLINICAL CORRELATIONS

As men age, the prostatic stroma and mucosal and submucosal glands begin to hypertrophy, a condition known as **benign prostatic hypertrophy.** The enlarged prostate partially strangulates the lumen of the urethra, resulting in difficulties with urination. At 50 years of age about 40% of the male population is afflicted with this condition; the percentage increases to 95% in 80-year-old men.

The second-most common form of cancer in men is **adenocarcinoma of the prostate.** It affects approximately 30% of the male population over the age of 75 years. Frequently the cancer cells enter the circulatory system and metastasize to bone. A simple blood test has been developed that may permit early detection of prostatic adenocarcinoma.

Bulbourethral Glands

The **bulbourethral glands (Cowper's glands)** are small, 3 to 5 mm in diameter, and they are located at the root of the penis just at the beginning of the membranous urethra (see Fig. 21-1). Their fibroelastic capsule has not only fibroblasts and smooth muscle cells but also skeletal muscle cells derived from the muscles of the urogenital diaphragm. Septa derived from the capsule divide this gland into several lobules. The epithelium of these compound tubuloalveolar glands varies from **simple cuboidal** to **simple columnar.**

The mucus produced by the bulbourethral glands is a thick, slippery fluid that probably functions to lubricate the lumen of the urethra. During the process of ejaculation this viscous fluid precedes the remainder of the semen.

Histophysiology of the Accessory Genital Glands

The bulbourethral glands produce a viscous slippery fluid that lubricates the lining of the urethra. It is the first of the glandular secretions to be released subsequent to erection of the penis. Just before ejaculation, secretions from the prostate are discharged into the urethra, as are the spermatozoa from the ampulla of the ductus deferens. The prostatic secretions apparently help the spermatozoa to achieve motility. The final secretions arise from the seminal vesicles, which are responsible for a significant increase in the volume of the semen. Their fructose-rich fluid is utilized by the spermatozoa for energy.

The ejaculate, known as **semen,** is about 3 ml in volume in humans and consists of secretions from the accessory glands and 200 to 300 million spermatozoa.

Penis

The **penis** functions both as an excretory organ for urine and as the male copulatory organ for the deposition of spermatozoa into the female reproductive tract. The penis is composed of three columns of **erectile tissue,** each enclosed by its own dense, fibrous connective tissue capsule, the **tunica albuginea** (Fig. 21-20).

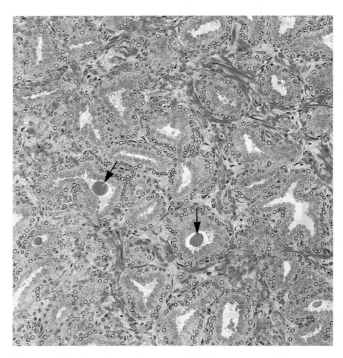

Figure 21-18. Photomicrograph of the prostate of a monkey. Prostatic concretions (*arrows*) (× 132).

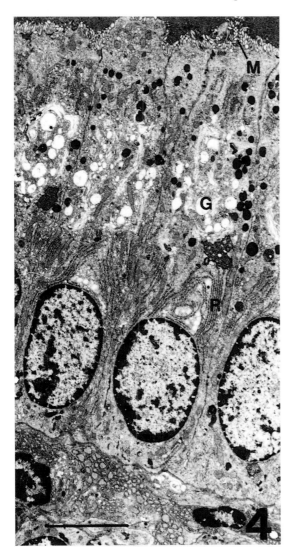

Figure 21–19. Electron micrograph of the hamster prostate. M, microvilli; G, Golgi apparatus; R, rough endoplasmic reticulum. Bar = 5 μm. (From Toma, J.G., and Buzzell, G.R.: Fine structure of the ventral and dorsal lobes of the prostate in the young adult Syrian hamster, Mesocricetus auratus. Am. J. Anat. **181**:132–140, 1988. Reprinted with permission of John Wiley & Sons, Inc.)

Two columns of erectile tissue, the **corpora cavernosa,** are positioned dorsally; their tunica albugineae are discontinuous in places, permitting communication between their erectile tissues. The third column of erectile tissue, the **corpus spongiosum,** is positioned ventrally. Because the corpus spongiosum houses the penile portion of the urethra, it is therefore also called the **corpus cavernosum urethrae.** The corpus spongiosum ends distally in an enlarged, bulbous portion, the **glans penis** (head of the penis). The tip of the glans penis is pierced by the end of the urethra as a vertical slit.

The three corpora are surrounded by a common loose connective tissue sheath, but no hypodermis, and are covered by thin skin. The skin of the proximal portion of the penis has coarse pubic hairs and numerous sweat and sebaceous glands. The distal portion of the penis is hairless and has only a few sweat glands. Skin continues distal to the glans penis to form a retractable sheath, the **prepuce,** which is lined by a mucous membrane, a moist, stratified squamous nonkeratinized epithelium.

Structure of Erectile Tissue

Erectile tissue of the penis contains numerous variably shaped, endothelially lined spaces that are separated from one another by trabeculae of connective tissue and smooth muscle cells. The vascular spaces of the corpora cavernosa are larger centrally and smaller peripherally near the tunica albuginea. However, the vascular spaces of the corpus spongiosum are similar in size throughout its extent. It is interesting to note that the trabeculae of the corpus spongiosum contain more elastic fibers and fewer smooth muscle cells than do those of the corpora cavernosa.

The erectile tissues of the corpora cavernosa receive blood from branches of the **deep** and **dorsal arteries of the penis** (see Fig. 21–20). These branches enter the walls of the trabeculae of the erectile tissue and either form capillary

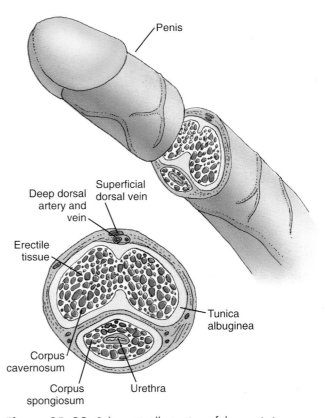

Figure 21–20. Schematic illustration of the penis in cross-section.

plexuses, which supply some blood flow into the vascular spaces, or form coiled arteries **(helical arteries),** which are important sources of blood to the vascular spaces during erection of the penis.

Venous drainage occurs via three groups of veins, which are drained by the **deep dorsal vein** (see Fig. 21–20). The three groups of veins arise from the base of the glans penis, from the dorsal aspect of the corpora cavernosa, and from the ventral aspect of the corpora cavernosa and the corpus spongiosum. Additionally some of the veins leave the erectile tissue at the root of the penis and drain into the plexus of veins that drain the prostate gland.

Mechanisms of Erection, Ejaculation, and Detumescence

When the penis is flaccid, the vascular spaces of the erectile tissue contain little blood. In this condition much of the arterial blood flow is diverted into arteriovenous anastomoses that connect the branches of the deep and dorsal arteries of the penis to veins that deliver their blood into the deep dor-

sal vein (Fig. 21–21A). Thus, the blood flow bypasses the vascular spaces of the erectile tissue. **Erection** occurs when blood flow is shifted to the vascular spaces of the erectile tissues (the corpora cavernosa and, to a limited extent, the corpus spongiosum), causing the penis to enlarge and become turgid (Fig. 21–21B). During erection the tunica albuginea surrounding the erectile tissues is stretched and decreases in thickness from 2 mm to 0.5 mm.

The shift in blood flow that leads to erection is controlled by the **parasympathetic** nervous system following sexual stimulation (e.g., pleasurable tactile, olfactory, visual, auditory, and psychological stimuli). The parasympathetic impulses trigger local release of **nitric oxide,** which causes relaxation of smooth muscles of the branches of the deep and dorsal arteries of the penis, increasing the flow of blood into the organ. Simultaneously, the arteriovenous anastomoses undergo constriction, diverting the flow of blood into the helical arteries of the erectile tissue. As these spaces become engorged with blood, the penis enlarges and becomes turgid, and erection ensues. The veins of the penis become compressed, and the blood is trapped in the vascular spaces

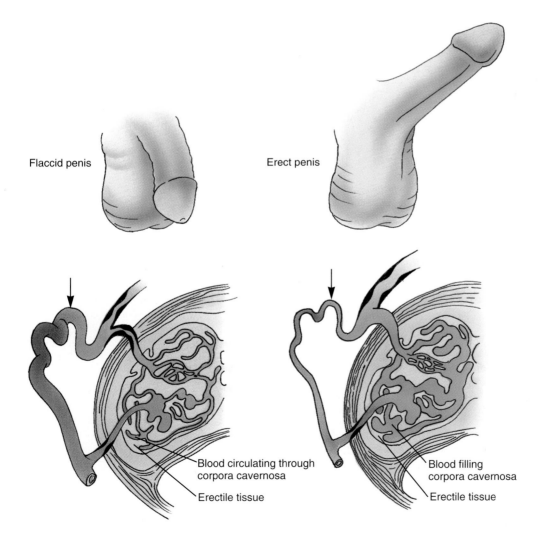

Figure 21–21. Schematic illustration of circulation in the flaccid and erect penis. Note that the arteriovenous anastomosis (*arrow*) in the flaccid penis is wide, diverting blood flow into the venous drainage, whereas in the erect penis the arteriovenous anastomosis is constricted and blood flow into the vascular spaces of the erectile tissue is increased, making the penis turgid with blood. (Adapted from Conti, G.: Acta Anat. **5:**217, 1952.)

Flaccid penis

Erect penis

Blood circulating through corpora cavernosa

Erectile tissue

Blood filling corpora cavernosa

Erectile tissue

of the erectile tissue, thus maintaining the penis in an erect condition (see Fig. 21–21).

Continued stimulation of the glans penis results in **ejaculation,** the forceful expulsion of **semen** from the male genital ducts. Each ejaculate, which has a volume of about 3 ml in humans, consists of secretions from the accessory genital glands and 200 to 300 million spermatozoa. Subsequent to erection, the bulbourethral glands release a viscous fluid that lubricates the lining of the urethra. Just before ejaculation, the prostate gland discharges its secretion into the urethra, and spermatozoa from the ampullae of the two ductus deferentes are released into the ejaculatory ducts. The prostatic secretion apparently helps the spermatozoa to achieve motility. The final secretion added to semen is a fructose-rich fluid, released from the seminal vesicles, that provides energy to the spermatozoa. This secretion forms much of the volume of the ejaculate.

CLINICAL CORRELATIONS

A single ejaculate normally contains approximately 50 to 100 million spermatozoa per milliliter. A man whose sperm count is less than 20 million spermatozoa per milliliter is considered **sterile.**

The inability to achieve erection is known as **impotence.** Temporary impotence can result from psychological factors or drugs (e.g., alcohol), whereas permanent impotence is caused by neurological or vascular pathologies.

Ejaculation, unlike erection, is regulated by the **sympathetic nervous system.** These impulses trigger the following sequence of events:

- Contraction of the smooth muscles of the genital ducts and accessory genital glands force the semen into the urethra.
- The sphincter muscle of the urinary bladder contracts, preventing the release of urine (or the entry of semen into the bladder).
- The bulbospongiosus muscle, which surrounds the proximal end of the corpus spongiosum (bulb of the penis), undergoes powerful, rhythmic contractions, resulting in forceful expulsion of semen from the urethra.

Ejaculation is followed by the cessation of parasympathetic impulses to the vascular supply of the penis. As a result, the atriovenous shunt is reopened, blood flow through the deep and dorsal arteries of the penis is diminished, and the vascular spaces of the erectile tissues are slowly emptied of blood by the venous drainage. As the blood leaves these vascular spaces, the penis undergoes **detumescence** and becomes flaccid.

Special Senses

22

Peripheral nerve terminals are of two structural types: (1) terminals of axons, which transmit impulses from the central nervous system (CNS) to skeletal and smooth muscles (**motor endings**) or to glands (**secretory endings**) and (2) terminals of dendrites, called **sensory endings** or **receptors,** which perceive various stimuli and transmit this sensory input to the CNS. These sensory receptors are classified into three types depending on the source of the stimulus— exteroceptors, proprioceptors, and interoceptors—and are components of the general or special somatic and visceral afferent pathways.

Exteroceptors, which are located near the body surface, are specialized to perceive stimuli from the external environment. Those receptors sensitive to temperature, touch, pressure, and pain are components of the **general somatic afferent** pathways; they are described in the first part of this chapter. Other exteroceptors are specialized for perceiving light (sense of vision) and sound (sense of hearing); these receptors, which are components of the **special somatic afferent** pathways, are discussed later in this chapter. Smell and taste stimuli are perceived by unique nerve endings in the viscera of the respiratory and digestive systems, respectively; these exteroceptors are classified as the **special visceral afferent** modality. The receptors for olfaction (sense of smell) are discussed in Chapter 15, and the receptors of taste are discussed in Chapter 16.

Proprioceptors are specialized receptors located in joint capsules, tendons, and intrafusal fibers within muscles (see Chapter 8). These **general somatic afferent** receptors transmit sensory input to the CNS, which is translated into information that relates to an awareness of the body in space and in movement. Certain receptors of the **vestibular** (balance) mechanism located within the inner ear are specialized in receiving stimuli related to motion vectors within the head; this input is transmitted to the brain for processing into awareness of motion for corrective balancing. The vestibular mechanisms are discussed later in this chapter.

Interoceptors are specialized receptors that perceive sensory information from within organs of the body; therefore, the modality serving this function is **general visceral afferent.**

Specialized Peripheral Receptors

The dendritic endings of certain sensory receptors located in various regions of the body, including muscles, tendons, skin, fascia, and joint capsules, are specialized to receive particular stimuli. These adaptations help the dendrite to respond to a particular stimulus. These receptors are classified into three types: **mechanoreceptors** that respond to touch (Fig. 22–1); **thermoreceptors** that respond to cold and warmth; and **nociceptors** that respond to pain due to mechanical stress, extremes of temperature differences, and chemical substances. Although these specialized receptors generally are triggered only by a particular stimulus, any stimulus that is intense enough will trigger any receptor.

Mechanoreceptors

Mechanoreceptors respond to mechanical stimuli that may deform the receptor or the tissues about the receptor. Stimuli that trigger the mechanoreceptors include touch, stretch, vibrations, and pressure.

Nonencapsulated Mechanoreceptors

Peritrical nerve endings, the simplest form of mechanoreceptors, are unmyelinated, lack Schwann cells, and are not covered by a connective tissue capsule. Such nerve endings are located in the epidermis of skin and in the cornea of the eye, where they respond to stimuli related to touch and pressure (see Fig. 22–1D). Still peritrical nerve endings are wrapped around the base and shaft of hair follicles. These function in touch perception related to the deformation of the hairs. Peritrical nerve endings are sensitive. A few naked nerve endings function as nociceptors or as thermoreceptors.

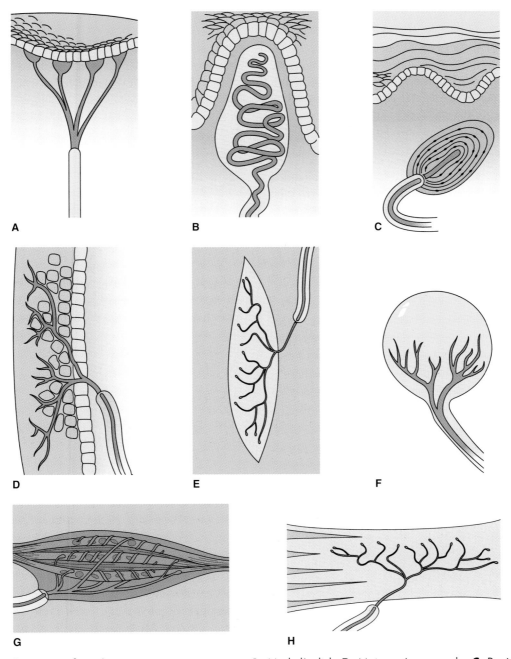

Figure 22–1. Diagram of various sensory receptors. A, Merkel's disk. **B,** Meissner's corpuscle. **C,** Pacinian corpuscle.
D, Peritricial (naked) nerve endings. **E,** Ruffini's corpuscle. **F,** Krause's end bulb. **G,** Neuromuscular spindle. **J,** Golgi tendon
organ.

Merkel's disks are slightly more complex mechanoreceptors (see Fig. 22–1A). Specialized for perceiving discriminatory touch, these receptors are composed of an expanded unmyelinated nerve terminal associated with **Merkel's cells,** specialized epithelial cells in the skin (see Fig. 14–1). These receptors are located mostly in nonhairy skin and regions of the body more sensitive to touch.

Encapsulated Mechanoreceptors

Several types of mechanoreceptors are encapsulated by a connective tissue capsule. These more complex receptors exhibit characteristic structures and location.

Meissner's corpuscles are encapsulated mechanoreceptors specialized for **tactile discrimination.** These receptors are located in the dermal papillae of the glabrous (nonhairy) portion of the fingers and palms of the hands, where they account for about half of the tactile receptors. They also are located in the skin of the foot, eyelids, lips, tongue, nipples, and forearm. Meissner's corpuscles, which measure 80 μm × 30 μm, are located in the dermal papillae with their long axis oriented perpendicular to the skin (see Fig. 22–1B). Each Meissner's corpuscle is formed by three or four nerve terminals and their associated Schwann cells, all of which are encapsulated by connective tissue. Contained within the capsule are stacks of epithelioid cells, possibly modified Schwann cells or fibroblasts, that serve to separate the branching nerve terminals. Meissner's corpuscles are especially sensitive to edges and points and to movements of these objects.

Pacinian corpuscles, another of the encapsulated mechanoreceptors, are located in the dermis and hypodermis in the digits of the hands and in the breasts, as well as in connective tissue of joints and the deep fascia about the mesenteries. These mechanoreceptors are specialized to perceive pressure, touch, and vibration. Pacinian corpuscles are large, ovoid receptors measuring 1 to 2 mm in length by 0.1 to 0.7 mm in diameter (see Fig. 22–1C). Each receptor is composed of a single unmyelinated fiber that courses the entire length of the corpuscle. The **core** of the corpuscle contains the nonmyelinated nerve terminal and its Schwann cells, surrounded by approximately 60 layers of modified fibroblasts, each layer separated from the next by a small fluid-filled space. An additional group of 30 less-dense modified fibroblasts surround the core and are in turn enveloped by connective tissue, forming the **capsule** around the core. The arrangement of the cells in the lamellae makes the histological section of a pacinian corpuscle resemble a sliced onion.

Ruffini's endings (corpuscles) are encapsulated endings located in the dermis of the skin, nail beds, and joint capsules. These large receptors, measuring 1 mm in length by 0.2 mm in diameter (see Fig. 22–1E), are composed of branched nonmyelinated terminals interspersed with collagen fibers and surrounded by four to five layers of modified fibroblasts. The connective tissue capsule surrounding each of these receptors is anchored at each end, which increases their sensibility to stretching and pressure in the skin and in the joint capsules.

Krause's end bulbs are spherical, encapsulated nerve endings located in the papillary region of the dermis (see Fig. 22–1F). Originally, they were thought to be receptors sensitive to cold, but present evidence does not support this concept. Their function is unknown.

Golgi tendon organs and **muscle spindle receptor organs** are both encapsulated mechanoreceptors involved in proprioception. Golgi tendon organs are stretch receptors located at the interface between the muscle and its tendon, where they perceive stretch and tension being exerted on the tendon (see Fig. 22–1H). Muscle spindle receptor organs, also called **neuromuscular spindles,** are specialized receptors located in skeletal muscle. These receptors are composed of from 3 to 12 small, intrafusal muscle fibers encapsulated by a collagenous sheath (see Fig. 22–1G). Both primary and secondary afferent fibers enter one end of the organ and become specialized into annulospiral endings and flower spray endings, receptors that react to changes in muscle tension and muscle length. Golgi tendon organs and muscle spindle receptor organs are discussed in Chapter 8.

Thermoreceptors

Thermoreceptors respond to temperature differences of about 2° C. They are grouped into three categories: warmth receptors, cold receptors, and temperature-sensitive nociceptors. Although specific receptors have not been identified for warmth, it is assumed that these receptors are naked endings of small nonmyelinated nerve fibers that respond to temperature increases. Cold receptors, on the other hand, are derived from naked nerve endings of myelinated fibers that branch and penetrate the epidermis. Because thermoreceptors are not activated by physical stimulation, they are thought to respond to differing rates of temperature-dependent biochemical reactions.

Nociceptors

Nociceptors are responsible for pain perception. These receptors are naked endings of myelinated nerve fibers that branch freely in the dermis before entering the epidermis. Nociceptors are divided into three groups: those that respond to mechanical stress or damage, those that respond to extremes in heat or cold, and those that respond to chemical compounds (e.g., bradykinin, serotonin, histamine).

Eye

The eyes (orbs), which measure about 24 mm in diameter, are located within the hollow bony orbits. They are the **photosensory organs** of the body. Light passes through the cornea, lens, and several refractory structures within the orb; light then is focused by the lens on a light-sensitive portion of the neural tunic of the eye, the **retina,** which contains the photosensitive **rods** and **cones.** Through a series of several layers of nerve cells and supporting cells, the visual information is transmitted by the optic nerve to the brain for processing.

The eyes begin to develop from three sources at about 4 weeks of embryonic development. Outgrowths of the forebrain, the future retina and optic nerve are the first to be observed. As a result of continued growth of this structure, the surface ectoderm is induced to develop into the lens and some of the accessory structures of the anterior portion of the eye. Later in development, adjacent mesenchyme condenses to form the tunics and associated structures of the orb.

The bulb of the eye is composed of three tunics (coats): a **fibrous tunic,** forming the tough outer coat of the eye; a

vascular tunic, the pigmented and vascular middle coat; and a **neural tunic,** the retina, composing the innermost coat (Fig. 22–2).

The fibrous tunic of the eye also receives insertions of the **extrinsic muscles** of the eye, which are responsible for coordinated movements of the eyes to gain access to various visual fields. Smooth muscles located within the orb accommodate focusing of the lens and control the aperture of the pupil. Located outside the orb, but still within the orbit, is the **lacrimal gland** (tear gland), which secretes **lacrimal fluid** (tears) that moisten the anterior surface of the eye. The lacrimal fluid moistens the eye and the inner surface of the eyelids by passing through the **conjunctiva,** a transparent membrane, which covers and protects the anterior surface of the eye.

Tunica Fibrosa

The external fibrous tunic of the eye, the **tunica fibrosa,** is divided into the **sclera** and the **cornea** (see Fig. 22–2). The white, opaque **sclera** covers the posterior five sixths of the orb, whereas the colorless, transparent **cornea** covers the anterior one sixth of the orb.

Sclera

The **sclera,** the white of the eye, is nearly devoid of blood vessels. It is a tough fibrous connective tissue layer about 1 mm thick posteriorly, thinning at the equator and then thickening again near its junction with the cornea. It consists of intersecting type I collagen bundles alternating with networks of elastic fibers; this arrangement gives form to the orb, which is maintained by intraocular pressure from the aqueous humor located anterior to the lens and the vitreous body located posterior to the lens.

Fibroblasts located in the connective tissue of the sclera are flat and elongated. Melanocytes are located in deeper regions of the sclera. Tendons of the extraocular muscles insert into the dense connective tissue surface layer of the sclera, which is covered by the **capsule of Tenon,** a fascial

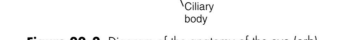

Figure 22–2. Diagram of the anatomy of the eye (orb).

sheath that covers the optic nerve and the orb as far anteriorly as the ciliary region. This sheath, which separates the orb from the periorbital fat, is connected to the sclera by a thin layer of loose connective tissue called the **episclera.**

Cornea

The **cornea** is the transparent, avascular, and highly innervated anterior portion of the fibrous tunic that bulges out anteriorly from the orb. It is slightly thicker than the sclera and is composed of five histologically distinct layers: corneal epithelium, membrane of Bowman, stroma, Descemet's membrane, and corneal endothelium.

The **corneal epithelium,** a continuation of the conjunctiva, is a stratified, squamous, nonkeratinized epithelium composed of five to seven layers of cells that covers the anterior surface of the cornea. The larger superficial cells have microvilli and exhibit zonulae occludentes. The remaining cells constituting this layer interdigitate and adhere to each other via desmosomes. Their cytoplasm contains the usual array of cytoplasmic organelles along with intermediate filaments. The corneal epithelium is highly innervated by numerous free nerve endings. Mitotic figures are observed mostly near the periphery. Damage to the cornea is repaired rapidly as cells migrate to the defect to cover the injured region. Subsequently, mitotic activity replaces the cells that migrated to the wound. The corneal epithelium also functions in transferring water and ions from the stroma into the conjunctival sac.

Bowman's membrane lies immediately deep to the corneal epithelium. Electron micrographs reveal it to be a fibrillar lamina, 6 to 9 μm thick, composed of type I collagen fibers arranged in an apparently random fashion. It is believed that Bowman's membrane is synthesized by both the corneal epithelium and cells of the underlying stroma. Sensory nerve fibers pass through this structure to enter the epithelium.

The transparent **stroma** is the thickest layer of the cornea, accounting for about 90% of its thickness. It is composed of collagenous connective tissue, consisting mostly of type I collagen fibers that are arranged in 200 to 250 lamellae. The collagen fibers within each lamella are arranged parallel to each other, but fiber orientation shifts in adjacent lamellae. The collagen fibers are interspersed with ground substance containing mostly chondroitin sulfate and keratan sulfate. Long, slender fibroblasts are also present among the collagen bundles. Lymphocytes and neutrophils are also abundant in this layer during inflammation. At the **limbus** (sclerocorneal junction) is a scleral sulcus whose inner aspect at the stroma is depressed and houses endothelial-lined spaces, known as the **trabecular meshwork,** that lead to the canal of Schlemm. The **canal of Schlemm** is the site of outflow of the aqueous humor from the anterior chamber of the eye to the venous system.

Descemet's membrane is a thick basement membrane interposed between the stroma and the underlying endothelium, which secreted it. Although this membrane is thin (5 μm at birth) and homogeneous in younger persons, electron microscopy has demonstrated that it becomes thicker (17 μm) and has cross-striations and hexagonal fiber patterns in older persons.

The **corneal endothelium,** which lines the internal (posterior) surface of the cornea, is formed of simple squamous epithelial cells. The corneal endothelium is also responsible for synthesis of proteins that may be necessary for maintaining Descemet's membrane. These cells exhibit numerous pinocytic vesicles, and their membranes have sodium pumps that transport Na$^+$ ions into the anterior chamber; these ions are passively followed by Cl$^-$ ions and water. Thus, excess fluid within the stroma is resorbed by the endothelium, keeping the stroma relatively dehydrated, a factor that contributes to maintaining the refractive quality of the cornea.

Tunica Vasculosa

The vascular middle tunic of the eye, the **tunica vasculosa (uvea),** is composed of three parts: the **choroid,** the **ciliary body,** and the **iris** (see Fig. 22–2).

Choroid

The **choroid** is the richly vascularized pigmented layer of the posterior wall of the orb that is loosely attached to the tunica fibrosa. It is composed of loose connective tissue containing numerous fibroblasts and a regular array of connective tissue containing numerous fibroblasts and a regular array of connective tissue cells, along with collagen, elastic fibers, and blood vessels. The black color of the choroid is due to the presence of melanocytes throughout it. Because of the abundance of small blood vessels in the inner surface of the choroid, that region is known as the **choriocapillary layer** and is responsible for providing nutrients to the retina. The choroid is separated from the retina by **Bruch's membrane,** a 1- to 4-μm-thick membrane composed of a network of elastic fibers located in the central region and flanked on either side by a layer of collagen fibers. The outer aspect of each collagen fiber layer is covered by a basal lamina—that of capillaries on one side and the pigment epithelium of the retina on the other side.

Ciliary Body

The **ciliary body** is the wedge-shaped extension of the choroid that rings the inner wall of the eye at the level of the lens, occupying the space between the ora serrata of the retina and the iris. One surface of the ciliary body abuts the sclera at the sclerocorneal junction, and another surface abuts the vitreous body; the medial surface projects toward the lens, forming short, finger-like projections known as the **ciliary processes.**

The ciliary body is composed of loose connective tissue containing numerous elastic fibers, blood vessels, and melanocytes. Its inner surface is lined by the **pars ciliaris of the retina,** a pigmented layer of the retina, which is composed of two cell layers. The outer layer, which faces the lumen of the orb, is nonpigmented ciliated columnar epithelium, although in the vicinity of the iris some of its cells may accumulate some pigment. The inner layer is composed of heavily **pigmented columnar epithelium** rich in melanin.

The anterior one third of the ciliary body has about 70 **ciliary processes,** which radiate out from a central core of connective tissue containing abundant fenestrated capillaries. Fibers, composed of fibrillin (zonule fibers), radiate from the ciliary processes to insert into the lens capsule, forming the **suspensory ligaments of the lens,** anchoring the lens in place.

The ciliary processes are covered by the same two layers of epithelia that cover the ciliary body. The inner nonpigmented layer has many interdigitations and enfoldings; its cells transport a protein-poor plasma filtrate into the posterior chamber of the eye, thus forming the **aqueous humor.** The aqueous humor flows from the posterior chamber into the anterior chamber by passing through the **pupillary aperture** between the iris and the lens. The aqueous humor exits the anterior chamber by passing into the trabecular meshwork near the limbus and finally into the canal of Schlemm, which leads directly to the venous system.

The bulk of the ciliary body is composed of three bundles of smooth muscle cells called the **ciliary muscle.** One bundle, because of its orientation, stretches the choroid, thus altering the opening of the canal of Schlemm for drainage of the aqueous humor. The remaining two muscle bundles, attached at the scleral spur, function in reducing tension on the zonulae. Contractions of this muscle, mediated by parasympathetic fibers of the oculomotor nerve (CN III), stretch the choroid body, thereby releasing tension on the suspensory ligaments of the lens. As a result, the lens becomes thicker and more convex. This action permits focusing on nearby objects, a process called **accommodation.**

CLINICAL CORRELATIONS

Glaucoma is a condition resulting from prolonged increased intraocular pressure caused by the failure of drainage of the aqueous humor from the anterior chamber of the eye. It is one of the world's leading causes of blindness. In **chronic glaucoma,** the most common condition, the continued increasing pressure causes progressive damage to the eye, particularly in the retina; if left untreated, it results in blindness.

Iris

The **iris,** the anterior-most extension of the choroid, lies between the posterior and anterior chambers of the eye, completely covering the lens except at the **pupillary aperture (pupil).** The iris is thickest in the middle, then thins toward its junction with the ciliary body and at the rim of the pupil. The anterior surface consists of two concentric rings: the **pupillary zone,** lying nearest the pupil, and the wider **ciliary zone.** The anterior surface of the iris is irregular, with trenches extending into it; it also contains contraction furrows, which are easily distinguished when the pupil is dilated. An incomplete layer of pigmented cells and fibroblasts covers the anterior surface of the iris. Deep to this layer is a stroma of poorly vascularized connective tissue containing numerous fibroblasts and melanocytes, which gives way to a well-vascularized, loose connective tissue zone.

The posterior surface of the iris is smooth and covered by the continuation of the two layers of epithelium that cover the ciliary body. The surface facing the lens is composed of heavily pigmented cells, which block the light from passing through the iris except at the pupil. Those epithelial cells facing the stroma of the iris have extensions that form the **dilatator pupillae muscle.** Hence, this muscle is myoepithelial in nature. Another muscle, the **sphincter pupillae muscle,** is located in a concentric ring around the pupil. Contractions of these smooth muscles alter the diameter of the pupil. The dilatator pupillae muscle, innervated by the sympathetic nervous system, dilates the pupil, whereas the sphincter pupillae muscle, innervated by parasympathetic fibers of the oculomotor nerve (CN III), constricts the pupil.

The abundant population of melanocytes located in the epithelium and stroma of the iris, in addition to blocking the passage of light into the eye, except at the pupil, also imparts color to the eyes. The eyes are dark when the number of melanocytes is large, whereas they are blue when the melanocyte number is low.

Lens

The lens of the eye is a flexible, biconvex, transparent disk composed of epithelial cells and their secreted products. The lens consists of three parts: lens capsule, subcapsular epithelium, and lens fibers (see Fig. 22–2).

The **lens capsule** is a basal lamina, 10 to 20 mm thick, containing mostly type IV collagen and glycoprotein covering the epithelial cells and surrounding the entire lens. This elastic, transparent, homogeneous structure, which refracts light, is thicker anteriorly than it is posteriorly.

The **subcapsular epithelium** is located only on the anterior surface of the lens, immediately deep to the lens capsule (Fig. 22–3). It is composed of a single layer of cuboidal cells, which communicate with each other via gap junctions. The apices of these cells are directed toward the lens fibers and interdigitate with them, especially in the vicinity of the equator, where they are more columnar and eventually become elongated.

The bulk of the lens is composed of approximately 2000 long cells known as **lens fibers.** These cells lie immediately

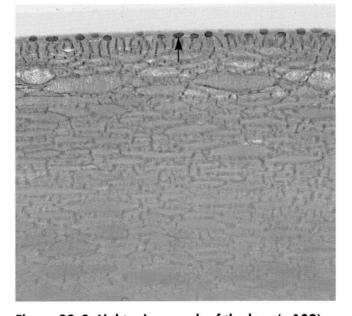

Figure 22–3. Light micrograph of the lens (× 132). Note the simple cuboidal epithelium (*arrow*) on the anterior surface.

deep to the subcapsular epithelium and lens capsule (Fig. 22–4). The cells of the subcapsular epithelium give rise to these highly differentiated lens fibers, which lose their nuclei and organelles and continue elongating to reach a length

of 7 to 10 mm as they mature. Eventually these long, hexagonal cells become filled with **crystallins,** lens proteins that increase the refractory index of the lens fibers.

CLINICAL CORRELATIONS

Presbyopia is the inability of the eye to focus on near objects (accommodation) and is caused by a decrease in the elasticity of the lens due to aging. As a result, the lens cannot become spherical for exact focusing. This condition can be corrected with glasses.

Cataract is usually an age-related condition in which the lens becomes opaque, thus impairing vision. This condition may be due to an accumulation of pigment or other substances and to excessive exposure to ultraviolet radiation. Although cataract does not usually respond to medication and will eventually lead to blindness, the opaque lens may be excised and replaced with a corrective lens.

VITREOUS BODY. The **vitreous body** is a transparent, refractile gel that fills the cavity of the eye (**vitreous cavity**) behind the lens. It is composed almost entirely of water (99%) containing a minute amount of electrolytes, collagen fibers, and hyaluronic acid. It adheres to the retina over its entire surface, especially at the ora serrata. Occasional macrophages and small cells called **hyalocytes** are observed at the periphery of the vitreous body; these are thought to synthesize collagen and hyaluronic acid. The fluid-filled

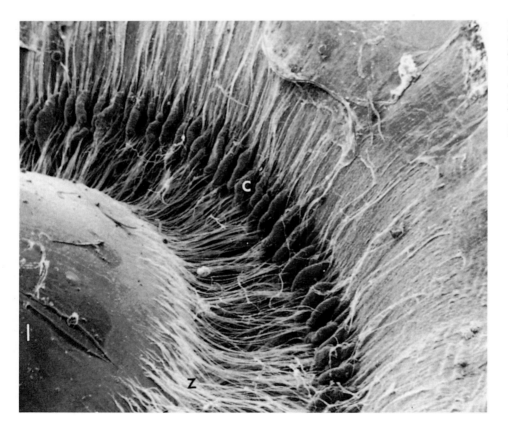

Figure 22–4. Scanning electron micrograph of the posterior surface of the lens (× 28). 1, lens; z, zonula fibers; c, ciliary body. (From Leeson, T.S., Leeson, C.R., and Paparo, A.A.: Text/Atlas of Histology. Philadelphia, W.B. Saunders, 1988.)

hyaloid canal, a narrow channel that was occupied by the hyaloid artery in the fetus, extends through the entire vitreous body from the posterior aspect of the lens to the optic disk.

RETINA (NEURAL TUNIC). The **retina,** the third and innermost tunic of the eye, is its neural portion, which contains the photoreceptor cells, known as rods and cones. The retina develops from the optic cup, an evagination of the prosencephalon, which gives rise to the primary optic vesicle. Later in development this structure invaginates to form a bilaminar secondary optic vesicle from which the retina develops, whereas the stalk of the optic cup becomes the optic nerve.

The retina is formed of an outer **pigmented layer** that develops from the outer wall of the optic cup, whereas the neural portion of the retina develops from the inner layer of the optic cup and is called the **retina proper.** It should be remembered that the cells composing the retina constitute a highly differentiated extension of the brain.

The **optic disk,** located on the posterior wall of the orb, is the exit site of the optic nerve. Because it contains no photoreceptor cells, it is insensitive to light and is therefore called the **"blind spot"** of the retina. Approximately 2.5 mm lateral to the **optic disk** is a yellow-pigmented zone in the retinal wall called the **macula lutea** (yellow spot). Located in the center of this spot is an oval depression, the **fovea centralis,** where visual acuity is greatest. The fovea is a specialized area of the retina containing only cones, which are packed tightly as the other layers of the retina are pushed aside. As distance from the fovea increases, the number of cones decreases, whereas the number of rods increases.

The portion of the retina that functions in photoreception lines the inner surface of the choroid layer from the optic disk to the ora serrata and is composed of 10 distinct layers (Figs. 22–5, 22–6). From outside, adjacent to the choroid, to inside, where they are continuous with the optic nerve, these layers are as follows:

1. Pigment epithelium
2. Layer of rods and cones
3. Outer limiting membrane
4. Outer nuclear layer
5. Outer plexiform layer
6. Inner nuclear layer
7. Inner plexiform layer
8. Ganglion cell layer
9. Optic nerve fiber layer
10. Inner limiting membrane

Pigment Epithelium

The pigment epithelium, derived from the outer layer of the optic cup, is composed of cuboidal to columnar cells (14 μm wide and 10 to 14 μm tall) whose nuclei are located basally. The cells are attached to Bruch's membrane, which is lo-

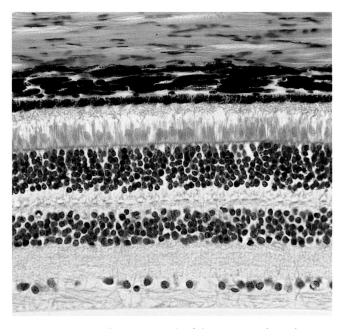

Figure 22–5. Light micrograph of the retina with its described 10 layers; the separation between the pigmented epithelium and the remainder of the retina is an artifact. (× 270).

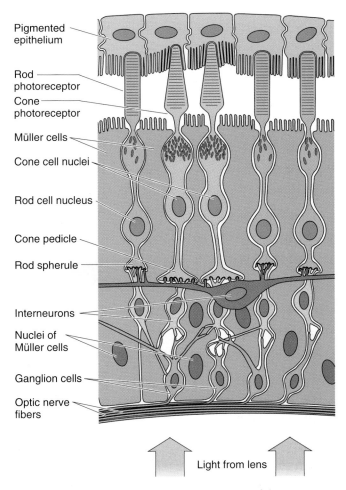

Figure 22–6. Diagram of the various layers of the retina.

cated between the choroid and the pigment cells. Mitochondria are especially abundant in the cytoplasm near the numerous cell invaginations with Bruch's membrane, suggesting transport in this region. Desmosomes, zonulae occludentes, and zonulae adherentes are present on the lateral cell membranes, forming the blood–retina barrier. Moreover, gap junctions on the lateral cell membranes permit intercellular communication. The cell apices exhibit microvilli and sleeve-like structures that surround the tips of the photoreceptor cells. Because these sleeve-like extensions merely surround the photoreceptor rod and cone tips, sudden hard jolts may disengage them, resulting in **detachment of the retina,** a common cause of partial blindness.

The most distinctive feature of the pigment cells is their abundance of melanin granules, which these cells synthesize and store in their apical portions. Also located there are the partially digested tips of the rods. Additionally, smooth endoplasmic reticulum, rough endoplasmic reticulum (RER), and Golgi apparatus are abundant in the cytoplasm.

The pigmented epithelium has several functions. Pigmented epithelial cells absorb light after it has passed through and stimulated the photoreceptors, thus preventing reflections from the tunics, which would impair focus. These pigmented cells continually phagocytize spent membranous disks from the tips of the photoreceptor rods. Pigment epithelial cells also play an active role in vision by esterifying vitamin A derivatives in their smooth endoplasmic reticulum.

Layer of Rods and Cones

The optical portion of the retina houses two distinct types of photoreceptor cells called **rods** and **cones.** Both rods and cones are polarized cells whose apical portions, known as the **outer segments,** are specialized dendrites. The outer segments of both rods and cones are surrounded by pigmented epithelial cells (see Fig. 22–6). The bases of the rod and cone cells form synapses with the underlying cells of the bipolar layer. It is estimated that there are approximately 100 to 120 million rods and 6 million cones.

RODS. Rods, which are activated in dim light only, are so sensitive that they can produce a signal from a single photon of light. On the other hand, they cannot mediate signals in bright light, and they cannot sense color.

Rods are elongated cells (50 μm × 3 μm) oriented parallel to each other but perpendicular to the retina. They are composed of **outer** and **inner segments,** a **nuclear region,** and a **synaptic region** (Fig. 22–7).

The **outer segment of the rod,** its dendritic end, presents several hundred flattened membranous lamellae oriented perpendicular to its long axis (Fig. 22–8). Each lamella represents an invagination of the plasmalemma, which is detached from the cell surface, thus forming a disk. Each disk is composed of two membranes separated from each other

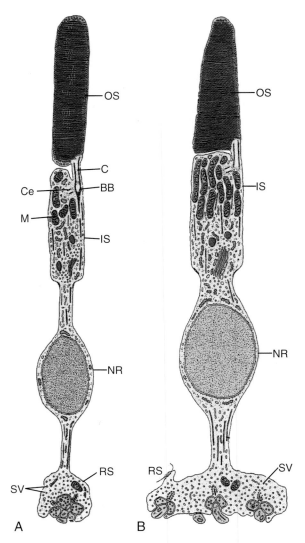

Figure 22–7. Diagram of the morphology of a rod (A) and cone (B). Abbreviations: outer segment (OS); connecting stalk (C); basal body (BB); centriole (Ce); inner segment (IS); mitochondria (M); synaptic region (RS); synaptic vesicles (SV); nuclear region (NR). From Lentz, T.L.: Cell Fine Structure. An Atlas of Drawings of Whole-Cell Structure. Philadelphia, W.B. Saunders Company, 1971.)

by an 8-nm space. The membranes contain **rhodopsin (visual purple),** a light-sensitive pigment.

The **inner segment of the rod** is separated from the outer segment by a constriction called the **connecting stalk.** Passing through the connecting stalk and into the outer segment of the rod is a modified cilium (lacking the central singlet microtubules) that arises from a basal body located at the apical end of the inner segment. Congregated near the interface with the connecting stalk are abundant mitochondria and cytoplasmic glycogen granules, both necessary for the production of energy for the visual process. The cytoplasm basal to the mitochondria is rich in microtubules, polysomes, smooth endoplasmic reticulum and RER, and Golgi

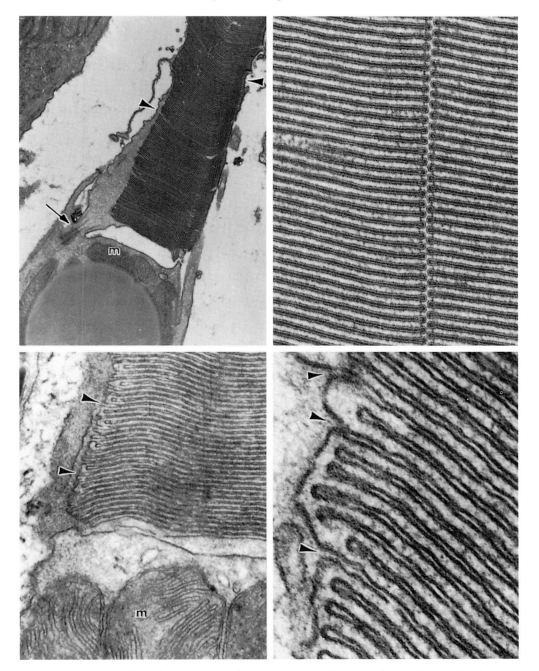

Figure 22–8. Electron micrographs of rods from the frog eye and cones from the squirrel eye. *Top left:* disks in the outer segment and mitochondria (m) in the inner segment of the frog rod; arrow points to a cilium connecting the inner and outer segments (× 18,000). *Top right:* higher magnification of the disks of the outer segment of the frog rod (× 85,000). *Bottom left:* junction of the outer and inner segments of the squirrel cone (× 32,000). *Bottom right:* higher magnification of the disks of the outer segment of the squirrel showing continuity of the lamellae with the plasmalemma (arrowheads) (× 92,000). (From Leeson, T.S., Leeson, C.R., and Paparo, A.A.: Text/Atlas of Histology. Philadelphia, W.B. Saunders, 1988.)

complexes. Proteins produced in the inner segment migrate to the outer segment, where they become incorporated into the disks. The disks gradually migrate to the apical end of the outer segment and are eventually shed into the sheaths of the pigment cells, where they will be phagocytized. The length of time from protein incorporation, through migra-

tion, and finally to shedding is less than 2 weeks.

Photoreception by rods begins with absorption of light by **rhodopsin,** which comprises the transmembrane protein **opsin** bound to *cis*-retinal, the aldehyde form of vitamin A. Absorption of light causes isomerization of the retinal moiety, which then dissociates from opsin. This **bleaching** yields activated opsin, which facilitates binding of guanosine triphosphate (GTP) to the α-subunit of a trimeric G protein called **transducin.** The resulting GTP-G$_\alpha$ activates cyclic guanosine monophosphate phosphodiesterase, an enzyme that catalyzes the breakdown of 3', 5'-cGMP. Rhodopsin is reassembled in an energy-consuming process assisted by **Müller cells** and **pigment cells.**

cGMP opens Na⁺ channels in the plasmalemma of rod cells. During the dark phase, Na⁺ ions are pumped out of the inner segment and enter the outer segment of the rods through gated Na⁺ channels. The presence of Na⁺ in the outer segment results in the release of neurotransmitter substance into the synapse with the bipolar cells. The light-induced activation of cGMP phosphodiesterase depletes cGMP levels; consequently, the gated Na⁺ channels close, and the rods become **hyperpolarized.** This event results in the inhibition of neurotransmitter release into the synapse with the bipolar cells. During the next dark phase the level of cGMP is regenerated, the Na⁺ ion channels are reopened, and the Na⁺ ion flow resumes as before.

It is interesting to note that the signal is not induced by depolarization, as it is in most cells; rather, light-induced hyperpolarization causes the signal to be transmitted through the various cell layers to the ganglion cells, where the signal generates an action potential along the axons to the brain.

CONES. Cones are activated in bright light and produce greater visual acuity than do rods. Cones are also elongated cells (60 μm × 1.5 μm), and their structure is similar to that of rods with the following few exceptions (see Fig. 22–7B; Figs. 22–8, 22–9):

- Their apical terminal (outer segment) is shaped more like a cone than a rod
- The disks of cones, although composed of lamellae of the plasmalemma, are attached to the plasma membrane, unlike the lamellae of the rods, which are separated from the plasma membrane
- Protein produced in the inner segment of cones migrates diffusely throughout the entire outer segment, whereas in rods, the protein is concentrated in the distal region of the outer segment
- Unlike rods, cones are sensitive to color

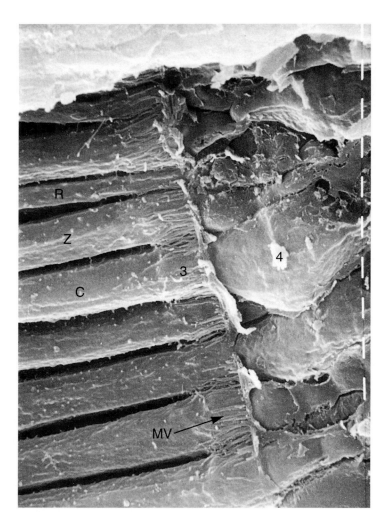

Figure 22–9. Scanning electron micrograph of the monkey retina displaying cones (C) and a few rods (R) (× 6300). (Z), inner segments; (3), external limiting membrane; (4), outer nuclear layer; (Mv), microvilli belonging to the Müller cells. (From Borwein, B., Borwein, D., Medeiros, J., and McGowan J.: The ultrastructure of monkey foveal photoreceptors, with special reference to the structure, shape, size, and spacing of the foveal cones. Am. J. Anat. **159:**125–146, 1980. Reprinted by permission of John Wiley & Sons, Inc.)

There are three types of cones, each containing a different variety of the photopigment **iodopsin.** Each variety of iodopsin has a maximum sensitivity to red, green, or blue.

The mode of function of the cones is similar to that of rods, except cones are sensitive to bright light and colors, so they provide the greatest visual acuity.

External Limiting Membrane

Although the term **external limiting membrane** is still used when describing the layers of the retina, it is not a membrane. Instead, electron micrographs have revealed this "layer" to be a row of zonulae adherentes between Müller cells and the photoreceptors. Distal to this, microvilli of the Müller cells project into the interstices between the inner segments of the rods and cones.

Outer Nuclear Layer

The **outer nuclear layer** consists of a zone mainly occupied by the nuclei of the rods and cones. In histological sections, the nuclei of rods are smaller, more rounded, and more darkly stained than cone nuclei.

Outer Plexiform Layer

Axodendritic synapses between the photoreceptor cells and other neuronal cells—including bipolar, amacrine, and horizontal cells—are located in the **outer plexiform layer.**

Inner Nuclear Layer

The nuclei of bipolar, amacrine, horizontal, and Müller cells compose the **inner nuclear layer.**

Inner Plexiform Layer

The processes of amacrine, bipolar, and ganglion cells are intermingled in the inner plexiform layer. **Axodendritic synapses** between axons of bipolar cells and the dendrites of ganglion cells also are located here.

Ganglion Cell Layer

Cell bodies of large multipolar neurons of the ganglion cells, up to 30 μm in diameter, are located in the **ganglion cell layer.** Axons of these neurons pass to the nerve fiber layer. Hyperpolarization of the rods and cones activates the ganglion cells, which then generate an action potential that is passed to the brain via the visual relay system.

Optic Nerve Fiber Layer

Optic nerve fibers are formed of unmyelinated axons of the ganglion cells in the **optic nerve fiber layer.** A myelin sheath is added as the nerve pierces the sclera.

Inner Limiting Membrane

Basal laminae of the Müller cells compose the **inner limiting membrane.**

Accessory Structures of the Eye

Conjunctiva

A transparent mucous membrane, known as the **conjunctiva,** lines the inner surface of the eyelids **(palpebral conjunctiva)** and covers the sclera of the anterior portion of the eye **(bulbar conjunctiva).** The conjunctiva is composed of a stratified columnar epithelium that contains goblet cells overlying a basal lamina and a lamina propria composed of loose connective tissue. Secretions of the goblet cells become a part of the **tear film,** which aids in lubricating and protecting the epithelium of the anterior eye. At the corneoscleral junction, where the cornea begins, the conjunctiva continues as the stratified squamous **corneal epithelium** and is devoid of goblet cells.

CLINICAL CORRELATIONS

Conjunctivitis is an inflammation of the conjunctiva usually associated with hyperemia and a discharge. It may be caused by a number of bacterial agents, viruses, allergens, and parasitic organisms. Some forms of conjunctivitis are extremely contagious, are damaging to the eye, and may cause blindness if untreated.

Eyelids

The eyelids are formed as folds of skin that cover the anterior surface of the developing eye. Accordingly, stratified squamous epithelium of skin covers their external surface, whereas at the **palpebral fissure,** palpebral conjunctiva covers their inner surface. The eyelids are supported by a framework of **tarsal plates.** Sweat glands are located in the skin of the eyelids, as are fine hairs and sebaceous glands. The dermis of the eyelids is generally thinner than in most skin, contains numerous elastic fibers, and is without fat. The margins of the eyelids contain **eyelashes** arranged in rows of three or four, but they are without arrector pili muscles. Modified sweat glands, called **glands of Moll,** form a simple spiral before opening into the eyelash follicles. **Meibomian glands,** modified sebaceous glands located in the tarsus of each lid, open on the free edge of the lids. The oily substance secreted by these glands becomes incorporated into the tear film and impedes evaporation of the tears. Other smaller modified sebaceous glands, the **glands of Zeis,** are associated with the eyelashes and secrete their product into the eyelash follicles.

Lacrimal Apparatus

The **lacrimal apparatus** includes the **lacrimal gland,** which secretes the **lacrimal fluid** (tears); the **lacrimal**

canaliculi, which carry the lacrimal fluid away from the surface of the eye; the **lacrimal sac,** a dilated portion of the ductal system; and the **nasolacrimal duct,** which delivers the lacrimal fluid to the nasal cavity.

The **lacrimal gland** lies in the lacrimal fossa located within the orbit, superior and lateral to the orb. It lies outside the conjunctival sac, although it communicates with the sac via 6 to 12 secretory ducts, which open into the sac at the lateral portion of the superior conjunctival fornix. The gland is a serous, compound tubuloalveolar gland that resembles the parotid gland. Myoepithelial cells completely surround the secretory portions.

Lacrimal fluid (tears) is composed mostly of water. This sterile fluid, containing **lysozyme,** an antibacterial agent, passes through the secretory ducts to enter the conjunctival sac. The upper eyelids, by blinking, wash the tears over the anterior portion of the sclera and cornea, thus keeping them moist and protected from dehydration. The lacrimal fluid is wiped in a medial direction and enters the **lacrimal puncta,** an aperture located in each of the medial margins of the superior and inferior eyelids. The puncta of each eyelid leads directly to **lacrimal canaliculi,** which join into a common conduit that leads to the lacrimal sac. The walls of the lacrimal canaliculi are lined by stratified squamous epithelium.

The **lacrimal sac** is the dilated superior portion of the nasolacrimal duct. It is lined by pseudostratified ciliated columnar epithelium.

The inferior continuation of the lacrimal sac is the **nasolacrimal duct,** also lined by pseudostratified ciliated colum-nar epithelium. This duct carries the lacrimal fluid into the inferior meatus located in the floor of the nasal cavity.

Ear (Vestibulocochlear Apparatus)

The ear—the organ of hearing as well as the organ of equilibrium or balance—is divisible into three parts: the external ear, middle ear (tympanic cavity), and the inner ear (Fig. 22–10). Sound waves received by the **external ear** are translated into mechanical vibrations by the tympanic membrane. These vibrations then are amplified by the bony ossicles in the **middle ear (tympanic cavity)** and transferred to the **inner ear.** The inner ear, a perilymph-filled bony labyrinth that ends in the cochlea and in which is suspended a membranous labyrinth housing the vestibular mechanism, is responsible for hearing and maintaining balance. Sensory input into the entire vestibulocochlear apparatus is transmitted to the brain by the acoustic nerve (CN VIII).

External Ear

The **external ear** is composed of the auricle (pinna), the external auditory meatus, and the tympanic membrane (see Fig. 22–10). The **auricle** develops from parts of the first and second branchial arches. Its general shape, size, and specific contours are usually distinctive for each individual with familial similarities. The pinna is composed of an irregularly shaped plate of elastic cartilage that is covered by thin skin, which adheres tightly to the cartilage. The cartilage of the

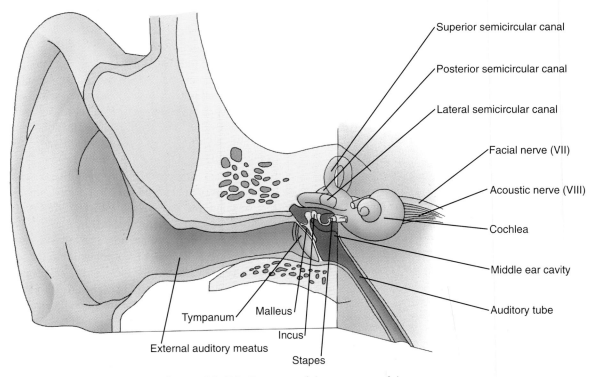

Figure 22–10. Diagram of the anatomy of the ear.

pinna is continuous with the cartilage lining the cartilaginous portion of the external auditory meatus.

The **external auditory meatus** is the canal that extends from the pinna into the temporal bone to the external surface of the tympanic membrane. Its superficial portion is composed of elastic cartilage, which is continuous with the cartilage of the pinna. Temporal bone replaces the cartilage as support in the inner two thirds of the meatus. The external auditory meatus is covered with skin containing hair follicles, sebaceous glands, and modified sweat glands known as **ceruminous glands,** which produce a waxy material called **cerumen** (earwax). Hair and the sticky wax help prevent objects from penetrating deeply into the meatus.

The **tympanic membrane** covers the deepest end of the external auditory meatus. It is the closing plate between the first pharyngeal groove and the first pharyngeal pouch, where ectoderm, mesoderm, and endoderm are in close proximity. The external surface of the tympanic membrane is covered by a thin epidermis derived from ectoderm, whereas its internal surface is composed of a simple squamous to cuboidal epithelium, derived from endoderm. A thin layer of mesodermal elements, including collagen fibers, elastic fibers, and fibroblasts, is interposed between the two surface layers of the tympanic membrane. This membrane receives sound waves transmitted to it by air through the external auditory meatus, which cause it to vibrate. In this fashion, the sound waves are converted into mechanical energy that is transmitted to the bony ossicles in the middle ear.

Middle Ear

The **middle ear,** or **tympanic cavity,** is an air-filled space located in the petrous portion of the temporal bone. This space communicates posteriorly with the mastoid air cells and anteriorly, via the **auditory tube (eustachian tube),** with the pharynx (see Fig. 22–10). The bony ossicles are housed in this space.

The tympanic cavity is lined by simple squamous epithelium, which is continuous with the internal lining of the tympanic membrane. However, in its deepest two thirds, the bone of the tympanic cavity gives way to cartilage. Its epithelial covering is a pseudostratified ciliated columnar epithelium as it approaches the auditory tube. The lamina propria over the bony wall adheres to it tightly and does not contain glands. The lamina propria overlying the cartilaginous portion, however, contains many mucous glands whose ducts open into the lumen of the tympanic cavity. Additionally, goblet cells and lymphoid tissue are found in the vicinity of the pharyngeal opening.

During swallowing and yawning, the orifice of the auditory tube at the pharynx opens, permitting an equalization of air pressure in the tympanic cavity with that of the external auditory meatus, located on the opposite side of the tympanic membrane. This is why swallowing or yawning relieves the "ear pressure" during rapid descent while flying.

Located within the medial wall of the tympanic cavity are the **oval** and **round windows,** which connect the middle ear cavity to the inner ear. These two openings are formed by membrane-covered voids in the bony wall. The **malleus, incus,** and **stapes**—the bony ossicles—are articulated in series by synovial joints lined with simple squamous epithelium. The malleus is attached to the tympanic membrane, with the incus interposed between it and the stapes, which, in turn, is attached to the oval window. Two small skeletal muscles, the **tensor tympani** and the **stapedius,** aid movements of the tympanic membrane and the bony ossicles.

Inner Ear

The **inner ear** is composed of the **bony labyrinth,** an irregular, hollowed-out cavity located within the petrous portion of the temporal bone, and the **membranous labyrinth,** which is suspended within the bony labyrinth (Fig. 22–11).

Bony Labyrinth

The **bony labyrinth** has three components: the **semicircular canals,** the **vestibule,** and the **cochlea.** It is lined with endosteum and is separated from the membranous labyrinth by the **perilymphatic space.** This space is filled with a clear fluid called the **perilymph,** within which the membranous labyrinth is suspended. The central region of the **bony labyrinth** is known as the **vestibule.**

The three **semicircular canals (superior, posterior,** and **lateral)** are oriented at 90 degrees to each other (see Fig. 22–11). One end of each canal is enlarged; this expanded region is called the **ampulla.** All three semicircular canals arise and return to the vestibule, except that one end of two of the canals share a common opening to the vestibule; consequently, there are only five orifices to the vestibule. Suspended within the canals are the **semicircular ducts,** which are regionally named continuations of the membranous labyrinth.

The **vestibule** is the central portion of the bony labyrinth located between the anteriorly placed cochlea and the posteriorly placed semicircular canals. Its lateral wall contains the **oval window (fenestra vestibuli),** covered by a membrane to which the footplate of the stapes is attached, and the **round window (fesnestra cochleae),** covered only by a membrane. The vestibule also houses specialized regions of the membranous labyrinth known as the utricle and the saccule.

The **cochlea** arises as a hollow bony spiral, which turns upon itself, like a snail's shell, $2\frac{1}{2}$ times around a central bony column, the **modiolus.** The modiolus projects into the spiraled cochlea with a shelf of bone called the **osseous spiral lamina,** through which traverse blood vessels and the **spiral ganglion,** the cochlear portion of the acoustic nerve.

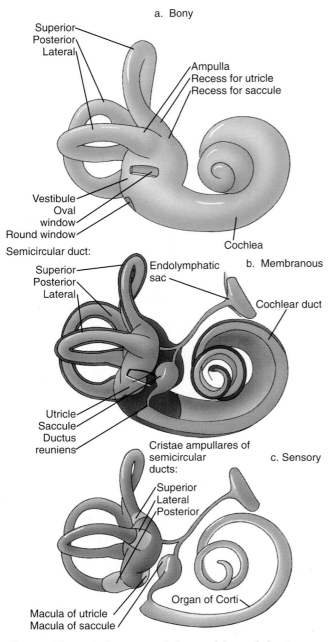

Semicircular canals:

a. Bony

Superior
Posterior
Lateral

Ampulla
Recess for utricle
Recess for saccule

Vestibule
Oval
window
Round window

Cochlea

Semicircular duct:

Superior
Posterior
Lateral

Endolymphatic
sac

b. Membranous

Cochlear duct

Utricle
Saccule
Ductus
reuniens

Cristae ampullares of
semicircular
ducts:

c. Sensory

Superior
Lateral
Posterior

Organ of Corti

Macula of utricle
Macula of saccule

Figure 22–11. Diagram of the cochlea of the inner ear. *Top:* anatomy of bony labyrinth. *Middle:* bony cochlea containing the membranous labyrinth. *Bottom:* anatomy of the membranous labyrinth.

Membranous Labyrinth

The **membranous labyrinth** is composed of an epithelium derived from the embryonic ectoderm, which invades the developing temporal bone and gives rise to two small sacs, the **utricle** and **saccule** (see Fig. 22–11). Circulating through the entire membranous labyrinth is **endolymph**, a viscous fluid that resembles intracellular fluid in its ionic composition (i.e., it is sodium-poor but potassium-rich).

Thin strands of connective tissue attached to the endosteum of the bony labyrinth pass through the perilymph to be inserted into the membranous labyrinth. In addition to anchoring the membranous labyrinth to the bony labyrinth, these connective tissue strands carry blood vessels that nourish the epithelia of the membranous labyrinth.

SACCULE AND UTRICLE. The **saccule** and the **utricle** are connected to each other by a small duct, the **ductus utriculosaccularis.** Additionally, small ducts from each join to form the **endolymphatic duct,** whose dilated blind end is known as the **endolymphatic sac.** Another small duct called the **ductus reuniens** joins the saccule with the duct of the cochlea.

The walls of the saccule and utricle are composed of a thin outer vascular layer of connective tissue and an inner layer of simple squamous to low cuboidal epithelium. Specialized regions of the saccule and utricle act as receptors for sensing orientation of the head relative to gravity and acceleration, respectively. These receptors are called the **macula of the saccule** and **macula of the utricle.**

The maculae of the saccule and utricle are located so that they are perpendicular to each other (i.e., the macula of the saccule is located predominantly in the wall, thus detecting linear vertical acceleration, whereas the macula of the utricle is located mostly in the floor, thus detecting linear horizontal acceleration. The epithelium of the nonreceptor regions of the saccule and utricle is composed of **light** and **dark cells.** Light cells have a few microvilli, and their cytoplasm contains a few pinocytotic vesicles, ribosomes, and only a small number of mitochondria. The cytoplasm of the dark cells, however, contains abundant coated vesicles, smooth vesicles, lipid droplets, and numerous elongated mitochondria located in compartments formed by enfoldings of the basal plasma membrane. Nuclei of the dark cells are irregular in shape and are often located apically. Although it is unclear how these two cell types function, it is speculated that the dark cells function in controlling endolymph composition.

These maculae are thickened areas of the epithelium, 2 to 3 mm in diameter. They are composed of two types of **neuroepithelial cells,** called **type I** and **type II hair cells,** and supporting cells which sit on a basal lamina (Fig 22–12). Nerve fibers from the vestibular portion of the acoustic nerve supply the neuroepithelial cells.

Each type I and type II hair cell has a single kinocilium and 50 to 100 stereocilia arranged in rows according to length, with the longest (10 μm) being nearest the kinocilium.

Type I hair cells are plump cells with a rounded base that narrow toward the neck (Fig. 22–13). Their cytoplasm contains occasional RER, a supranuclear Golgi complex, and numerous small vesicles. Each stereocilium, which is anchored in a dense terminal web, is a long microvillus with a core of many actin filaments cross-linked by **fimbrin.** The filamentous core imparts rigidity to the stereocilia, so that bending can occur only in the neck region, near their site of origin from the apical plasma membrane.

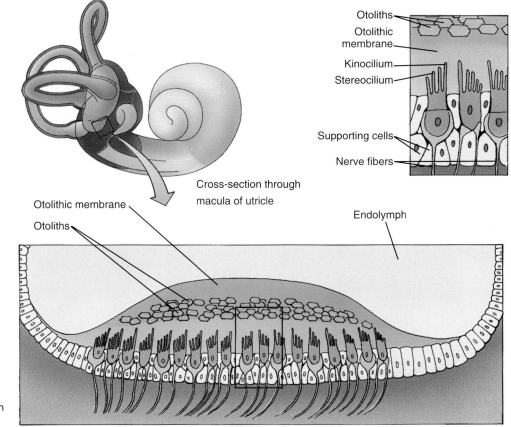

Figure 22-12. Diagram of hair cells and supporting cells in the macula of the utricle.

Type II hair cells are similar to type I hair cells with regard to the stereocilia and kinocilium, but their shape is more columnar and their cytoplasm contains a larger Golgi complex and more vesicles (see Fig. 22–13).

Supporting cells of the maculae, which are interposed between both types of hair cells, have a few microvilli. Thick junctional complexes bind these cells to each other and to the hair cells. They exhibit a well-developed Golgi complex and secretory granules, suggesting that they may help maintain the hair cells or that they may contribute to the production of endolymph.

Innervation of the hair cells is derived from the vestibular portion of the acoustic nerve. The rounded bases of the type I hair cells are almost entirely surrounded by a cup-shaped afferent nerve fiber. Type II hair cells exhibit many afferent fibers synapsing on the basal area of the cell. Structures resembling **synaptic ribbons** are present near the bases of type I and type II hair cells. The synaptic ribbons of the type II hair cells appear to function in synapses with efferent nerves, which are thought to be responsible for modulating sensitivity. The function of the synaptic ribbons of the type I hair cells is unclear.

The stereocilia of the neurepithelial hair cells are covered by and embedded in a thick, gelatinous, glycoprotein mass, the **otolithic membrane.** The surface region of this membrane contains small calcium carbonate crystals known as **otoliths** or **otoconia** (see Fig. 22–13).

SEMICIRCULAR DUCTS. Each **semicircular duct,** a continuation of the membranous labyrinth arising from the utricle, is housed within its semicircular canal and thus conforms to its shape. Each of the three ducts is dilated at its lateral end (near the utricle). These expanded regions, called the **ampullae,** contain the **cristae ampullares,** which are specialized receptor areas. Each crista ampullaris is composed of a ridge whose free surface is covered by sensory epithelium consisting of **neuroepithelial hair cells** and **supporting cells** (Fig. 22–14). The supporting cells sit on the basal lamina, whereas the hair cells do not; rather, the hair cells are cradled between the supporting cells. The neuroepithelial cells are also known as type I and type II hair cells and exhibit the same morphology as the hair cells of the maculae. The **cupula,** a gelatinous glycoprotein mass overlying the cristae ampulares, is similar to the otolithic membrane in structure and function, except that it is cone-shaped and does not contain otoliths.

COCHLEAR DUCT AND ORGAN OF CORTI. The **cochlear duct,** a diverticulum of the saccule, is another regionally named portion of the membranous labyrinth. The

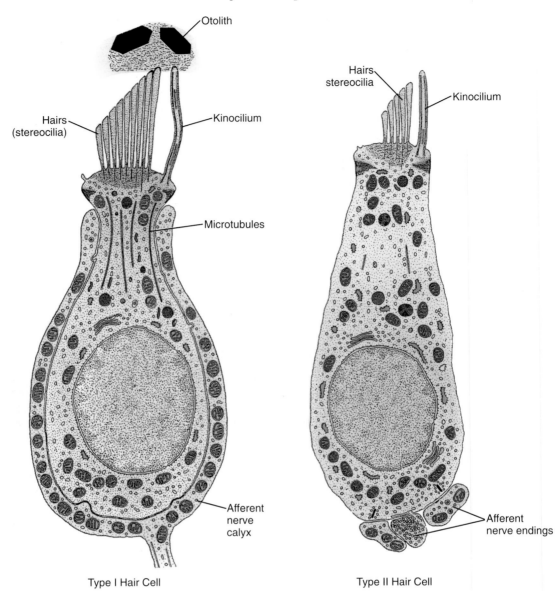

Type I Hair Cell   Type II Hair Cell

Figure 22–13. Diagram demonstrating the morphology of type I and type II neuroepithelial (hair) cells of the maculae of the saccule and utricle. (From Lentz, T.L.: Cell Fine Structure. An Atlas of Drawings of Whole-Cell Structure. Philadelphia, W.B. Saunders Company, 1971.)

cochlear duct is a wedge-shaped receptor organ housed in the bony cochlea and surrounded on two sides by perilymph but separated from it by two membranes (Figs. 22–15, 22–16). The roof of the **scala media (cochlear duct)** is the **vestibular (Reissner's) membrane,** whereas the floor of the scala media is the **basilar membrane.** The perilymph-filled compartment lying above the vestibular membrane is called the **scala vestibuli,** whereas the perilymph-filled compartment lying below the basilar membrane is the **scala tympani.** Both of these compartments communicate at the **helicotrema** near the apex of the cochlea.

The **vestibular membrane** is composed of two layers of squamous epithelium separated from each other by a basal

lamina. The inner layer is the lining cells of the scala media, whereas the outer layer is the lining cells of the scala vestibuli. Numerous tight junctions seal both layers of cells, thus ensuring a high ionic gradient across the membrane. The **basilar membrane,** extending from the spiral lamina at the modiolus to the lateral wall, supports the organ of Corti and is composed of two zones, **zona arcuata** and **zona pectinata.** The zona arcuata is thinner, lies more medial, and supports the organ of Corti. The zona pectinata is similar to a fibrous meshwork containing a few fibroblasts.

The lateral wall of the cochlear duct, extending between the vestibular membrane and the spiral prominence, is covered by a pseudostratified epithelium called the **stria vascu-**

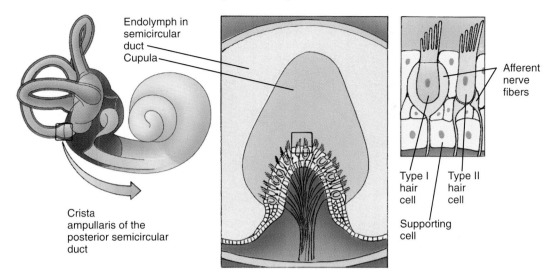

Figure 22–14. Diagram of the hair cells and supporting cells in one of the cristae ampullares of the semicircular canals.

laris. Unlike most epithelia, it contains an *intraepithelial plexus of capillaries.* Although the stria vascularis is reported to be composed of three cell types—**basal, intermediate,** and **marginal cells**—the three cell types greatly resemble each other in electron micrographs.

Dark-staining **marginal cells** have abundant microvilli on their free surface. Their dense cytoplasm contains numerous mitochondria and small vesicles. Labyrinthine, narrow cell processes containing elongated mitochondria are abundant on the basilar portion of the cells.

Light-staining **basal** and **intermediate cells** have less-dense cytoplasm containing only few mitochondria. Both have cytoplasmic processes that radiate out from the cell surfaces to interdigitate with the cell processes of the marginal cells and with other intermediate cells. Basal cells also have cellular processes that ascend around the bases of the marginal cells, forming cup-like structures that isolate and support the marginal cells. **Intraepithelial capillaries** are positioned such that they are surrounded by basal processes of the marginal cells and the ascending processes of the basal and intermediate cells.

It is suggested that the marginal cells are responsible for the maintenance of the ionic composition of the endolymph.

The **spiral prominence** is also located on the inferior portion of the lateral wall of the cochlear duct. It is a small protuberance that juts out from the periosteum of the cochlea into the cochlear duct, throughout its entire length. The basal cells of the stria vascularis are continuous with the vascular layer of cells covering the prominence. Inferiorly, these cells are reflected into the spiral sulcus, where they become cuboidal. Other cells of this layer continue onto the basilar lamina as the **cells of Claudius,** which overlie the smaller **cells of Boettcher.** The latter cells are located only in the basilar turns of the cochlea. It is unclear how the cells of Claudius and Boettcher function.

At the narrowest portion of the cochlear duct, where the vestibular and basilar membranes meet, periosteum covering the spiral lamina bulges out into the scala media, forming the **limbus of the spiral lamina.** Part of the limbus projects over the **internal spiral sulcus (tunnel).** The upper portion of the limbus is the **vestibular lip,** and the lower portion is called the **tympanic lip** of the limbus, a continuation of the basilar membrane. Numerous perforations in the tympanic lip accommodate branches of the cochlear division of the acoustic nerve. **Interdental cells** located within the body of the spiral limbus secrete the **tectorial membrane,** a proteoglycan-rich gelatinous mass containing numerous fine keratin-like filaments, overlying the organ of Corti. Stereocilia of specialized receptor hair cells of the organ of Corti are embedded in the tectorial membrane.

The **organ of Corti,** the specialized receptor organ for hearing, lies on the basilar membrane and is composed of neuroepithelial hair cells and several types of supporting cells. Although the supporting cells of the organ of Corti have different characteristics, they all originate on the basilar membrane and contain bundles of microtubules and microfilaments, and their apical surfaces are all interconnected at the free surface of the organ of Corti. Supporting cells include **pillar cells, phalangeal cells, border cells,** and **cells of Hensen** (see Figs. 22–15, 22–16).

Supporting Cells of the Organ of Corti. Inner and **outer pillar cells** are tall cells with wide bases and apical ends; thus they are shaped like an elongated "I." They are attached to the basilar membrane, and each one arises from a broad base. The central portions of both inner and outer pillar cells are deflected to form the walls of the **inner tunnel,** where the inner pillar cell forms the medial wall of the tunnel and the outer pillar cells form the lateral wall of the tunnel. At their apices, both inner and outer pillar cells are again in

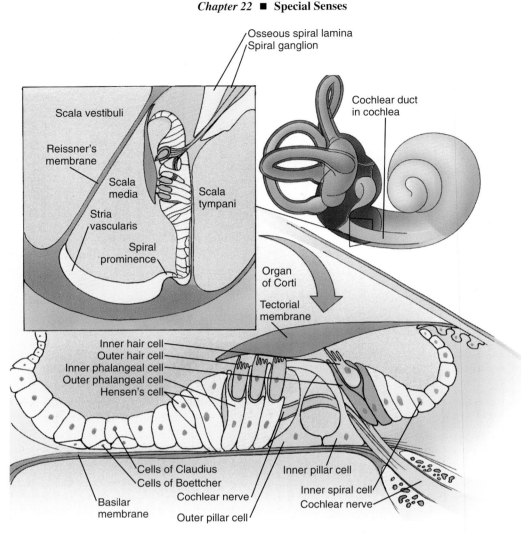

Figure 22–15. Diagram of the organ of Corti.

contact with each other. Their cytoplasm contains bundles of microfilaments and microtubules. Inner pillar cells outnumber outer pillar cells, with three inner pillar cells usually abutting two outer pillar cells. The pillar cells support the hair cells of the organ of Corti.

Outer phalangeal cells are tall columnar cells that are attached to the basilar membrane. Their apical portions are cup-shaped to support the basilar portions of the outer hair cells along with bundles of efferent and afferent nerve fibers, which pass between them on their way to the hair cells. Because their cup-shaped apices cradle the hair cells, these cells do not reach the free surface of the organ of Corti. However, originating from the lateral aspect of these cells is a small **phalangeal process** that extends to the reticular lamina. Microtubules and microfilaments within the phalangeal process add to its rigidity. The distal, flattened end of the phalangeal process is in contact with its cradled hair cell and an adjacent hair cell. There is a fluid-filled gap around unsupported regions of the outer hair cells. This space is called the **space of Nuel,** and it communicates with the inner tunnel.

Inner phalangeal cells are located deep to the inner pillar cells; unlike the outer phalangeal cells, they completely surround the inner hair cells they support.

Border cells delineate the inner border of the organ of Corti. They are slender cells that support the inner aspects of the organ of Corti.

Cells of Hensen define the outer border of the organ of Corti. They are tall cells that are located between the outer phalangeal cells and the shorter cells of Claudius, which rest on the underlying **cells of Boettcher.** All of these cells support the outer aspects of the organ of Corti.

Neuroepithelial Cells (Hair Cells) of the Organ of Corti.
Neuroepithelial hair cells are specialized for transducing impulses for the organ of hearing. Depending on their locations, these cells are called **inner hair cells** and **outer hair cells.**

Inner hair cells, a single row of cells that extends the entire length of the organ of Corti, are located near the inner limit of that organ. They are supported by inner phalangeal

Outer hair cells, located near the outer limit of the organ of Corti, are arranged in rows of three (or four) along the entire length of this organ. They are supported throughout most of their length by outer phalangeal cells. The outer hair cells are elongated cylindrical cells whose nuclei are located near their bases. Their cytoplasm contains abundant RER, and their mitochondria are located basally. The cytoplasm of those cells just beneath the lateral walls contains a **cortical lattice,** composed of 5- to 7-nm filaments cross-linked by thinner filaments, that appears to support the cell and resist deformation. Afferent and efferent fibers synapse on the basilar portion of the hair cells. Extending from the apical surface of the outer hair cells are as many as 100 stereocilia arranged in a W shape. These stereocilia vary in length and are arranged in ordered gradation. Like the inner hair cells, the outer hair cells do not have a kinocilium, but a basal body is present.

Vestibular Function

The sense of position in space and in movement is essential to activate and deactivate certain muscles that function in accommodating the body for balance. The sensory mechanism for this function is the **vestibular apparatus** located in the inner ear. This apparatus comprises the utricle, saccule, and semicircular ducts.

Stereocilia of neuroepithelial hair cells located in the ampullae of the utricle and saccule are embedded in the otolithic membrane. **Linear movements** of the head cause displacement of the endolymph, which disturbs the positioning of the otoliths within the otolithic membrane and consequently the membrane itself, thereby bending the stereocilia of the hair cells. Movements of the stereocilia are transduced into action potentials, which are conducted by synapses to the vestibular portion of the acoustic nerve for transmittal to the brain.

Circular movements of the head are sensed by receptor sites in the semicircular ducts housed within the semicircular canals. Stereocilia of the neuroepithelial hair cells of the cristae ampullares are embedded in the cupula. Movements of the endolymph within the semicircular ducts disturb the orientation of the cupula, which subsequently distorts the stereocilia of the hair cells. This mechanical stimulus is transduced to an electrical impulse that is transferred by synapse to branches of the vestibular portion of the acoustic nerve for transmission to the brain.

Information concerning the linear and circular movements of the head, recognized by receptors of the inner ear, are transmitted to the brain via the acoustic nerve. There it is interpreted, and adjustments to the balance are initiated by activating specific muscle masses responsible for posture.

Cochlear Function

Sound waves collected by the external ear pass into the external auditory meatus and are received by the tympanic

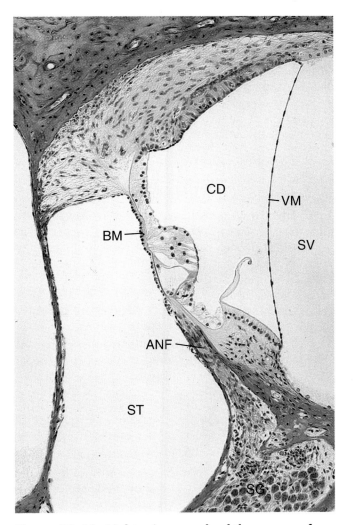

Figure 22–16. Light micrograph of the organ of Corti sitting on the basilar membrane (BM) within the cochlea (× 211). The cochlear duct (CD), containing endolymph, is limited by the vestibular membrane (VM) and the basilar membrane (BM). The scala vestibuli (SV) and the scala tympani (ST) contain perilymph. Observe the spiral ganglion (SG) and the acoustic nerve fibers (ANF) coming from the hair cells of the organ of Corti.

cells throughout their entire length. Inner hair cells are short and exhibit a centrally located nucleus, numerous mitochondria (especially, beneath the terminal web), RER and smooth endoplasmic reticulum, and small vesicles. Their basal aspect also contains microtubules. The apical surface contains 50 to 60 stereocilia arranged in a V shape. The core of the stereocilium contains microfilaments, cross-linked with fimbrin, similar to the type I hair cells of the vestibular labyrinth. The microfilaments of the stereocilia merge with those of the terminal web. Although a kinocilium is not present in inner hair cells, a basal body and centriole are both evident in the apical region of these cells. The basal aspects of these cells synapse with afferent fibers of the cochlear portion of the acoustic nerve.

membrane, which is set into motion. Functionally, the tympanic membrane converts the sound waves into mechanical energy. Vibrations of the tympanic membrane set the malleus, and consequently the remaining two ossicles, into motion. Because of a mechanical advantage rendered by the articulations of the three bony ossicles, the mechanical energy is amplified about 20 times when it reaches the footplate of the stapes, where it impinges on the membrane of the fenestra vestibuli (oval window). Movements of the oval window initiate pressure waves in the perilymph within the scala vestibuli. Because fluid (in this instance, perilymph) is incompressible, the wave is passed through the scala vestibuli, through the helicotrema, into the scala tympani. The pressure wave in the perilymph of the scala tympani causes the basilar membrane to vibrate. Because the organ of Corti is firmly attached to the basilar membrane, a rocking motion within the basilar membrane is translated into a shearing motion on the stereocilia of the hair cells that are embedded in the overlying rigid tectorial membrane. When the shearing force produces a deflection of the stereocilia toward the taller stereocilia, the cell becomes depolarized, thus generating an impulse that is transmitted through synapses into the afferent nerve fibers (Fig. 22–17).

How differences in sound frequency or pitch are distinguished is not understood. It has long been thought that the basilar membrane, which becomes shorter with each turn of the cochlea, vibrates at different frequencies relative to its width. Therefore, low-frequency sounds would be detected near the base of the cochlea, whereas high-frequency sounds would be detected near the apex of the cochlea, whereas high-frequency sounds would be detected near the base of the cochlea. Recent evidence suggests that efferent input to the hair cells cause them to vary their length, which alters their response to different frequencies.

CLINICAL CORRELATIONS

Conductive deafness may be caused by any condition that impedes the conduction of the sound waves from the external ear through the middle ear and into the organ of Corti of the inner ear. Conditions that can lead to conductive deafness include the presence of foreign bodies, **otitis media** (constriction of the movements of the bony ossicles), and **otosclerosis** (fixation of footplate of the stapes in the oval window).

Nerve deafness usually results from a disease process that interrupts transmission of the nerve impulse. The interruption may be located anywhere in the cochlear division of the acoustic nerve from the organ of Corti to the brain. Disease processes that can lead to nerve deafness include rubella, tumors of the nerve, and nerve degeneration.

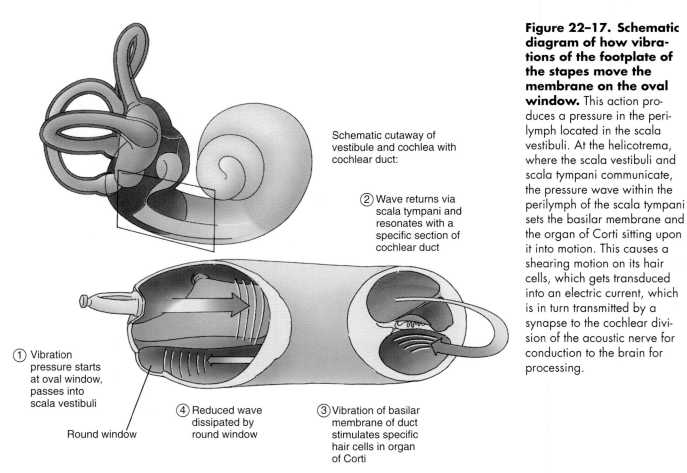

Schematic cutaway of vestibule and cochlea with cochlear duct:

② Wave returns via scala tympani and resonates with a specific section of cochlear duct

① Vibration pressure starts at oval window, passes into scala vestibuli

Round window

④ Reduced wave dissipated by round window

③ Vibration of basilar membrane of duct stimulates specific hair cells in organ of Corti

Figure 22–17. Schematic diagram of how vibrations of the footplate of the stapes move the membrane on the oval window. This action produces a pressure in the perilymph located in the scala vestibuli. At the helicotrema, where the scala vestibuli and scala tympani communicate, the pressure wave within the perilymph of the scala tympani sets the basilar membrane and the organ of Corti sitting upon it into motion. This causes a shearing motion on its hair cells, which gets transduced into an electric current, which is in turn transmitted by a synapse to the cochlear division of the acoustic nerve for conduction to the brain for processing.

Index

Note: Page numbers in *italics* refer to illustrations; page numbers followed by t refer to tables.

Neuron(s) *(Continued)*
mitochondria of, 159
motor (efferent), 140–141, 145–146, *145, 157,* 162
multipolar, *156, 158,* 162
Nissl bodies of, *10,* 158, *159*
nucleus of, 158
olfactory cells as, 285
polarization of, 167–168, *168, 169*
postganglionic, 178
preganglionic, 178
pseudounipolar, *158,* 162
Purkinje, *158*
pyramidal, *158*
receptors on, 155
sensory (afferent), 155, 162
size of, 156
somatic, 175–176, *176*
structure of, 156–161, *156–161*
support cells (neuroglia) for, 39t, 103, 155, 162–167, *162–167*
synapses of, 168–172
function of, 141–142, *144*
morphology of, 169, *170,* 171–172, *171*
types of, 169, *169*
trophic relationships of, 161
unipolar, *158,* 162
α-Neurons, myelinated axons of, 141
Neuropeptides, as neurotransmitters, 172, 173t
Neuropil, 179
Neurophysin, 257
Neurotendinous spindles (Golgi tendon organs), 146, *423,* 424
Neurotensin, 321t
Neurotoxins, action of, 143
eosinophil-derived, 193
Neurotransmission, 141–143, *142–144*
disorders of, 143
Neurotransmitters, actions of, 141–142, *144,* 172, 173t
disorders of, 172
in ion channel gating, 16
in signaling, 17
in synaptic vesicles, 171
receptors for, 172
release of, 169
types of, 172, 173t
Neutral proteases, in mast cells, 97, 101, 101t
Neutrophil(s), defects of, 193
formation of, *204,* 206–208, *209,* 211t
functions of, 191, *194,* 192t
granules of, 191, *193,* 211t
in connective tissue, 103
in phagocytosis, 26
margination of, 207
morphology of, *186, 188,* 191, 192t, *193*
origin of, *93*

Neutrophil chemotactic factor, in mast cells, 97, 100, 101t, 102
Nexin, of cilia, 77
Nexus junctions. See *Gap junctions.*
Nicotinamide adenine dinucleotide, in oxidative phosphorylation, 34
Nicotinamide adenine dinucleotide dehydrogenase complex, 33
Nidi of crystallization, in bone calcification, 126
Nipple, 400
Nissl bodies, *10,* 158, *159*
Nitric oxide, as neurotransmitter, 172
in blood pressure regulation, 219
in penile function, 420
in signaling, 18
Nociceptors, 424
Node(s), atrioventricular, 226, *226*
lymph. See *Lymph nodes.*
of Ranvier, *157,* 165, *166, 174*
conduction at, 174
sinoatrial, 226, *226*
Nodule(s), lymphoid, 241–242, *241*
of bronchi, 292
of small intestine, *326*
of spleen, 244, *244*
of tonsils, 248–249, *249*
Peyer's patches as, 248, 330
Nonkeratinized epithelia, 71t, 72, *72, 74*
Nonpolar fatty acyl tails, of cell membrane, *13,* 14
Norepinephrine, 173t
action of, 176, 267
in fat release, 97
in melatonin release, 267
in smooth muscle function, 152
in vasoconstriction, 214
synthesis of, 262, *263,* 266, 267
Nostrils (nares), 284
Notochord, 155
Nuclear bag fibers, 145, *145*
Nuclear chain fibers, 145, *145*
Nuclear layers, of retina, *432,* 433
Nuclear pore complex, 44–45, *45, 46*
Nuclear region, of retinal rods and cones, 430, *430*
Nucleolus, *11, 12, 43, 44,* 51–52
definition of, 42
matrix of, 51–52
organizing regions of, 52
Nucleoplasm, 42, 50–51
Nucleosomes, 46–47, *47*
Nucleotides, in ion channel gating, 16
Nucleus (brain), 179
paraventricular, *252,* 257
supraoptic, *252,* 257
visceromotor, of cranial nerves, 178
Nucleus (cell), *12,* 42–57
cell cycle and, 52–54, *52–55*
chromatin of, 46–47, *47*

Nucleus (cell) *(Continued)*
chromosomes in, 47–50, *48, 49, 51*
components of, 41
envelope of, *11,* 42, *43–46*
lamina of, 39t, 44, *44*
matrix of, 51
meiosis and, 55–57, *56–57*
membranes of, 42, *43,* 44, *44, 46*
nucleolus of, *11, 12, 43, 44,* 51–52
nucleoplasm of, 42, 50–51
of astrocytes, *163*
of hepatocytes, 351, *351, 352*
of leukocytes, 192t
of muscle cells, 153t
of neuron, 158
of oligodendrocytes, *165*
pores of, 42, *43,* 44–45, *44–46*
shape of, 41
Nucleus pulposus, 113–114
Nuel, space of, 440
Null cells, 196, 197
Nurse cells, in erythropoiesis, 206
Nutrient arteries, to bone marrow, 200
Nutrition, bone growth and, 129–130, 129t

O

Obesity, 107
Objective lens, of light microscope, 3, *3*
Oblique layer, of muscularis externa, of stomach, 320
Obstructive jaundice, 352
Occluding junctions, of epithelia, 79–80, *80–82,* 82
Oddi, sphincter of, 357, 357t
Odontoblasts, 304, 305, 307, *307*
Odontoclasts, 305
Odontogenesis, 305–308, *306, 307*
Odor receptor molecule, 287
Olfactory cells, 285, *286*
Olfactory epithelium, 285, *285–287*
Olfactory region, of nasal cavity, 285–287, *285–287*
Olfactory vesicles, 285, *286, 287*
Oligodendrocytes, *162,* 164, *165*
Oligodendroglioma, 162
Oncogenes, 54
Oocytes, *383,* 384, *384–386*
fertilization of, 394–395, *395, 396*
Oogonia, 384
Open circulation theory, of spleen function, 243, *245*
Opsin, 431–432
Opsonization, 246
Optic disk, 429
Optic nerve, *425, 429,* 433
Ora serrata, *425,* 428
Oral cavity, 302–311

Thyroid-stimulating hormone (thyrotropin), 252, 255
  action of, 254t, 257, 259–260
Thyrotrophs, 255
Thyrotropin. See *Thyroid-stimulating hormone (thyrotropin).*
Thyroxine (T₄), 268t
  abnormal levels of, 260–261
  action of, 257, 260–261
  release of, 259–260, *260*
  storage of, 258
  synthesis of, 259–260, *260*
  T lymphocyte effects of, 240
Tight junctions, of epithelia, 79–80, *80–82,* 82
Tissue(s), composition of, 58
  connective. See *Connective tissue.*
  definition of, 9
  epithelial. See also *Epithelium (epithelia); Gland(s).*
    functions of, 70
    fluid flow in, 58, *58*
      edema and, 105
    mucous, 104
    preparation of, for light microscopy, 1–3, 2t
Tissue fluid, composition of, 187
Tissue thromboplastin, in coagulation, 198
Titin, in skeletal muscle, 136, *138,* 140t
Tolerance, immunological, 231
  to drugs, liver function and, 354–355
Toluidine blue, 2–3
Tomes process, in odontogenesis, 307
Tongue, 309–311, *309–311*
Tonofibrils, in epidermis, 271
Tonofilaments, 39t
  of epidermis, 271
  of epithelia, 85
Tonsils, 248–249, *249*
Tooth. See *Teeth.*
Tooth germ, 306
Trabeculae, of bone, 118
  in endochondral bone formation, 123
  in intramembranous bone formation, 121, *122*
  of lymph nodes, 240, *241*
  of spleen, 243, *244, 245*
Trabecular arteries, of spleen, 243, *245*
Trabecular cells, of arachnoid, 181
Trabecular meshwork, 426
Trabecular vein, *244, 245*
Trachea, 288–290, *289, 290,* 299t
Trafficking, membrane, 27, *27*
trans Golgi face, 24, *24*
trans Golgi network, 24, *24, 25,* 26
Transcription, 49, *49,* 50
  hormones in, 18
  in protein synthesis, 20
Transcytosis, in capillaries, 223, *224*
  in small intestine, 330

Transducin, of retina, 432
Transduction, in signaling, 18
Transfer RNA. See under *RNA.*
Transferrin, in iron transport, 247
  receptors for, antibodies to, blood–brain barrier permeability and, 182
  testicular, synthesis of, 405
Transforming growth factor, in keratinocyte growth, 275
Trans-Golgi network, in spermiogenesis, 408
Transient cells, in connective tissue, 94, 103–104, *103–105*
Transitional epithelia. See under *Epithelium (epithelia).*
Translation, in protein synthesis, 20–23, *21–23*
Transmembrane junctional proteins, of epithelia, 80, *80,* 82, *84*
Transmembrane linker proteins, integrins as, 68–69
  of epithelia, 82, 85
Transmembrane proteins, of cell membrane, 14
Transmission, volume, in brain cells, 172
Transmission electron microscopy, 6, 7
  equipment for, *3*
Transneuronal degeneration, 185
Transplantation, of bone marrow, 203
Transport, active, 15, *16,* 17
  antiport, *16,* 17
  axonal, 160–161
  coupled, *16,* 17
  nuclear pore, 45
  passive, 15, *16,* 17
  receptor-mediated, in nuclear pore, 45
    of blood–brain barrier, 182
  symport, *16,* 17
  transcellular, epithelial tissues in, 70
  types of, 15, *16*
  uniport, *16,* 17
Transport proteins, of cell membrane, 14–15, *16*
Transport vesicles, for proteins, 23–24, *24,* 26
Transporter (hub), of nuclear pore complex, 44, *46*
Transverse (T) tubules, of cardiac muscle, 147, 153t
  of skeletal muscle, 132, 134, *136, 137,* 153t
Trauma, nerve, regeneration in, 184–185, *185*
Triads, of skeletal muscle, 134, *135, 137*
  portal, 346, *347*
Tricarboxylic acid cycle, 34
Trichohyalin granules, 280
Tricuspid valve, 226
Trigger proteins, in cell cycle regulation, 52

Triglycerides, formation of, in fat metabolism, 97
  transport of, 97, *99*
Trigone, of bladder, 380
Trigonum fibrosum, of cardiac skeleton, 228
Triiodothyronine (T₃), 268t
  abnormal levels of, 260–261
  action of, 257, 260–261
  release of, 259–260, *260*
  storage of, 258
  synthesis of, 259–260, *260*
Triskelions, clathrin, 25, 26
Trisomy 21 (Down syndrome), 48
Tritium, in autoradiography, 5–6, *6, 7*
Trophic influence, in nerve regeneration, 185
Trophic relationships, of neurons, 161
Trophoblasts, *395, 396*
Tropinin, 138, *138,* 140t
  absence of, in smooth muscle, 151
Tropocollagen, 62, *63,* 64, *66,* 94
Tropomyosin, 137, *138,* 140t
  in smooth muscle, 151
Trunk, pulmonary, 214, 226
Trypsin inhibitor, 342
TSH. See *Thyroid-stimulating hormone (thyrotropin).*
Tubular glands, 89, *89*
  coiled, 276–277, *276, 277*
Tubular myelin, of pneumocytes, 297
Tubules, dentinal, 304
  kidney. See *Kidney, tubules of; Nephron(s).*
  of platelets, 197–198, *198,* 200t
  seminiferous. See *Seminiferous tubules.*
  surface-opening (connecting), of platelets, 197, *198,* 200t
  transverse (T), of cardiac muscle, 147, 153t
    of skeletal muscle, 132, 134, *136, 137,* 153t
Tubuli recti, of testis, 404, 412
Tubulins, dimers of, in axonal transport, 161
  of cytoskeleton, *37*
Tubuloacinar glands, 89, *89*
Tubuloalveolar gland(s), mammary glands as, 399
  prostate as, 417
  salivary glands as, 338
Tubulovesicular system, of parietal cells, 317–318, *319,* 324, *324*
Tumor(s), benign, in epithelial cell transformation, 86
  malignant. See *Cancer.*
  of adipose tissue, 108
  of central nervous system, 161–162
  of pituitary gland, 257
Tumor necrosis factor-α, in phagocytosis, 237, *237*
Tunic, neural. See *Retina.*